# The Rise of Mitochondria in Medicine

# The Rise of Mitochondria in Medicine

Editor
**Loredana Moro**

MDPI • Basel • Beijing • Wuhan • Barcelona • Belgrade • Manchester • Tokyo • Cluj • Tianjin

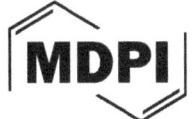

*Editor*
Loredana Moro
National Research Council
Italy

*Editorial Office*
MDPI
St. Alban-Anlage 66
4052 Basel, Switzerland

This is a reprint of articles from the Special Issue published online in the open access journal *Journal of Clinical Medicine* (ISSN 2077-0383) (available at: https://www.mdpi.com/journal/jcm/special_issues/Mitochondria_Medicine).

For citation purposes, cite each article independently as indicated on the article page online and as indicated below:

LastName, A.A.; LastName, B.B.; LastName, C.C. Article Title. *Journal Name* **Year**, *Article Number*, Page Range.

**ISBN 978-3-03936-918-8 (Pbk)**
**ISBN 978-3-03936-919-5 (PDF)**

Cover image courtesy of Loredana Moro.

© 2020 by the authors. Articles in this book are Open Access and distributed under the Creative Commons Attribution (CC BY) license, which allows users to download, copy and build upon published articles, as long as the author and publisher are properly credited, which ensures maximum dissemination and a wider impact of our publications.

The book as a whole is distributed by MDPI under the terms and conditions of the Creative Commons license CC BY-NC-ND.

# Contents

**About the Editor** . . . . . . . . . . . . . . . . . . . . . . . . . . . . . . . . . . . . . . . . . . . . . . . . vii

**Loredana Moro**
Mitochondria at the Crossroads of Physiology and Pathology
Reprinted from: *J. Clin. Med.* **2020**, *9*, 1971, doi:10.3390/jcm9061971 . . . . . . . . . . . . . . . . . 1

**Giampaolo Morciano, Simone Patergnani, Massimo Bonora, Gaia Pedriali, Anna Tarocco, Esmaa Bouhamida, Saverio Marchi, Gina Ancora, Gabriele Anania, Mariusz R. Wieckowski, Carlotta Giorgi and Paolo Pinton**
Mitophagy in Cardiovascular Diseases
Reprinted from: *J. Clin. Med.* **2020**, *9*, 892, doi:10.3390/jcm9030892 . . . . . . . . . . . . . . . . . 9

**Sonia Missiroli, Ilaria Genovese, Mariasole Perrone, Bianca Vezzani, Veronica A. M. Vitto and Carlotta Giorgi**
The Role of Mitochondria in Inflammation: From Cancer to Neurodegenerative Disorders
Reprinted from: *J. Clin. Med.* **2020**, *9*, 740, doi:10.3390/jcm9030740 . . . . . . . . . . . . . . . . . 35

**Jubert Marquez, Jessa Flores, Amy Hyein Kim, Bayalagmaa Nyamaa, Anh Thi Tuyet Nguyen, Nammi Park and Jin Han**
Rescue of TCA Cycle Dysfunction for Cancer Therapy
Reprinted from: *J. Clin. Med.* **2019**, *8*, 2161, doi:10.3390/jcm8122161 . . . . . . . . . . . . . . . . . 61

**Mégane Pizzimenti, Marianne Riou, Anne-Laure Charles, Samy Talha, Alain Meyer, Emmanuel Andres, Nabil Chakfé, Anne Lejay and Bernard Geny**
The Rise of Mitochondria in Peripheral Arterial Disease Physiopathology: Experimental and Clinical Data
Reprinted from: *J. Clin. Med.* **2019**, *8*, 2125, doi:10.3390/jcm8122125 . . . . . . . . . . . . . . . . . 79

**Maria Favia, Lidia de Bari, Antonella Bobba and Anna Atlante**
An Intriguing Involvement of Mitochondria in Cystic Fibrosis
Reprinted from: *J. Clin. Med.* **2019**, *8*, 1890, doi:10.3390/jcm8111890 . . . . . . . . . . . . . . . . . 93

**Lilach Simchi, Julia Panov, Olla Morsy, Yonatan Feuermann and Hanoch Kaphzan**
Novel Insights into the Role of UBE3A in Regulating Apoptosis and Proliferation
Reprinted from: *J. Clin. Med.* **2020**, *9*, 1573, doi:10.3390/jcm9051573 . . . . . . . . . . . . . . . . . 123

**Anna Picca, Flora Guerra, Riccardo Calvani, Federico Marini, Alessandra Biancolillo, Giovanni Landi, Raffaella Beli, Francesco Landi, Roberto Bernabei, Anna Rita Bentivoglio, Maria Rita Lo Monaco, Cecilia Bucci and Emanuele Marzetti**
Mitochondrial Signatures in Circulating Extracellular Vesicles of Older Adults with Parkinson's Disease: Results from the EXosomes in PArkiNson's Disease (EXPAND) Study
Reprinted from: *J. Clin. Med.* **2020**, *9*, 504, doi:10.3390/jcm9020504 . . . . . . . . . . . . . . . . . 147

**Clara Berenguer-Escuder, Dajana Grossmann, Francois Massart, Paul Antony, Lena F. Burbulla, Enrico Glaab, Sophie Imhoff, Joanne Trinh, Philip Seibler, Anne Grünewald and Rejko Krüger**
Variants in Miro1 Cause Alterations of ER-Mitochondria Contact Sites in Fibroblasts from Parkinson's Disease Patients
Reprinted from: *J. Clin. Med.* **2019**, *8*, 2226, doi:10.3390/jcm8122226 . . . . . . . . . . . . . . . . . 163

Jack C. Morton, Jane A. Armstrong, Ajay Sud, Alexei V. Tepikin, Robert Sutton and David N. Criddle
Altered Bioenergetics of Blood Cell Sub-Populations in Acute Pancreatitis Patients
Reprinted from: *J. Clin. Med.* **2019**, *8*, 2201, doi:10.3390/jcm8122201 . . . . . . . . . . . . . . . . . 181

Ivana Kurelac, Ander Abarrategi, Moira Ragazzi, Luisa Iommarini, Nikkitha Umesh Ganesh, Thomas Snoeks, Dominique Bonnet, Anna Maria Porcelli, Ilaria Malanchi and Giuseppe Gasparre
A Humanized Bone Niche Model Reveals Bone Tissue Preservation Upon Targeting Mitochondrial Complex I in Pseudo-Orthotopic Osteosarcoma
Reprinted from: *J. Clin. Med.* **2019**, *8*, 2184, doi:10.3390/jcm8122184 . . . . . . . . . . . . . . . . . 195

Lucia Trisolini, Nicola Gambacorta, Ruggiero Gorgoglione, Michele Montaruli, Luna Laera, Francesco Colella, Mariateresa Volpicella, Anna De Grassi and Ciro Leonardo Pierri
FAD/NADH Dependent Oxidoreductases: From Different Amino Acid Sequences to Similar Protein Shapes for Playing an Ancient Function
Reprinted from: *J. Clin. Med.* **2019**, *8*, 2117, doi:10.3390/jcm8122117 . . . . . . . . . . . . . . . . . 209

Maria Antonietta Ajmone-Cat, Chiara Spinello, Daniela Valenti, Francesca Franchi, Simone Macrì, Rosa Anna Vacca and Giovanni Laviola
Brain-Immune Alterations and Mitochondrial Dysfunctions in a Mouse Model of Paediatric Autoimmune Disorder Associated with Streptococcus: Exacerbation by Chronic Psychosocial Stress
Reprinted from: *J. Clin. Med.* **2019**, *8*, 1514, doi:10.3390/jcm8101514 . . . . . . . . . . . . . . . . . 239

Irene Bravo-Alonso, Rosa Navarrete, Ana Isabel Vega, Pedro Ruíz-Sala, María Teresa García Silva, Elena Martín-Hernández, Pilar Quijada-Fraile, Amaya Belanger-Quintana, Sinziana Stanescu, María Bueno, Isidro Vitoria, Laura Toledo, María Luz Couce, Inmaculada García-Jiménez, Ricardo Ramos-Ruiz, Miguel Ángel Martín, Lourdes R. Desviat, Magdalena Ugarte, Celia Pérez-Cerdá, Begoña Merinero, Belén Pérez and Pilar Rodríguez-Pombo
Genes and Variants Underlying Human Congenital Lactic Acidosis—From Genetics to Personalized Treatment
Reprinted from: *J. Clin. Med.* **2019**, *8*, 1811, doi:10.3390/jcm8111811 . . . . . . . . . . . . . . . . . 265

Rocio Rius, Nicole J. Van Bergen, Alison G. Compton, Lisa G. Riley, Maina P. Kava, Shanti Balasubramaniam, David J. Amor, Miriam Fanjul-Fernandez, Mark J. Cowley, Michael C. Fahey, Mary K. Koenig, Gregory M. Enns, Simon Sadedin, Meredith J Wilson, Tiong Y. Tan, David R. Thorburn and John Christodoulou
Clinical Spectrum and Functional Consequences Associated with Bi-Allelic Pathogenic *PNPT1* Variants
Reprinted from: *J. Clin. Med.* **2019**, *8*, 2020, doi:10.3390/jcm8112020 . . . . . . . . . . . . . . . . . 285

Loredana Moro
Mitochondrial Dysfunction in Aging and Cancer
Reprinted from: *J. Clin. Med.* **2019**, *8*, 1983, doi:10.3390/jcm8111983 . . . . . . . . . . . . . . . . . 297

# About the Editor

**Loredana Moro** is a Researcher of the Institute of Biomembranes, Bioenergetics, and Molecular Biotechnologies at the Italian National Research Council. She earned her PhD in Biochemistry and Molecular Biology in 2003 from the University of Bari. She has worked at Yale University, University of Rochester Medical Center, University of Texas Southwestern Medical Center, and NYU Langone Medical Center. She currently investigates the molecular basis of cancer development and progression, with a focus on the mechanisms of invasion and metastasis.

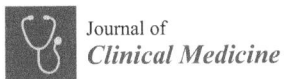 

*Editorial*

# Mitochondria at the Crossroads of Physiology and Pathology

Loredana Moro

Institute of Biomembranes, Bioenergetics and Molecular Biotechnologies, National Research Council, Via Amendola 122/O, 70126 Bari, Italy; l.moro@ibiom.cnr.it

Received: 19 June 2020; Accepted: 22 June 2020; Published: 24 June 2020

**Abstract:** Mitochondria play a crucial role in cell life and death by regulating bioenergetic and biosynthetic pathways. They are able to adapt rapidly to different microenvironmental stressors by accommodating the metabolic and biosynthetic needs of the cell. Mounting evidence places mitochondrial dysfunction at the core of several diseases, notably in the context of pathologies of the cardiovascular and central nervous system. In addition, mutations in some mitochondrial proteins are *bona fide* cancer drivers. Better understanding of the functions of these multifaceted organelles and their components may finetune our knowledge on the molecular bases of certain diseases and suggest new therapeutic avenues.

**Keywords:** mitochondria; mitochondrial dysfunction; neurodegenerative diseases; cancer; aging; inflammation; infection; cardiovascular diseases

## 1. Introduction

Mitochondria are semi-autonomous organelles with a double membrane system, namely the inner and the outer mitochondrial membrane that delimit the intermembrane space. The inner mitochondrial membrane demarcates the matrix, a viscous microenvironment that contains several enzymes catalyzing a plethora of anabolic and catabolic reactions. Mitochondria contain their own genome, the mitochondrial DNA (mtDNA), a circular double-stranded DNA molecule of 16,569 bp in humans, which encodes only 13 mitochondrial proteins belonging to the electron transport chain (ETC), 22 transfer RNAs and 2 ribosomal RNAs needed to carry out the mitochondrial protein synthesis. All the other mitochondrial components are encoded by the nuclear genome.

Mitochondria are the energy powerhouses of the cell, being responsible for 90% of energy production in the form of ATP by coupling the flux of electrons throughout the mitochondrial respiratory complexes I-IV with oxidative phosphorylation (OXPHOS). In brief, complete oxidation of nutrients through the tricarboxylic acid cycle (TCA) within mitochondria produces reduced coenzymes (NADH, FADH2) that act as electron donors. The flux of electrons through the mitochondrial respiratory chain complexes produces an electrochemical gradient used by the mitochondrial respiratory Complex V to generate ATP. Notably, the function of mitochondria in cell physiology goes beyond their role as energy producers and metabolic regulators. Indeed, these multifaceted organelles play a pivotal role in the modulation of cell death pathways and intracellular signaling [1]. The ETC is also the main cellular source of reactive oxygen species (ROS), owing to an incomplete reduction of oxygen by Complex I and Complex III. Mitochondrial ROS production can lead to oxidative damage to proteins, membranes and DNA, thus impairing the ability of mitochondria to carry out their biosynthetic and catabolic reactions, including the TCA cycle, heme synthesis, fatty acid oxidation, the urea cycle and amino acid metabolism [2]. Mitochondrial oxidative damage can also promote permeabilization of the mitochondrial outer membrane (MOMP), resulting in release of intermembrane space proteins, such as cytochrome c, and activation of the mitochondrial apoptotic pathway. Furthermore, mitochondrial

ROS production promotes the opening of the mitochondrial permeability transition pore (mPTP), leading to permeabilization of the inner mitochondrial membrane to small molecules in pathological conditions, such as during ischaemia (loss of blood flow) and subsequent reperfusion [3].

Two mitochondria quality control mechanisms are in place to meet the functional needs of any given cell under different physiological and pathological conditions: (a) mitochondrial biogenesis, fusion and fission [4–6]; (b) mitophagy [7,8]. The first mechanism is a balanced process that allows maintenance of the physiological mitochondrial homeostasis when cells face metabolic or microenvironmental stresses [9]. Mitochondrial fission guarantees an adequate distribution of mitochondria in dividing cells. Mitochondrial fusion allows complementation between dysfunctional mitochondria within the cell to maximize mitochondrial performance in response to stress. Three GTPases, mitofusin 1 (Mfn1), Mfn2, and optic atrophy 1 (Opa1), are primarily involved in the regulation of mitochondrial fusion. Instead, mitochondrial fission is mainly controlled by the GTPase dynamin-related protein 1 (Drp1) [10]. Disruption of the balance between fusion and fission is associated with neurodegenerative diseases, such as Parkinson's, and cancer [9,10]. The second mechanism, mitophagy, is a specific form of autophagy that removes damaged mitochondria and reduces the mitochondrial mass upon microenvironmental stresses, such as hypoxia and nutrient starvation, promoting cell survival [11]. Mitophagy dysregulation has been implicated in cancer development and progression [12], neurodegeneration [13] and cardiovascular diseases [7].

Mitochondrial dysfunction can lead to an array of diseases. Depending on the nature of the defect leading to mitochondrial dysfunction, primary and secondary mitochondrial diseases can be distinguished. Primary mitochondrial diseases develop as a consequence of germline mutations in mtDNA and/or nuclear DNA genes that encode proteins affecting mitochondrial functionality and energy production, including ETC proteins and proteins involved in mtDNA replication, such as POLG. The first primary mitochondrial disease was described in 1962 [14] and involved a 35-year-old woman displaying excessive perspiration, polyphagia, polydipsia without polyuria, asthenia and decreased body weight, symptoms that started when she was seven years old. In addition, her basal metabolic rate was +172%, and she presented with creatinuria, myopathy and pathological cardiomyogram. She was diagnosed with a disorder of the enzymatic organization of the mitochondria. Studies with mitochondria isolated from the skeletal muscle of this hypermetabolic patient revealed OXPHOS uncoupling [14]. Since then, a range of primary mitochondrial diseases has been described (reviewed in [15]). Secondary mitochondrial defects can be caused by germline mutations in genes not involved in respiration/oxidative phosphorylation or can be acquired during the lifetime upon environmental insults. Notably, environmental stress can induce mtDNA alterations leading to mitochondrial dysfunction during aging, inflammatory response, etc. [16,17]. From a pathological point of view, primary and secondary mitochondrial diseases can cause very similar symptoms, sometimes making diagnosis difficult.

At the molecular level, mitochondrial dysfunction can affect the levels of key intracellular signaling regulators, such as ROS and $Ca^{2+}$, that can be transmitted to the nucleus (mitochondria-to-nucleus signaling or retrograde signaling) resulting in changes in gene expression and modulation of a range of cellular functions [1,18–20]. In addition, the release of mtDNA and peptides from the mitochondrial matrix can activate an immune response that promotes a pro-inflammatory cascade [21]. Mitochondrial metabolites can also act as signaling molecules and epigenetic modulators. In this context, citrate, an intermediate of the TCA cycle, represents the major source of acetyl-CoA for protein acetylation, a co- and post-translational modification that regulates protein levels and intracellular signaling in physiological and pathological conditions [22]. Emerging data have also provided new evidences of connections between mitochondrial dynamics and physical contacts among mitochondria and the endoplasmic reticulum (ER), known as mitochondrial-associated ER membranes (MAMs), which can finetune the mechanisms of regulation of energy production, $Ca^{2+}$ homeostasis, survival and apoptosis [23]. Here, a synthetic overview of the role of mitochondria in specific physiopathological conditions is provided (Figure 1).

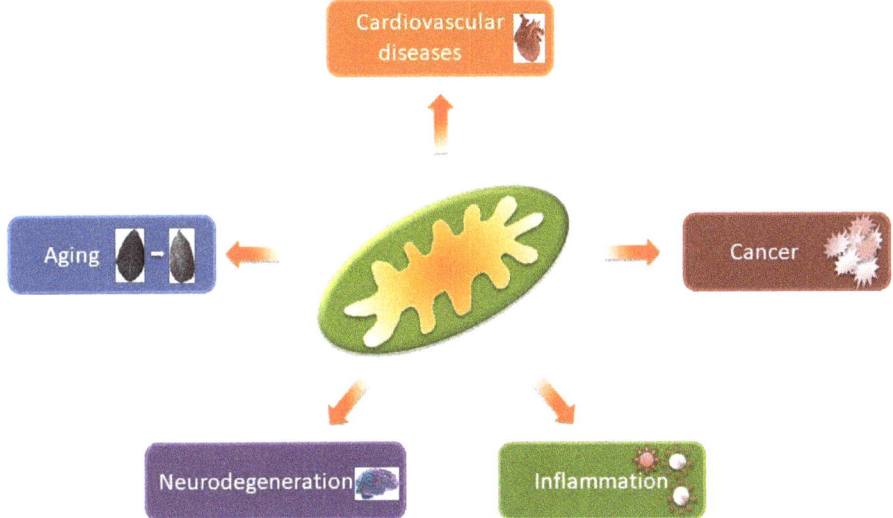

**Figure 1.** Involvement of mitochondria in different pathological conditions.

## 2. Cardiovascular Diseases

Cardiovascular diseases are a leading cause of death worldwide. This class of diseases comprises several pathologies, including ischemic heart disease, peripheral vascular disease, cardiac arrest, heart failure, cardiomyopathies, hypertension, atherosclerosis, and arrhythmia. Mitochondria have been involved at various degrees in the pathological aspects of these diseases. Notably, mitochondrial dysfunction of muscle cells represents a key event in the prognosis of peripheral arterial disease. Reduced OXPHOS activity due to ETC impairment increases ROS levels and $Ca^{2+}$ release from mitochondria, causing apoptosis [24]. However, if ROS levels remain below a threshold, the cells activate a defense program involving production of antioxidants and increased mitochondrial biogenesis. These mechanisms, known as mitohormesis, can limit the damage caused by repeated cycles of ischemia-reperfusion in peripheral arterial disease [24]. Pharmacological treatments that can improve mitohormesis might be a promising therapeutic approach for peripheral arterial disease and other cardiovascular diseases. Disruption of mitophagy also exacerbates the development of cardiovascular diseases [7]. Growing evidence indicates that the pharmacological targeting of the mitochondria with drugs/natural compounds able to modulate mitophagy can ameliorate cardiovascular disorders in patients and be cardioprotective [7,25]. Future studies that aim at a better understanding the pathogenesis of some cardiovascular diseases are crucial to develop mitochondria-targeting drugs in the clinic.

## 3. Inflammation

Inflammation is a complex, protective body response to infections and tissue damage. The inflammatory response signals the immune system to repair damaged tissue and defend against pathogens (viruses, bacteria, etc.) or other harmful stimuli through secretion of specific mediators. However, when inflammation persists, it may drive various diseases and tissue damage. Mitochondrial-derived ROS play a key role in the inflammatory response. Notably, mitochondria are considered the main drivers of the NLRP3 (NOD-, LRR- and pyrin domain-containing 3) inflammasome [26–29], representing a central hub that controls innate immunity and response to inflammation.

Among various inflammatory conditions, mitochondria are involved in the hyper-inflammatory response, also reported as cytokine storm, caused by the SARS-CoV-2 (COVID-19) respiratory infection ([30] and references therein). When macrophages and other immune cells detect viruses, they start secreting cytokines and chemokines to communicate with other immune cells [31]. Strikingly, Wuhan's Covid-19 patients with severe clinical symptoms requiring ICU admission displayed higher levels of the cytokines/chemokines CCL2, TNF-α and CXCL10 compared to individuals with less severe symptoms [32]. The release of large quantities of pro-inflammatory cytokines and chemokines by overdriven immune effector cells sustains an aberrant systemic inflammatory response that results in the immune system attacking the body, which in turn causes the acute respiratory distress syndrome [33]. Immune cells under a hyper-inflammatory state metabolically adapt to this stress condition by favoring aerobic glycolysis over OXPHOS for energy production. This metabolic rewiring allows macrophages to become more phagocytic and favors anabolic reactions for the synthesis and secretion of cytokines and chemokines in a vicious cycle ([30] and references therein). Side by side, many biosynthetic reactions occurring in mitochondria of hyper-activated macrophages are inhibited as a consequence of OXPHOS and TCA cycle inhibition. Melatonin's synthesis is among these reactions: acetyl-CoA, a cofactor in the rate-limiting reaction for melatonin synthesis, lacks due to the TCA cycle inhibition [30]. Thus, melatonin cannot be synthetized. Notably, melatonin is a potent anti-inflammatory and anti-oxidant and its administration to COVID-19 patients has been recently proposed as potential adjuvant treatment strategy to reduce the severity of the COVID-19 pandemic [34–36]. Though clinical evidences are not yet available, several scientific data supports the potential utility of melatonin to attenuate the worst symptoms of COVID-19 infection [37,38].

## 4. Aging

Mitochondrial dysfunction has long been recognized as a driver of the aging process. Early studies have linked accumulation of mitochondrial DNA mutations and the concomitant decline in ETC and OXPHOS activity to aging [29,39]. Furthermore, genetic studies in mice support a causal relation between mtDNA depletion and aging [40]. Recent evidences have confirmed that healthy centenarians retain more "intact" mtDNA copies than old people and frail centenarians [40], suggesting that "healthy" mtDNA is a hallmark of healthy aging. Besides the mtDNA status, activation of mitochondria-to-nucleus signaling pathways, particularly the mitochondrial unfolded protein response (UPR$^{mt}$), has been implicated in aging. UPR$^{mt}$ activation promotes transcription of several nuclear genes, such as those encoding antioxidant proteins and enzymes, which support survival, gain of the mitochondrial functionality and, thus, longevity and lifespan [41]. It should be noted that if a heteroplasmic mtDNA pool is present, UPR$^{mt}$ activation could exacerbate mitochondrial dysfunction as it may lead to accumulation of mutant mtDNA [42].

Alterations in the removal of damaged mitochondria through mitophagy have also been implicated in aging. Mitophagy markedly decreases during aging in mammalian tissues and organs [43,44] and this may be responsible for the known accumulation of damaged mitochondria in aging tissues. Notably, genetic manipulations in C. elegans that increase mitophagy also extend the organismal lifespan [45], strengthening the connection between altered mitophagy and aging.

## 5. Neurodegeneration

Neurodegenerative diseases are characterized by changes in mitochondrial morphology and biochemical activity. Alzheimer's (AD) and Parkinson's (PD) disease are the most diffuse neurodegenerative illnesses among older adults. Brain cells from AD and PD patients show reduced respiratory activity and mitochondrial biogenesis [46,47]. A prominent pathological feature of AD is the impaired cerebral glucose metabolism, which is reduced by 45% in the early stages, preceding neurological impairment and atrophy, and further declines in the late stages of the disease [48]. The decrease in glucose metabolism is associated with reduced expression and activity of mitochondrial enzymes, including pyruvate dehydrogenase, isocitrate dehydrogenase and α-ketoglutarate dehydrogenase, three enzymes of the TCA cycle [49]. In addition, reduced activity of the mitochondrial respiratory complexes I, II, III and IV has also been documented [46]. Somatic mutations in the mitochondrial genome have been detected in postmortem brain tissue from AD patients, at levels higher than in healthy brains [50]. These mutations may not only affect the ETC but also trigger other neuropathological consequences, such as increased ROS production and oxidative stress in neurons and promotion of amyloidogenic processing of the amyloid precursor protein. Mitophagy is also diminished in AD's neurons, and this may contribute to the etiopathogenesis of AD. Indeed, mitophagy was able to prevent or reverse the cognitive impairment in several AD models [51], confirming the critical involvement of mitochondria in AD.

Mutations in nuclear genes encoding mitochondrial proteins important for the proper function of mitochondria have been directly linked to PD. Notably, mutations in proteins involved in mitochondrial quality control, such as PINK1, Parkin and LRRK2, are a frequent cause of monogenic PD [52]. Loss or impaired functionality of these proteins results in mitochondrial fragmentation, dysregulation of calcium homeostasis and changes in mitochondria-endoplasmic reticulum contact sites (MERCs). Recently, mutations in Miro1, a protein important for the regulation of the structure and function of MERCs, have been causally linked to PD establishing that variants in the gene encoding for Miro1 represent rare genetic risk factors for neurodegenerative diseases like PD ([53] and references therein).

Although there is no doubt about the involvement of mitochondrial dysfunction in AD and PD, still more research is required to identify therapeutic targets that could improve mitochondrial activity and reduce oxidative stress in neurons in the early stages of these neurodegenerative diseases. Future studies should be aimed at investigating the chronological sequence of molecular events involved in the pathogenesis of these diseases. Further investigations are also needed to assess whether mitochondrial dysfunction represents a primary cause of AD or a consequence of other molecular/genetic events.

## 6. Cancer

Mitochondrial dysfunction has been involved in different aspects of the pathogenesis of cancer, from the early steps of cancer development to cancer progression to a metastatic phenotype, and resistance to anti-cancer drugs [1,19,29]. In this context, mutations in three TCA cycle enzymes, namely succinate dehydrogenase, fumarate hydratase and isocitrate dehydrogenase, have been shown to play a causal role in carcinogenesis [54,55], thus providing compelling evidence for the involvement of mitochondrial metabolic alterations as cancer drivers. Indeed, mutations in succinate dehydrogenase predispose to hereditary paragangliomas, pheochromocytomas, neuroblastomas, gastrointestinal tumors, renal cell cancers and thyroid tumors [54]. Sporadic and hereditary mutations of fumarate hydratase trigger accumulation of an oncogenic metabolite, i.e., fumarate, that favors development of hereditary leiomyomatosis and renal cell carcinoma, Ewing sarcoma and osteosarcoma, adrenocortical carcinoma, pheochromocytoma, glioma, neuroblastoma, paraganglioma, and ependymoma [55]. Mutations in isocitrate dehydrogenase are only somatic and have been detected in about 20% of patients with acute myeloid leukemia or angioimmunoblastic T-cell lymphoma, and at lower frequencies in patients with thyroid, prostate, colorectal cancer and B-cell acute lymphoblastic leukemia [54,56].

Besides mutations in nuclear-encoded mitochondrial proteins, mutations in mtDNA-encoded proteins have also been implicated in the pathogenesis of cancer. The spectrum of somatic mtDNA mutations varies among different tissues, and increasing evidence shows that the load of mtDNA mutations could have prognostic value. The majority of cancer-related mtDNA mutations have been found in prostate cancer, with a total of more than 700 unique somatic mtDNA mutations associated with this cancer [57]. There is increasing evidence that mtDNA mutations/depletion may favor cancer progression to a metastatic and drug-resistant phenotype through increased production of ROS and/or activation of a mitochondria-to-nucleus signaling that leads to expression of pro-metastatic and pro-survival nuclear genes [20,29,58–60]. Although mtDNA damage may not be the first driver of cancer progression, it is likely that it represents a "supporter" event that facilitates and accelerates different steps of the metastatic cascade, probably within a precise time window that remains to be identified.

## 7. Conclusions

Mitochondrial dysfunction is implicated in several pathological conditions, ranging from neurodegenerative and cardiovascular diseases, to aging, cancer and inflammation. Each of these conditions shows a peculiar involvement of mitochondria. For example, up to 94% of PD patients show a defect in Miro1 function, because this protein, located on the mitochondrial surface, fails to detach from depolarized mitochondria resulting in defective mitochondrial locomotion and clearance by mitophagy [61]. These new results suggest that Miro1-based therapeutic strategies may provide new avenues to a personalized medicine for PD.

The role of mitochondrial dysfunction in other diseases is still somehow controversial. In some cases, it may represent a driver event, like for mutations in the TCA cycle enzymes succinate dehydrogenase, fumarate hydratase and isocitrate dehydrogenase that predispose to certain types of tumors. In other cases, a transient mitochondrial dysfunction may support a metabolic rewiring needed by the cells to adapt and survive to microenvironmental stressors.

**Conflicts of Interest:** The author declares no conflict of interest.

## References

1. Guerra, F.; Arbini, A.; Moro, L. Mitochondria and cancer chemoresistance. *Biochim. Biophys. Acta (BBA) Bioenerg.* **2017**, *1858*, 686–699. [CrossRef] [PubMed]
2. Murphy, M.P. How mitochondria produce reactive oxygen species. *Biochem. J.* **2008**, *417*, 1–13. [CrossRef] [PubMed]
3. Halestrap, A.P.; Pasdois, P. The role of the mitochondrial permeability transition pore in heart disease. *Biochim. Biophys. Acta (BBA) Bioenerg.* **2009**, *1787*, 1402–1415. [CrossRef] [PubMed]
4. Jornayvaz, F.R.; Shulman, G.I. Regulation of mitochondrial biogenesis. *Essays Biochem.* **2010**, *47*, 69–84. [CrossRef]
5. Tahrir, F.G.; Langford, D.; Amini, S.; Ahooyi, T.M.; Khalili, K. Mitochondrial quality control in cardiac cells: Mechanisms and role in cardiac cell injury and disease. *J. Cell. Physiol.* **2018**, *234*, 8122–8133. [CrossRef]
6. Morciano, G.; Pedriali, G.; Sbano, L.; Iannitti, T.; Giorgi, C.; Pinton, P. Intersection of mitochondrial fission and fusion machinery with apoptotic pathways: Role of Mcl-1. *Biol. Cell* **2016**, *108*, 279–293. [CrossRef]
7. Morciano, G.; Patergnani, S.; Bonora, M.; Pedriali, G.; Tarocco, A.; Bouhamida, E.; Marchi, S.; Ancora, G.; Anania, G.; Wieckowski, M.R.; et al. Mitophagy in Cardiovascular Diseases. *J. Clin. Med.* **2020**, *9*, 892. [CrossRef]
8. Ding, W.-X.; Yin, X.-M. Mitophagy: Mechanisms, pathophysiological roles, and analysis. *Biol. Chem.* **2012**, *393*, 547–564. [CrossRef]
9. Youle, R.J.; Van Der Bliek, A.M. Mitochondrial Fission, Fusion, and Stress. *Science* **2012**, *337*, 1062–1065. [CrossRef]
10. Dai, W.; Jiang, L. Dysregulated Mitochondrial Dynamics and Metabolism in Obesity, Diabetes, and Cancer. *Front. Endocrinol.* **2019**, *10*, 570. [CrossRef]
11. Chourasia, A.H.; Boland, M.L.; MacLeod, K. Mitophagy and cancer. *Cancer Metab.* **2015**, *3*, 4. [CrossRef] [PubMed]
12. Bernardini, J.P.; Lazarou, M.; Dewson, G. Parkin and mitophagy in cancer. *Oncogene* **2016**, *36*, 1315–1327. [CrossRef]
13. Fivenson, E.M.; Lautrup, S.H.; Sun, N.; Scheibye-Knudsen, M.; Stevnsner, T.V.; Nilsen, H.; A Bohr, V.; Fang, E.F. Mitophagy in neurodegeneration and aging. *Neurochem. Int.* **2017**, *109*, 202–209. [CrossRef] [PubMed]
14. Luft, R.; Ikkos, D.; Palmieri, G.; Ernster, L.; Afzelius, B. A Case of Severe Hypermetabolism Of Nonthyroid Origin With A Defect In The Maintenance of Mitochondrial Respiratory Control: A Correlated Clinical, Biochemical, and Morphological Study. *J. Clin. Investig.* **1962**, *41*, 1776–1804. [CrossRef] [PubMed]
15. Schapira, A.H. Mitochondrial diseases. *Lancet* **2012**, *379*, 1825–1834. [CrossRef]
16. Circu, M.L.; Moyer, M.P.; Harrison, L.; Aw, T.Y. Contribution of glutathione status to oxidant-induced mitochondrial DNA damage in colonic epithelial cells. *Free Radic. Biol. Med.* **2009**, *47*, 1190–1198. [CrossRef]

17. Rachek, L.I.; Yuzefovych, L.V.; LeDoux, S.P.; Julie, N.L.; Wilson, G.L. Troglitazone, but not rosiglitazone, damages mitochondrial DNA and induces mitochondrial dysfunction and cell death in human hepatocytes. *Toxicol. Appl. Pharmacol.* **2009**, *240*, 348–354. [CrossRef]
18. Tait, S.W.; Green, D.R. Mitochondria and cell signalling. *J. Cell Sci.* **2012**, *125*, 807–815. [CrossRef]
19. Guerra, F.; Guaragnella, N.; Arbini, A.; Bucci, C.; Giannattasio, S.; Moro, L. Mitochondrial Dysfunction: A Novel Potential Driver of Epithelial-to-Mesenchymal Transition in Cancer. *Front. Oncol.* **2017**, *7*, 295. [CrossRef]
20. Srinivasan, S.; Guha, M.; Kashina, A.; Avadhani, N.G. Mitochondrial dysfunction and mitochondrial dynamics-The cancer connection. *Biochim. Biophys. Acta (BBA) Bioenerg.* **2017**, *1858*, 602–614. [CrossRef]
21. Chandel, N.S. Evolution of Mitochondria as Signaling Organelles. *Cell Metab.* **2015**, *22*, 204–206. [CrossRef]
22. Drazic, A.; Myklebust, L.M.; Ree, R.; Arnesen, T. The world of protein acetylation. *Biochim. Biophys. Acta (BBA) Proteins Proteom.* **2016**, *1864*, 1372–1401. [CrossRef] [PubMed]
23. Lee, S.; Min, K.-T. The Interface Between ER and Mitochondria: Molecular Compositions and Functions. *Mol. Cells* **2018**, *41*, 1000–1007. [PubMed]
24. Pizzimenti, M.; Riou, M.; Charles, A.-L.; Talha, S.; Meyer, A.; Andrès, E.; Chakfé, N.; Lejay, A.; Geny, B. The Rise of Mitochondria in Peripheral Arterial Disease Physiopathology: Experimental and Clinical Data. *J. Clin. Med.* **2019**, *8*, 2125. [CrossRef] [PubMed]
25. Bonora, M.; Wieckowski, M.R.; Sinclair, D.A.; Kroemer, G.; Pinton, P.; Galluzzi, L. Targeting mitochondria for cardiovascular disorders: Therapeutic potential and obstacles. *Nat. Rev. Cardiol.* **2018**, *16*, 33–55. [CrossRef] [PubMed]
26. Rimessi, A.; Previati, M.; Nigro, F.; Wieckowski, M.R.; Pinton, P. Mitochondrial reactive oxygen species and inflammation: Molecular mechanisms, diseases and promising therapies. *Int. J. Biochem. Cell Biol.* **2016**, *81*, 281–293. [CrossRef]
27. Zitvogel, L.; Kepp, O.; Galluzzi, L.; Kroemer, G. Inflammasomes in carcinogenesis and anticancer immune responses. *Nat. Immunol.* **2012**, *13*, 343–351. [CrossRef]
28. Missiroli, S.; Genovese, I.; Perrone, M.; Vezzani, B.; Vitto, V.A.M.; Giorgi, C. The Role of Mitochondria in Inflammation: From Cancer to Neurodegenerative Disorders. *J. Clin. Med.* **2020**, *9*, 740. [CrossRef]
29. Moro, L. Mitochondrial Dysfunction in Aging and Cancer. *J. Clin. Med.* **2019**, *8*, 1983. [CrossRef]
30. Reiter, R.J.; Sharma, R.; Ma, Q.; Dominquez-Rodriguez, A.; Marik, P.E.; Abreu-Gonzalez, P. Melatonin Inhibits COVID-19-induced Cytokine Storm by Reversing Aerobic Glycolysis in Immune Cells: A Mechanistic Analysis. *Med. Drug Discov.* **2020**, *6*, 100044. [CrossRef]
31. Zhang, J.-M.; An, J. Cytokines, Inflammation, and Pain. *Int. Anesthesiol. Clin.* **2007**, *45*, 27–37. [CrossRef] [PubMed]
32. Huang, C.; Wang, Y.; Li, X.; Ren, L.; Zhao, J.; Hu, Y.; Zhang, L.; Fan, G.; Xu, J.; Gu, X.; et al. Clinical features of patients infected with 2019 novel coronavirus in Wuhan, China. *Lancet* **2020**, *395*, 497–506. [CrossRef]
33. Coperchini, F.; Chiovato, L.; Croce, L.; Magri, F.; Rotondi, M. The cytokine storm in COVID-19: An overview of the involvement of the chemokine/chemokine-receptor system. *Cytokine Growth Factor Rev.* **2020**, *53*, 25–32. [CrossRef] [PubMed]
34. Zhou, G.; Li, S.; Xia, J. Network-Based Approaches for Multi-omics Integration. *Methods Mol. Biol.* **2020**, *2104*, 469–487. [CrossRef]
35. Shneider, A.; Kudriavtsev, A.; Vakhrusheva, A. Can melatonin reduce the severity of COVID-19 pandemic? *Int. Rev. Immunol.* **2020**, 1–10. [CrossRef]
36. Zhang, R.; Wang, X.; Ni, L.; Di, X.; Ma, B.; Niu, S.; Liu, C.; Reiter, R. COVID-19: Melatonin as a potential adjuvant treatment. *Life Sci.* **2020**, *250*, 117583. [CrossRef]
37. Salles, C. Correspondence COVID-19: Melatonin as a potential adjuvant treatment. *Life Sci.* **2020**, *253*, 117716. [CrossRef]
38. Herrera, E.A.; Gonzalez-Candia, A. Comment on Melatonin as a potential adjuvant treatment for COVID-19. *Life Sci.* **2020**, *253*, 117739. [CrossRef]
39. Sun, N.; Youle, R.J.; Finkel, T. The Mitochondrial Basis of Aging. *Mol. Cell* **2016**, *61*, 654–666. [CrossRef]
40. O'Hara, R.; Tedone, E.; Ludlow, A.T.; Huang, E.; Arosio, B.; Mari, D.; Shay, J.W. Quantitative mitochondrial DNA copy number determination using droplet digital PCR with single-cell resolution. *Genome Res.* **2019**, *29*, 1878–1888. [CrossRef]

41. Zhao, Q.; Wang, J.; Levichkin, I.V.; Stasinopoulos, S.; Ryan, M.T.; Hoogenraad, N. A mitochondrial specific stress response in mammalian cells. *EMBO J.* **2002**, *21*, 4411–4419. [CrossRef] [PubMed]
42. Melber, A.; Haynes, C.M. UPRmt regulation and output: A stress response mediated by mitochondrial-nuclear communication. *Cell Res.* **2018**, *28*, 281–295. [CrossRef] [PubMed]
43. Sun, N.; Yun, J.; Liu, J.; Malide, D.; Liu, C.; Rovira, I.I.; Holmström, K.; Fergusson, M.M.; Yoo, Y.H.; Combs, C.A.; et al. Measuring In Vivo Mitophagy. *Mol. Cell* **2015**, *60*, 685–696. [CrossRef] [PubMed]
44. García-Prat, L.; Martínez-Vicente, M.; Perdiguero, E.; Ortet, L.; Rodríguez-Ubreva, J.; Rebollo, E.; Ruiz-Bonilla, V.; Gutarra, S.; Ballestar, E.; Serrano, A.L.; et al. Autophagy maintains stemness by preventing senescence. *Nature* **2016**, *529*, 37–42. [CrossRef]
45. Palikaras, K.; Lionaki, E.; Tavernarakis, N. Coordination of mitophagy and mitochondrial biogenesis during ageing in C. elegans. *Nature* **2015**, *521*, 525–528. [CrossRef] [PubMed]
46. Onyango, I.G. Mitochondria in the pathophysiology of Alzheimer s and Parkinson s diseases. *Front. Biosci.* **2017**, *22*, 854–872. [CrossRef]
47. Hirai, K.; Aliev, G.; Nunomura, A.; Fujioka, H.; Russell, R.L.; Atwood, C.S.; Johnson, A.B.; Kress, Y.; Vinters, H.V.; Tabaton, M.; et al. Mitochondrial Abnormalities in Alzheimer's Disease. *J. Neurosci.* **2001**, *21*, 3017–3023. [CrossRef]
48. Chen, Z.; Zhong, C. Decoding Alzheimer's disease from perturbed cerebral glucose metabolism: Implications for diagnostic and therapeutic strategies. *Prog. Neurobiol.* **2013**, *108*, 21–43. [CrossRef]
49. Henchcliffe, C.; Beal, M.F. Mitochondrial biology and oxidative stress in Parkinson disease pathogenesis. *Nat. Clin. Pract. Neurol.* **2008**, *4*, 600–609. [CrossRef]
50. Lin, M.T.; Simon, D.K.; Ahn, C.H.; Kim, L.M.; Beal, M.F. High aggregate burden of somatic mtDNA point mutations in aging and Alzheimer's disease brain. *Hum. Mol. Genet.* **2002**, *11*, 133–145. [CrossRef]
51. Fang, E.F. Mitophagy and NAD+ inhibit Alzheimer disease. *Autophagy* **2019**, *15*, 1112–1114. [CrossRef] [PubMed]
52. Truban, D.; Hou, X.; Caulfield, T.R.; Fiesel, F.C.; Springer, W. PINK1, Parkin, and Mitochondrial Quality Control: What can we Learn about Parkinson's Disease Pathobiology? *J. Park. Dis.* **2017**, *7*, 13–29. [CrossRef] [PubMed]
53. Berenguer-Escuder, C.; Grossmann, D.; Massart, F.; Antony, P.M.; Burbulla, L.F.; Glaab, E.; Imhoff, S.; Trinh, J.; Seibler, P.; Grünewald, A.; et al. Variants in Miro1 Cause Alterations of ER-Mitochondria Contact Sites in Fibroblasts from Parkinson's Disease Patients. *J. Clin. Med.* **2019**, *8*, 2226. [CrossRef] [PubMed]
54. Cardaci, S.; Ciriolo, M.R. TCA Cycle Defects and Cancer: When Metabolism Tunes Redox State. *Int. J. Cell Biol.* **2012**, *2012*, 161837. [CrossRef]
55. Schmidt, C.; Sciacovelli, M.; Frezza, C. Fumarate hydratase in cancer: A multifaceted tumour suppressor. *Semin. Cell Dev. Biol.* **2020**, *98*, 15–25. [CrossRef]
56. Marquez, J.; Flores, J.; Kim, A.H.; Nyamaa, B.; Nguyen, A.T.T.; Park, N.; Han, J. Rescue of TCA Cycle Dysfunction for Cancer Therapy. *J. Clin. Med.* **2019**, *8*, 2161. [CrossRef]
57. Kalsbeek, A.M.F.; Chan, E.; Corcoran, N.M.; Hovens, C.M.; Hayes, V.M. Mitochondrial genome variation and prostate cancer: A review of the mutational landscape and application to clinical management. *Oncotarget* **2017**, *8*, 71342–71357. [CrossRef]
58. Ishikawa, K.; Takenaga, K.; Akimoto, M.; Koshikawa, N.; Yamaguchi, A.; Imanishi, H.; Nakada, K.; Honma, Y.; Hayashi, J.-I. ROS-Generating Mitochondrial DNA Mutations Can Regulate Tumor Cell Metastasis. *Science* **2008**, *320*, 661–664. [CrossRef]
59. Moro, L.; Arbini, A.A.; Yao, J.L.; Di Sant'Agnese, P.A.; Marra, E.; Greco, M. Mitochondrial DNA depletion in prostate epithelial cells promotes anoikis resistance and invasion through activation of PI3K/Akt2. *Cell Death Differ.* **2009**, *16*, 571–583. [CrossRef]
60. Arbini, A.; Guerra, F.; Greco, M.; Marra, E.; Gandee, L.; Xiao, G.; Lotan, Y.; Gasparre, G.; Hsieh, J.-T.; Moro, L. Mitochondrial DNA depletion sensitizes cancer cells to PARP inhibitors by translational and post-translational repression of BRCA2. *Oncogenesis* **2013**, *2*, e82. [CrossRef]
61. Hsieh, C.-H.; Li, L.; Vanhauwaert, R.; Nguyen, K.T.; Davis, M.D.; Bu, G.; Wszolek, Z.K.; Wang, X. Miro1 Marks Parkinson's Disease Subset and Miro1 Reducer Rescues Neuron Loss in Parkinson's Models. *Cell Metab.* **2019**, *30*, 1131–1140. [CrossRef] [PubMed]

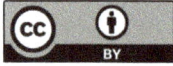

© 2020 by the author. Licensee MDPI, Basel, Switzerland. This article is an open access article distributed under the terms and conditions of the Creative Commons Attribution (CC BY) license (http://creativecommons.org/licenses/by/4.0/).

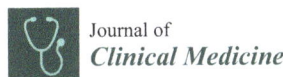 

Review

# Mitophagy in Cardiovascular Diseases

Giampaolo Morciano [1,2], Simone Patergnani [1,2], Massimo Bonora [2], Gaia Pedriali [1,2], Anna Tarocco [2,3], Esmaa Bouhamida [2], Saverio Marchi [4], Gina Ancora [5], Gabriele Anania [6], Mariusz R. Wieckowski [7], Carlotta Giorgi [2] and Paolo Pinton [1,2,*]

1. Maria Cecilia Hospital, GVM Care & Research, Via Corriera 1, Cotignola, 48033 Ravenna, Italy; mrcgpl@unife.it (G.M.); simone.patergnani@unife.it (S.P.); pdrgai@unife.it (G.P.)
2. Department of Medical Sciences, Laboratory for Technologies of Advanced Therapies (LTTA), University of Ferrara, 44121 Ferrara, Italy; bnrmsm1@unife.it (M.B.); trcnna@unife.it (A.T.); esmaa.bouhamida@unife.it (E.B.); grgclt@unife.it (C.G.)
3. Neonatal Intensive Care Unit, University Hospital S. Anna Ferrara, 44121 Ferrara, Italy
4. Department of Clinical and Molecular Sciences, Marche Polytechnic University, 60126 Ancona, Italy; s.marchi@staff.univpm.it
5. Neonatal Intensive Care Unit, Infermi Hospital Rimini, 47923 Rimini, Italy; gina.ancora@auslromagna.it
6. Department of Medical Sciences, Section of General and Thoracic Surgery, University of Ferrara, 44121 Ferrara, Italy; gabriele.anania@unife.it
7. Laboratory of Mitochondrial Biology and Metabolism, Nencki Institute of Experimental Biology of the Polish Academy of Sciences, 3 Pasteur Str., 02-093 Warsaw, Poland; m.wieckowski@nencki.edu.pl
* Correspondence: paolo.pinton@unife.it

Received: 5 March 2020; Accepted: 15 March 2020; Published: 24 March 2020

**Abstract:** Cardiovascular diseases are one of the leading causes of death. Increasing evidence has shown that pharmacological or genetic targeting of mitochondria can ameliorate each stage of these pathologies, which are strongly associated with mitochondrial dysfunction. Removal of inefficient and dysfunctional mitochondria through the process of mitophagy has been reported to be essential for meeting the energetic requirements and maintaining the biochemical homeostasis of cells. This process is useful for counteracting the negative phenotypic changes that occur during cardiovascular diseases, and understanding the molecular players involved might be crucial for the development of potential therapies. Here, we summarize the current knowledge on mitophagy (and autophagy) mechanisms in the context of heart disease with an important focus on atherosclerosis, ischemic heart disease, cardiomyopathies, heart failure, hypertension, arrhythmia, congenital heart disease and peripheral vascular disease. We aim to provide a complete background on the mechanisms of action of this mitochondrial quality control process in cardiology and in cardiac surgery by also reviewing studies on the use of known compounds able to modulate mitophagy for cardioprotective purposes.

**Keywords:** mitophagy; cardiovascular diseases; mitochondria; autophagy

## 1. Fundamental Aspects of Mitophagy

Recent decades have been characterized by robust success in efforts to reduce mortality due to heart disease; however, heart disease remains one of the leading causes of death. Every year, approximately 18 million people around the globe die from cardiovascular diseases (CVDs) [1]. Advances in clinical care and the identification of novel pathogenetic mechanisms and new drug targets are necessary to reduce the acutely lethal manifestations of heart disease. Several areas of challenge have emerged as possible platforms for designing innovative therapeutic approaches. For example, pathways involving mitochondria play major roles in heart physiology [2]. Indeed, mitochondria constitute approximately 30–40% of the cardiomyocyte volume [3], and cardiomyocyte function is closely associated with mitochondrial status; thus, CVDs have unsurprisingly been linked to mitochondrial dysfunction [4–6].

Mitochondria are considered the "energy powerhouses of cells". Within these organelles, a large proportion of cellular adenosine triphosphate (ATP) is generated from the degradation of sugars and long-chain fatty acids (FAs) and from the metabolism of amino acids and lipids. Cardiac mitochondria use 60% to 90% of the energy originating from FA oxidation (FAO) as their primary energy source (they also use glucose, pyruvate, and lactate) to improve cardiac function, whereas most other organs use glucose as the major energy substrate [7]. Mitochondria are deeply involved in calcium ($Ca^{2+}$) handling [8–10]. Recent advances in the identification of the molecular partners regulating $Ca^{2+}$ dynamics in the mitochondrial compartment have helped elucidate the critical contributions of mitochondria to (patho) physiological conditions that rely on mitochondrial $Ca^{2+}$ oscillations [11]. Mitochondria are also the primary sources of intracellular reactive oxygen species (ROS) [12]. These dangerous species are produced in the electron transport chain (ETC) due to the partial reduction of oxygen to superoxide by complex I and complex III and are very harmful to cells. Accordingly, ROS activate several cell death pathways, including necrosis and apoptosis pathways; more importantly, they also cause severe damage to DNA [13]. Mitochondria possess their own DNA (mtDNA), which is almost exclusively maternally inherited [14,15] and consists of base pairs that constitute 37 genes encoding 13 polypeptides essential for oxidative phosphorylation (OXPHOS) plus 22 tRNAs and two rRNAs. Unlike nuclear DNA (nDNA), mtDNA has rudimentary DNA repair mechanisms and is not protected by histones. Hence, mtDNA is more susceptible to ROS-induced damage than nDNA. Indeed, the mutation rate of mtDNA has been estimated to be approximately 15-fold higher than that of nDNA [16].

Clearly, these elements highlight the importance of preserving mitochondrial integrity. Mitochondrial dysfunction can impact various aspects of normal cell life and ultimately induce severe alterations that can lead to the death of the cell itself. Mitochondria have developed two different mechanisms to maintain a healthy status and guarantee an active quality control system. In the first mechanism, biogenesis, fission and fusion cooperate with each other to increase the mitochondrial population under conditions of high energetic demand or to permit a damaged organelle to fuse with a healthy mitochondrion and replace its damaged or lost components [17,18]. In brief, biogenesis is regulated by a series of transcription factors like Transcription Factor A, Mitochondrial (TFAM), Transcription Factor B2, Mitochondrial (TFB2M), Nuclear Respiratory Factor 1 (NRF1), Nuclear Factor, Erythroid 2 Like 2 (NRF2), Estrogen Receptor-related Receptor-alpha (ERRs) and Peroxisome proliferator-activated receptor Gamma Coactivator 1-alpha (PGC-1α) that ensure the maintenance of mitochondrial mass and positively regulate other genes involved in OXPHOS, heme biosynthesis and the import of proteins into mitochondria. Instead, fission and fusion rely on a pool of proteins mainly localized in mitochondria, such as mitofusin (MFN) 1 and 2 in the outer mitochondrial membrane (OMM) and optic atrophy 1 (OPA1) in the inner mitochondrial membrane (IMM), which are needed for the fusion of mitochondrial membranes and mtDNA exchange, and dynamin-related protein 1 (DRP1) and fission mitochondrial 1 (FIS1), which allow mitochondrial division, especially for the transmission of mitochondria to daughter cells in mitosis. In healthy cells, the mitochondrial network is highly interconnected, and there is a balance between the two mechanisms: impaired fusion leads to mitochondrial fragmentation, and unbalanced fission leads to mitochondrial elongation.

In contrast, the second mechanism is expected to remove damaged organelles. This mainly occurs through a cellular mechanism referred to as mitochondrial autophagy (mitophagy, Figure 1) [19].

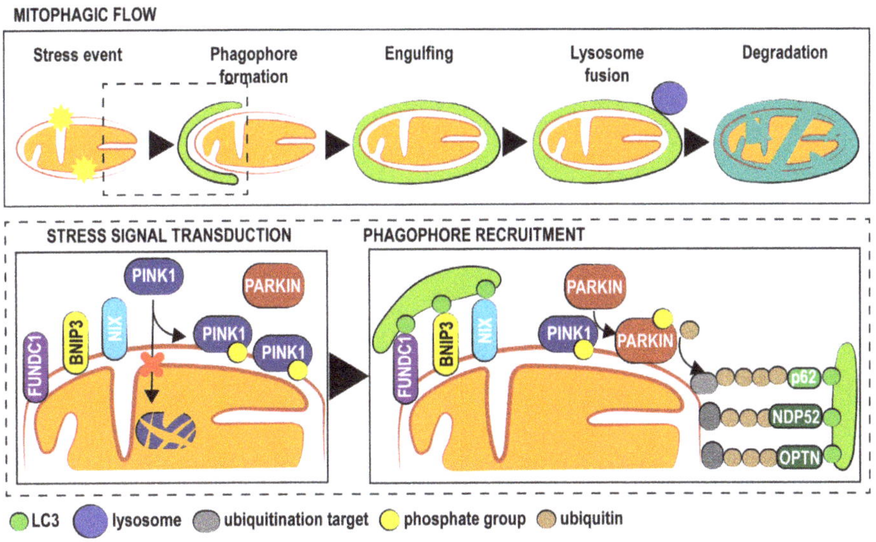

**Figure 1.** Molecular routes of mitophagy. Schematic representation of mitochondrial fate during mitophagy (upper panel). Representation of rearrangements of effectors onto the OMM in response to stress stimuli (lower left panel) and participants in the recruitment of the phagophore around the OMM (lower right panel) during mitophagy. OMM, outer mitochondrial membrane; FUNDC1, FUN14 Domain Containing 1; BNIP3, BCL2/adenovirus E1B 19 kDa protein-interacting protein 3; NIX, NIP-3-Like Protein X; PINK1, PTEN-induced kinase 1; PARKIN, Parkin RBR E3 Ubiquitin Protein Ligase; NDP52, Nuclear Domain 10 Protein 52; OPTN, Optineurin; LC3, Microtubule Associated Protein 1 Light Chain 3.

First described over 50 years ago, autophagy is responsible for the sequestration and degradation of cytosolic components via the lysosomal pathway. During this conserved and physiologic process, a double-membrane vesicle (autophagosome) engulfs cellular material and then fuses with a lysosome to degrade it [20]. When discovered, autophagy was thought to be a nonspecific process in which cytosolic material was randomly sequestered. Autophagy has also been described as a selective mechanism capable of targeting viruses and bacteria (xenophagy), portions of the endoplasmic reticulum (ER; reticulophagy), peroxisomes (pexophagy) and mitochondria (mitophagy) [21].

Among the types of autophagy, mitophagy has become the most described and studied. Several conditions (cellular differentiation, fertilization, oxygen deprivation) and molecules (drugs and proteins) modulate this process. Furthermore, variations in the levels of mitophagy have been found in a diverse array of human pathologies, including cancer, neurodegeneration and CVDs [22].

Mitophagy was first observed in yeast, when two independent research groups screened for mitophagy-deficient mutants and identified the autophagy-related gene 32 (Atg32), which is essential for mitophagy. Previous studies have suggested that the gene products of Aup1p and Uth1p are involved in the autophagic degradation of mitochondria [23,24]; however, these factors were not identified during genomic screening. In mammals, the first observation of mitophagy was made during the maturation of reticulocytes. Mature red blood cells are devoid of mitochondria because immature red blood cells lose their mitochondria via mitophagy during differentiation. This event is mediated by the OMM protein BCL2/Adenovirus E1B 19 KDa Protein-Interacting Protein 3-Like (BNIP3L; also known as NIP-3-Like Protein X, NIX), whose expression increases during maturation. NIX contains a motif required for binding to microtubule-associated protein 1 (MAP1) light chain 3 (LC3) [25,26], which is localized on the surface of the autophagosomal membrane and mediates the sequestration of mitochondria into autophagic vesicles. Subsequent studies have found that

Nix/BNIP3L shares 50% homology with BCL2 Interacting Protein 3 (BNIP3) [27]. Interestingly, this factor is involved in autophagy and mitophagy under hypoxic conditions both in cancer and during myocardial ischemia/reperfusion (I/R) injury (IRI) [28,29]. These findings suggest that mitophagy in mammals may be a mechanism conserved across various cell types and not only in reticulocytes. Accordingly, mitophagic elements have been unveiled in all human tissues, and a specific molecular mechanism governing mitophagy has been found. The discovery of this cellular pathway arose from research on Parkinson's disease [30,31], which revealed a particular form of recessive Parkinsonism characterized by mutation in two genes: Parkin RBR E3 Ubiquitin Protein Ligase (PARK2), which codes for a cytosolic E3 ubiquitin ligase named Parkin, and PTEN-induced kinase 1 (PINK1), whose protein product is a kinase localized on the mitochondrial surface [32,33].

Normally, PINK1 enters mitochondria through the activity of translocase of the outer membrane (TOM) and reaches the mitochondrial inner membrane through the activity of translocase of the inner membrane (TIM), which recognizes an amino-terminal mitochondrial targeting sequence. During these importing steps, PINK1 is subjected to a series of proteolytic cleavage events by the intermembrane serine protease presenilin-associated rhomboid-like protein (PARL), and the full-length form of 64 kDa is sequentially cleaved into fragments of 60 kDa and 52 kDa [34,35]. Once released in the cytosol, the 52-kDa fragment is then degraded by the proteasome [36]. Overall, these mechanisms permit the maintenance of very low levels of PINK1 during unstressed conditions.

When a mitochondrial population becomes damaged, the mitochondrial import of full-length PINK1 throughout the TIM/TOM complex is disrupted; PINK1 then accumulates on the OMMs of only injured mitochondria and is stabilized in a complex composed of TOM7, TOM40, TOM70, TOM20 and TOM22 [37,38]. PINK1 mediates two different phosphorylation events aimed at converting the autoinhibited E3-ubiquitin (Ub) ligase Parkin into an active phospho-Ub-dependent enzyme. The first step involves autophosphorylation at S402, S228 and T257. Interestingly, mutations in these residues abolish both PINK1 activity and Parkin recruitment at the mitochondrial surface [39]. The second event is the direct phosphorylation of Parkin at S65 in the N-terminal Ubl domain, which increases its E3 ligase activity [40]. Finally, PINK1 provokes the addition of a phosphate onto S65 of Ub. As a result of this complex regulatory mechanism, the E3 ligase activity of Parkin is activated, allowing it to ubiquitinate mitochondrial proteins via direct interaction with phospho-Ub conjugates on the mitochondria. The presence of these poly-Ub chains promotes the recruitment of specific Ub-binding autophagy receptors to connect damaged mitochondria to LC3-positive phagosomes for clearance in lysosomes. Initial studies suggested that p62/sequestosome 1 (p62/SQSTM1) was the main receptor involved in mitophagy [41]. Subsequent studies have demonstrated that in addition to p62, at least four other receptors, neighbor of Brca1 (NBR1), nuclear dot protein 52 (NDP52), optineurin (OPTN) and TAX1BP1 (TBK1), are involved during the selective removal of damaged mitochondria. Despite the large number of studies, which adaptor is effectively essential for mitophagy remains unclear [42]. Experiments performed on cell lines with penta-knockout (KO) for all five receptors have suggested that only Nuclear Domain 10 Protein 52 (NDP52) and OPTN are effectively required for mitophagy. However, these experiments were performed on a single cell line, and not all cell types and tissues have comparable levels of these molecules [43].

## 2. Mitophagy in Cardiovascular Diseases

### 2.1. Atherosclerosis

Atherosclerosis (AS) is a chronic inflammatory disease that is very prevalent in industrialized nations. The interplay among lipid accumulation, increased vascular smooth muscle cell (VSMC) proliferation, matrix turnover, calcification and inflammation cause a significant narrowing of the arteries because of plaque buildup inside the artery lumen. In the last 10 years, various methods have been applied to assess autophagy in cells that form atherosclerotic plaques (VSMCs, endothelial cells, macrophages), including electron microscopy, fluorescence microscopy and western blot approaches [44,45]. Studies conducted on human specimens and mouse models of AS have reported either dysfunctional or decreased autophagy based on detection of the autophagic markers p62 and LC3-II in cells isolated from plaques [46–48]. Indeed, a strong decrease in LC3-II expression has been reported in patients with unstable plaques compared to those with stable plaques [48]; such decreases would enable dead cell accumulation in the artery wall and subsequent plaque destabilization (Figure 2). A dysfunction in the autophagic process, caused by either autophagy related 7 (ATG7) deletion in VSMCs [49,50] or a macrophage-specific ATG5-null mutant mouse model [46], has been linked to atheroma development in AS. In the latter, cholesterol crystals are not removed from plaques and trigger an increased secretion of interleukin (IL)-1β after macrophage inflammasome hyperactivation [46]. In humans and animals, complete loss of autophagy (like ATG5-null cells) is incompatible with life, and according to some authors, a slight decrease in autophagy is not always associated with experimental atherosclerosis [46]; therefore, further severe dysfunctions would be expected to occur in this pathway. One of these could be progressive lysosomal impairment with a concomitant accumulation of p62, a protein responsible for bringing polyubiquitinated proteins to the autophagosome for lysosome-dependent degradation.

Much less is known about mitophagy in the context of AS than about mitophagy in a general sense. Overall, mitophagy, together with fission and fusion dynamics, helps clear damaged mitochondria by optimizing the function of the total mitochondrial population inside cells [51]. Given that ROS and inflammation play pivotal roles in the progression of disease, activation of mitophagy by oxidized low-density lipoprotein (ox-LDL, an atherosclerotic agent) [52] and through exogenous melatonin administration [53] counteracts AS progression by stabilizing atherosclerotic plaques (Table 1). Indeed, melatonin was able to modulate mitophagy via a SIRT3/FOXO3a/Parkin-dependent signaling pathway and to attenuate IL-1β secretion.

Table 1. Summary of literature describing mitophagic pathways in cardiovascular diseases.

| Pathology | Mechanism of Action | References |
|---|---|---|
| Atherosclerosis | Atherosclerotic plaque stabilization mediated by ox-LDL. | [52] |
| | NLRP3 inflammasome activation by the SIRT3/FOXO3a/Parkin signaling pathway. | [53] |
| Ischemic heart disease | Mitophagy is an adaptive metabolic response to hypoxia mediated by BNIP3, Beclin-1 and ATG5. | [54] |
| | Pigment epithelium-derived factor (PEDF) protects hypoxic cardiomyocytes in a rat model through the PEDF/PEDF-R/PA/DAG/PKC-α/ULK1/FUNDC1 pathway. | [55] |
| | Fundc1-knockout (KO) platelets present impaired mitochondria, which cause more I/R heart injury. | [56] |
| | FUNDC1 loss of function through CK2α-mediated phosphorylation leads to the development of cardiac I/R injury in mice. | [57] |
| | HMGB1 treatment in a murine model inhibits apoptosis via mTORC1 inhibition. | [58] |
| Cardiomyopathies and heart failure | Inhibition of the dynamic process through the expression of dominant-negative Drp1 (Drp1$^{K38A}$) results in disruption of mitophagy. C452F Drp1 mutation causes spontaneous development of monogenic dilated CM. | [59] |
| | Mice lacking transferrin receptor (Tfrc) develop lethal CM and drastically ineffective mitophagy due to altered expression of proteins involved in mitophagy. | [60] |
| | Enhancement of mitophagy by TAT-Beclin1 attenuates the development of DCM. | [61] |
| | Melatonin inhibits Mst1 phosphorylation, increases LC3-II levels and enhances Parkin activity in mice with CM. | [62] |
| | Parkin-deficient mice are more sensitive to MI, developing larger infarcts and exhibiting reduced survival. | [63] |
| | An increase in BNIP3 expression is detected in adult rat hearts with chronic HF. | [64] |
| | Tamoxifen-inducible cardiac-specific Drp1-KO mice present cardiac dysfunction and increased susceptibility to I/R linked to an accumulation of damaged mitochondria (due to mitophagy inhibition). | [65] |
| | Phosphorylation of Ser495 in PINK1 by AMPKα2 prevents the progression of HF. | [66] |
| | Cytosolic p53 binding to Parkin prevents its translocation to damaged mitochondria, modulating cardiac dysfunction in HF. | [67] |

**Table 1.** *Cont.*

| Pathology | Mechanism of Action | References |
|---|---|---|
| Hypertension | The coexistence of obesity and HT aggravates mitochondrial dysfunction; RAAS activation inhibits mitochondrial biogenesis. | [68] |
| | Spermidine assumption leads to a delayed onset of HT in wild-type animals by stimulating mitophagy in cardiomyocytes, but these effects are abolished in ATG5-KO mice. | [69] |
| | EPCs in HT patients present mitochondrial dysfunctions linked to impairment of the CXCR4/JAK2/SIRT5 signaling pathway and failure of angiogenic capacity. | [70] |
| Arrhythmia | Decrease in mitophagy leads to pro-arrhythmic spontaneous $Ca^{2+}$ release via oxidized RyR2s by mito-ROS. | [71] |
| Peripheral vascular disease | PVD fibers present an accumulation of LC3 that is not completely colocalized with LAMP2. | [72] |
| Mitophagy in cardiac surgery | Post-cardiopulmonary bypass samples display decreased levels of mitophagy adapters NDP52 and OPTN, decreased expression of the long form of Opa1, and translocation of Parkin to the mitochondrial fraction. | [73] |
| | Reperfusion after CABG surgery induces FUNDC1 dephosphorylation and mitophagy activation, causing platelet aggregation and increased risk of thrombosis. | [74] |

Ox-LDL: oxidized low-density lipoprotein; NLRP3: Nucleotide-binding domain, leucine-rich-containing family, pyrin domain-containing-3; SIRT3: Sirtuin 3; FOXO3a: Forkhead Box O3; Parkin: Parkin RBR E3 Ubiquitin Protein Ligase; BNIP3: BCL2 Interacting Protein 3; ATG5: Autophagy related 5; PEDF: Pigment epithelial-derived factor; PEDF-R: PEDF receptor; PA: palmitic acid; DAG: diacylglycerol; PKC-α: protein kinase C alpha; ULK1: Unc-51 Like Autophagy Activating Kinase 1; FUNDC1: FUN14 Domain Containing 1; CK2α: protein kinase CK2 alpha; I/R: ischemia/reperfusion; HMGB1: High Mobility Group Box 1; mTORC1: mammalian target of rapamycin complex 1; CM: cardiomyopathy; TAT_Beclin1: Trans-Activator of Transcription-Beclin1; DCM: diabetic cardiomyopathy; LC3-II: Microtubule Associated Protein 1 Light Chain 3 II; MI: myocardial infarction; HF: heart failure; PINK1: PTEN Induced Kinase 1; AMPKα2: adenosine monophosphate protein kinase alpha 2; RAAS: renin–angiotensin–aldosterone system; ATG5-KO: autophagy related 5-knock out; CXCR4: C-X-C Motif Chemokine Receptor 4; JAK2: Janus Kinase 2; SIRT5: Sirtuin 5; RYR2: Ryanodine Receptor 2; mito-ROS: mitochondrial reactive oxygen species; PVD: peripheral vascular disease; LAMP2: Lysosomal Associated Membrane Protein 2; NDP52: Nuclear Domain 10 Protein 52; OPTN: optineurin; CABG: Coronary Artery Bypass Graft.

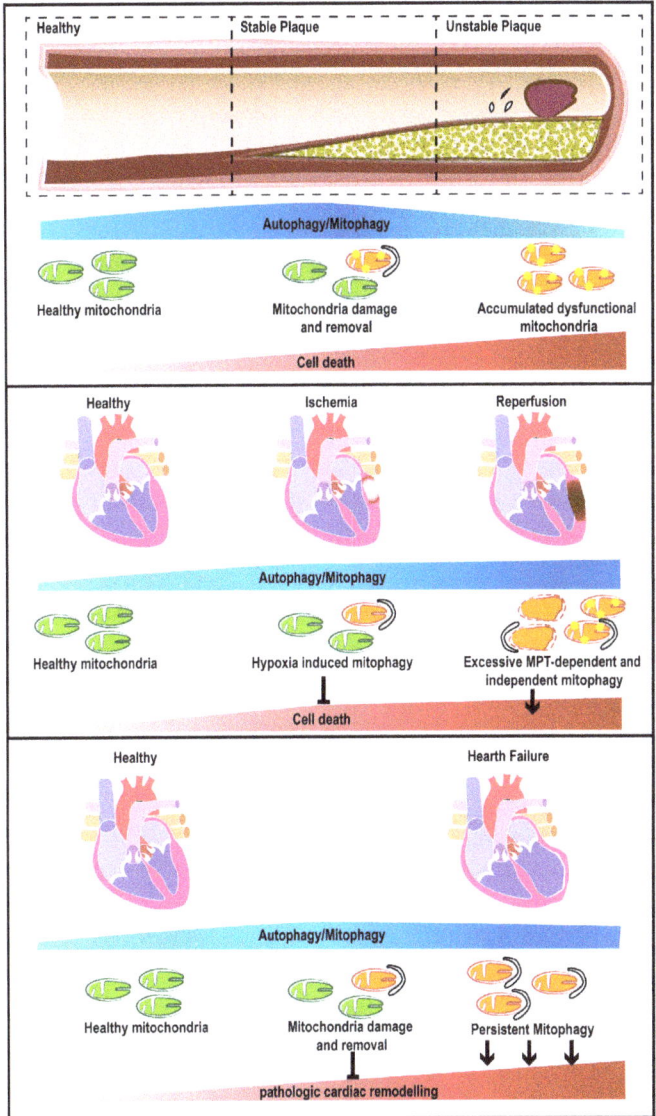

**Figure 2.** Involvement of mitophagy in major CVDs. Schematic representation of tissue remodeling during atherosclerosis (AS) (upper panel), I/R (middle panel) and heart failure (HF; lower panel) with related alterations in mitophagy extent, cell death or tissue remodeling. CVDs, cardiovascular diseases; I/R, ischemia/reperfusion; MPT, mitochondrial permeability transition; HF, heart failure.

## 2.2. Ischemic Heart Disease

A consequence of AS is ischemic heart disease (IHD), where the full or partial recovery of myocardial function is always difficult to achieve due to severe mitochondrial impairment [75,76]. Events consisting of I/R phases are accompanied by oxidative stress, pH changes, and cytosolic and mitochondrial $Ca^{2+}$ overload, which lead to the opening of the mitochondrial permeability transition pore complex (PTPC) and contribute to cardiomyocyte death [12,77–80].

Autophagy (which is activated by increased cytosolic $Ca^{2+}$ concentrations [81]) and mitophagy are known to be features of I/R-related diseases, and ex vivo experiments on cardiac ischemia, such as those performed with the Langendorff system, have made great contributions to these findings. Lysosomal alterations were first observed in perfused rabbit hearts in 1980; after 40 min of ischemia, the number of autophagosomes increases and peaks during reperfusion, suggesting that both ischemia and reperfusion can induce autophagy [82]. These findings have also been replicated in the mouse heart in vivo [83]. I/R-dependent upregulation of autophagy has been assessed by the detection of increased LC3-II and Beclin1 protein expression in association with Bcl-2-associated athanogene (BAG-1), a multifunctional prosurvival molecule [84]. Enhanced autophagy has also been detected after hypoxia treatment combined with glucose deprivation and subsequent reperfusion in fetal mouse hearts; localized lysosomal digestion limits injury to the entire cell, suggesting a role for the autophagic process in the repair of sublethal injury [85]. Thus, autophagy appears to be an important mechanism in cardiac tissue protection during and after hypoxia; indeed, inhibition of autophagy in animals through wortmannin treatment impairs the induction of LC3-II formation and Beclin1 overexpression, limiting cardioprotection [84].

In cultured cardiomyocytes, ischemia and glucose deprivation cause significant reductions in the levels of ATP that coincide with the upregulation of adenosine monophosphate-activated protein kinase (AMPK)-dependent autophagy and the inhibition of the mammalian target of rapamycin (mTOR) pathway. Accordingly, transgenic mice overexpressing dominant-negative AMPK display a diminished induction of autophagy following ischemia [83]. At the time of reperfusion, when physiological conditions are restored, AMPK is no longer activated; thus, considering previous findings, autophagy likely proceeds through an AMPK-independent mechanism, and some data have suggested that it occurs via Beclin1 overexpression [83].

Statistically, autophagy and mitophagy may be classified as protective mechanisms, but this could be an oversimplification. Under conditions in which the heart experiences energy loss, such as ischemia, the autophagic pathway may be protective, as it preserves basal metabolic requirements; however, induction of autophagy under other circumstances, such as at the time of reperfusion, may be detrimental. In agreement with this hypothesis, inhibition of Beclin1 has been reported to protect against myocyte death in vivo [83]. Other evidence has come from the use of urocortin, an endogenous cardiac peptide previously shown to reduce other forms of myocyte cell death induced by I/R; urocortin downregulates Beclin1 expression by activating the phosphoinositide 3 (PI3) kinase/Akt pathway [86].

Reperfusion of the heart is well accepted to lead to the opening of the PTPC [87,88]; however, the link between the PTPC and autophagy (or mitophagy) activation is poorly understood, and the literature remains controversial. As PTPC opening leads to mitochondrial membrane potential loss and mitochondria depolarization, the mitophagic pathway is expected to be activated. Indeed, mitophagic pathway activation is ascribed to PTPC opening in hepatocytes of rats and mice and in livers of human patients [89,90], where PTPC opening also plays a role in starvation-induced mitophagy [91]. Accordingly, blockade of pore opening with the known inhibitor cyclosporine A (CsA) has been found to prevent both mitochondrial swelling and autophagy caused by calpain 10 overexpression [92]. Moreover, overexpression of PINK1 in cardiac cells protects the cells from death by significantly delaying the onset of PTPC opening [93]; if PINK1 is depleted, as is the case in KO animals, the heart becomes increasingly vulnerable to ex vivo IRI. Between PTPC activity and autophagy/mitophagy, a feedback loop may exist where each pathway, in turn, controls the other one. PTPC opening can give rise to an autophagic-dependent cell repair mechanism when few mitochondria are involved during a moderate insult, but this process may become inadequate under extensive damage where cells tend to die.

On the other hand, a study headed by Gustafsson AB suggested that BNIP3-dependent mitophagy (induced upon hypoxia and in failing hearts [94,95]) in adult cardiomyocytes does not depend on PTPC opening [96] but only requires BNIP3 and constitutively expressed Beclin1 and autophagy related 5 (ATG5) [97].

Additionally, ER stress and the unfolded protein response (UPR) have been associated with the induction of autophagy and mitophagy [54,98,99]. Studies performed on both cultured neonatal rat and adult mouse ventricular myocytes have shown activation of ER stress and UPR processes under I/R conditions [100–102]. Indeed, hypoxia activates the UPR in surviving myocytes in the border zones of infarcted hearts [103]. Furthermore, activation of the ER stress response was found to be involved in the development of IHD in a predisposed transgenic murine model [104].

I/R reportedly induces excessive mitochondrial fission; this pathway can lead to the generation of two mitochondrial populations with either increased or decreased membrane potential. Most of the time, the depolarized population is not able to fuse and undergoes mitophagy-dependent removal. Thus, mitophagy is dependent on mitochondrial fission; inhibition of the dynamic process through the expression of dominant-negative Drp1$^{K38A}$ or through Fis1 RNA interference results in disruption of mitophagy and subsequent accumulation of dysfunctional mitochondria [105]. Before Drp1 moves to mitochondria to allow fission, "marked" organelles are subjected to early-stage constriction at the mitochondria-associated membranes (MAMs), highlighting an active role for these microdomains in the choice of division sites, the recruitment of proteins and adaptors and the fulfillment of that process [18,106,107]. Further evidence derives from the study of inverted formin 2 (INF2), an ER-localized protein that orchestrates upstream Drp1, actin filament rearrangement and calcium fluxes at MAMs from the ER to mitochondria, which are essential to guarantee mitochondrial fission [108,109].

Other evidence of the cardioprotective roles of mitophagy has been described; for example, Fun14 domain-containing protein 1 (FUNDC1), a mitophagy receptor that interacts with LC3, is able to mediate the process in response to hypoxia [55,57] and has been found to regulate mitochondrial homeostasis, protecting the heart from IRI, in a mouse model [56]. Indeed, FUNDC1 loss of function through casein kinase 2α (CK2α)-mediated phosphorylation leads to inhibition of mitophagy and significant enhancement of tissue damage [110].

During in vivo acute myocardial infarction (MI) induced by permanent ligation of the left coronary artery in transgenic mice, autophagy is enhanced to preserve cellular ATP levels and protect cardiomyocytes from ischemic death [111] (Figure 2).

High-mobility group box-1 protein (HMGB1) is able to migrate to mitochondria and bind with mitophagy-related proteins after exogenous administration. In vivo evidence has shown that HMGB1 treatment in a murine model of acute MI might induce cardiomyocyte survival, protecting infarcted hearts [58]. Attenuation of apoptosis has been ascribed to the induced activation of AMPK and inhibition of mTOR complex 1 (mTORC1) [58]. Experiments on transgenic mice with cardiac-specific overexpression of HMGB1 have shown that the protein enhances angiogenesis, restores cardiac function, and improves survival after myocardial infarction (MI) [112]. Autophagy inhibition in the heart, similar to that observed upon macrophage-stimulating 1 (Mst1, a proapoptotic kinase) activation, has been associated with p62 accumulation and aggregate formation accompanied by the disappearance of autophagosomes and cardiac dysfunction in mice subjected to MI [113].

As introduced previously, a fine balance between all mitochondrial quality control mechanisms is required for cell homeostasis. In IHD, a prominent role is played by mitochondrial biogenesis, the impairment of which is responsible for the altered energy production in the heart [114]. If mitophagy can be positively modulated (as described in Section 4) to rescue the phenotype of cardiomyocytes, peroxisome-proliferator-activated receptor coactivator (PGC)-1α may be strongly reactivated upon long-term exercise training to restore metabolism, although only partially [114].

*2.3. Cardiomyopathies*

Cardiomyopathy (CM) is a muscle-specific disorder of the heart characterized by abnormal myocardial structure and function occurring independently of any demonstrable CVDs, such as coronary artery disease (CAD), uncontrolled hypertension (HT), significant valvular heart disease, and congenital heart disorders. The prevalence of CM is 3% in the global population and increases to 12% in diabetic patients, leading to increased risks of HF and mortality [115]. Hyperglycemia, systemic and cardiac insulin resistance, increased free fatty acid (FFA) levels, renin-angiotensin-aldosterone system (RAAS) activation, sympathetic dysfunction, myocardial inflammation, oxidative stress, remodeling and fibrosis are factors that contribute to the development of CM. However, the exact pathophysiological mechanisms remain unclear [116].

Diabetic hearts have decreased rates of glucose oxidation and increased rates of FAO, resulting in oxidative stress, impaired OXPHOS, and eventually mitochondrial dysfunction. The increased FAO capacity is energetically detrimental and is mediated by the enhanced activity of peroxisome proliferator-activated receptor (PPAR)-α [117,118]. Additionally, metabolic stress-induced mitochondrial dysfunction, enhanced ROS production and increased $Ca^{2+}$ overload-induced PTPC opening result in cardiomyocyte necrosis. Although increasing evidence has indicated that mitochondria are pivotal players in the pathophysiology and development of CM, the mechanism still remains to be investigated [119].

Efficient clearance of dysfunctional mitochondria through mitophagy is crucial for mitochondrial quality control and thus for the maintenance of cardiomyocyte viability [120]. Alterations in both autophagy and mitophagy have been extensively documented to be involved in the pathogenesis of several CMs [121]. Notably, several studies have revealed that the process of autophagy is inhibited in the hearts of type 1 and 2 diabetic mice, suggesting that inhibition of this process may contribute to diabetic CM (DCM) [122–124]. Interestingly, PINK1 and Parkin protein levels are significantly lower in type 1 diabetic hearts than in healthy hearts, leading to decreased cardiac mitophagy; this decrease in cardiac mitophagy is correlated with reduced expression of the small GTPase Rab9, which is involved in a noncanonical alternative selective autophagic pathway and is responsible for mitochondrial degradation during erythrocyte maturation in the absence of ATG5 [124–126]. Recent evidence has shown that mitochondrial dynamics play essential roles in the formation and maintenance of cardiomyocytes [127]. One role is linked to the importance of Drp1, the small GTPase involved in mitochondrial fission at the OMM, which is crucial for cardiac function and in response to energy stress [59,127–129]. Indeed, Drp1 deletion in cardiomyocytes results in decreased mitophagy and cardiac dysfunction, enhancing the risk of IRI [65,128].

Cahill TJ et al. reported that a single C452F mutation in Drp1 causes spontaneous development of monogenic dilated CM along with a wide variety of abnormal mitochondrial defects, including defective mitophagy [59] (Table 1). This missense mutation has been described as an enhancer of Drp1 GTPase activity that fails to guarantee the disassembly of the protein after oligomerization, thus causing it to become a partially dysfunctional protein. In the so-called Python heart, energetic failure may be ascribed to reduced mitochondrial $Ca^{2+}$ uptake (as a consequence of ATPase Sarcoplasmic/Endoplasmic Reticulum Ca2+ Transporting 2 (SERCA2) inactivation) and to elevated numbers of inefficient mitochondria [59]. However, interruption of mitochondrial fusion is also related to rapid dilated CM onset, as observed in the adult heart upon ablation of both mitofusin 1 (MFN1) and 2 [130]. This deleterious effect is mainly attributable to a lack of fusion rather than to mitophagy dysfunction. In addition, mice bearing heart-specific deletion of either Mfn2 [131] or Park2 with concomitant expression of one Mfn2 mutant (a nonphosphorylatable form) [132] are predisposed to perinatal progressive CM and death within a few weeks after birth.

Many other studies on the importance of mitophagy in CM are present in the literature. For example, mitophagy can be considered a valid therapeutic target for transferrin receptor (*Tfrc*)-dependent CM, in which mice lacking this receptor develop lethal CM and drastically ineffective mitophagy [60]. During mitophagy, mtDNA is also degraded by DNase II in lysosomes. Incomplete digestion of mtDNA stimulates inflammation in cardiac tissue and is able to cause HF [133]. Recently, Tong M and associates demonstrated that during high-fat diet consumption, suppression of mitophagy increases the accumulation of lipids in the heart. The same study revealed that enhancement of mitophagy by Trans-Activator of Transcription (TAT)-Beclin1 tends to inhibit the development of CM [61] (Table 1). In a recent investigation, Wang S. et al. reported that mitophagy could be a target of melatonin treatment. Indeed, melatonin inhibits Mst1 phosphorylation, increases LC3-II levels and enhances Parkin-mediated mitochondrial removal to counteract the negative effects of CM [63]. In line with these observations, chronic treatment with metformin (classified as an antidiabetic and a potent inducer of autophagy), heme oxygenase-1 (HO-1) or mitochondrial aldehyde dehydrogenase (ALDH2) prevents CM by activating AMPK, normalizing cardiac autophagic activity, and inhibiting cardiomyocyte apoptosis through stimulation of Mitogen-Activated Protein Kinase 8 (JNK)-Bcl-2 signaling, thereby promoting the disruption of the Bcl-2-Beclin1 complex in diabetic heart tissue [123,134,135]. An additional downstream event is downregulation of nucleotide-binding domain, leucine-rich-containing family, pyrin domain-containing-3 (NLRP3) inflammasome levels in diabetic mice [136]. Interestingly, the NLRP3 inflammasome is considered a novel molecular marker in DCM that is activated by high FFA levels, hyperglycemia, and impaired insulin metabolic signaling.

Activation of the RAAS is considered a primary event in the etiology of both diabetes and HT (see below). RAAS activation contributes to insulin resistance in humans and correlates with increased levels of oxidative stress and cell death in affected hearts. Consistent with these effects and associations, the RAAS has been found to be upregulated during the pathogenesis of DCM. However, insulin signaling seems to have an additional role, especially at birth: inhibiting autophagy when a newborn starts to feed. Indeed, deletion of insulin receptor genes induces excessive organelle removal, contributing to myocyte loss and HF [137]. Overall, these findings support the importance of auto/mitophagy in ensuring the existence of a functional network of mitochondria and suggest that they provide cardioprotection.

## 2.4. Heart Failure

The 2016 European Society of Cardiology (ESC) guidelines for the diagnosis and treatment of acute and chronic HF state that "HF is a clinical syndrome characterized by typical symptoms (i.e., breathlessness, ankle swelling and fatigue) that may be accompanied by signs (i.e., elevated jugular venous pressure, pulmonary crackles and peripheral oedema) caused by a structural and/or functional cardiac abnormality, resulting in a reduced cardiac output and/or elevated intracardiac pressures at rest or during stress" [138].

This clinical scenario is strictly associated with mitochondrial function. To date, few studies have focused on the specific role of mitophagy in the heart, but emerging evidence supports a protective action for mitophagy in response to stress. Cardiomyocytes have been demonstrated to undergo caspase-independent cell death in the context of HF, and apoptosis, oncosis, and autophagy act simultaneously but play different roles in HF in humans [139,140].

In detail, failing hearts present impaired morphology of mitochondrial cristae, with disorganization and reduced cristae density [141]. These structural changes have also been detected in the hearts of Parkin-deficient mice, which exhibit disorganized mitochondrial networks and significantly reduced mitochondrial sizes; these mice are more sensitive to MI than their wild-type littermates, developing larger infarcts and exhibiting reduced survival. Parkin-KO cardiomyocytes present reduced mitophagy linked to dysfunctional mitochondria after MI [62] (Table 1). Moreover, evidence from ATG5-deficient mice has indicated that constitutive autophagy in the normal heart is a homeostatic mechanism for maintaining cardiomyocyte size and global cardiac structure and function, while upregulation of autophagy under HF conditions is an adaptive response to protect the heart from hemodynamic stress [142].

As introduced in the first section and as remarked upon previously, BNIP3 is a mediator of mitophagy and is activated during hypoxia; its effects have also been observed in an in vivo model of chronic HF [64]. In myocytes, mitophagy is a protective response in which Drp1-mediated mitochondrial fission and the recruitment of Parkin collaborate [143]. If disruption of Drp1 occurs, mitochondrial elongation increases with concomitant inhibition of mitophagy, promoting cardiac dysfunction and increased susceptibility to I/R. Similar evidence has also been obtained with tamoxifen-inducible cardiac-specific Drp1-KO mice [65]. In pig hearts, repetitive myocardial stunning induces autophagy as a homeostatic mechanism in which apoptosis is inhibited and tissue damage is limited. In fact, in this model, heart function fully recovers after normalization of coronary flow, suggesting that autophagy may promote the survival of hibernating myocardium [144].

A recent study has also suggested a role of mitophagy in HF pathogenesis (Figure 2). By using heart samples from HF patients and AMPKα2 genetically modified mouse models with transverse aortic constriction (TAC), researchers have found a serine residue (S495) in PINK1 that undergoes phosphorylation after exposure to AMPKα2 upon dissipation of the mitochondrial membrane potential in cardiomyocytes. This process has been found to be essential for the efficient translocation of Parkin to the mitochondria to increase the rate of mitophagy during HF [66] (Table 1). Moreover, PINK1 protein levels are markedly reduced in cases of end-stage human HF, indicating inefficient mitophagy [145].

In 2013, Hoshino A demonstrated that the impairment of mitophagy by cytosolic p53 facilitates HF in mice through binding of p53 to Parkin and subsequent p53 sequestration. This process impairs the reuse of dysfunctional mitochondria and subsequently induces the development of cardiac dysfunction [67] (Table 1). Recent studies on KO mouse models have also highlighted a role for Ulk1-dependent mitophagy in the protection of the heart against pressure overload-induced HF [146].

Coupled with impaired mitophagy, defects in mitochondrial biogenesis (and thus mtDNA depletion) occur due to downregulation of PGC-1α in the early stages of HF [147]. Moreover, failing hearts have been found to express depleted levels of nuclear respiratory factor 1 (NRF1), mitochondrial transcription factor A (TFAM) and estrogen-related receptor α (ERRα), and this reduction in expression has been demonstrated to negatively impact disease progression [148].

Most of the literature considers autophagy and mitophagy to be mediators of cardioprotection, especially when mitophagy removes damaged mitochondria; however, paradoxically, as observed in other heart diseases, several reports have described these pathways as degenerative processes in the context of HF, since their activation triggers a switch from compensated cardiac hypertrophy to HF with fibrosis onset [149]. In addition, stress-induced mitophagy in the failing heart is similar to a maladaptive response to hemodynamic parameters such as pressure overload and contributes to negative remodeling of the myocardium [150]. This process is mainly mediated by Beclin1 expression, as heterozygous disruption of Beclin1 in transgenic mice diminishes pathological remodeling.

## 2.5. Hypertension

HT is a multifactorial disease resulting from multiple causes and mechanisms controlling blood pressure, as Dr. Irvine H. proposed in a theory named the "mosaic of arterial hypertension" in 1967 [151]. Addressing HT is crucial because it remains a pivotal risk factor for CVDs.

Few studies have focused on mitophagy behavior in hypertensive hearts. In 2015, a study indicated that the coexistence of obesity and HT aggravates mitochondrial dysfunction, worsening left ventricular ejection fraction and general clinical outcomes in young animals. In this context, RAAS activation plays a dual role: it inhibits mitochondrial biogenesis by decreasing PGC-1α, NRF1 and TFAM and mediates the excessive clearance of mitochondria via mitophagy. The latter may occur following drastic changes in mitochondrial fission/fusion balance, where the cleavage of OPA1 (increased ratio of short isoform to long isoform) and the concomitant downregulation of MFN1 enhance mitochondrial fragmentation. Consequently, these dramatic modifications in mitochondrial turnover aggravate cell injury [68]. Taken together, these findings suggest that mitophagy may contribute to the development of hypertensive hearts, and further studies may provide new insights into these mechanisms. Further evidence derives from a murine model of HT induced by feeding mice a high-salt diet [69]. Spermidine assumption led to a delayed onset of HT in wild-type animals by stimulating autophagy and mitophagy in cardiomyocytes; however, spermidine had no beneficial effects in ATG5 KO mice, which lacked LC3-II and expressed high levels of p62/ Sequestosome 1 (SQSTM1) [69] (Table 1).

In addition to defects in this mitochondrial quality control system, general organelle dysfunction has been reported to be involved during HT [70,152,153]. At the level of the microvasculature of HT patients, capillary rarefaction is an important clinical sign to be evaluated. Capillary rarefaction may be counteracted by the action of endothelial progenitor cells (EPCs) strongly involved in angiogenesis, but mitochondrial dysfunction in these cells leads to a significant imbalance between microvasculature resistance and new vessel formation. Downregulation of the C-X-C motif chemokine receptor 4 (CXCR4)/Janus kinase 2 (JAK2)/sirtuin 5 (SIRT5) signaling pathway is responsible for EPC dysfunction exacerbating HT in patients; indeed, CXCR4, which is depleted in HT samples, is able to improve SIRT5-dependent mitochondrial function via JAK2 phosphorylation [70] (Table 1).

We aimed to provide a general overview of mitophagy/autophagy in HT diseases; however, we found conflicting evidence when considering pulmonary HT (PH), as further summarized in [153]. Briefly, increased levels of LC3-II were detected in almost all disease models (human, rat, mouse). The role of this increase is controversial, and the upstream (or downstream) mechanism remains unknown. In two cases, autophagy was considered cardioprotective by reducing vascular remodeling [154,155]. On the basis of other experimental data, autophagy was classified as detrimental since its ablation promoted angiogenesis and attenuated HF and HT [156,157].

### 2.6. Arrhythmia

Arrhythmia is a condition in which electric signals that allow the heart to beat do not work properly. Since electrical propagation supports proper cardiac function, arrhythmia can be fatal in some circumstances [158]. Thus far, there is no direct evidence linking defective mitophagy to the onset of this pathology, but mitochondria play key functional roles that depend on the amounts of ATP and ROS produced. Indeed, decreased ATP content and increased ROS generation negatively affect the electrical conduction of the heart through intracellular ion balance disruption [159], introducing heterogeneity in cardiac action potentials. The first link between mitophagy and proarrhythmic disturbances was revealed in 2019 in a study by Murphy KR and colleagues, who found that decreases in mitophagy due to aging lead to mitochondrial depolarization, ROS overproduction and consequent ryanodine receptor 2 (RyR2) oxidation; these changes induce altered and increased spontaneous $Ca^{2+}$ waves (SCWs), enhancing the probability of arrhythmia [71] (Table 1). These findings have been further confirmed by the findings that ATG7 overexpression and Torin1 treatment restored mitochondrial polarization, normal ROS production and normal SCWs. For this reason, proper activation of the mitophagic (or autophagic) pathway could eliminate damaged organelles by preserving cell homeostasis.

### 2.7. Congenital Heart Disease

The incidence of moderate-to-severe structural congenital heart disease (CHD) in liveborn infants is 6 to 8 per 1000 live births; 3 per 1000 live births have heart disease that results in death or requires cardiac catheterization or surgery during the first year of life.

Recently, some authors [160,161] have found that anomalies in cilia function are implicated in CHDs. Cilia are hair-like organelles that can be found on the surfaces of different types of cells. They perform various functions, such as functions related to cell signaling, extracellular fluid propulsion and cell cycle control. The literature reports that motile and immotile cilia are required to establish left-right identity in developing embryos. During heart development, the most important role for cilia is establishing left-right asymmetry and determining the direction of heart looping [161]. Burkhalter MD reported a link between cilia and mitochondrial function during the development of heterotaxy syndromes. Impairment of mitochondrial function results in longer cilia, while shorter cilia are generated when organelle activity is enhanced. Interestingly, he also found a significant reduction in mtDNA in a cohort of heterotaxy patients [160]. Some important reports have provided proof of an association between autophagy and cilia length; in detail, cilia elongation depends on mTOR pathway suppression and thus autophagy activation, which enables suppression of proteasomal degradation of the proteins that constitute cilia [162–164].

Since autophagy is known to be involved in cardiomyocyte differentiation [165], impairment of this process may be the cause of some CHDs.

## 2.8. Peripheral Vascular Disease

Peripheral vascular disease (PVD) is a disorder of arteries and veins that causes pain and fatigue, often during physical exercise; however, damage to the vessel structure does not necessarily occur. VSMCs are the primary constituents of blood vessels, and they play very important roles, of which their capacity to transform into macrophage-like and osteochondrogenic-like cells is especially important. Several lines of evidence support the hypothesis that genetic reprogramming in VSMCs occurs when peripheral vessels become damaged [166]. VSMCs are currently believed to be exposed to autophagic stimuli such as oxidants, cytokines, ox-LDL and growth factors during PVD (i.e., after percutaneous coronary intervention) and that this molecular cascade determines the conversion of these cells to a macrophage-like phenotype, while the osteochondrogenic type is suppressed [167]. Thus, autophagy appears to be a regulator of the cell response to injury. In the most common PVD, deep venous thrombosis (DVT), ATG5 plays a critical role in the progression of the pathology since it mediates thrombus recanalization, acting mainly on endothelial cells. In this context, ATG5 activates Akt phosphorylation, which is counteracted by the use of 3-methyladenine (3-MA); 3-MA inhibits autophagy by lowering ATG5 levels and concomitantly inhibiting endothelial cell migration and tube formation [168]. Strong evidence of the role of autophagy in promoting angiogenesis has also been derived from other studies on pathologies requiring considerable tissue-remodeling programs, such as cancers, and from findings following the pharmacological inhibition of this pathway. Indeed, the enhanced presence of lysosome-associated membrane protein (LAMP) and cathepsin D drives robust angiogenesis in the context of infantile hemangioma [169,170]. Otherwise, chronic expression of ATG5 induces cell death.

Patients with peripheral artery disease usually present with decreased mobility, which cannot be explained only by ischemia-related events or pain. Many reports that have focused on muscle fiber types and their distributions in PVD patients compared to non-PVD participants have reported impaired mitochondrial respiration, enhanced oxidative stress and loss of intermyofibrillar mitochondria [72]. In addition, excessive mitophagy has been detected in parallel with the loss of compensatory mechanisms, such as PGC-1α overexpression. This uncontrolled and dysfunctional mitochondrial removal is independent of age and has been evaluated by direct assessment of LC3-II increases in fibers [72] (Table 1). Although further experiments are needed to fully address the causes and consequences associated with mitophagy, the findings thus far may help to guide research towards new treatments for this group of diseases. For further details, please also refer to [121].

## 2.9. Mitophagy in Human Cardiac Surgery

Nevertheless, many people are subjected to cardiac surgery involving coronary artery bypass grafting (CABG), and despite the use of cardioplegic solutions to preserve heart function, I/R remains one of the main challenges in this periprocedural setting.

In 2013, a descriptive paper reported that the heart of patients undergoing CABG activates the homeostatic intracellular repair response (HIR) program, a prevailing aspect of which is autophagy activation [171]. In heart samples from 19 patients, p62, Beclin1, ATG5 and LC3-II degradation were recorded, suggesting an increased autophagic flux [171]. The same authors later asserted that mitophagy and mitochondrial biogenesis also take part in the HIR program by increasing their activation following cardiac surgery [73]. Despite the innovative approach and use of human samples in these studies, additional studies should further confirm this evidence because autophagy and mitophagy are complex and difficult to assess in tissues. For example, the low levels of LC3-II detected in the first study [171] indicate both low autophagy induction and increased flux without protein replacement. In the second paper [73], mitophagy activation was inferred from Parkin translocation from the cytosol to mitochondria in heart samples before and after surgery and from decreased levels in optineurin (OPTN) and NDP52 receptors in the total homogenate; however, the translocation of these proteins into mitochondria and their clustering should be evaluated. Notably, a high percentage of patients being analyzed might be under statin treatment, which induces autophagy itself [172].

Nevertheless, mitophagy activation during CABG, assessed by FUNDC1 dephosphorylation, has also been reported by a second independent group, but this was described as a deleterious event in the follow-up of patients as it caused platelet aggregation and increased risk of thrombosis [74].

## 3. Targeting Mitophagy for Cardioprotection

As a mechanism critical for mitochondrial quality control, mitophagy is essential for the establishment of a healthy mitochondrial population inside cells. We have discussed how disruption of mitophagic and autophagic pathways exacerbates the development of heart diseases, but it is important to understand how these pathways modulate heart diseases for therapeutic purposes.

Various chemical reagents, drugs and natural compounds are able to modulate mitophagy (Table 2), and studies on their use in therapies are in progress.

**Table 2.** Summary of compounds that provide significant cardioprotection via mitophagy regulation.

| Compound | Target/Mechanism of Action | Cardiovascular Effect |
| --- | --- | --- |
| TEMPOL | SOD mimetic/reduces ROS and counteracts age-related mitophagy | Improves preconditioning after hypoxia/reoxygenation in aged cultured cardiomyocytes |
| Simvastatin | mTOR-dependent activation of mitophagy through Parkin and p62/SQSTM1 | Improves cardioprotection during left ventricular artery occlusion and reperfusion |
| Zinc | Favors SOD activity and activates PINK1/Beclin1-dependent mitophagy | Improves the recovery of cultured cardiomyocytes after hypoxia/reoxygenation |
| Liraglutide | Agonist of GLP1, stimulates SIRT1 and promotes Parkin-mediated mitophagy | Promotes recovery after left ventricular artery ligation-induced ischemia |
| Melatonin | Inhibits Mst1 phosphorylation, increases LC3-II levels and enhances Parkin-mediated mitophagy | Counteracts diabetic CM |
| Metformin | Activates autophagy by disrupting the Bcl2-Beclin1 complex | Inhibits cardiomyocyte apoptosis in diabetic heart |

TEMPOL: 4-hydroxy-2,2,6,6-tetramethylpiperidin-1-oxyl; SOD: superoxide dismutase 1; ROS: reactive oxygen species; SQSTM1: Sequestosome 1; PINK1: PTEN Induced Kinase 1; GLP1: Glucagon Like Peptide 1; SIRT1: Sirtuin 1; LC3-II: Microtubule Associated Protein 1 Light Chain 3 II; CM: cardiomyopathy.

Polyphenols are plant-derived compounds that offer many health benefits. Recent studies have revealed the ability of these compounds to alter mitophagy via different signaling pathways; for example, resveratrol and quercetin act on FOXO3a signaling and promote PINK1 and Parkin overexpression [173], curcumin regulates transcription factor EB (TFEB) activity via the inhibition of mTORC1 [174], and melanoidin activates mitophagy by increasing the levels of Beclin1 [175]. The mTOR pathway is also the target of a drug belonging to the statin class, simvastatin, which inhibits cholesterol biosynthesis. Simvastatin acts on the mitochondrial translocation of Parkin and p62/SQSTM1 to increase mitophagy and autophagy [172], which is required for cardioprotection.

On the other hand, also excessive and persistent mitophagy can also be deleterious; in this context, Parkin, PINK1 and Beclin1 proteins may be upregulated. This upregulation can be counteracted by multiple types of treatments, such as those involving the use of the superoxide dismutase (SOD) mimetic 4-hydroxy-2,2,6,6-tetramethylpiperidin-1-oxyl (TEMPOL) and mitoTEMPOL [176,177], which counteract age-related mitophagy impairment associated with diseases. Other modulators of mitophagy mediators are zinc [178] and liraglutide [179]. Zinc is able to ensure proper mitophagic pathway signaling through PINK1 and Beclin1 by limiting ROS generation and mitochondrial membrane potential dissipation, while liraglutide, an agonist of the glucagon-like peptide 1 (GLP1) receptor, upregulates the sirtuin 1 (SIRT1) pathway, promoting Parkin-mediated mitophagy, and has already been validated as a molecule useful for the repair of infarcted hearts. Another SIRT1 activator with similar effects related to mitophagy and cardioprotection is nicotinamide [180].

Among all the antioxidants mentioned so far, melatonin plays a very important role in cardioprotection. Although melatonin is known to be a master regulator of cell death and inflammation [181], a few studies have reported its roles in inducing autophagy [182,183] and mitophagy during CVDs. In addition to the two studies mentioned in the "Atherosclerosis" and "Cardiomyopathies" sections [53,63], other studies have been conducted on ischemia and reperfusion conditions, during which mitochondrial fission is activated and the PTPC is in its open state [184]. Another study reported upregulation of the PINK1/Parkin pathway and cell death mediated by mitophagy [185]. These (perhaps apparently) controversial results require further research in the field to clearly evaluate the molecular mechanisms associated with cardioprotection. Similarly, the link between PTPC activity and mitophagy/autophagy has not yet been fully addressed [91,186]. Mitochondrial dynamics are strongly linked to mitophagy; consequently, therapies targeting proteins involved in fission or fusion may also act on mitophagy. Mfn2, which is essential for mitochondrial fusion, has also been found to be a receptor for Parkin recruitment to mitochondria that should undergo mitophagy [131]; this process is regulated by PINK1 phosphorylation involving the T111/S442 residues, the simultaneous mutation of which prevents functional interactions between Mfn2 and Parkin. The absence of Mfn2 prevented Parkin translocation and thus mitophagy [131]. Mfn2 mutations are reportedly able to cause diseases such as the neurodegenerative Charcot Marie Tooth type 2A, and the use of agonists to improve Mfn2 actions reverses mitochondrial dysfunction [187]. Mfn2 can also be phosphorylated at S378 by PINK1, and this phosphorylation site is essential to its functions. Therefore, Mfn2 agonists may also act on mitophagy as well as mitochondrial fusion to counteract the negative effects of the disease.

## 4. Future Perspectives and Conclusions

The crucial role of mitochondria in cardiac function is well established; thus, a fine balance between the removal of dysfunctional mitochondria and their replacement with new organelles is needed. Overall, induction of mitophagy is seen as a cardioprotective mechanism started by the heart to protect itself from different types of damage, but to what extent (coupled to the setting) mitophagy may be beneficial and the circumstances in which it can be considered detrimental are not yet clear. In addition, the heart is characterized by three different mitochondrial subpopulations, and it would be interesting to understand whether there are differences in mitophagy among these subpopulations and the purpose of these differences. Therefore, a threefold evaluation of mitochondrial dynamics, biogenesis and PTPC opening should be considered when examining mitophagy.

The proper use of disease animal models combined with cardiac-specific deletion of proteins involved in such pathways and in-depth analysis of human samples may provide further insights to address conflicting evidence and unanswered questions. Recent important findings highlight the role of microRNA (miR)-dependent regulation of gene expression in cardiac protection and repair [188]. An interesting association between miRs and mitophagy has also been reported. Under experimental I/R conditions, upregulation of miR-410 and concomitant loss of mitophagy have been found to occur [189]; under these circumstances, miR-410 was associated with decreased cell viability and severe mitochondrial impairment, which may occur via direct interaction with HMGB1 and subsequent mitophagy inhibition. A second miR (miR-137) has also been detected to be overexpressed under the same conditions; this miR is able to downregulate Nix and FUNDC1, impairing mitophagy [190]. Therefore, controlling and monitoring the expression of miRs may be an added value for cardioprotective therapies.

**Author Contributions:** G.M. conceived, planned, wrote and corrected the review; S.P. wrote the introduction section; M.B. conceived figures and tables; G.P. wrote Ischemia Heart Disease paragraph and conceived tables; A.T. wrote Congenital Heart Disease and Peripheral Heart Disease paragraphs; E.B. wrote Hypertension chapter; S.M. corrected the review; G.A. (Gina Ancora) wrote Congenital Heart Disease paragraph; G.A. (Gabriele Anania) helped to refine the draft of the review; M.R.W. helped to refine the draft of the review; C.G. corrected the review and the abstract and P.P. conceived and corrected the review. All authors have read and agreed to the published version of the manuscript.

**Acknowledgments:** PP is grateful to Camilla degli Scrovegni for continuous support. The Signal Transduction Laboratory is supported by the Italian Association for Cancer Research (AIRC, IG-23670), Telethon (GGP11139B),

Progetti di Rilevante Interesse Nazionale (PRIN, 2017 E5L5P3) and local funds from the University of Ferrara to PP. CG is supported by local funds from the University of Ferrara, the Italian Association for Cancer Research (AIRC: IG-19803), the Italian Ministry of Health (GR-2013-02356747), by a Fondazione Cariplo grant, the European Research Council (ERC, 853057—InflaPML) and Progetti di Rilevante Interesse Nazionale (PRIN, 2017 7E9EPY). MRW is supported by the National Science Centre, Poland (UMO-2018/29/B/NZ1/00589). Moreover, MRW gratefully acknowledge the financial support for this research from the FOIE GRAS and mtFOIE GRAS projects. These projects received funding from the European Union's Horizon 2020 Research and Innovation Programme under the Marie Skłodowska-Curie grant agreement No. 722619 (FOIE GRAS) and grant agreement No. 734719 (mtFOIE GRAS).

**Conflicts of Interest:** The authors declare no conflicts of interest.

## References

1. Benjamin, E.J.; Blaha, M.J.; Chiuve, S.E.; Cushman, M.; Das, S.R.; Deo, R.; de Ferranti, S.D.; Floyd, J.; Fornage, M.; Gillespie, C.; et al. Heart Disease and Stroke Statistics-2017 Update: A Report From the American Heart Association. *Circulation* **2017**, *135*, 146–603. [CrossRef]
2. Siasos, G.; Tsigkou, V.; Kosmopoulos, M.; Theodosiadis, D.; Simantiris, S.; Tagkou, N.M.; Tsimpiktsioglou, A.; Stampouloglou, P.K.; Oikonomou, E.; Mourouzis, K.; et al. Mitochondria and cardiovascular diseases-from pathophysiology to treatment. *Ann. Transl. Med.* **2018**, *6*, 256. [CrossRef]
3. Harris, D.A.; Das, A.M. Control of mitochondrial ATP synthesis in the heart. *Biochem. J.* **1991**, *280*, 561–573. [CrossRef] [PubMed]
4. Bonora, M.; Wieckowski, M.R.; Sinclair, D.A.; Kroemer, G.; Pinton, P.; Galluzzi, L. Targeting mitochondria for cardiovascular disorders: Therapeutic potential and obstacles. *Nat. Rev. Cardiol.* **2019**, *16*, 33–55. [CrossRef] [PubMed]
5. Brown, D.A.; Perry, J.B.; Allen, M.E.; Sabbah, H.N.; Stauffer, B.L.; Shaikh, S.R.; Cleland, J.G.; Colucci, W.S.; Butler, J.; Voors, A.A.; et al. Expert consensus document: Mitochondrial function as a therapeutic target in heart failure. *Nat. Rev. Cardiol.* **2017**, *14*, 238–250. [CrossRef] [PubMed]
6. Piquereau, J.; Caffin, F.; Novotova, M.; Lemaire, C.; Veksler, V.; Garnier, A.; Ventura-Clapier, R.; Joubert, F. Mitochondrial dynamics in the adult cardiomyocytes: Which roles for a highly specialized cell? *Front. Physiol.* **2013**, *4*, 102. [CrossRef] [PubMed]
7. Fernandez-Vizarra, E.; Enriquez, J.A.; Perez-Martos, A.; Montoya, J.; Fernandez-Silva, P. Tissue-specific differences in mitochondrial activity and biogenesis. *Mitochondrion* **2011**, *11*, 207–213. [CrossRef] [PubMed]
8. Rimessi, A.; Pedriali, G.; Vezzani, B.; Tarocco, A.; Marchi, S.; Wieckowski, M.R.; Giorgi, C.; Pinton, P. Interorganellar calcium signaling in the regulation of cell metabolism: A cancer perspective. *Semin. Cell Dev. Biol.* **2019**. [CrossRef]
9. Giorgi, C.; Danese, A.; Missiroli, S.; Patergnani, S.; Pinton, P. Calcium Dynamics as a Machine for Decoding Signals. *Trends Cell Biol.* **2018**, *28*, 258–273. [CrossRef]
10. Pinton, P.; Leo, S.; Wieckowski, M.R.; Di Benedetto, G.; Rizzuto, R. Long-term modulation of mitochondrial $Ca^{2+}$ signals by protein kinase C isozymes. *J. Cell Biol.* **2004**, *165*, 223–232. [CrossRef]
11. Granatiero, V.; De Stefani, D.; Rizzuto, R. Mitochondrial Calcium Handling in Physiology and Disease. *Adv. Exp. Med. Biol.* **2017**, *982*, 25–47. [CrossRef] [PubMed]
12. Giorgi, C.; Marchi, S.; Simoes, I.C.M.; Ren, Z.; Morciano, G.; Perrone, M.; Patalas-Krawczyk, P.; Borchard, S.; Jedrak, P.; Pierzynowska, K.; et al. Mitochondria and Reactive Oxygen Species in Aging and Age-Related Diseases. *Int. Rev. Cell Mol. Biol.* **2018**, *340*, 209–344. [CrossRef] [PubMed]
13. Jezek, J.; Cooper, K.F.; Strich, R. Reactive Oxygen Species and Mitochondrial Dynamics: The Yin and Yang of Mitochondrial Dysfunction and Cancer Progression. *Antioxidants* **2018**, *7*, 13. [CrossRef] [PubMed]
14. Luo, S.; Valencia, C.A.; Zhang, J.; Lee, N.C.; Slone, J.; Gui, B.; Wang, X.; Li, Z.; Dell, S.; Brown, J.; et al. Biparental Inheritance of Mitochondrial DNA in Humans. *Proc. Natl. Acad. Sci. USA* **2018**, *115*, 13039–13044. [CrossRef]
15. Rius, R.; Cowley, M.J.; Riley, L.; Puttick, C.; Thorburn, D.R.; Christodoulou, J. Biparental inheritance of mitochondrial DNA in humans is not a common phenomenon. *Genet. Med.* **2019**. [CrossRef]
16. Richter, C.; Park, J.W.; Ames, B.N. Normal oxidative damage to mitochondrial and nuclear DNA is extensive. *Proc. Natl. Acad. Sci. USA* **1988**, *85*, 6465–6467. [CrossRef]

17. Tahrir, F.G.; Langford, D.; Amini, S.; Mohseni Ahooyi, T.; Khalili, K. Mitochondrial quality control in cardiac cells: Mechanisms and role in cardiac cell injury and disease. *J. Cell. Physiol.* **2019**, *234*, 8122–8133. [CrossRef]
18. Morciano, G.; Pedriali, G.; Sbano, L.; Iannitti, T.; Giorgi, C.; Pinton, P. Intersection of mitochondrial fission and fusion machinery with apoptotic pathways: Role of Mcl-1. *Biol. Cell* **2016**, *108*, 279–293. [CrossRef]
19. Patergnani, S.; Pinton, P. Mitophagy and mitochondrial balance. *Methods Mol. Biol.* **2015**, *1241*, 181–194. [CrossRef]
20. Galluzzi, L.; Vitale, I.; Aaronson, S.A.; Abrams, J.M.; Adam, D.; Agostinis, P.; Alnemri, E.S.; Altucci, L.; Amelio, I.; Andrews, D.W.; et al. Molecular mechanisms of cell death: Recommendations of the Nomenclature Committee on Cell Death 2018. *Cell Death Differ.* **2018**, *25*, 486–541. [CrossRef]
21. Gatica, D.; Lahiri, V.; Klionsky, D.J. Cargo recognition and degradation by selective autophagy. *Nat. Cell Biol.* **2018**, *20*, 233–242. [CrossRef]
22. Um, J.H.; Yun, J. Emerging role of mitophagy in human diseases and physiology. *BMB Rep.* **2017**, *50*, 299–307. [CrossRef] [PubMed]
23. Kissova, I.; Deffieu, M.; Manon, S.; Camougrand, N. Uth1p is involved in the autophagic degradation of mitochondria. *J. Biol. Chem.* **2004**, *279*, 39068–39074. [CrossRef] [PubMed]
24. Tal, R.; Winter, G.; Ecker, N.; Klionsky, D.J.; Abeliovich, H. Aup1p, a yeast mitochondrial protein phosphatase homolog, is required for efficient stationary phase mitophagy and cell survival. *J. Biol. Chem.* **2007**, *282*, 5617–5624. [CrossRef] [PubMed]
25. Schwarten, M.; Mohrluder, J.; Ma, P.; Stoldt, M.; Thielmann, Y.; Stangler, T.; Hersch, N.; Hoffmann, B.; Merkel, R.; Willbold, D. Nix directly binds to GABARAP: A possible crosstalk between apoptosis and autophagy. *Autophagy* **2009**, *5*, 690–698. [CrossRef] [PubMed]
26. Schweers, R.L.; Zhang, J.; Randall, M.S.; Loyd, M.R.; Li, W.; Dorsey, F.C.; Kundu, M.; Opferman, J.T.; Cleveland, J.L.; Miller, J.L.; et al. NIX is required for programmed mitochondrial clearance during reticulocyte maturation. *Proc. Natl. Acad. Sci. USA* **2007**, *104*, 19500–19505. [CrossRef] [PubMed]
27. Zhang, J.; Ney, P.A. Mechanisms and biology of B-cell leukemia/lymphoma 2/adenovirus E1B interacting protein 3 and Nip-like protein X. *Antioxid. Redox Signal.* **2011**, *14*, 1959–1969. [CrossRef]
28. Chourasia, A.H.; Macleod, K.F. Tumor suppressor functions of BNIP3 and mitophagy. *Autophagy* **2015**, *11*, 1937–1938. [CrossRef]
29. Hamacher-Brady, A.; Brady, N.R.; Logue, S.E.; Sayen, M.R.; Jinno, M.; Kirshenbaum, L.A.; Gottlieb, R.A.; Gustafsson, A.B. Response to myocardial ischemia/reperfusion injury involves Bnip3 and autophagy. *Cell Death Differ.* **2007**, *14*, 146–157. [CrossRef]
30. Kitada, T.; Asakawa, S.; Hattori, N.; Matsumine, H.; Yamamura, Y.; Minoshima, S.; Yokochi, M.; Mizuno, Y.; Shimizu, N. Mutations in the parkin gene cause autosomal recessive juvenile parkinsonism. *Nature* **1998**, *392*, 605–608. [CrossRef]
31. Valente, E.M.; Abou-Sleiman, P.M.; Caputo, V.; Muqit, M.M.; Harvey, K.; Gispert, S.; Ali, Z.; Del Turco, D.; Bentivoglio, A.R.; Healy, D.G.; et al. Hereditary early-onset Parkinson's disease caused by mutations in PINK1. *Science* **2004**, *304*, 1158–1160. [CrossRef] [PubMed]
32. Narendra, D.; Tanaka, A.; Suen, D.F.; Youle, R.J. Parkin is recruited selectively to impaired mitochondria and promotes their autophagy. *J. Cell Biol.* **2008**, *183*, 795–803. [CrossRef] [PubMed]
33. Narendra, D.P.; Jin, S.M.; Tanaka, A.; Suen, D.F.; Gautier, C.A.; Shen, J.; Cookson, M.R.; Youle, R.J. PINK1 is selectively stabilized on impaired mitochondria to activate Parkin. *PLoS Biol.* **2010**, *8*, e1000298. [CrossRef] [PubMed]
34. Deas, E.; Plun-Favreau, H.; Gandhi, S.; Desmond, H.; Kjaer, S.; Loh, S.H.; Renton, A.E.; Harvey, R.J.; Whitworth, A.J.; Martins, L.M.; et al. PINK1 cleavage at position A103 by the mitochondrial protease PARL. *Hum. Mol. Genet.* **2011**, *20*, 867–879. [CrossRef]
35. Jin, S.M.; Lazarou, M.; Wang, C.; Kane, L.A.; Narendra, D.P.; Youle, R.J. Mitochondrial membrane potential regulates PINK1 import and proteolytic destabilization by PARL. *J. Cell Biol.* **2010**, *191*, 933–942. [CrossRef]
36. Yamano, K.; Youle, R.J. PINK1 is degraded through the N-end rule pathway. *Autophagy* **2013**, *9*, 1758–1769. [CrossRef]
37. Hasson, S.A.; Kane, L.A.; Yamano, K.; Huang, C.H.; Sliter, D.A.; Buehler, E.; Wang, C.; Heman-Ackah, S.M.; Hessa, T.; Guha, R.; et al. High-content genome-wide RNAi screens identify regulators of parkin upstream of mitophagy. *Nature* **2013**, *504*, 291–295. [CrossRef]

38. Lazarou, M.; Jin, S.M.; Kane, L.A.; Youle, R.J. Role of PINK1 binding to the TOM complex and alternate intracellular membranes in recruitment and activation of the E3 ligase Parkin. *Dev. Cell* **2012**, *22*, 320–333. [CrossRef]
39. Okatsu, K.; Oka, T.; Iguchi, M.; Imamura, K.; Kosako, H.; Tani, N.; Kimura, M.; Go, E.; Koyano, F.; Funayama, M.; et al. PINK1 autophosphorylation upon membrane potential dissipation is essential for Parkin recruitment to damaged mitochondria. *Nat. Commun.* **2012**, *3*, 1016. [CrossRef]
40. Kondapalli, C.; Kazlauskaite, A.; Zhang, N.; Woodroof, H.I.; Campbell, D.G.; Gourlay, R.; Burchell, L.; Walden, H.; Macartney, T.J.; Deak, M.; et al. PINK1 is activated by mitochondrial membrane potential depolarization and stimulates Parkin E3 ligase activity by phosphorylating Serine 65. *Open Biol.* **2012**, *2*, 120080. [CrossRef]
41. Geisler, S.; Holmstrom, K.M.; Skujat, D.; Fiesel, F.C.; Rothfuss, O.C.; Kahle, P.J.; Springer, W. PINK1/Parkin-mediated mitophagy is dependent on VDAC1 and p62/SQSTM1. *Nat. Cell Biol.* **2010**, *12*, 119–131. [CrossRef] [PubMed]
42. Pickles, S.; Vigie, P.; Youle, R.J. Mitophagy and Quality Control Mechanisms in Mitochondrial Maintenance. *Curr. Biol.* **2018**, *28*, R170–R185. [CrossRef] [PubMed]
43. Lazarou, M.; Sliter, D.A.; Kane, L.A.; Sarraf, S.A.; Wang, C.; Burman, J.L.; Sideris, D.P.; Fogel, A.I.; Youle, R.J. The ubiquitin kinase PINK1 recruits autophagy receptors to induce mitophagy. *Nature* **2015**, *524*, 309–314. [CrossRef] [PubMed]
44. Liu, H.; Cao, Y.; Tong, T.; Shi, J.; Zhang, Y.; Yang, Y.; Liu, C. Autophagy in atherosclerosis: A phenomenon found in human carotid atherosclerotic plaques. *Chin. Med. J.* **2015**, *128*, 69–74. [CrossRef]
45. Perrotta, I. The use of electron microscopy for the detection of autophagy in human atherosclerosis. *Micron* **2013**, *50*, 7–13. [CrossRef]
46. Razani, B.; Feng, C.; Coleman, T.; Emanuel, R.; Wen, H.; Hwang, S.; Ting, J.P.; Virgin, H.W.; Kastan, M.B.; Semenkovich, C.F. Autophagy links inflammasomes to atherosclerotic progression. *Cell Metab.* **2012**, *15*, 534–544. [CrossRef]
47. Sergin, I.; Bhattacharya, S.; Emanuel, R.; Esen, E.; Stokes, C.J.; Evans, T.D.; Arif, B.; Curci, J.A.; Razani, B. Inclusion bodies enriched for p62 and polyubiquitinated proteins in macrophages protect against atherosclerosis. *Sci. Signal.* **2016**, *9*. [CrossRef]
48. Swaminathan, B.; Goikuria, H.; Vega, R.; Rodriguez-Antiguedad, A.; Lopez Medina, A.; Freijo Mdel, M.; Vandenbroeck, K.; Alloza, I. Autophagic marker MAP1LC3B expression levels are associated with carotid atherosclerosis symptomatology. *PLoS ONE* **2014**, *9*, e115176. [CrossRef]
49. Grootaert, M.O.; da Costa Martins, P.A.; Bitsch, N.; Pintelon, I.; De Meyer, G.R.; Martinet, W.; Schrijvers, D.M. Defective autophagy in vascular smooth muscle cells accelerates senescence and promotes neointima formation and atherogenesis. *Autophagy* **2015**, *11*, 2014–2032. [CrossRef]
50. Nahapetyan, H.; Moulis, M.; Grousset, E.; Faccini, J.; Grazide, M.H.; Mucher, E.; Elbaz, M.; Martinet, W.; Vindis, C. Altered mitochondrial quality control in Atg7-deficient VSMCs promotes enhanced apoptosis and is linked to unstable atherosclerotic plaque phenotype. *Cell Death Dis.* **2019**, *10*, 119. [CrossRef]
51. Swiader, A.; Nahapetyan, H.; Faccini, J.; D'Angelo, R.; Mucher, E.; Elbaz, M.; Boya, P.; Vindis, C. Mitophagy acts as a safeguard mechanism against human vascular smooth muscle cell apoptosis induced by atherogenic lipids. *Oncotarget* **2016**, *7*, 28821–28835. [CrossRef] [PubMed]
52. Kattoor, A.J.; Pothineni, N.V.K.; Palagiri, D.; Mehta, J.L. Oxidative Stress in Atherosclerosis. *Curr. Atheroscler. Rep.* **2017**, *19*, 42. [CrossRef] [PubMed]
53. Ma, S.; Chen, J.; Feng, J.; Zhang, R.; Fan, M.; Han, D.; Li, X.; Li, C.; Ren, J.; Wang, Y.; et al. Melatonin Ameliorates the Progression of Atherosclerosis via Mitophagy Activation and NLRP3 Inflammasome Inhibition. *Oxid. Med. Cell. Longev.* **2018**, *2018*, 9286458. [CrossRef] [PubMed]
54. Kouroku, Y.; Fujita, E.; Tanida, I.; Ueno, T.; Isoai, A.; Kumagai, H.; Ogawa, S.; Kaufman, R.J.; Kominami, E.; Momoi, T. ER stress (PERK/eIF2alpha phosphorylation) mediates the polyglutamine-induced LC3 conversion, an essential step for autophagy formation. *Cell Death Differ.* **2007**, *14*, 230–239. [CrossRef] [PubMed]
55. Li, Y.; Liu, Z.; Zhang, Y.; Zhao, Q.; Wang, X.; Lu, P.; Zhang, H.; Wang, Z.; Dong, H.; Zhang, Z. PEDF protects cardiomyocytes by promoting FUNDC1mediated mitophagy via PEDF-R under hypoxic condition. *Int. J. Mol. Med.* **2018**, *41*, 3394–3404. [CrossRef] [PubMed]
56. Zhang, W.; Siraj, S.; Zhang, R.; Chen, Q. Mitophagy receptor FUNDC1 regulates mitochondrial homeostasis and protects the heart from I/R injury. *Autophagy* **2017**, *13*, 1080–1081. [CrossRef]

57. Liu, L.; Feng, D.; Chen, G.; Chen, M.; Zheng, Q.; Song, P.; Ma, Q.; Zhu, C.; Wang, R.; Qi, W.; et al. Mitochondrial outer-membrane protein FUNDC1 mediates hypoxia-induced mitophagy in mammalian cells. *Nat. Cell Biol.* **2012**, *14*, 177–185. [CrossRef] [PubMed]
58. Foglio, E.; Puddighinu, G.; Germani, A.; Russo, M.A.; Limana, F. HMGB1 Inhibits Apoptosis Following MI and Induces Autophagy via mTORC1 Inhibition. *J. Cell. Physiol.* **2017**, *232*, 1135–1143. [CrossRef] [PubMed]
59. Cahill, T.J.; Leo, V.; Kelly, M.; Stockenhuber, A.; Kennedy, N.W.; Bao, L.; Cereghetti, G.M.; Harper, A.R.; Czibik, G.; Liao, C.; et al. Resistance of dynamin-related protein 1 oligomers to disassembly impairs mitophagy, resulting in myocardial inflammation and heart failure. *J. Biol. Chem.* **2016**, *291*, 25762. [CrossRef] [PubMed]
60. Xu, W.; Barrientos, T.; Mao, L.; Rockman, H.A.; Sauve, A.A.; Andrews, N.C. Lethal Cardiomyopathy in Mice Lacking Transferrin Receptor in the Heart. *Cell Rep.* **2015**, *13*, 533–545. [CrossRef] [PubMed]
61. Tong, M.; Saito, T.; Zhai, P.; Oka, S.I.; Mizushima, W.; Nakamura, M.; Ikeda, S.; Shirakabe, A.; Sadoshima, J. Mitophagy Is Essential for Maintaining Cardiac Function During High Fat Diet-Induced Diabetic Cardiomyopathy. *Circ. Res.* **2019**, *124*, 1360–1371. [CrossRef] [PubMed]
62. Kubli, D.A.; Zhang, X.; Lee, Y.; Hanna, R.A.; Quinsay, M.N.; Nguyen, C.K.; Jimenez, R.; Petrosyan, S.; Murphy, A.N.; Gustafsson, A.B. Parkin protein deficiency exacerbates cardiac injury and reduces survival following myocardial infarction. *J. Biol. Chem.* **2013**, *288*, 915–926. [CrossRef] [PubMed]
63. Wang, S.; Zhao, Z.; Feng, X.; Cheng, Z.; Xiong, Z.; Wang, T.; Lin, J.; Zhang, M.; Hu, J.; Fan, Y.; et al. Melatonin activates Parkin translocation and rescues the impaired mitophagy activity of diabetic cardiomyopathy through Mst1 inhibition. *J. Cell. Mol. Med.* **2018**, *22*, 5132–5144. [CrossRef] [PubMed]
64. Regula, K.M.; Ens, K.; Kirshenbaum, L.A. Inducible expression of BNIP3 provokes mitochondrial defects and hypoxia-mediated cell death of ventricular myocytes. *Circ. Res.* **2002**, *91*, 226–231. [CrossRef]
65. Ikeda, Y.; Shirakabe, A.; Maejima, Y.; Zhai, P.; Sciarretta, S.; Toli, J.; Nomura, M.; Mihara, K.; Egashira, K.; Ohishi, M.; et al. Endogenous Drp1 mediates mitochondrial autophagy and protects the heart against energy stress. *Circ. Res.* **2015**, *116*, 264–278. [CrossRef]
66. Wang, B.; Nie, J.; Wu, L.; Hu, Y.; Wen, Z.; Dong, L.; Zou, M.H.; Chen, C.; Wang, D.W. AMPKalpha2 Protects Against the Development of Heart Failure by Enhancing Mitophagy via PINK1 Phosphorylation. *Circ. Res.* **2018**, *122*, 712–729. [CrossRef]
67. Hoshino, A.; Mita, Y.; Okawa, Y.; Ariyoshi, M.; Iwai-Kanai, E.; Ueyama, T.; Ikeda, K.; Ogata, T.; Matoba, S. Cytosolic p53 inhibits Parkin-mediated mitophagy and promotes mitochondrial dysfunction in the mouse heart. *Nat. Commun.* **2013**, *4*, 2308. [CrossRef]
68. Zhang, X.; Li, Z.L.; Eirin, A.; Ebrahimi, B.; Pawar, A.S.; Zhu, X.Y.; Lerman, A.; Lerman, L.O. Cardiac metabolic alterations in hypertensive obese pigs. *Hypertension* **2015**, *66*, 430–436. [CrossRef]
69. Eisenberg, T.; Abdellatif, M.; Schroeder, S.; Primessnig, U.; Stekovic, S.; Pendl, T.; Harger, A.; Schipke, J.; Zimmermann, A.; Schmidt, A.; et al. Cardioprotection and lifespan extension by the natural polyamine spermidine. *Nat. Med.* **2016**, *22*, 1428–1438. [CrossRef]
70. Yu, B.B.; Zhi, H.; Zhang, X.Y.; Liang, J.W.; He, J.; Su, C.; Xia, W.H.; Zhang, G.X.; Tao, J. Mitochondrial dysfunction-mediated decline in angiogenic capacity of endothelial progenitor cells is associated with capillary rarefaction in patients with hypertension via downregulation of CXCR4/JAK2/SIRT5 signaling. *EBioMedicine* **2019**, *42*, 64–75. [CrossRef]
71. Murphy, K.R.; Baggett, B.; Cooper, L.L.; Lu, Y.J.O.U.; Sedivy, J.M.; Terentyev, D.; Koren, G. Enhancing Autophagy Diminishes Aberrant Ca(2+) Homeostasis and Arrhythmogenesis in Aging Rabbit Hearts. *Front. Physiol.* **2019**, *10*, 1277. [CrossRef] [PubMed]
72. White, S.H.; McDermott, M.M.; Sufit, R.L.; Kosmac, K.; Bugg, A.W.; Gonzalez-Freire, M.; Ferrucci, L.; Tian, L.; Zhao, L.; Gao, Y.; et al. Walking performance is positively correlated to calf muscle fiber size in peripheral artery disease subjects, but fibers show aberrant mitophagy: An observational study. *J. Transl Med.* **2016**, *14*, 284. [CrossRef] [PubMed]
73. Andres, A.M.; Tucker, K.C.; Thomas, A.; Taylor, D.J.; Sengstock, D.; Jahania, S.M.; Dabir, R.; Pourpirali, S.; Brown, J.A.; Westbrook, D.G.; et al. Mitophagy and mitochondrial biogenesis in atrial tissue of patients undergoing heart surgery with cardiopulmonary bypass. *JCI Insight* **2017**, *2*, e89303. [CrossRef] [PubMed]
74. Zhou, H.; Li, D.; Zhu, P.; Hu, S.; Hu, N.; Ma, S.; Zhang, Y.; Han, T.; Ren, J.; Cao, F.; et al. Melatonin suppresses platelet activation and function against cardiac ischemia/reperfusion injury via PPARgamma/FUNDC1/mitophagy pathways. *J. Pineal Res.* **2017**, *63*. [CrossRef] [PubMed]

75. Tonet, E.; Bernucci, D.; Morciano, G.; Campo, G. Pharmacological protection of reperfusion injury in ST-segment elevation myocardial infarction. Gone with the wind? *Postepy Kardiol Interwencyjnej* **2018**, *14*, 5–8. [CrossRef] [PubMed]
76. Hausenloy, D.J.; Yellon, D.M. Ischaemic conditioning and reperfusion injury. *Nat. Rev. Cardiol.* **2016**, *13*, 193–209. [CrossRef]
77. Ong, S.B.; Samangouei, P.; Kalkhoran, S.B.; Hausenloy, D.J. The mitochondrial permeability transition pore and its role in myocardial ischemia reperfusion injury. *J. Mol. Cell. Cardiol.* **2015**, *78*, 23–34. [CrossRef]
78. Bonora, M.; Morganti, C.; Morciano, G.; Pedriali, G.; Lebiedzinska-Arciszewska, M.; Aquila, G.; Giorgi, C.; Rizzo, P.; Campo, G.; Ferrari, R.; et al. Mitochondrial permeability transition involves dissociation of F1FO ATP synthase dimers and C-ring conformation. *EMBO Rep.* **2017**, *18*, 1077–1089. [CrossRef]
79. Campo, G.; Morciano, G.; Pavasini, R.; Bonora, M.; Sbano, L.; Biscaglia, S.; Bovolenta, M.; Pinotti, M.; Punzetti, S.; Rizzo, P.; et al. Fo ATP synthase C subunit serum levels in patients with ST-segment Elevation Myocardial Infarction: Preliminary findings. *Int. J. Cardiol.* **2016**, *221*, 993–997. [CrossRef]
80. Bonora, M.; Pinton, P. A New Current for the Mitochondrial Permeability Transition. *Trends Biochem. Sci.* **2019**, *44*, 559–561. [CrossRef]
81. Hoyer-Hansen, M.; Bastholm, L.; Szyniarowski, P.; Campanella, M.; Szabadkai, G.; Farkas, T.; Bianchi, K.; Fehrenbacher, N.; Elling, F.; Rizzuto, R.; et al. Control of macroautophagy by calcium, calmodulin-dependent kinase kinase-beta, and Bcl-2. *Mol. Cell* **2007**, *25*, 193–205. [CrossRef] [PubMed]
82. Decker, R.S.; Wildenthal, K. Lysosomal alterations in hypoxic and reoxygenated hearts. I. Ultrastructural and cytochemical changes. *Am. J. Pathol.* **1980**, *98*, 425–444. [PubMed]
83. Matsui, Y.; Takagi, H.; Qu, X.; Abdellatif, M.; Sakoda, H.; Asano, T.; Levine, B.; Sadoshima, J. Distinct roles of autophagy in the heart during ischemia and reperfusion: Roles of AMP-activated protein kinase and Beclin 1 in mediating autophagy. *Circ. Res.* **2007**, *100*, 914–922. [CrossRef]
84. Gurusamy, N.; Lekli, I.; Gorbunov, N.V.; Gherghiceanu, M.; Popescu, L.M.; Das, D.K. Cardioprotection by adaptation to ischaemia augments autophagy in association with BAG-1 protein. *J. Cell. Mol. Med.* **2009**, *13*, 373–387. [CrossRef] [PubMed]
85. Sybers, H.D.; Ingwall, J.; DeLuca, M. Autophagy in cardiac myocytes. *Recent Adv. Stud. Cardiac Struct. Metab.* **1976**, *12*, 453–463. [PubMed]
86. Valentim, L.; Laurence, K.M.; Townsend, P.A.; Carroll, C.J.; Soond, S.; Scarabelli, T.M.; Knight, R.A.; Latchman, D.S.; Stephanou, A. Urocortin inhibits Beclin1-mediated autophagic cell death in cardiac myocytes exposed to ischaemia/reperfusion injury. *J. Mol. Cell. Cardiol.* **2006**, *40*, 846–852. [CrossRef]
87. Griffiths, E.J.; Halestrap, A.P. Mitochondrial non-specific pores remain closed during cardiac ischaemia, but open upon reperfusion. *Biochem. J.* **1995**, *307*, 93–98. [CrossRef]
88. Morciano, G.; Bonora, M.; Campo, G.; Aquila, G.; Rizzo, P.; Giorgi, C.; Wieckowski, M.R.; Pinton, P. Mechanistic Role of mPTP in Ischemia-Reperfusion Injury. *Adv. Exp. Med. Biol.* **2017**, *982*, 169–189. [CrossRef]
89. Elmore, S.P.; Qian, T.; Grissom, S.F.; Lemasters, J.J. The mitochondrial permeability transition initiates autophagy in rat hepatocytes. *FASEB J.* **2001**, *15*, 2286–2287. [CrossRef]
90. Teckman, J.H.; An, J.K.; Blomenkamp, K.; Schmidt, B.; Perlmutter, D. Mitochondrial autophagy and injury in the liver in alpha 1-antitrypsin deficiency. *Am. J. Physiol. Gastrointest. Liver Physiol.* **2004**, *286*, G851–G862. [CrossRef]
91. Carreira, R.S.; Lee, Y.; Ghochani, M.; Gustafsson, A.B.; Gottlieb, R.A. Cyclophilin D is required for mitochondrial removal by autophagy in cardiac cells. *Autophagy* **2010**, *6*, 462–472. [CrossRef] [PubMed]
92. Arrington, D.D.; Van Vleet, T.R.; Schnellmann, R.G. Calpain 10: A mitochondrial calpain and its role in calcium-induced mitochondrial dysfunction. *Am. J. Physiol. Cell Physiol.* **2006**, *291*, C1159–C1171. [CrossRef] [PubMed]
93. Siddall, H.K.; Yellon, D.M.; Ong, S.B.; Mukherjee, U.A.; Burke, N.; Hall, A.R.; Angelova, P.R.; Ludtmann, M.H.; Deas, E.; Davidson, S.M.; et al. Loss of PINK1 increases the heart's vulnerability to ischemia-reperfusion injury. *PLoS ONE* **2013**, *8*, e62400. [CrossRef]
94. Bruick, R.K. Expression of the gene encoding the proapoptotic Nip3 protein is induced by hypoxia. *Proc. Natl. Acad. Sci. USA* **2000**, *97*, 9082–9087. [CrossRef] [PubMed]

95. Kubasiak, L.A.; Hernandez, O.M.; Bishopric, N.H.; Webster, K.A. Hypoxia and acidosis activate cardiac myocyte death through the Bcl-2 family protein BNIP3. *Proc. Natl. Acad. Sci. USA* **2002**, *99*, 12825–12830. [CrossRef] [PubMed]
96. Quinsay, M.N.; Thomas, R.L.; Lee, Y.; Gustafsson, A.B. Bnip3-mediated mitochondrial autophagy is independent of the mitochondrial permeability transition pore. *Autophagy* **2010**, *6*, 855–862. [CrossRef]
97. Zhang, H.; Bosch-Marce, M.; Shimoda, L.A.; Tan, Y.S.; Baek, J.H.; Wesley, J.B.; Gonzalez, F.J.; Semenza, G.L. Mitochondrial autophagy is an HIF-1-dependent adaptive metabolic response to hypoxia. *J. Biol. Chem.* **2008**, *283*, 10892–10903. [CrossRef]
98. Ogata, M.; Hino, S.; Saito, A.; Morikawa, K.; Kondo, S.; Kanemoto, S.; Murakami, T.; Taniguchi, M.; Tanii, I.; Yoshinaga, K.; et al. Autophagy is activated for cell survival after endoplasmic reticulum stress. *Mol. Cell. Biol.* **2006**, *26*, 9220–9231. [CrossRef]
99. Yorimitsu, T.; Nair, U.; Yang, Z.; Klionsky, D.J. Endoplasmic reticulum stress triggers autophagy. *J. Biol. Chem.* **2006**, *281*, 30299–30304. [CrossRef]
100. Qi, X.; Vallentin, A.; Churchill, E.; Mochly-Rosen, D. deltaPKC participates in the endoplasmic reticulum stress-induced response in cultured cardiac myocytes and ischemic heart. *J. Mol. Cell. Cardiol.* **2007**, *43*, 420–428. [CrossRef]
101. Szegezdi, E.; Duffy, A.; O'Mahoney, M.E.; Logue, S.E.; Mylotte, L.A.; O'Brien, T.; Samali, A. ER stress contributes to ischemia-induced cardiomyocyte apoptosis. *Biochem. Biophys. Res. Commun.* **2006**, *349*, 1406–1411. [CrossRef] [PubMed]
102. Terai, K.; Hiramoto, Y.; Masaki, M.; Sugiyama, S.; Kuroda, T.; Hori, M.; Kawase, I.; Hirota, H. AMP-activated protein kinase protects cardiomyocytes against hypoxic injury through attenuation of endoplasmic reticulum stress. *Mol. Cell. Biol.* **2005**, *25*, 9554–9575. [CrossRef] [PubMed]
103. Severino, A.; Campioni, M.; Straino, S.; Salloum, F.N.; Schmidt, N.; Herbrand, U.; Frede, S.; Toietta, G.; Di Rocco, G.; Bussani, R.; et al. Identification of protein disulfide isomerase as a cardiomyocyte survival factor in ischemic cardiomyopathy. *J. Am. Coll. Cardiol.* **2007**, *50*, 1029–1037. [CrossRef] [PubMed]
104. Azfer, A.; Niu, J.; Rogers, L.M.; Adamski, F.M.; Kolattukudy, P.E. Activation of endoplasmic reticulum stress response during the development of ischemic heart disease. *Am. J. Physiol. Heart Circ. Physiol.* **2006**, *291*, H1411–H1420. [CrossRef]
105. Twig, G.; Elorza, A.; Molina, A.J.; Mohamed, H.; Wikstrom, J.D.; Walzer, G.; Stiles, L.; Haigh, S.E.; Katz, S.; Las, G.; et al. Fission and selective fusion govern mitochondrial segregation and elimination by autophagy. *EMBO J.* **2008**, *27*, 433–446. [CrossRef] [PubMed]
106. Friedman, J.R.; Lackner, L.L.; West, M.; DiBenedetto, J.R.; Nunnari, J.; Voeltz, G.K. ER tubules mark sites of mitochondrial division. *Science* **2011**, *334*, 358–362. [CrossRef]
107. Westermann, B. Organelle dynamics: ER embraces mitochondria for fission. *Curr. Biol.* **2011**, *21*, R922–R924. [CrossRef]
108. Korobova, F.; Ramabhadran, V.; Higgs, H.N. An actin-dependent step in mitochondrial fission mediated by the ER-associated formin INF2. *Science* **2013**, *339*, 464–467. [CrossRef]
109. Wales, P.; Schuberth, C.E.; Aufschnaiter, R.; Fels, J.; Garcia-Aguilar, I.; Janning, A.; Dlugos, C.P.; Schafer-Herte, M.; Klingner, C.; Walte, M.; et al. Calcium-mediated actin reset (CaAR) mediates acute cell adaptations. *Elife* **2016**, *5*. [CrossRef]
110. Zhou, H.; Zhu, P.; Wang, J.; Zhu, H.; Ren, J.; Chen, Y. Pathogenesis of cardiac ischemia reperfusion injury is associated with CK2alpha-disturbed mitochondrial homeostasis via suppression of FUNDC1-related mitophagy. *Cell Death Differ.* **2018**, *25*, 1080–1093. [CrossRef]
111. Kanamori, H.; Takemura, G.; Goto, K.; Maruyama, R.; Ono, K.; Nagao, K.; Tsujimoto, A.; Ogino, A.; Takeyama, T.; Kawaguchi, T.; et al. Autophagy limits acute myocardial infarction induced by permanent coronary artery occlusion. *Am. J. Physiol. Heart Circ. Physiol.* **2011**, *300*, H2261–H2271. [CrossRef] [PubMed]
112. Kitahara, T.; Takeishi, Y.; Harada, M.; Niizeki, T.; Suzuki, S.; Sasaki, T.; Ishino, M.; Bilim, O.; Nakajima, O.; Kubota, I. High-mobility group box 1 restores cardiac function after myocardial infarction in transgenic mice. *Cardiovasc. Res.* **2008**, *80*, 40–46. [CrossRef] [PubMed]
113. Maejima, Y.; Kyoi, S.; Zhai, P.; Liu, T.; Li, H.; Ivessa, A.; Sciarretta, S.; Del Re, D.P.; Zablocki, D.K.; Hsu, C.P.; et al. Mst1 inhibits autophagy by promoting the interaction between Beclin1 and Bcl-2. *Nat. Med.* **2013**, *19*, 1478–1488. [CrossRef] [PubMed]

114. Tao, L.; Bei, Y.; Lin, S.; Zhang, H.; Zhou, Y.; Jiang, J.; Chen, P.; Shen, S.; Xiao, J.; Li, X. Exercise Training Protects Against Acute Myocardial Infarction via Improving Myocardial Energy Metabolism and Mitochondrial Biogenesis. *Cell. Physiol. Biochem.* **2015**, *37*, 162–175. [CrossRef]
115. Dandamudi, S.; Slusser, J.; Mahoney, D.W.; Redfield, M.M.; Rodeheffer, R.J.; Chen, H.H. The prevalence of diabetic cardiomyopathy: A population-based study in Olmsted County, Minnesota. *J. Card Fail.* **2014**, *20*, 304–309. [CrossRef]
116. Paolillo, S.; Marsico, F.; Prastaro, M.; Renga, F.; Esposito, L.; De Martino, F.; Di Napoli, P.; Esposito, I.; Ambrosio, A.; Ianniruberto, M.; et al. Diabetic Cardiomyopathy: Definition, Diagnosis, and Therapeutic Implications. *Heart Fail. Clin.* **2019**, *15*, 341–347. [CrossRef]
117. Duncan, J.G.; Finck, B.N. The PPARalpha-PGC-1alpha Axis Controls Cardiac Energy Metabolism in Healthy and Diseased Myocardium. *PPAR Res.* **2008**, *2008*, 253817. [CrossRef]
118. Finck, B.N.; Kelly, D.P. Peroxisome proliferator-activated receptor alpha (PPARalpha) signaling in the gene regulatory control of energy metabolism in the normal and diseased heart. *J. Mol. Cell. Cardiol.* **2002**, *34*, 1249–1257. [CrossRef] [PubMed]
119. Schilling, J.D. The mitochondria in diabetic heart failure: From pathogenesis to therapeutic promise. *Antioxid. Redox Signal.* **2015**, *22*, 1515–1526. [CrossRef] [PubMed]
120. Tong, M.; Sadoshima, J. Mitochondrial autophagy in cardiomyopathy. *Curr. Opin. Genet. Dev.* **2016**, *38*, 8–15. [CrossRef]
121. Bravo-San Pedro, J.M.; Kroemer, G.; Galluzzi, L. Autophagy and Mitophagy in Cardiovascular Disease. *Circ. Res.* **2017**, *120*, 1812–1824. [CrossRef] [PubMed]
122. He, C.; Bassik, M.C.; Moresi, V.; Sun, K.; Wei, Y.; Zou, Z.; An, Z.; Loh, J.; Fisher, J.; Sun, Q.; et al. Exercise-induced BCL2-regulated autophagy is required for muscle glucose homeostasis. *Nature* **2012**, *481*, 511–515. [CrossRef] [PubMed]
123. Xie, Z.; Lau, K.; Eby, B.; Lozano, P.; He, C.; Pennington, B.; Li, H.; Rathi, S.; Dong, Y.; Tian, R.; et al. Improvement of cardiac functions by chronic metformin treatment is associated with enhanced cardiac autophagy in diabetic OVE26 mice. *Diabetes* **2011**, *60*, 1770–1778. [CrossRef] [PubMed]
124. Xu, X.; Kobayashi, S.; Chen, K.; Timm, D.; Volden, P.; Huang, Y.; Gulick, J.; Yue, Z.; Robbins, J.; Epstein, P.N.; et al. Diminished autophagy limits cardiac injury in mouse models of type 1 diabetes. *J. Biol. Chem.* **2013**, *288*, 18077–18092. [CrossRef]
125. Kobayashi, S.; Liang, Q. Autophagy and mitophagy in diabetic cardiomyopathy. *Biochim. Biophys. Acta* **2015**, *1852*, 252–261. [CrossRef] [PubMed]
126. Nishida, Y.; Arakawa, S.; Fujitani, K.; Yamaguchi, H.; Mizuta, T.; Kanaseki, T.; Komatsu, M.; Otsu, K.; Tsujimoto, Y.; Shimizu, S. Discovery of Atg5/Atg7-independent alternative macroautophagy. *Nature* **2009**, *461*, 654–658. [CrossRef]
127. Ikeda, Y.; Shirakabe, A.; Brady, C.; Zablocki, D.; Ohishi, M.; Sadoshima, J. Molecular mechanisms mediating mitochondrial dynamics and mitophagy and their functional roles in the cardiovascular system. *J. Mol. Cell. Cardiol.* **2015**, *78*, 116–122. [CrossRef]
128. Kageyama, Y.; Hoshijima, M.; Seo, K.; Bedja, D.; Sysa-Shah, P.; Andrabi, S.A.; Chen, W.; Hoke, A.; Dawson, V.L.; Dawson, T.M.; et al. Parkin-independent mitophagy requires Drp1 and maintains the integrity of mammalian heart and brain. *EMBO J.* **2014**, *33*, 2798–2813. [CrossRef]
129. Ishihara, T.; Ban-Ishihara, R.; Maeda, M.; Matsunaga, Y.; Ichimura, A.; Kyogoku, S.; Aoki, H.; Katada, S.; Nakada, K.; Nomura, M.; et al. Dynamics of mitochondrial DNA nucleoids regulated by mitochondrial fission is essential for maintenance of homogeneously active mitochondria during neonatal heart development. *Mol. Cell. Biol.* **2015**, *35*, 211–223. [CrossRef]
130. Chen, Y.; Liu, Y.; Dorn, G.W. Mitochondrial fusion is essential for organelle function and cardiac homeostasis. *Circ. Res.* **2011**, *109*, 1327–1331. [CrossRef]
131. Chen, Y.; Dorn, G.W. PINK1-phosphorylated mitofusin 2 is a Parkin receptor for culling damaged mitochondria. *Science* **2013**, *340*, 471–475. [CrossRef] [PubMed]
132. Gong, G.; Song, M.; Csordas, G.; Kelly, D.P.; Matkovich, S.J.; Dorn, G.W. Parkin-mediated mitophagy directs perinatal cardiac metabolic maturation in mice. *Science* **2015**, *350*. [CrossRef] [PubMed]
133. Oka, T.; Hikoso, S.; Yamaguchi, O.; Taneike, M.; Takeda, T.; Tamai, T.; Oyabu, J.; Murakawa, T.; Nakayama, H.; Nishida, K.; et al. Mitochondrial DNA that escapes from autophagy causes inflammation and heart failure. *Nature* **2012**, *485*, 251–255. [CrossRef] [PubMed]

134. He, C.; Zhu, H.; Li, H.; Zou, M.H.; Xie, Z. Dissociation of Bcl-2-Beclin1 complex by activated AMPK enhances cardiac autophagy and protects against cardiomyocyte apoptosis in diabetes. *Diabetes* **2013**, *62*, 1270–1281. [CrossRef]
135. Zhao, Y.; Zhang, L.; Qiao, Y.; Zhou, X.; Wu, G.; Wang, L.; Peng, Y.; Dong, X.; Huang, H.; Si, L.; et al. Heme oxygenase-1 prevents cardiac dysfunction in streptozotocin-diabetic mice by reducing inflammation, oxidative stress, apoptosis and enhancing autophagy. *PLoS ONE* **2013**, *8*, e75927. [CrossRef]
136. Yang, F.; Qin, Y.; Wang, Y.; Meng, S.; Xian, H.; Che, H.; Lv, J.; Li, Y.; Yu, Y.; Bai, Y.; et al. Metformin Inhibits the NLRP3 Inflammasome via AMPK/mTOR-dependent Effects in Diabetic Cardiomyopathy. *Int. J. Biol. Sci.* **2019**, *15*, 1010–1019. [CrossRef]
137. Riehle, C.; Wende, A.R.; Sena, S.; Pires, K.M.; Pereira, R.O.; Zhu, Y.; Bugger, H.; Frank, D.; Bevins, J.; Chen, D.; et al. Insulin receptor substrate signaling suppresses neonatal autophagy in the heart. *J. Clin. Investig.* **2013**, *123*, 5319–5333. [CrossRef]
138. Ponikowski, P.; Voors, A.A.; Anker, S.D.; Bueno, H.; Cleland, J.G.F.; Coats, A.J.S.; Falk, V.; Gonzalez-Juanatey, J.R.; Harjola, V.P.; Jankowska, E.A.; et al. 2016 ESC Guidelines for the diagnosis and treatment of acute and chronic heart failure: The Task Force for the diagnosis and treatment of acute and chronic heart failure of the European Society of Cardiology (ESC)Developed with the special contribution of the Heart Failure Association (HFA) of the ESC. *Eur. Heart J.* **2016**, *37*, 2129–2200. [CrossRef]
139. Knaapen, M.W.; Davies, M.J.; De Bie, M.; Haven, A.J.; Martinet, W.; Kockx, M.M. Apoptotic versus autophagic cell death in heart failure. *Cardiovasc. Res.* **2001**, *51*, 304–312. [CrossRef]
140. Kostin, S.; Pool, L.; Elsasser, A.; Hein, S.; Drexler, H.C.; Arnon, E.; Hayakawa, Y.; Zimmermann, R.; Bauer, E.; Klovekorn, W.P.; et al. Myocytes die by multiple mechanisms in failing human hearts. *Circ. Res.* **2003**, *92*, 715–724. [CrossRef]
141. Bugger, H.; Schwarzer, M.; Chen, D.; Schrepper, A.; Amorim, P.A.; Schoepe, M.; Nguyen, T.D.; Mohr, F.W.; Khalimonchuk, O.; Weimer, B.C.; et al. Proteomic remodelling of mitochondrial oxidative pathways in pressure overload-induced heart failure. *Cardiovasc. Res.* **2010**, *85*, 376–384. [CrossRef] [PubMed]
142. Nakai, A.; Yamaguchi, O.; Takeda, T.; Higuchi, Y.; Hikoso, S.; Taniike, M.; Omiya, S.; Mizote, I.; Matsumura, Y.; Asahi, M.; et al. The role of autophagy in cardiomyocytes in the basal state and in response to hemodynamic stress. *Nat. Med.* **2007**, *13*, 619–624. [CrossRef] [PubMed]
143. Lee, Y.; Lee, H.Y.; Hanna, R.A.; Gustafsson, A.B. Mitochondrial autophagy by Bnip3 involves Drp1-mediated mitochondrial fission and recruitment of Parkin in cardiac myocytes. *Am. J. Physiol. Heart Circ. Physiol.* **2011**, *301*, H1924–H1931. [CrossRef] [PubMed]
144. Yan, L.; Vatner, D.E.; Kim, S.J.; Ge, H.; Masurekar, M.; Massover, W.H.; Yang, G.; Matsui, Y.; Sadoshima, J.; Vatner, S.F. Autophagy in chronically ischemic myocardium. *Proc. Natl. Acad. Sci. USA* **2005**, *102*, 13807–13812. [CrossRef] [PubMed]
145. Billia, F.; Hauck, L.; Konecny, F.; Rao, V.; Shen, J.; Mak, T.W. PTEN-inducible kinase 1 (PINK1)/Park6 is indispensable for normal heart function. *Proc. Natl. Acad. Sci. USA* **2011**, *108*, 9572–9577. [CrossRef]
146. Saito, T.; Nah, J.; Oka, S.I.; Mukai, R.; Monden, Y.; Maejima, Y.; Ikeda, Y.; Sciarretta, S.; Liu, T.; Li, H.; et al. An alternative mitophagy pathway mediated by Rab9 protects the heart against ischemia. *J. Clin. Investig.* **2019**, *129*, 802–819. [CrossRef]
147. Barger, P.M.; Brandt, J.M.; Leone, T.C.; Weinheimer, C.J.; Kelly, D.P. Deactivation of peroxisome proliferator-activated receptor-alpha during cardiac hypertrophic growth. *J. Clin. Investig.* **2000**, *105*, 1723–1730. [CrossRef]
148. Pisano, A.; Cerbelli, B.; Perli, E.; Pelullo, M.; Bargelli, V.; Preziuso, C.; Mancini, M.; He, L.; Bates, M.G.; Lucena, J.R.; et al. Impaired mitochondrial biogenesis is a common feature to myocardial hypertrophy and end-stage ischemic heart failure. *Cardiovasc. Pathol.* **2016**, *25*, 103–112. [CrossRef]
149. Hein, S.; Arnon, E.; Kostin, S.; Schonburg, M.; Elsasser, A.; Polyakova, V.; Bauer, E.P.; Klovekorn, W.P.; Schaper, J. Progression from compensated hypertrophy to failure in the pressure-overloaded human heart: Structural deterioration and compensatory mechanisms. *Circulation* **2003**, *107*, 984–991. [CrossRef]
150. Zhu, H.; Tannous, P.; Johnstone, J.L.; Kong, Y.; Shelton, J.M.; Richardson, J.A.; Le, V.; Levine, B.; Rothermel, B.A.; Hill, J.A. Cardiac autophagy is a maladaptive response to hemodynamic stress. *J. Clin. Investig.* **2007**, *117*, 1782–1793. [CrossRef]
151. Page, I.H. The mosaic theory of arterial hypertension–its interpretation. *Perspect. Biol. Med.* **1967**, *10*, 325–333. [CrossRef] [PubMed]

152. Marshall, J.D.; Bazan, I.; Zhang, Y.; Fares, W.H.; Lee, P.J. Mitochondrial dysfunction and pulmonary hypertension: Cause, effect, or both. *Am. J. Physiol. Lung Cell. Mol. Physiol.* **2018**, *314*, L782–L796. [CrossRef] [PubMed]
153. Aggarwal, S.; Mannam, P.; Zhang, J. Differential regulation of autophagy and mitophagy in pulmonary diseases. *Am. J. Physiol. Lung Cell. Mol. Physiol.* **2016**, *311*, L433–L452. [CrossRef] [PubMed]
154. Lahm, T.; Albrecht, M.; Fisher, A.J.; Selej, M.; Patel, N.G.; Brown, J.A.; Justice, M.J.; Brown, M.B.; Van Demark, M.; Trulock, K.M.; et al. 17beta-Estradiol attenuates hypoxic pulmonary hypertension via estrogen receptor-mediated effects. *Am. J. Respir. Crit. Care Med.* **2012**, *185*, 965–980. [CrossRef] [PubMed]
155. Lee, S.J.; Smith, A.; Guo, L.; Alastalo, T.P.; Li, M.; Sawada, H.; Liu, X.; Chen, Z.H.; Ifedigbo, E.; Jin, Y.; et al. Autophagic protein LC3B confers resistance against hypoxia-induced pulmonary hypertension. *Am. J. Respir. Crit. Care Med.* **2011**, *183*, 649–658. [CrossRef] [PubMed]
156. Rawat, D.K.; Alzoubi, A.; Gupte, R.; Chettimada, S.; Watanabe, M.; Kahn, A.G.; Okada, T.; McMurtry, I.F.; Gupte, S.A. Increased reactive oxygen species, metabolic maladaptation, and autophagy contribute to pulmonary arterial hypertension-induced ventricular hypertrophy and diastolic heart failure. *Hypertension* **2014**, *64*, 1266–1274. [CrossRef]
157. Teng, R.J.; Du, J.; Welak, S.; Guan, T.; Eis, A.; Shi, Y.; Konduri, G.G. Cross talk between NADPH oxidase and autophagy in pulmonary artery endothelial cells with intrauterine persistent pulmonary hypertension. *Am. J. Physiol. Lung Cell. Mol. Physiol.* **2012**, *302*, L651–L663. [CrossRef]
158. Waldmann, V.; Marijon, E. Cardiac arrhythmias: Diagnosis and management. *Rev. Med. Interne* **2016**, *37*, 608–615. [CrossRef]
159. Yang, K.C.; Bonini, M.G.; Dudley, S.C., Jr. Mitochondria and arrhythmias. *Free Radic. Biol. Med.* **2014**, *71*, 351–361. [CrossRef]
160. Burkhalter, M.D.; Sridhar, A.; Sampaio, P.; Jacinto, R.; Burczyk, M.S.; Donow, C.; Angenendt, M.; Competence Network for Congenital Heart Defects, I.; Hempel, M.; Walther, P.; et al. Imbalanced mitochondrial function provokes heterotaxy via aberrant ciliogenesis. *J. Clin. Investig.* **2019**, *129*, 2841–2855. [CrossRef]
161. Zaidi, S.; Brueckner, M. Genetics and Genomics of Congenital Heart Disease. *Circ. Res.* **2017**, *120*, 923–940. [CrossRef] [PubMed]
162. Pampliega, O.; Cuervo, A.M. Autophagy and primary cilia: Dual interplay. *Curr. Opin. Cell Biol.* **2016**, *39*, 1–7. [CrossRef] [PubMed]
163. Tang, Z.; Lin, M.G.; Stowe, T.R.; Chen, S.; Zhu, M.; Stearns, T.; Franco, B.; Zhong, Q. Autophagy promotes primary ciliogenesis by removing OFD1 from centriolar satellites. *Nature* **2013**, *502*, 254–257. [CrossRef] [PubMed]
164. Wang, S.; Livingston, M.J.; Su, Y.; Dong, Z. Reciprocal regulation of cilia and autophagy via the MTOR and proteasome pathways. *Autophagy* **2015**, *11*, 607–616. [CrossRef] [PubMed]
165. Zhang, J.; Liu, J.; Liu, L.; McKeehan, W.L.; Wang, F. The fibroblast growth factor signaling axis controls cardiac stem cell differentiation through regulating autophagy. *Autophagy* **2012**, *8*, 690–691. [CrossRef]
166. Lacolley, P.; Regnault, V.; Nicoletti, A.; Li, Z.; Michel, J.B. The vascular smooth muscle cell in arterial pathology: A cell that can take on multiple roles. *Cardiovasc. Res.* **2012**, *95*, 194–204. [CrossRef] [PubMed]
167. Salabei, J.K.; Hill, B.G. Implications of autophagy for vascular smooth muscle cell function and plasticity. *Free Radic. Biol. Med.* **2013**, *65*, 693–703. [CrossRef]
168. Hu, N.; Kong, L.S.; Chen, H.; Li, W.D.; Qian, A.M.; Wang, X.Y.; Du, X.L.; Li, C.L.; Yu, X.B.; Li, X.Q. Autophagy protein 5 enhances the function of rat EPCs and promotes EPCs homing and thrombus recanalization via activating AKT. *Thromb. Res.* **2015**, *136*, 642–651. [CrossRef]
169. Sarafian, V.; Dikov, D.; Karaivanov, M.; Belovejdov, V.; Stefanova, P. Differential expression of ABH histo-blood group antigens and LAMPs in infantile hemangioma. *J. Mol. Histol.* **2005**, *36*, 455–460. [CrossRef]
170. Kroemer, G.; Jaattela, M. Lysosomes and autophagy in cell death control. *Nat. Rev. Cancer* **2005**, *5*, 886–897. [CrossRef]
171. Jahania, S.M.; Sengstock, D.; Vaitkevicius, P.; Andres, A.; Ito, B.R.; Gottlieb, R.A.; Mentzer, R.M., Jr. Activation of the homeostatic intracellular repair response during cardiac surgery. *J. Am. Coll. Surg.* **2013**, *216*, 719–726. [CrossRef] [PubMed]
172. Andres, A.M.; Hernandez, G.; Lee, P.; Huang, C.; Ratliff, E.P.; Sin, J.; Thornton, C.A.; Damasco, M.V.; Gottlieb, R.A. Mitophagy is required for acute cardioprotection by simvastatin. *Antioxid. Redox Signal.* **2014**, *21*, 1960–1973. [CrossRef] [PubMed]

173. Das, S.; Mitrovsky, G.; Vasanthi, H.R.; Das, D.K. Antiaging properties of a grape-derived antioxidant are regulated by mitochondrial balance of fusion and fission leading to mitophagy triggered by a signaling network of Sirt1-Sirt3-Foxo3-PINK1-PARKIN. *Oxid. Med. Cell Longev.* **2014**, *2014*, 345105. [CrossRef] [PubMed]
174. Zhang, J.; Wang, J.; Xu, J.; Lu, Y.; Jiang, J.; Wang, L.; Shen, H.M.; Xia, D. Curcumin targets the TFEB-lysosome pathway for induction of autophagy. *Oncotarget* **2016**, *7*, 75659–75671. [CrossRef]
175. Yang, L.; Wang, X.; Yang, X. Possible antioxidant mechanism of melanoidins extract from Shanxi aged vinegar in mitophagy-dependent and mitophagy-independent pathways. *J. Agric. Food Chem.* **2014**, *62*, 8616–8622. [CrossRef]
176. Ma, L.; Zhu, J.; Gao, Q.; Rebecchi, M.J.; Wang, Q.; Liu, L. Restoring Pharmacologic Preconditioning in the Aging Heart: Role of Mitophagy/Autophagy. *J. Gerontol. A Biol. Sci. Med. Sci.* **2017**, *72*, 489–498. [CrossRef]
177. Thangaraj, A.; Periyasamy, P.; Guo, M.L.; Chivero, E.T.; Callen, S.; Buch, S. Mitigation of cocaine-mediated mitochondrial damage, defective mitophagy and microglial activation by superoxide dismutase mimetics. *Autophagy* **2019**, 1–24. [CrossRef]
178. Bian, X.; Teng, T.; Zhao, H.; Qin, J.; Qiao, Z.; Sun, Y.; Liun, Z.; Xu, Z. Zinc prevents mitochondrial superoxide generation by inducing mitophagy in the setting of hypoxia/reoxygenation in cardiac cells. *Free Radic. Res.* **2018**, *52*, 80–91. [CrossRef]
179. Qiao, H.; Ren, H.; Du, H.; Zhang, M.; Xiong, X.; Lv, R. Liraglutide repairs the infarcted heart: The role of the SIRT1/Parkin/mitophagy pathway. *Mol. Med. Rep.* **2018**, *17*, 3722–3734. [CrossRef]
180. Jang, S.Y.; Kang, H.T.; Hwang, E.S. Nicotinamide-induced mitophagy: Event mediated by high NAD+/NADH ratio and SIRT1 protein activation. *J. Biol. Chem.* **2012**, *287*, 19304–19314. [CrossRef]
181. Tarocco, A.; Caroccia, N.; Morciano, G.; Wieckowski, M.R.; Ancora, G.; Garani, G.; Pinton, P. Melatonin as a master regulator of cell death and inflammation: Molecular mechanisms and clinical implications for newborn care. *Cell Death Dis.* **2019**, *10*, 317. [CrossRef] [PubMed]
182. Carloni, S.; Favrais, G.; Saliba, E.; Albertini, M.C.; Chalon, S.; Longini, M.; Gressens, P.; Buonocore, G.; Balduini, W. Melatonin modulates neonatal brain inflammation through endoplasmic reticulum stress, autophagy, and miR-34a/silent information regulator 1 pathway. *J. Pineal Res.* **2016**, *61*, 370–380. [CrossRef] [PubMed]
183. Carloni, S.; Riparini, G.; Buonocore, G.; Balduini, W. Rapid modulation of the silent information regulator 1 by melatonin after hypoxia-ischemia in the neonatal rat brain. *J. Pineal Res.* **2017**, *63*. [CrossRef] [PubMed]
184. Morciano, G.; Giorgi, C.; Bonora, M.; Punzetti, S.; Pavasini, R.; Wieckowski, M.R.; Campo, G.; Pinton, P. Molecular identity of the mitochondrial permeability transition pore and its role in ischemia-reperfusion injury. *J. Mol. Cell Cardiol.* **2015**, *78*, 142–153. [CrossRef]
185. Zhou, H.; Zhang, Y.; Hu, S.; Shi, C.; Zhu, P.; Ma, Q.; Jin, Q.; Cao, F.; Tian, F.; Chen, Y. Melatonin protects cardiac microvasculature against ischemia/reperfusion injury via suppression of mitochondrial fission-VDAC1-HK2-mPTP-mitophagy axis. *J. Pineal Res.* **2017**, *63*. [CrossRef]
186. Kim, I.; Rodriguez-Enriquez, S.; Lemasters, J.J. Selective degradation of mitochondria by mitophagy. *Arch. Biochem. Biophys.* **2007**, *462*, 245–253. [CrossRef]
187. Rocha, A.G.; Franco, A.; Krezel, A.M.; Rumsey, J.M.; Alberti, J.M.; Knight, W.C.; Biris, N.; Zacharioudakis, E.; Janetka, J.W.; Baloh, R.H.; et al. MFN2 agonists reverse mitochondrial defects in preclinical models of Charcot-Marie-Tooth disease type 2A. *Science* **2018**, *360*, 336–341. [CrossRef]
188. Gabisonia, K.; Prosdocimo, G.; Aquaro, G.D.; Carlucci, L.; Zentilin, L.; Secco, I.; Ali, H.; Braga, L.; Gorgodze, N.; Bernini, F.; et al. MicroRNA therapy stimulates uncontrolled cardiac repair after myocardial infarction in pigs. *Nature* **2019**, *569*, 418–422. [CrossRef]
189. Yang, F.; Li, T.; Dong, Z.; Mi, R. MicroRNA-410 is involved in mitophagy after cardiac ischemia/reperfusion injury by targeting high-mobility group box 1 protein. *J. Cell Biochem.* **2018**, *119*, 2427–2439. [CrossRef]
190. Li, W.; Zhang, X.; Zhuang, H.; Chen, H.G.; Chen, Y.; Tian, W.; Wu, W.; Li, Y.; Wang, S.; Zhang, L.; et al. MicroRNA-137 is a novel hypoxia-responsive microRNA that inhibits mitophagy via regulation of two mitophagy receptors FUNDC1 and NIX. *J. Biol. Chem.* **2014**, *289*, 10691–10701. [CrossRef]

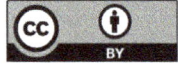 © 2020 by the authors. Licensee MDPI, Basel, Switzerland. This article is an open access article distributed under the terms and conditions of the Creative Commons Attribution (CC BY) license (http://creativecommons.org/licenses/by/4.0/).

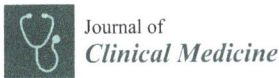

Review

# The Role of Mitochondria in Inflammation: From Cancer to Neurodegenerative Disorders

Sonia Missiroli, Ilaria Genovese, Mariasole Perrone, Bianca Vezzani, Veronica A. M. Vitto and Carlotta Giorgi *

Department of Medical Sciences, Laboratory for Technologies of Advanced Therapies (LTTA), University of Ferrara, 44121 Ferrara, Italy; msssno@unife.it (S.M.); ilaria.genovese@unife.it (I.G.); prrmsl@unife.it (M.P.); vzzbnc@unife.it (B.V.); vttvnc@unife.it (V.A.M.V.)
* Correspondence: grgclt@unife.it

Received: 21 January 2020; Accepted: 6 March 2020; Published: 9 March 2020

**Abstract:** The main features that are commonly attributed to mitochondria consist of the regulation of cell proliferation, ATP generation, cell death and metabolism. However, recent scientific advances reveal that the intrinsic dynamicity of the mitochondrial compartment also plays a central role in proinflammatory signaling, identifying these organelles as a central platform for the control of innate immunity and the inflammatory response. Thus, mitochondrial dysfunctions have been related to severe chronic inflammatory disorders. Strategies aimed at reestablishing normal mitochondrial physiology could represent both preventive and therapeutic interventions for various pathologies related to exacerbated inflammation. Here, we explore the current understanding of the intricate interplay between mitochondria and the innate immune response in specific inflammatory diseases, such as neurological disorders and cancer.

**Keywords:** mitochondria; inflammation; neurodegenerative diseases; cancer

## 1. Introduction

In addition to their role as cellular powerhouses by coupling metabolite oxidation through the tricarboxylic acid (TCA) cycle to the production of high amounts of adenosine triphosphate (ATP) by the electron transport chain (ETC), mitochondria are multifaceted organelles that execute a wide array of functions, including regulation of calcium ($Ca^{2+}$) homeostasis, orchestration of apoptosis and differentiation [1].

Mitochondria contain their own DNA genome (mtDNA) that is expressed and replicated by nucleus-encoded factors imported into the organelle. mtDNA encodes thirteen proteins necessary for oxidative phosphorylation as well as the ribosomal and transfer RNAs needed for their translation. Mitochondria are functionally versatile organelles, which continuously elongate (by fusion), undergo fission to form new mitochondria or undergo controlled turnover (by mitophagy). These processes represent a fundamental framework of mitochondrial dynamics determining mitochondria morphology and volume and allow their immediate adaptation to energetic needs. Thus, mitochondria change their shape and number in response to physiological or metabolic conditions and guard against deleterious stresses that preserve cellular homeostasis.

Mitochondria are also the primary source of cellular reactive oxygen species (ROS) and are therefore highly involved in oxidative stress [2]. Under physiological conditions, ROS act as mitogen signals that provide many cellular functions; however, ROS overproduction leads to uncontrolled reactions with proteins, mtDNA and lipids, resulting in cell dysfunction and/or death.

In addition to their dynamic behavior in programmed cell death and metabolism, mitochondria are now considered central hubs in regulating innate immunity and inflammatory responses [3].

For decades, it has been observed that during the activation phase of an immune response, immune cells shift from a state of relative quiescence to a highly active metabolic state, which usually consists of a transition to a robust anabolic condition aimed at sustaining cell proliferation [4].

As a consequence, mitochondria have emerged as being necessary for both the establishment and maintenance of innate and adaptive immune cell responses [5,6]. Moreover, mitochondrial metabolism helps to control the function of immune cells beyond its role in generating ATP or metabolites that support macromolecule synthesis (for more details see [3])

Inflammation is a complex organismal response to infection and/or tissue damage in which various secreted mediators coordinate defense and repair and avoid further cell or tissue injury. Inflammation also stimulates tissue repair and regeneration to restore homeostasis and organismal health. Nevertheless, when the inflammatory process persists, it acquires new characteristics and drives various diseases in which inflammation and tissue damage/stress self-sustain each other [7].

An abundance of evidence points to a role for ROS generated by mitochondria (mROS) in regulating inflammatory signaling; thus, it is not surprising that mitochondria have been implicated in multiple aspects of the inflammatory response [8].

In general, inflammation induced by oxidative stress acts as a feedback system sustaining a stressful condition that could result in severe tissue damage and trigger chronic inflammation. This process is mainly orchestrated by the activation of the NOD-, LRR- and pyrin domain-containing 3 (NLRP3) inflammasome, currently the most fully characterized inflammasome [9] (see the text for further details). Thus, mitochondria can be considered the principal drivers of NLRP3-mediated inflammation as they can modulate innate immunity via redox-sensitive inflammatory pathways or directly activate the inflammasome complex. In line with this notion, (i) mitochondria represent a checkpoint of the intracellular cascades of numerous downstream pattern recognition receptors (PRRs); (ii) mitochondria have been recently identified as the major site for the generation of damage-associated molecular patterns (DAMPs), which are molecules recognized by the innate immune system that can polarize the fate of the inflammatory response by modulating the energetic level of immune cells in a NLRP3-dependent manner; and (iii) mtDNA has been implicated in NLRP3 inflammasome activation, inducing the release of proinflammatory cytokines so strongly that it can be considered a trigger of neurodegeneration [10].

In this review, we aim to discuss the role of the mitochondria in coordinating proinflammatory signaling, starting from their key role in modulating the innate immunity response and further focusing on mitochondrial dysfunction in two pathologies known to be supported and promoted by inflammation: neurodegenerative diseases and cancer. Nevertheless, we will briefly describe actual therapies aimed at targeting the mitochondria-driven inflammatory response.

## 2. Mitochondria: Key Players in Innate Immunity

In recent years, studies on mitochondrial control of immunity have expanded drastically, and they have increasingly identified mitochondria as key hubs in the innate immune system, acting as signaling platforms as well as mediators in effector responses. The first line of defense against dangerous stimuli is represented by the innate immune response [10]. Recognition of pathogens is predominantly arbitrated by a set of germline-encoded molecules on innate immune cells that are denoted to as PRRs. PRRs are able to perceive and distinguish conserved microbial structures, pathogen-associated molecular patterns (PAMPs) like lipoproteins, carbohydrate, microbial nucleic acids, or endogenous DAMPs including ATP, mtDNA, and cardiolipin, which are released by the cells of the host in response to injury or necrotic cell death [11].

These molecules often are similar to PAMPs both in terms of their structures and specific locations and can be exposed to PRRs during pathological conditions or failure of homeostasis.

Among the PRRs, the membrane-bound Toll-like receptors (TLRs), nucleotide-binding oligomerization domain-like receptors (NLRs), C-type lectin receptors (CLRs), AIM2-like receptor (ALR) and retinoic acid-inducible gene I (RIG-I)-like receptor (RLR) activate the immune system and trigger a response against a pathogen, resulting in the activation of different intracellular signaling cascades, such as the activation of nuclear factor NF-kB (nuclear factor kappa-light-chain-enhancer of activated B cells) or the cellular kinase c-Jun amino-terminal kinase (JNK) [12], and the release of proinflammatory cytokines, chemokines and adhesion molecules, thereby accelerating the inflammatory response [13].

This section focuses on the key role of mitochondria in modulating innate immune responses after viral infection, NLRP3 inflammasome activation or bacterial exposure (Figure 1).

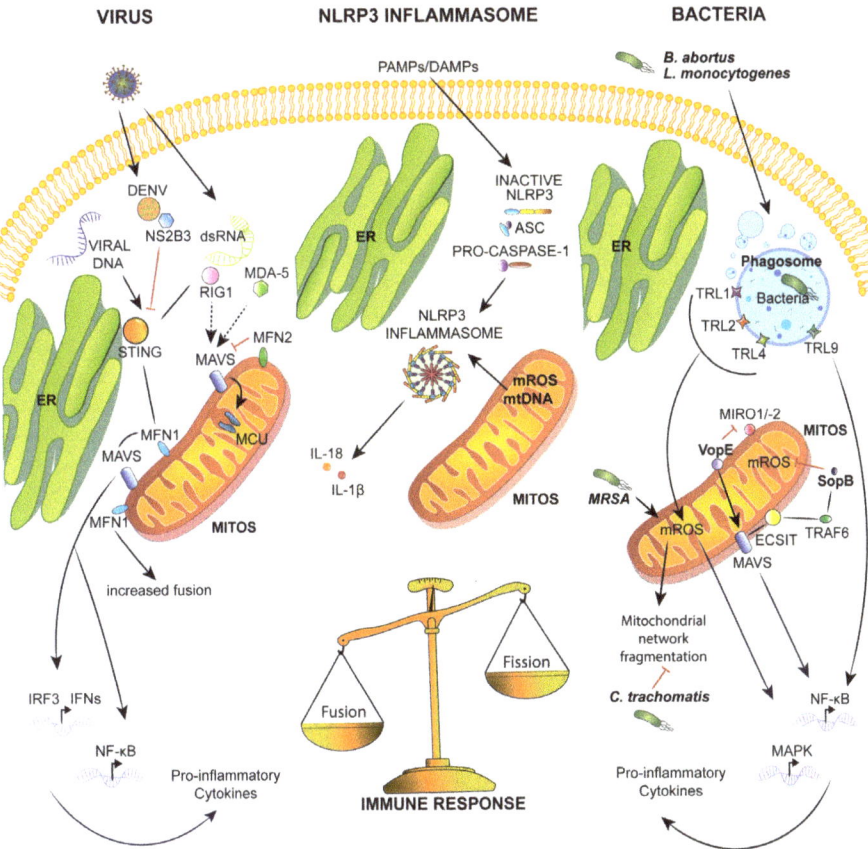

**Figure 1.** Schematic representation of the role of mitochondria in innate immunity. Viral infection, exposure to PAMPs/DAMPs or exposure to bacteria can activate the immune response, altering mitochondrial dynamics and functions. Upon viral infection, MAVS plays a key role in activation of the innate immune response, activating NF-kB and IRF-3 (interferon regulatory factor 3) signaling and inducing proinflammatory cytokine and type I interferon release. Moreover, mitochondria are a key source of DAMPs that are able to activate the NLRP3 inflammasome, leading to proinflammatory cytokine release such as IL-1β and IL-18. Several bacteria manipulate mitochondria during infection. See text for further details. DAMPs: damage-associated molecular patterns; DENV: dengue virus; ER: endoplasmic reticulum; NLRP3: NOD-, LRR- and pyrin domain-containing 3; MCU: mitochondrial calcium uniporter; MDA-5: melanoma differentiation-associated gene 5; MFN: mitofusin; mROS: mitochondrial reactive oxygen species; PAMPs: pathogen-associated molecular patterns; RIG-1: retinoic acid-inducible gene I; TLRs: Toll-like receptors; TRAF6: tumor necrosis factor receptor associated factor 6.

## 2.1. Mitochondrial Dynamics During Viral Infection

Throughout viral infection, the immune response can be mediated by two receptors of the RLR pathway, melanoma differentiation–associated gene 5 (MDA-5) and the RIG-I, which detect cytoplasmic, virus-derived dsRNA [14]. These two pathways merge at the point of transcriptional activation, leading to the production of type I interferons (IFN-α and IFN-β). Notably, both RIG-I and MDA-5 contain two caspase recruitment domains (CARDs) that permit them to interact with the CARD domain of the mitochondrial antiviral signaling (MAVS) protein.

The identification of the MAVS protein initiated research on the role and function of mitochondria in the activation of innate immune pathways [15]. MAVS is embedded on the outer mitochondrial membrane (OMM) via its C-terminal transmembrane domain. MAVS is a pivotal signaling adaptor that activates NF-kB and IRF-3 signaling, inducing antiviral and inflammatory pathways for the production of proinflammatory cytokines and IFN-I during the development of innate immune responses to RNA viruses [16]. Intriguingly, it has been demonstrated that MAVS interacts with mitofusin-2 (MFN2) via a central 4,3 hydrophobic heptad region (HR1) [17]. In particular, a large amount of MFN2 sequesters MAVS in a nonproductive state, reducing both endogenous transcription factor interferon regulatory factor 3 (IRF-3) dimerization and NF-kB expression. On the other hand, the loss of endogenous MFN2 increases the production of IFN-β following a viral infection, which decreases viral replication. It is speculated that MFN2 inhibits dimerization at the CARD domain of MAVS [17]. Interestingly, similar results have not been obtained by modulating MFN1 expression levels, suggesting that MFN2 has a single role in regulating MAVS signaling, independent of its function in mitochondrial fusion. Noteworthy, cells deficient in both mitofusins lack the ability to undergo mitochondrial fusion and display a reduced MMP correlated to a defective cellular antiviral immune responses [18]. The dissipation of MMP has no effect on the activation of IRF-3 downstream of MAVS, suggesting that MMP and MAVS are involved in the same stage of RLR signaling pathway [18].

Moreover, MAVS interacts with stimulator of interferon genes (STING), a protein localized at the endoplasmic reticulum (ER) and involved in the antiviral cell response [19]. Upon infection with DNA viruses, STING is activated downstream of cGAMP synthase (cGAS) to induce IFN-I. STING interacts with RIG-1, stabilizing it, and activates both the IRF3 and NF-kB transcription pathways and the subsequent release of cytokines and proteins, such as the type I IFN, which exert its antipathogenic activities [20,21]. A growing body of literature has demonstrated that mitochondrial dynamics modulate antiviral RLR signaling, adding a new layer of complexity to mitochondrial antiviral immune responses [22,23].

Castanier and colleagues demonstrated that RLR activation promotes mitochondrial network elongation [24]. In an elegant way, they showed that MAVS binds MFN1 (functioning as a negative regulator of MAVS) and STING at the ER-mitochondrial interface, regulates mitochondrial morphology and facilitates the mitochondria–ER association required for signal transduction. Moreover, cytomegalovirus (CMV) infection impedes signaling downstream from MAVS and reduces the MAVS-STING association. [24]. Finally, they stated that mitochondrial fusion is required for efficient RLR signaling, as inhibition of fusion by knockdown of either MFN1 or optic atrophy 1 (OPA1) decreased virus-induced NF-kB and IRF3 activation [24]. On the other hand, cells depleted of dynamin-related protein 1 (DRP1) and FIS1, proteins involved in mitochondrial fission, displayed elongated mitochondrial networks and increased RLR signaling.

A recent study found that evolutionarily conserved signaling intermediate in Toll pathways (ECSIT) localizes at the mitochondrial surface with MAVS protein and mediates bridging of the MAVS protein to RIG-I or MDA5. In turn, ECSIT induces the activation of the antiviral response via upregulation of IRF3 and increasing the expression of IFN-β during viral infection [25].

Another example of how viral infection could modulate mitochondrial dynamics is represented by dengue virus (DENV) infection. DENV protease NS2B3 cleaves MFN1 and MFN2, which participate in host defense in different ways: MFN1 fosters MAVS-mediated IFN production and caspase activation, while MFN2 attenuates DENV-induced cell death acting on mitochondrial membrane potential (MMP) [26].

The findings regarding the role of proteins implicated in fission and fusion are controversial, but it is quite apparent that MFN1 and MFN2 interact with MAVS during RLR signaling, and further studies should clarify the exact roles of MFNs in this process. Taken together, these studies reveal as the mitochondrial fusion process is required for a proper ER-mitochondria connection and RLR-MAVS signalosome formation.

Furthermore, upon viral infection, the mitochondrial calcium uniporter (MCU) complex amplifies the RLR signaling activation interacting with MAVS complexes at mitochondria and positively regulates the release of the proinflammatory cytokine IFN-β [27]. IFN-I production by the RLR pathway controls numerous IFN-stimulated genes (ISGs) by binding to interferon-α/β receptor 1 (IFNAR1) and activating downstream signaling via ER stress [27].

Emerging evidence has demonstrated that influenza A virus infection promotes mROS production, which drives innate immune inflammation and worsens viral pathogenesis. Pharmacological inhibition of mROS with the specific scavenger mitoTEMPO reduces airway and lung inflammation in an in vivo model and alleviates influenza virus pathology (31190565).

## 2.2. Mitochondrial Dynamics in NLRP3 Inflammasome Activation

In the last few decades, inflammasomes have been increasingly recognized as playing an important role in innate immune and inflammatory responses. Among the several inflammasomes, the NLRP3 inflammasome has been the most studied and well characterized. The NLRP3 inflammasome is a multiprotein complex that consists of the scaffold protein NLRP3, the adaptor protein ASC (or PYCARD), and the enzyme caspase-1. NLRP3 is a molecular platform activated upon signs of cellular 'danger' to trigger innate immune defenses through the release of proinflammatory cytokines such as interleukin (IL)-1β and IL-18 [28].

A variety of endogenous and exogenous stimuli, such as extracellular ATP, microbial infection, bacterial pore-forming toxins and monosodium urate, asbestos and the adjuvant alum, are able to activate the NLRP3 inflammasome [29], but the mechanisms of activation are currently unclear.

Furthermore, it has been proposed that ROS are responsible for NLRP3 inflammasome activation. The cellular sources of the ROS responsible for NLRP3 inflammasome activation need careful clarification, although numerous studies have convincingly excluded the NADPH oxidase isoforms NOX1, NOX2 and NOX4 [30,31]. Moreover, electron transport through mitochondrial oxidative phosphorylation (OXPHOS) is an important source of cellular ROS that, in turn, can damage cellular proteins, lipids, and nucleic acids via oxidation but can also be a critical second messenger in various redox-sensitive signaling pathways [32,33].

In this context, a great relevance has been attributed to the plethora of activities that takes place at mitochondria-associated ER membranes (MAMs), formed by the close apposition between the ER and mitochondria membranes (principally OMM) [34,35]. This defined region of the cell displays specific properties and a distinct set of proteins [36,37] that allows its purification by biochemical procedures [38]. It is well established that MAMs control several signaling pathways, from the regulation of lipid transfer to $Ca^{2+}$ signaling [39], as well as coordination of ROS homeostasis and inflammation [40]. Thus, MAMs do not only serve as structural base for the localization of multiple molecular players, but also as a strategic platform for the decoding of signals of various nature.

A decade ago, Zhou and colleagues demonstrated that mROS can trigger NLRP3 inflammasome activation [41]. Under resting conditions, NLRP3 localizes to the cytosol, but once activated, NLRP3 relocates into mitochondria and MAMs together with its partner ASC in a ROS-dependent manner [41]. NLRP3 inflammasome activation is impaired by the inhibition of complex I or III of the mitochondrial respiratory chain or by the inhibition of the voltage-dependent anionic channel (VDAC), known to promote ROS generation [41]. Moreover, thioredoxin (TRX)-interacting protein (TXNIP), a protein involved in type 2 diabetes, redistributes to MAMs/mitochondria upon NLRP3 inflammasome activation in a ROS-dependent manner [42].

Furthermore, mROS, through the modulation of the NLRP3 inflammasome, can activate innate immunity [41,43].

In addition to alteration of inflammatory signaling pathways regulated by mROS, several studies have demonstrated that $Ca^{2+}$-signaling is also important during NLRP3-mediated inflammation [44].

As in many other settings involving $Ca^{2+}$ signaling, $Ca^{2+}$ appears to be mobilized from the extracellular space as well as intracellular stores. Different hypotheses have been proposed for the role of $Ca^{2+}$-signaling in NLRP3 activation [45], one of which is based on the role that $Ca^{2+}$ sensing receptor (CASR) may have in the activation of NLRP3 by either increasing intracellular $Ca^{2+}$ or decreasing cAMP [46]. Another model proposed that $Ca^{2+}$ flux, through ER $Ca^{2+}$ release channels, promotes mitochondrial $Ca^{2+}$ overload and destabilization [47]. Supporting evidence by Misawa et al. reports that, during inflammasome formation, microtubules enhance the perinuclear migration of mitochondria, favoring the juxtaposition of all components for NLRP3 assembly between ER and the mitochondria [48]. These data suggest that the proximity between mitochondria and ER facilitates the transmission and propagation of $Ca^{2+}$ signals between the two organelles, promoting the inflammatory response.

No less important, mtDNA has been demonstrated to mediate the inflammatory response and to be important for caspase-1 activation. In response to LPS and ATP, inhibition of autophagic proteins leads to dysfunctional mitochondria and cytosolic translocation of mtDNA; in turn, cytosolic mtDNA contributes to downstream activation of caspase-1 [49]. Corroborating these results, Shimada and colleagues stated that oxidized mtDNA binds and activates the NLRP3 inflammasome [50].

Moreover, mitochondrial dynamics also are able to modulate NLRP3 inflammasome activation. In fact, knockdown of *Drp1* induces an increased mitochondrial elongation, which leads to NLRP3-dependent caspase-1 activation and IL-1β production in mouse bone marrow-derived macrophages [51]. In addition, chemical stimulators of mitochondrial fission, like carbonyl cyanide m-chlorophenyl hydrazine, clearly reduce NLRP3 inflammasome assembly and activation [51]. Recently, SESN2 (sestrin 2), known as stress-inducible protein, has been shown to induce mitophagy that removes the damaged mitochondria repressing prolonged NLRP3 inflammasome activation [52].

## 2.3. Mitochondrial Dynamics during Bacterial Infection

As already mentioned, mitochondria are the target of choice for viruses, but also several bacteria have been reported to manipulate mitochondria during infection.

Mitochondrial Rho GTPases (Miro1 and Miro2) have been reported to regulate mitochondrial dynamics and in turn the mitochondria-dependent immune response during bacterial infection. During infection, a *Vibrio cholerae* Type 3 secretion system effector (VopE) localizes to the mitochondria, thanks to membrane potential, and acts as a specific GTPase-activating protein, which interferes with Miro1 and 2 [53]. Intriguingly, VopE increases MAVS aggregation and induces NF-kB signaling [53].

Furthermore, infection with *Brucella abortus* leads to altered mitochondrial energy production due to a metabolic shift to a Warburg-like state [54] and induces DRP1-independent mitochondrial fragmentation [55].

An example of how bacteria exploit the mitochondrial network to promote their own replication is infection with *Listeria monocytogenes*, which severely alters mitochondrial dynamics by causing mitochondrial network fragmentation and loss of MMP [56]

To favor its own replication, *Legionella pneumophila* interacts with mitochondria, inducing mitochondria fragmentation that finally leads to altered mitochondrial metabolism [57].

Another example of how bacteria create a favorable niche for their replication is *Chlamydia trachomatis*, an obligate intracellular human pathogen, which preserves mitochondrial integrity by inhibiting fragmentation and reducing DRP1 expression [58]. Furthermore, *C. trachomatis* initially takes advantage of host ATP mitochondrial production and then generates a sodium gradient to sustain its energetic demand [59].

Emerging evidence has demonstrated that mROS also facilitate antibacterial innate immune signaling and phagocyte bactericidal activity.

The SopB effector protein of *Salmonella typhimurium* suppresses mROS generation in response to infection to dampen the host immune response and to facilitate its establishment into the host cell [60]. SopB binds to cytosolic tumor necrosis factor receptor associated factor 6 (TRAF6), prevents its recruitment to mitochondria and inhibits apoptosis [60].

Infection of macrophages with methicillin-resistant *Staphylococcus aureus* (MRSA) induces mROS production that is IRE1α-dependent and triggers the generation of Parkin-dependent mitochondrial-derived vesicles (MDVs), which contribute to mitochondrial-peroxide accumulation in the bacteria-containing phagosome [61].

West et al. demonstrated that the mitochondrial adaptor protein ECSIT interacts with TRAF6 to upregulate mROS production in macrophages, which is essential for bactericidal activity following TLR1, TLR2 or TLR4 ligation [62].

Additionally, bacterial DNA is recognized by TLR9, a member of the highly conserved PRRs known as TLR. TLR9 recognizes unmethylated CpG dinucleotides, which are abundant in prokaryotic DNA and yet are rare in eukaryotic DNA. Nevertheless, mtDNA could be considered a ligand of TLR9 [63].

Taken together, these data pinpointed that, in addition to their well-established roles in the control of apoptosis and cellular metabolism, mitochondria are also intertwined in the innate immune response to cellular damage and appear to be pivotal hubs for innate immune signaling and the consequent generation of effector responses.

## 3. Role of Mitochondria and Neuroinflammation in Neurodegenerative Diseases

Neurodegeneration is a pathological condition characterized by the progressive degeneration and loss of neurons and synapses in a particular area of the central nervous system (CNS). This degenerative process is based on a multifactorial mechanism, which involves genetics, aging, endogenous and environmental factors. Even if the basic molecular mechanisms beyond neurodegeneration are still not fully understood, neurodegenerative disorders (NDDs) can be grouped according to common pathogenic mechanisms: aberrant protein dynamics (misfolding, defective degradation, proteasomal dysfunction), oxidative stress and excessive ROS production, impaired bioenergetics with mitochondrial dysfunction and DNA damage, neutrophil dysfunction and neuroinflammatory processes [64].

In this review, we are going to focus on the impact of mitochondrial dysfunction and neuroinflammation in the development of NDDs from a clinical point of view.

Notably, local sterile inflammation has been shown to be finely linked with the development and the progression of different NDDs, such as Alzheimer's disease (AD), Parkinson's disease (PD), amyotrophic lateral sclerosis (ALS) and multiple sclerosis (MS) [65,66]. Neuroinflammation is commonly driven through the abnormal activation of brain immune cells, namely, microglia and astrocytes, by DAMP molecules released from damaged and necrotic cells [67,68]. Microglia cells represent the macrophage counterpart in the brain. They are responsible for the removal of damaged neurons and for monitoring pathogens. On the other hand, astrocytes account for the maintenance of brain structure and regulation of synapses and represent neuronal metabolic support [67]. Dysregulated activation of microglia and astrocytes results in persistent inflammasome activation, which, together with an increased level of DAMPs, leads to the establishment of low-grade chronic inflammation and thus to the development of age-related pathological processes [69]. Noticeably, neuroinflammation drives the increased secretion of cytokines and chemokines not only within the brain, but also systemically [70] and, in some cases, might lead to blood brain barrier disruption with the consequent infiltration of peripheral immune cells [67]. Accordingly, neuroinflammatory processes have been associated with metabolism alterations, such as obesity and type 2 diabetes [71,72]. At the molecular level, neuroinflammation is mainly triggered by redox status [73]: ROS are produced by microglia upon their activation by intrinsic or extrinsic factors (reviewed in [74]) and are released in the extracellular space. Uncontrolled ROS production might affect intracellular redox balance, thus inducing the expression of proinflammatory genes by acting as second messengers [75]. Consequently, abnormal activation of microglia leads to the release of reactive oxygen intermediates, proinflammatory cytokines, complement proteins and proteinases, driving a chronic inflammatory state responsible for triggering or maintaining neurodegenerative processes [76]. It is important to underline that redox-dependent pathways not only control inflammation but also are involved in different cellular functions, such as the regulation of metabolism, aging, proliferation, differentiation and apoptosis [77]. As already mentioned, the major players involved in these processes are mitochondria, as they are responsible for both generating ROS and responding to ROS-induced cellular changes [78]. Hence, mitochondrial dysfunction can be both the leading cause of neuroinflammation and can be induced by it. It is well known that mitochondria represent the cellular energy supply, and since the primary source of energy for the brain is glucose, alterations of neuronal glucose metabolism, mainly supported by mitochondria, lead to impaired cognitive functions [78]. The brain uses approximately 25% of the total glucose required by the body [79]; this is because neurons depend on OXPHOS to support their functions, like synaptic transmission and maintenance of neuronal potential [68,80,81].

Briefly, the OXPHOS pathway generates ATP using nicotinamide adenine dinucleotide (NADH) and flavin adenine dinucleotide (FADH2) produced by the TCA cycle. Therefore, due to the restricted ability of neurons to enhance glycolysis or to counteract oxidative stress, mitochondrial dysfunction leading to energy failure and oxidative damage is considered the basis of neuronal cell loss in neuroinflammation [82,83]. Consequently, prolonged inflammation, due to microglial inflammasome activation, oxidants and cytokine secretion (as $H_2O_2$, IL-1β and IL-18), combined with the alteration of neuronal cell metabolism are the triggering causes of neurodegeneration (Figure 2) [68]. Interestingly, aberrant activity of TCA enzymes, such as alpha-ketoglutarate dehydrogenase (KGDH), and pyruvate dehydrogenase (PDH) have been observed in the brain tissue of patients with AD [84,85].

More complex is the scenario in MS, where cellular metabolism varies according to the activity of the disease. Specifically, in active MS demyelinating lesions, characterized by the presence of activated microglia and macrophages, increased levels of PDH complex, malate dehydrogenase (MDH) and KGDH were detected compared to normal white matter, indicating that glycolytic and TCA cycle pathways were increased [86]. On the contrary, in demyelinated axons, namely, inside the inactive lesion (plaque), KGDH activity was reduced, thus correlating with terminal axonal damage [86]. These findings suggest that the TCA cycle is definitely altered in NDDs, but upregulation or downregulation of its enzymes might change according to the type of disease and the type of cells involved.

Oxidative stress and mitochondrial metabolism are finely linked in NDDs: myeloperoxidase activity has been shown to be upregulated in the microglia of patients with AD and the brains of patients with MS [87,88], and myeloperoxidase products, namely, hypochlorous acid and chloramine, can inhibit KGDH activity, thus revealing its sensitivity to inflammatory ROS.

Administration of glutathione, a well-known antioxidant, was able to restore KGDH activity after peroxynitrite treatment in neuroblastoma cell cultures [89]. Taken together, these results suggest that during neuroinflammation, TCA cycle enzyme activity is affected, indicating the possible involvement of inflammatory mediators (as ROS) in altering mitochondrial metabolism.

This hypothesis is supported by studies conducted on different cell types and tissues, such as cardiomyocytes, fibroblasts, skeletal muscle and liver, in which inflammatory cytokines have been shown to influence TCA cycle components, mainly reducing PDH activity and therefore acetyl-CoA production via glycolysis.

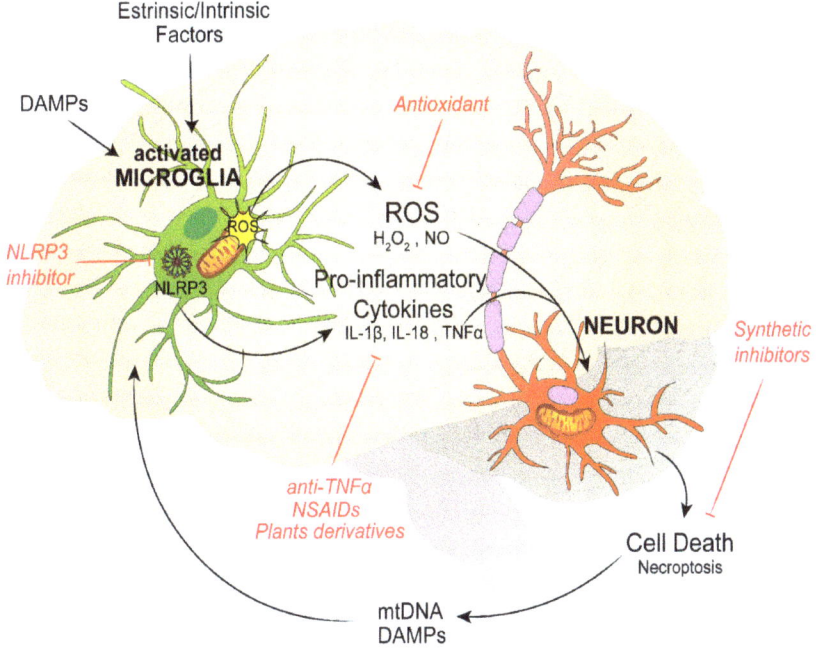

**Figure 2.** Involvement of mitochondrial dysfunction and neuroinflammation in the development of neurodegenerative diseases. DAMPs or extrinsic/intrinsic factors activate microglia that lead to ROS production and proinflammatory cytokines release that in turn alter neuronal functions and induce cell death. This creates a vicious cycle that favors mtDNA and DAMP production, activating the NLRP3 inflammasome. Selective NLRP3 inhibitors, antioxidants, specific inhibitors that block the necroptotic pathway, anti-TNFα, NSAIDs and plant derivatives can prevent this mechanism. DAMPs: damage-associated molecular patterns; NLRP3: NOD-, LRR- and pyrin domain-containing 3; NSAID: nonsteroidal anti-inflammatory drugs; mtDNA: mitochondrial DNA; ROS: reactive oxygen species.

Interestingly, genes encoding ETC complexes have been shown to be downregulated in patients presenting mild cognitive impairment, AD or MS. In AD patients, upregulation of immune genes was reported, confirming the correlation between impaired cell metabolism and inflammation [90]. In both AD and MS, microglia are persistently activated with the consequent release of inflammatory mediators, such as ROS, cytokines and chemokines, which leads to OXPHOS impairment in neurons and other glial cells [83]. Several studies have shown how TNFα bursts, either induced by lipopolysaccharide (LPS) or by direct TNFα administration, affect OXPHOS complexes in the liver, primary neuronal cell culture and cardiac muscle [91–95]. At the same time, TNFα inhibition restored complex III and ATP synthase activity [96]. TNFα is a pleiotropic cytokine that is able to induce cell death by binding to the p55 receptor (TNF receptor 1). Interestingly, it has been shown that in the neurodegenerative context, TNFα induces neuronal cell death by silencing survival signals (SOSS), such as phosphatidylinositol 3' kinase, indicating SOSS inhibition as a possible treatment for neurodegenerative disorders [97]. Noticeably, TNFα treatment promotes mitophagy in neuro-blastoma cells [98]. TNFα exerts its proinflammatory role also by reducing peroxisome proliferator-activated receptor (PPAR)-γ coactivator 1α (PGC-1α) expression [99] and by increasing mitochondrial fragmentation acting on OPA1 isoform balance [100], even if these effects have not been investigated in nervous tissue yet.

However, PGC-1α has been found to be downregulated in NDD neurons, and IL-1β has been shown to induce mitochondrial fragmentation and to impair the respiration rate in astrocytes, underlying the role of proinflammatory cytokines in regulating mitochondria dynamics in the CNS [101].

Damaged mitochondria trigger the process of mitochondrial membrane permeabilization, known to be the starting point of both apoptosis and necrosis. Apoptosis is essential for nervous system development, whereas adult neurons are resistant to this form of cell death [102]. Recently, different studies have shown how necroptosis, a form of regulated necrotic cell death induced by TNFα, is highly activated in NDDs [102–104]. Briefly, necroptosis is a form of programed cell death coordinated by receptor-interacting kinases 1 (RIPK1) and RIPK3 and mixed lineage kinase domain-like protein (MLKL) under caspase-8 deficient conditions. Necroptosis can be stimulated by TNF, other members of the TNF death ligand family, interferons, Toll-like receptor signaling and viral infection [105]. In MS patients, the RIPK1-RIPK3-MLKL pathway is activated, and experiments in animal models showed that oligodendrocytes necroptosis could be blocked by RIPK1 inhibition [66,106].

Lastly, as previously mentioned, accumulation of damaged mitochondria can activate NLRP3 inflammasome-dependent inflammation in microglia. Moreover, damaged neurons are responsible for releasing DAMPs, such as mtDNA, in the extracellular environment, eliciting local inflammation [49] by increasing inflammasome activation, and thus IL-1β secretion, and also binding to microglial toll-like receptor-9, inducing TNFα and nitric oxide (NO) production [107].

In conclusion, neuroinflammation affects many mitochondrial processes such as TCA, OXPHOS, fusion and fission, membrane permeabilization, and mitophagy and might also induce the accumulation of mtDNA mutations, impairing energy production and thus distressing cognitive ability, even if a direct correlation between alterations of these cellular functions and patient clinical outcomes is still under investigation. Moreover, extracellular release of mitochondrial components (mtDNA or proteins) acts as an inflammatory boost, leading to a vicious inflammatory cycle. Therefore, from a therapeutic point of view, suppression of microglia-mediated inflammation can be considered an important curative strategy for NDDs. Accordingly, different nonsteroidal anti-inflammatory drugs (NSAID) repress microglial activation, targeting cyclooxygenase (COX) or PPAR-γ and exerting neuroprotective effects in the CNS [76,108]. Several studies suggested inhibition of Rho kinase (ROCK) signaling, shown to be involved in mitochondrial fission, as a promising treatment option for NDD [109]. Interestingly, a recent study revealed that curcumin, the main curcuminoid isolated from *Curcuma longa* (turmeric), significantly reduced TNFα, prostaglandin E2 (PGE2), and NO secretion in in vitro lipoteichoic acid-activated microglial cells. Curcumin also inhibited NO synthases (iNOS) and COX-2 expression [110]. Similarly, the ent-kauranoid diterpenoid glaucocalyxin B, isolated from the aerial parts of *Rabdosia japonica*, decreased NO, TNFα, IL-1β, COX-2 and iNOS in LPS-activated microglia cells [111]. These plant derivatives might represent a promising approach in targeting neuroinflammation, and different studies are aiming to define their optimal bioavailability, even if their use in clinic has yet to be defined [112,113]. Another therapeutic approach to reduce neuroinflammation is blocking necroptotic pathways with synthetic inhibitors (RIP1 inhibitors, RIP3 inhibitors, MLKL inhibitors) to mitigate NDD progression [114]. Drug treatments aimed at manipulating inflammasome assembly therapeutically are currently used in clinic [115], but, despite their promising efficacy, they still do not resolve the disease. The low efficacy of actual therapies in treating NDDs might be due to the complexity of neurodegenerative processes, which involve neuroinflammation but also have roots in genetic predisposition and environmental factors. Nevertheless, reduction in inflammation ameliorates disease progression, therefore representing a fundamental complementary therapy. Since neuroinflammation is one of the triggering causes of NDDs, therapies aimed at reducing the inflammatory process result in a reduction in disease progression, therefore representing a fundamental complementary therapy.

## 4. Inflammation-Related Mitochondrial Dysfunction in Cancer: A Negative Loop

In 1893, Rudolf Virchow was the first to hypothesize that chronic inflammation and tumorigenesis were connected [116]. This assumption was deduced from the presence of leukocytes in cancerous lesions and from the idea that inflammation caused by injuries and irritants can contribute to cell proliferation.

Further studies indicated that inflammation represents a potential risk factor for tumorigenesis; indeed, some inflammatory conditions are related to malignant transformation. Some examples of this correlation can be found in *Helicobacter pylori*-caused gastritis and gastric cancer, gut pathogens involved in inflammatory bowel diseases and colon rectal cancer, or human Papilloma virus' cervicitis and cervical cancer, but also in chemical/physical irritants such as asbestos fibers that lead to asbestosis and mesothelioma or UV rays that cause sunburns and melanoma, as well as tobacco and alcohol, which cause bronchitis or pancreatitis, respectively, leading to lung cancer and pancreatic/liver cancer [117].

Recent studies demonstrated that approximately 25% of tumor malignancies are related to chronic inflammation and pathogen infection [118]. As a matter of fact, cancer-related inflammation is the 7th hallmark in tumor development [119].

Hanahan and Weinberg reviewed that cancer-related chronic inflammation drives unlimited proliferative potential, independence from growth factors, enhanced angiogenesis, metastasis, escape from apoptosis and resistance to growth inhibition [120].

Further evidence demonstrated that the tumor microenvironment, rich in inflammatory cells, fosters proliferation, survival and migration of tumors. Moreover, cancer cells appropriate some of the signaling molecules of innate immunity to promote invasiveness and proliferation [121].

To summarize, deficient pathogen eradication or recurring injuries, as well as prolonged inflammatory signaling, support cancer development, so that tumors can be considered a failed wound-healing process [117].

It is largely known that mitochondria regulate the metabolic needs of cells and decide between life and death upon different conditions. Recently, it has been demonstrated that MOM permeabilization exposes cells to considerable proinflammatory effects; among these, the release of mtDNA from the mitochondria leads to the IFN-I response and NF-kB proinflammatory signaling via the IAP-regulated mechanism [122].

Otto Warburg, in the 1930s, was the first to link mitochondrial dysfunctions to cancer. Indeed, he observed that tumor cells display an increased rate of aerobic glycolysis; from this evidence, he speculated that the production of ATP via glycolysis instead of oxidative phosphorylation might be explained by mitochondrial respiratory capacity impairment.

Moreover, several studies have proposed that altered cancer cell metabolism, defined as acidic and/or ischemic, that enables survival in a hostile environment represents a strategy of evasion from the attack of immune system cells, thus reinforcing cancer stem cell resistance [123].

In past decades, a large amount of data has been collected on the possible mitochondrial defects that can lead to cancer, such as alteration in the activity and expression of the mitochondrial respiration complex (MRC) and mtDNA mutations [124].

Of note, dysfunction in MRC Complex I is associated with Hürtle cell tumors of the thyroid [125], and a decrease in Complex III activity can be linked to breast cancer, [126] and Hürtle cell tumors [127,128]. Moreover, decreased activity of Complex II, III, and IV is associated with the aggressiveness of renal cell tumors [129].

Regarding mtDNA, many lines of evidence show correlation between mutations and ovarian, kidney, thyroid, liver, gastric, colon, lung, head and neck, brain, breast, and bladder cancers and leukemia [130].

Even though the link between key mitochondrial players and cancer is quite well established, the connection between MRC dysfunction and mtDNA mutations in cancer and inflammation remains to be fully elucidated. In a vicious cycle, the impairment of respiratory chain proteins and mitochondrial genes causes an increase in mitochondrial ROS production, as these species are the cause of damage.

Among mitochondrial dysfunctions, it is well established that ROS are important signaling molecules that participate in cell migration and invasiveness, proliferation, migration and gene transcription. In addition, ROS levels increase upon mitochondrial malfunction, as tumor cells usually have higher ROS production compared to normal cells [2].

Intriguingly, a connection between ROS and hypoxia-inducible factor (HIF) has been reported. HIF is a crucial transcription factor for cancer metabolism and metastasis, and it is activated upon hypoxic conditions. ROS, though, are able to stabilize HIF even under a normal oxygen concentration, thus promoting tumorigenesis [131].

Moreover, lack of succinate dehydrogenase (Complex I) and fumarate hydratase in tumors is related to difficulty in HIF degradation [132].

Additionally, a ROS increase results in activation of the NLRP3 inflammasome and release of proinflammatory cytokines, such as IL-1β, that suppress immune-surveillance, enabling tumor progression [9].

Thus, chronic inflammation diseases are characterized by an overproduction of free radicals, often concomitant with a decreased capacity to scavenge them [133]. When ROS reach a dangerous level, cancer cells increase mitochondrial production of NADPH to diminish the effect of ROS to evade apoptosis [134].

ROS represent a threat to all biological macromolecules in the cell; in particular, they cause oxidation to the fatty acids of plasma membranes, proteins and genes, causing mutations and cancer-related alterations [135].

Upon the activation of innate immune cells, there is secretion of proinflammatory soluble molecules, cytokines and chemokines that induce ROS production (Figure 3). In a chronic inflammation context, ROS production from immune system cells can drive to cell damage or hyperplasia [136]; for instance, IL-1, IL-6, TNFα and IFN-γ induce ROS production in nonphagocytic cells as well.

Indeed, in the inflammatory process, TNFα activates the transcription factor NF-kB, which in turn induces the expression of genes involved in cell proliferation, carcinogenesis and blockage of apoptosis, as well as the production of proinflammatory cytokines to potentiate the response. In this context, ROS have a dual role: (i) they can be considered a potential threat when overproduced by mitochondria in tumorigenesis, as well as enhancers of cancer proliferation through the activation of proliferation pathways via the innate immune system, together with the inactivation immune surveillance; and (ii) they can sustain a chronic innate immune response.

As stated, nucleic acids can be severely damaged by free radicals, especially mtDNA, since they lack the protection of histone proteins. In a dangerous loop reaction, ROS induce mutations in mtDNA, leading to dysfunction in the production of proteins of the respiratory chain, thus enhancing the production of ROS [137]. An alternative study conducted by Trifunovic and collaborators reported that mtDNA mutator mice, an aging model, did not show either an increase in ROS production or an increased sensitivity to oxidative stress-induced cell death despite the accumulation of mtDNA mutations in a linear manner, even in the presence of severe respiratory chain impairment [138]. Even though this study gives an alternative point of view on mtDNA mutation-dependent ROS production, it would be interesting to understand which mitochondrial genes are more susceptible to mutation in order to define whether there can be a direct correlation between mtDNA mutations and ROS production.

Although mtDNA is the most harmed macromolecule, it fulfills a double role in cancer-related inflammation. Recently, several pieces of evidence showed a horizontal transfer of mitochondria between tumor cells and surrounding nontumor cells, so it has been hypothesized that this transfer is a strategy that cancer cells adopt to counteract mitochondrial dysfunction and satisfy high metabolic requirements [139]. Tan and collaborators have demonstrated that when there is a lack of mtDNA, there is a decrease in tumor growth, so tumor cells start to acquire mtDNA molecules from healthy surrounding cells, restoring their metabolic functions and their tumorigenic potential, most likely with the aid of the mitochondria themselves [140].

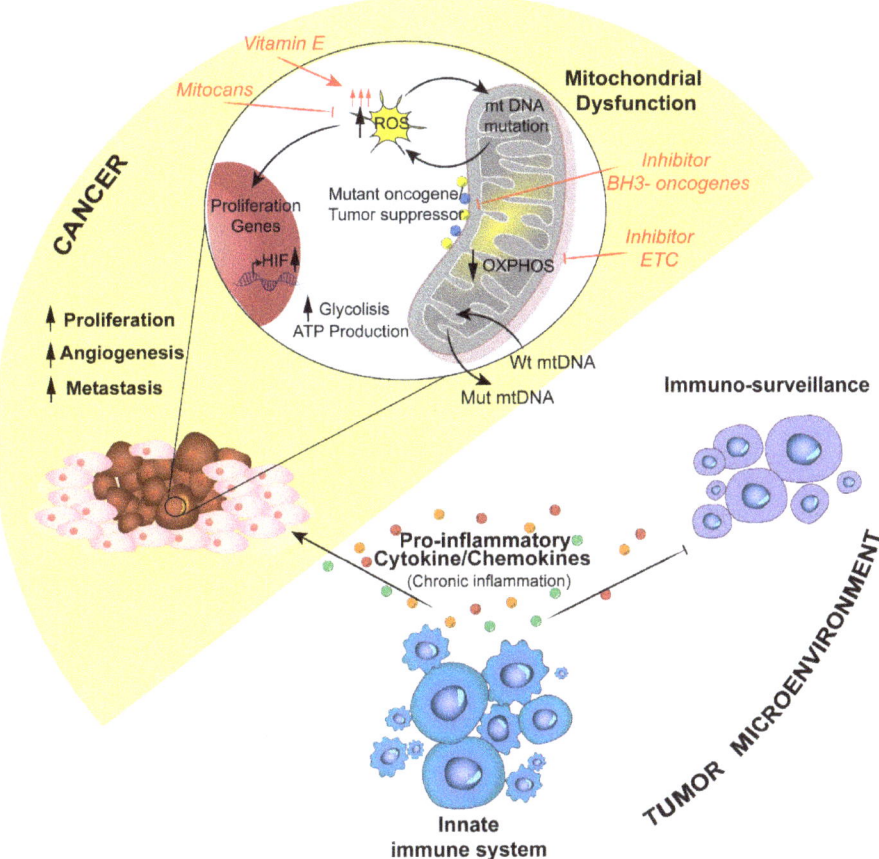

**Figure 3.** Schematic representation of how mitochondrial dysfunctions, which alter the inflammatory response, can promote cancer. In cancer, mitochondrial dysfunctions lead to increased ROS production, which can have a dual role that is either dangerous or prosurvival. On the one hand, mitochondrial ROS (mROS) can accumulate DNA mutations; on the other hand, mROS can increase cytokine inflammatory release from the innate immune system. A strategy that cancer cells can adopt to survive the increased rate of mutations is represented by the horizontal transfer of wild-type mtDNA molecules from surrounding healthy cells. The inflammatory response by the innate immune system can sustain cell tumor growth instead of counteracting it, altering the immune-surveillance and STING pathways (see text for further details). The main clinical strategy could be the selective inhibition of mROS production. ETC: electron transport chain; MOMP: mitochondrial outer membrane permeabilization; mtDNA: mitochondrial DNA; OXPHOS: mitochondrial oxidative phosphorylation; PKM2: pyruvate kinase M2; ROS: reactive oxygen species.

To date, it remains undefined how this phenomenon is triggered and how healthy cells can be persuaded. Some in vitro evidence has shown that solid tumor cell lines are able to acquire healthy mitochondria from MSCs (mesenchymal stem cells) and endothelial cells, possibly suggesting the participation of the circulatory system in this process. For a complete overview on the topic and possible strategies for mtDNA transfer, we suggest the review by Berridge and collaborators [141].

It has been reported that cancer progression is promoted by mtDNA molecules in the surrounding microenvironment and circulating system, which in turn regulates the production of proinflammatory cytokines suppressing antitumor effects exerted by the immune system. Dendritic cells, through STING signaling, recognize circulating mtDNA activating lymphocytes to trigger tumor suppression, but the inappropriate sensing of mtDNA results in a deficiency of cancer cell clearance by those cells [142]. Furthermore, mtDNA transfer from cancer cells to the microenvironment enriched in immune cells, such as monocytes and natural killer cells, leads to their dysfunction and apoptosis, thus reinforcing tumor progression; for a complete overview refer to Liu et al. [143].

Thus, mutated mtDNA can either be the victim or the inducer of ROS production (from both mitochondria and the innate immune system), possibly representing a risk or an advantage for cancer proliferation. However, circulating wild-type mtDNA transferred by surrounding cells can provide mutations in cancer cells, resulting in evasion of death.

Mitochondrial dysregulation does not involve only free radical production or mtDNA mutation and/or transfer; indeed, the literature is full of evidence showing the involvement of $Ca^{2+}$ homeostasis alterations in cancer. This occurs also at MAMs, which provide the allocation of important oncogenes or oncosuppressors, such as p53, PML, PTEN, kRAS, Bcl-2, and Bcl-Xl [144–147], all of which are known to reduce mitochondrial $Ca^{2+}$ uptake, thus blocking apoptosis in cancer models.

As stated, cancer cells are marked by a defective metabolism, so therapies targeting glycolysis, pyruvate oxidation and glutamine metabolism would have a protective effect from chronic inflammation as well [148].

Targeting metabolic traits can be tricky though, since immune and cancer cells have some metabolic differences, and tumor metabolic pathways must be shut down in order to trigger the apoptotic event. Moreover, cancer and immune infiltrating cells reside together in a microenvironment where signaling molecules influence the metabolic choices of both [149]. Tumor-associated macrophages (TAMs) are the best example of metabolic reprogramming exerted by cancer cells because this promotes the increase in protumoral factor production, fostering protumorigenic inflammation conditions that favor the proliferation and metastasis of cancer. TAMs are essentially "educated" by the tumor to let them deliver essential molecules to sustain their proliferation [150].

Together with TAMs, in infiltrating tumor cells it is possible to find several populations of T lymphocytes, particularly T helper 17 cells (Th17) [151] inhibited by the tumor itself. Indeed, it has been proposed that their suppression corresponds to the promotion of regulatory suppressive Treg cells, a population associated with tumorigenesis boost [152]. The impairment of mitochondrial metabolism and failure of immunosurveillance create the conditions for immune-associated diseases, and it is clear by now that cancer is one of these [152] (Figure 3).

The relationship between inflammation and cancer is thus established as a vicious cycle in the mitochondria, where infiltrating immune cells are recruited upon proinflammatory signaling aiming at the eradication of cancer, which is recognized as an inflammatory disease; at the same time, the tumor mass can take advantage of the inflammatory microenvironment to sustain its metabolism. ROS have a crucial role throughout the whole process. Indeed, ROS produced by the immune response aid tumor growth, while on the other hand, cancer cells with impaired mitochondria increase ROS production as well, leading to potential harm that can be evaded through horizontal mtDNA transfer and the upregulation of detoxifying systems.

Recent research showed that the Warburg effect is favorable to tumor cells because it upregulates antioxidant enzymes such as glutathione reductase, superoxide dismutase, catalase, peroxiredoxin, and thioredoxin to diminish the overproduction of ROS [153] that harm mitochondrial macromolecules (i.e., mtDNA and protein), as previously stated.

Another enzyme that plays an important role in this process is the glycolytic enzyme pyruvate kinase M2; cancer cells express the embryonic isoform (PKM2) [154]. The increase in ROS inhibits PKM2 leading to a switch from glycolysis to pentose phosphate metabolism to produce reducing equivalents (NADPH), which are essential to maintain antioxidant molecule activity and necessary for ROS detoxification [155]. In this way, the regulation of PKM2 gives cancer the capability to resist the increase in mtROS production [153].

Fortunately, much effort has been expended in developing therapies against this vicious cycle, all of them targeting apoptosis induction; these therapies are grouped in a category of molecules called mitocans (mitochondrial targeted anticancer drugs).

A group of them includes vitamin E analogs that enhance ROS production in the mitochondria, favoring the induction of apoptosis specifically in cancer cells because they are under greater oxidative stress compared to normal cells [124,156]. These mitocans can also be designed for specific mitochondrial targets, for example components of the OMM, inter-membrane space, *cristae* or the matrix. Specifically, these targets, such as hexokinase (HK), VDAC and adenine nucleotide translocase (ANT), can be involved in the production and shuttling of ADP/ATP; mitocans against these proteins disrupt the main metabolic processes and the antioxidative capability of the tumor [157].

There is also clinical approval for BH3 mimetics that target antiapoptotic proteins of the Bcl-2 family [158,159] for chronic lymphocytic leukemia [160].

ETC is another powerful target for specific inhibitors since its disruption impairs oxidative phosphorylation [161].

Moreover, a novel mitochondrial inhibitor named CPI-613 has been approved for a phase I clinical study with pancreatic cancer patients. This compound blocks two enzymes, pyruvate dehydrogenase and a-ketoglutarate dehydrogenase [162,163], and was administered in combination with modified FOLFIRINOX; the combination has given improved outcomes [164,165].

Nevertheless, other molecules are undergoing optimization processes, and these are compounds that can hinder mitochondrial transmembrane potential, such as lipophilic cations [152]; the Krebs cycle, consequently affecting ECT and OXPHOS [166]; inhibitors against the conversion of pyruvate to AcCoA, hindering the Krebs cycle [167]; or inhibitors that interfere with DNA polymerase, which influences mtDNA transcription, with consequent effects on the mitochondrial protein pool [168,169].

All of this evidence supports mitochondria as new pharmacological targets for patients with cancer. Obviously, more work is necessary to shed light on how mitochondrial dysfunction modulates the inflammatory response associated with tumor development.

## 5. Conclusions

Besides their ancestral function as the powerhouse of eukaryotic cells, mitochondria have gained attention as principal intracellular signaling platforms associated with innate immunity and inflammation. It is now clear that mitochondrial derangement can be considered a crucial pathogenic mechanism of several diseases characterized by chronic inflammation, including neurodegenerative diseases, cancer, rheumatoid and metabolic disorders.

Mitochondrial defects that are able to trigger inflammation are not only limited to metabolic variation or imbalance of the physiological mechanisms that control shape and number but could also be extended to other mitochondrial pathways. As an example, chronic stresses capable of increasing mitochondrial $Ca^{2+}$ entry induce sustained inflammation, and MCU-mediated $Ca^{2+}$ overload is essential for triggering NLRP3-mediated inflammation in patients with cystic fibrosis during infection with *Pseudomonas aeruginosa* [170]. Together with the role of MCU in the regulation of decreasing IFN-β levels induced by viral infection discussed above [27], these observations suggest that the MCU complex could be identified as a potential target in the treatment of inflammation-associated diseases. Future work is required to evaluate if other components of the mitochondrial $Ca^{2+}$ machinery, for example the $Ca^{2+}$ efflux system [171], are involved in the control of inflammation.

Nevertheless, other important issues remain to be clarified. As the interface between mitochondria and MAMs has an important role in controlling the inflammation response [172], it is tempting to speculate that other mitochondrial molecules can regulate MAVS signaling and/or be critical for RLR signaling. Do the mitochondria also translate other innate immunity signaling?

Therapies that target mitochondria-NLRP3 inflammasome activation or mitochondrial dysfunction affecting immune cell function may hold great promise in the treatment of diverse inflammation-mediated diseases. Therefore, answers to these questions may provide new pharmacological targets for the treatment of acute and chronic pathological and inflammatory disorders.

**Author Contributions:** S.M. and C.G. conceived the article; S.M., I.G., M.P. and B.V. wrote the manuscript with input from C.G.; V.A.M.V. prepared display items under supervision from S.M. and C.G. All authors have read and agreed to the published version of the manuscript.

**Funding:** This work was supported by the Italian Association for Cancer Research (AIRC), the Italian Ministry of Health and ERC-STG (Project: 853057—InflaPML) to C.G. I.G. was supported by a research fellowship: AIRC "Acqua Vitasnella" id. 22552.

**Conflicts of Interest:** The authors declare no conflicts of interest.

## Abbreviations

| | |
|---|---|
| AD | Alzheimer's disease; |
| ALR | AIM2-like receptor; |
| ALS | amyotrophic lateral sclerosis; |
| ANT | adenine nucleotide translocase; |
| ATP | adenosine triphosphate; |
| $Ca^{2+}$ | calcium ion; |
| CARDs | caspase recruitment domains; |
| CASR | $Ca^{2+}$ sensing receptor; |
| CLRs | C-type lectin receptors; |
| COX | cyclooxygenase; |
| CMV | cytomegalovirus; |
| DAMPs | damage-associated molecular patterns; |
| DENV | dengue virus; |
| ETC | electron transport chain; |
| ER | endoplasmic reticulum; |
| FADH2 | flavin adenine dinucleotide; |
| HIF | hypoxia-inducible factors; |
| HK | hexokinase; |
| IFN | type I interferon |
| IL-1β | interleukin-1beta; |
| IRF-3 | interferon regulatory factor 3; |
| JNK | c-Jun amino-terminal kinase; |
| KGDH | alpha-ketoglutarate dehydrogenase; |
| MAMs | mitochondria associated ER membranes; |
| MAVS | mitochondrial antiviral signaling; |
| MCU | mitochondrial calcium uniporter; |
| MDA-5 | melanoma differentiation-associated gene 5; |
| MDVs | mitochondrial-derived vesicles; |
| MFN1 | mitofusin-1; |
| MFN2 | mitofusin-2; |
| MMP | mitochondrial membrane potential; |
| mROS | mitochondrial reactive oxygen species; |
| mtDNA | mitochondrial DNA; |
| MRC | mitochondrial respiration complex; |
| MS | multiple sclerosis; |
| NADH | nicotinamide adenine dinucleotide; |
| NDDs | neurodegenerative disorders; |
| NF-kB | nuclear factor kappa-light-chain-enhancer of activated B cells |
| NSAID | nonsteroidal anti-inflammatory drugs; |
| NO | nitric oxide; |
| NLRs | nucleotide-binding oligomerization domain-like receptors; |

| | |
|---|---|
| NLRP3 | NOD-, LRR- and pyrin domain containing 3; |
| OMM | outer mitochondrial membrane; |
| OPA1 | optic atrophy 1; |
| OXPHOS | mitochondrial oxidative phosphorylation; |
| PAMPs | pathogen-associated molecular patterns; |
| PD | Parkinson's disease; |
| PDH | pyruvate dehydrogenase; |
| PKM2 | pyruvate kinase M2; |
| PRRs | pattern recognition receptor; |
| RIG-1 | retinoic acid-inducible gene I; |
| RIPK1 | receptor-interacting kinases 1; |
| RLR | RIG-I-like receptor; |
| ROS | reactive oxygen species; |
| SOSS | silencing of survival signals; |
| STING | stimulator of interferon genes; |
| TAMs | tumor-associated macrophages; |
| TCA | tricarboxylic acid cycle; |
| TLRs | Toll-like receptors; |
| TRAF6 | tumor necrosis factor receptor associated factor 6; |
| VDAC | voltage-dependent anionic channel; |
| VopE | Type 3 secretion system effector. |

## References

1. Giorgi, C.; Marchi, S.; Pinton, P. The machineries, regulation and cellular functions of mitochondrial calcium. *Nat. Rev. Mol. Cell Biol.* **2018**, *19*, 713–730. [CrossRef]
2. Marchi, S.; Giorgi, C.; Suski, J.M.; Agnoletto, C.; Bononi, A.; Bonora, M.; De Marchi, E.; Missiroli, S.; Patergnani, S.; Poletti, F.; et al. Mitochondria-ros crosstalk in the control of cell death and aging. *J. Signal Transduct.* **2012**, *2012*, 329635. [CrossRef] [PubMed]
3. Mohanty, A.; Tiwari-Pandey, R.; Pandey, N.R. Mitochondria: The indispensable players in innate immunity and guardians of the inflammatory response. *J. Cell Commun. Signal* **2019**, *13*, 303–318. [CrossRef] [PubMed]
4. Pearce, E.L.; Pearce, E.J. Metabolic pathways in immune cell activation and quiescence. *Immunity* **2013**, *38*, 633–643. [CrossRef] [PubMed]
5. Sandhir, R.; Halder, A.; Sunkaria, A. Mitochondria as a centrally positioned hub in the innate immune response. *Biochim. Biophys. Acta Mol. Basis Dis.* **2017**, *1863*, 1090–1097. [CrossRef] [PubMed]
6. Weinberg, S.E.; Sena, L.A.; Chandel, N.S. Mitochondria in the regulation of innate and adaptive immunity. *Immunity* **2015**, *42*, 406–417. [CrossRef] [PubMed]
7. Medzhitov, R. Origin and physiological roles of inflammation. *Nature* **2008**, *454*, 428–435. [CrossRef]
8. Rimessi, A.; Previati, M.; Nigro, F.; Wieckowski, M.R.; Pinton, P. Mitochondrial reactive oxygen species and inflammation: Molecular mechanisms, diseases and promising therapies. *Int. J. Biochem. Cell Biol.* **2016**, *81*, 281–293. [CrossRef]
9. Zitvogel, L.; Kepp, O.; Galluzzi, L.; Kroemer, G. Inflammasomes in carcinogenesis and anticancer immune responses. *Nat. Immunol.* **2012**, *13*, 343–351. [CrossRef] [PubMed]
10. Mathew, A.; Lindsley, T.A.; Sheridan, A.; Bhoiwala, D.L.; Hushmendy, S.F.; Yager, E.J.; Ruggiero, E.A.; Crawford, D.R. Degraded mitochondrial DNA is a newly identified subtype of the damage associated molecular pattern (DAMP) family and possible trigger of neurodegeneration. *J. Alzheimers Dis.* **2012**, *30*, 617–627. [CrossRef]
11. Kawai, T.; Akira, S. TLR signaling. *Cell Death Differ.* **2006**, *13*, 816–825. [CrossRef] [PubMed]
12. Nguyen, M.T.; Satoh, H.; Favelyukis, S.; Babendure, J.L.; Imamura, T.; Sbodio, J.I.; Zalevsky, J.; Dahiyat, B.I.; Chi, N.W.; Olefsky, J.M. JNK and tumor necrosis factor-alpha mediate free fatty acid-induced insulin resistance in 3T3-L1 adipocytes. *J. Biol. Chem.* **2005**, *280*, 35361–35371. [CrossRef] [PubMed]
13. Garlanda, C.; Dinarello, C.A.; Mantovani, A. The interleukin-1 family: Back to the future. *Immunity* **2013**, *39*, 1003–1018. [CrossRef] [PubMed]
14. Kawai, T.; Akira, S. Innate immune recognition of viral infection. *Nat. Immunol.* **2006**, *7*, 131–137. [CrossRef]

15. Seth, R.B.; Sun, L.; Ea, C.K.; Chen, Z.J. Identification and characterization of MAVS, a mitochondrial antiviral signaling protein that activates NF-kappaB and IRF 3. *Cell* **2005**, *122*, 669–682. [CrossRef]
16. Jacobs, J.L.; Coyne, C.B. Mechanisms of MAVS regulation at the mitochondrial membrane. *J. Mol. Biol.* **2013**, *425*, 5009–5019. [CrossRef]
17. Yasukawa, K.; Oshiumi, H.; Takeda, M.; Ishihara, N.; Yanagi, Y.; Seya, T.; Kawabata, S.; Koshiba, T. Mitofusin 2 inhibits mitochondrial antiviral signaling. *Sci. Signal* **2009**, *2*, ra47. [CrossRef]
18. Koshiba, T.; Yasukawa, K.; Yanagi, Y.; Kawabata, S. Mitochondrial membrane potential is required for MAVS-mediated antiviral signaling. *Sci. Signal* **2011**, *4*, ra7. [CrossRef]
19. Choi, H.J.; Park, A.; Kang, S.; Lee, E.; Lee, T.A.; Ra, E.A.; Lee, J.; Lee, S.; Park, B. Human cytomegalovirus-encoded US9 targets MAVS and STING signaling to evade type I interferon immune responses. *Nat. Commun.* **2018**, *9*, 125. [CrossRef]
20. Abe, T.; Barber, G.N. Cytosolic-DNA-mediated, STING-dependent proinflammatory gene induction necessitates canonical NF-kappaB activation through TBK1. *J. Virol.* **2014**, *88*, 5328–5341. [CrossRef]
21. Ishikawa, H.; Barber, G.N. STING is an endoplasmic reticulum adaptor that facilitates innate immune signalling. *Nature* **2008**, *455*, 674–678. [CrossRef] [PubMed]
22. Arnoult, D.; Soares, F.; Tattoli, I.; Girardin, S.E. Mitochondria in innate immunity. *EMBO Rep.* **2011**, *12*, 901–910. [CrossRef] [PubMed]
23. West, A.P.; Shadel, G.S.; Ghosh, S. Mitochondria in innate immune responses. *Nat. Rev. Immunol.* **2011**, *11*, 389–402. [CrossRef] [PubMed]
24. Castanier, C.; Garcin, D.; Vazquez, A.; Arnoult, D. Mitochondrial dynamics regulate the RIG-I-like receptor antiviral pathway. *EMBO Rep.* **2010**, *11*, 133–138. [CrossRef]
25. Lei, C.Q.; Zhang, Y.; Li, M.; Jiang, L.Q.; Zhong, B.; Kim, Y.H.; Shu, H.B. ECSIT bridges RIG-I-like receptors to VISA in signaling events of innate antiviral responses. *J. Innate Immun.* **2015**, *7*, 153–164. [CrossRef]
26. Yu, C.Y.; Liang, J.J.; Li, J.K.; Lee, Y.L.; Chang, B.L.; Su, C.I.; Huang, W.J.; Lai, M.M.; Lin, Y.L. Dengue Virus Impairs Mitochondrial Fusion by Cleaving Mitofusins. *PLoS Pathog.* **2015**, *11*, e1005350. [CrossRef]
27. Cheng, J.; Liao, Y.; Zhou, L.; Peng, S.; Chen, H.; Yuan, Z. Amplified RLR signaling activation through an interferon-stimulated gene-endoplasmic reticulum stress-mitochondrial calcium uniporter protein loop. *Sci. Rep.* **2016**, *6*, 20158. [CrossRef]
28. Schroder, K.; Zhou, R.; Tschopp, J. The NLRP3 inflammasome: A sensor for metabolic danger? *Science* **2010**, *327*, 296–300. [CrossRef]
29. Tschopp, J.; Schroder, K. NLRP3 inflammasome activation: The convergence of multiple signalling pathways on ROS production? *Nat. Rev. Immunol.* **2010**, *10*, 210–215. [CrossRef]
30. Meissner, F.; Molawi, K.; Zychlinsky, A. Superoxide dismutase 1 regulates caspase-1 and endotoxic shock. *Nat. Immunol.* **2008**, *9*, 866–872. [CrossRef]
31. Van Bruggen, R.; Koker, M.Y.; Jansen, M.; van Houdt, M.; Roos, D.; Kuijpers, T.W.; van den Berg, T.K. Human NLRP3 inflammasome activation is Nox1-4 independent. *Blood* **2010**, *115*, 5398–5400. [CrossRef] [PubMed]
32. Hamanaka, R.B.; Chandel, N.S. Mitochondrial reactive oxygen species regulate cellular signaling and dictate biological outcomes. *Trends Biochem. Sci.* **2010**, *35*, 505–513. [CrossRef] [PubMed]
33. Shadel, G.S.; Horvath, T.L. Mitochondrial ROS signaling in organismal homeostasis. *Cell* **2015**, *163*, 560–569. [CrossRef] [PubMed]
34. Rizzuto, R.; Pinton, P.; Carrington, W.; Fay, F.S.; Fogarty, K.E.; Lifshitz, L.M.; Tuft, R.A.; Pozzan, T. Close contacts with the endoplasmic reticulum as determinants of mitochondrial Ca2+ responses. *Science* **1998**, *280*, 1763–1766. [CrossRef] [PubMed]
35. Vance, J.E. Phospholipid synthesis in a membrane fraction associated with mitochondria. *J. Biol. Chem.* **1990**, *265*, 7248–7256. [PubMed]
36. Poston, C.N.; Krishnan, S.C.; Bazemore-Walker, C.R. In-depth proteomic analysis of mammalian mitochondria-associated membranes (MAM). *J. Proteom.* **2013**, *79*, 219–230. [CrossRef]
37. Zhang, A.; Williamson, C.D.; Wong, D.S.; Bullough, M.D.; Brown, K.J.; Hathout, Y.; Colberg-Poley, A.M. Quantitative proteomic analyses of human cytomegalovirus-induced restructuring of endoplasmic reticulum-mitochondrial contacts at late times of infection. *Mol. Cell Proteom.* **2011**, *10*. [CrossRef]
38. Wieckowski, M.R.; Giorgi, C.; Lebiedzinska, M.; Duszynski, J.; Pinton, P. Isolation of mitochondria-associated membranes and mitochondria from animal tissues and cells. *Nat. Protoc.* **2009**, *4*, 1582–1590. [CrossRef]

39. Missiroli, S.; Danese, A.; Iannitti, T.; Patergnani, S.; Perrone, M.; Previati, M.; Giorgi, C.; Pinton, P. Endoplasmic reticulum-mitochondria Ca(2+) crosstalk in the control of the tumor cell fate. *Biochim. Biophys. Acta Mol. Cell Res.* **2017**, *1864*, 858–864. [CrossRef]
40. Giorgi, C.; Missiroli, S.; Patergnani, S.; Duszynski, J.; Wieckowski, M.R.; Pinton, P. Mitochondria-associated membranes: Composition, molecular mechanisms, and physiopathological implications. *Antioxid Redox Signal* **2015**, *22*, 995–1019. [CrossRef]
41. Zhou, R.; Yazdi, A.S.; Menu, P.; Tschopp, J. A role for mitochondria in NLRP3 inflammasome activation. *Nature* **2011**, *469*, 221–225. [CrossRef] [PubMed]
42. Zhou, R.; Tardivel, A.; Thorens, B.; Choi, I.; Tschopp, J. Thioredoxin-interacting protein links oxidative stress to inflammasome activation. *Nat. Immunol.* **2010**, *11*, 136–140. [CrossRef] [PubMed]
43. Heid, M.E.; Keyel, P.A.; Kamga, C.; Shiva, S.; Watkins, S.C.; Salter, R.D. Mitochondrial reactive oxygen species induces NLRP3-dependent lysosomal damage and inflammasome activation. *J. Immunol.* **2013**, *191*, 5230–5238. [CrossRef] [PubMed]
44. Giorgi, C.; Danese, A.; Missiroli, S.; Patergnani, S.; Pinton, P. Calcium Dynamics as a Machine for Decoding Signals. *Trends Cell Biol.* **2018**, *28*, 258–273. [CrossRef] [PubMed]
45. Horng, T. Calcium signaling and mitochondrial destabilization in the triggering of the NLRP3 inflammasome. *Trends Immunol.* **2014**, *35*, 253–261. [CrossRef] [PubMed]
46. Lee, G.S.; Subramanian, N.; Kim, A.I.; Aksentijevich, I.; Goldbach-Mansky, R.; Sacks, D.B.; Germain, R.N.; Kastner, D.L.; Chae, J.J. The calcium-sensing receptor regulates the NLRP3 inflammasome through Ca2+ and cAMP. *Nature* **2012**, *492*, 123–127. [CrossRef] [PubMed]
47. Murakami, T.; Ockinger, J.; Yu, J.; Byles, V.; McColl, A.; Hofer, A.M.; Horng, T. Critical role for calcium mobilization in activation of the NLRP3 inflammasome. *Proc. Natl. Acad. Sci. USA* **2012**, *109*, 11282–11287. [CrossRef]
48. Misawa, T.; Takahama, M.; Kozaki, T.; Lee, H.; Zou, J.; Saitoh, T.; Akira, S. Microtubule-driven spatial arrangement of mitochondria promotes activation of the NLRP3 inflammasome. *Nat. Immunol.* **2013**, *14*, 454–460. [CrossRef]
49. Nakahira, K.; Haspel, J.A.; Rathinam, V.A.; Lee, S.J.; Dolinay, T.; Lam, H.C.; Englert, J.A.; Rabinovitch, M.; Cernadas, M.; Kim, H.P.; et al. Autophagy proteins regulate innate immune responses by inhibiting the release of mitochondrial DNA mediated by the NALP3 inflammasome. *Nat. Immunol.* **2011**, *12*, 222–230. [CrossRef]
50. Shimada, K.; Crother, T.R.; Karlin, J.; Dagvadorj, J.; Chiba, N.; Chen, S.; Ramanujan, V.K.; Wolf, A.J.; Vergnes, L.; Ojcius, D.M.; et al. Oxidized mitochondrial DNA activates the NLRP3 inflammasome during apoptosis. *Immunity* **2012**, *36*, 401–414. [CrossRef]
51. Park, S.; Won, J.H.; Hwang, I.; Hong, S.; Lee, H.K.; Yu, J.W. Defective mitochondrial fission augments NLRP3 inflammasome activation. *Sci. Rep.* **2015**, *5*, 15489. [CrossRef] [PubMed]
52. Kim, M.J.; Bae, S.H.; Ryu, J.C.; Kwon, Y.; Oh, J.H.; Kwon, J.; Moon, J.S.; Kim, K.; Miyawaki, A.; Lee, M.G.; et al. SESN2/sestrin2 suppresses sepsis by inducing mitophagy and inhibiting NLRP3 activation in macrophages. *Autophagy* **2016**, *12*, 1272–1291. [CrossRef] [PubMed]
53. Suzuki, M.; Danilchanka, O.; Mekalanos, J.J. Vibrio cholerae T3SS effector VopE modulates mitochondrial dynamics and innate immune signaling by targeting Miro GTPases. *Cell Host Microbe* **2014**, *16*, 581–591. [CrossRef] [PubMed]
54. Czyz, D.M.; Willett, J.W.; Crosson, S. Brucella abortus Induces a Warburg Shift in Host Metabolism That Is Linked to Enhanced Intracellular Survival of the Pathogen. *J. Bacteriol.* **2017**, *199*. [CrossRef] [PubMed]
55. Lobet, E.; Willemart, K.; Ninane, N.; Demazy, C.; Sedzicki, J.; Lelubre, C.; De Bolle, X.; Renard, P.; Raes, M.; Dehio, C.; et al. Mitochondrial fragmentation affects neither the sensitivity to TNFalpha-induced apoptosis of Brucella-infected cells nor the intracellular replication of the bacteria. *Sci. Rep.* **2018**, *8*, 5173. [CrossRef] [PubMed]
56. Stavru, F.; Bouillaud, F.; Sartori, A.; Ricquier, D.; Cossart, P. Listeria monocytogenes transiently alters mitochondrial dynamics during infection. *Proc. Natl. Acad. Sci. USA* **2011**, *108*, 3612–3617. [CrossRef] [PubMed]
57. Escoll, P.; Song, O.R.; Viana, F.; Steiner, B.; Lagache, T.; Olivo-Marin, J.C.; Impens, F.; Brodin, P.; Hilbi, H.; Buchrieser, C. Legionella pneumophila Modulates Mitochondrial Dynamics to Trigger Metabolic Repurposing of Infected Macrophages. *Cell Host Microbe* **2017**, *22*, 302–316. [CrossRef]

58. Chowdhury, S.R.; Reimer, A.; Sharan, M.; Kozjak-Pavlovic, V.; Eulalio, A.; Prusty, B.K.; Fraunholz, M.; Karunakaran, K.; Rudel, T. Chlamydia preserves the mitochondrial network necessary for replication via microRNA-dependent inhibition of fission. *J. Cell Biol.* **2017**, *216*, 1071–1089. [CrossRef]
59. Liang, P.; Rosas-Lemus, M.; Patel, D.; Fang, X.; Tuz, K.; Juarez, O. Dynamic energy dependency of Chlamydia trachomatis on host cell metabolism during intracellular growth: Role of sodium-based energetics in chlamydial ATP generation. *J. Biol. Chem.* **2018**, *293*, 510–522. [CrossRef]
60. Ruan, H.; Zhang, Z.; Tian, L.; Wang, S.; Hu, S.; Qiao, J.J. The Salmonella effector SopB prevents ROS-induced apoptosis of epithelial cells by retarding TRAF6 recruitment to mitochondria. *Biochem. Biophys. Res. Commun.* **2016**, *478*, 618–623. [CrossRef]
61. Abuaita, B.H.; Schultz, T.L.; O'Riordan, M.X. Mitochondria-Derived Vesicles Deliver Antimicrobial Reactive Oxygen Species to Control Phagosome-Localized Staphylococcus aureus. *Cell Host Microbe* **2018**, *24*, 625–636. [CrossRef] [PubMed]
62. West, A.P.; Brodsky, I.E.; Rahner, C.; Woo, D.K.; Erdjument-Bromage, H.; Tempst, P.; Walsh, M.C.; Choi, Y.; Shadel, G.S.; Ghosh, S. TLR signalling augments macrophage bactericidal activity through mitochondrial ROS. *Nature* **2011**, *472*, 476–480. [CrossRef] [PubMed]
63. Zhang, Q.; Raoof, M.; Chen, Y.; Sumi, Y.; Sursal, T.; Junger, W.; Brohi, K.; Itagaki, K.; Hauser, C.J. Circulating mitochondrial DAMPs cause inflammatory responses to injury. *Nature* **2010**, *464*, 104–107. [CrossRef] [PubMed]
64. Jellinger, K.A. Basic mechanisms of neurodegeneration: A critical update. *J. Cell Mol. Med.* **2010**, *14*, 457–487. [CrossRef]
65. Lin, M.T.; Beal, M.F. Mitochondrial dysfunction and oxidative stress in neurodegenerative diseases. *Nature* **2006**, *443*, 787–795. [CrossRef]
66. Patergnani, S.; Fossati, V.; Bonora, M.; Giorgi, C.; Marchi, S.; Missiroli, S.; Rusielewicz, T.; Wieckowski, M.R.; Pinton, P. Mitochondria in Multiple Sclerosis: Molecular Mechanisms of Pathogenesis. *Int. Rev. Cell Mol. Biol.* **2017**, *328*, 49–103. [CrossRef]
67. Wilkins, H.M.; Weidling, I.W.; Ji, Y.; Swerdlow, R.H. Mitochondria-Derived Damage-Associated Molecular Patterns in Neurodegeneration. *Front. Immunol.* **2017**, *8*, 508. [CrossRef]
68. Yin, F.; Sancheti, H.; Patil, I.; Cadenas, E. Energy metabolism and inflammation in brain aging and Alzheimer's disease. *Free Radic. Biol. Med.* **2016**, *100*, 108–122. [CrossRef]
69. Kapetanovic, R.; Bokil, N.J.; Sweet, M.J. Innate immune perturbations, accumulating DAMPs and inflammasome dysregulation: A ticking time bomb in ageing. *Ageing Res. Rev.* **2015**, *24*, 40–53. [CrossRef]
70. Licastro, F.; Pedrini, S.; Caputo, L.; Annoni, G.; Davis, L.J.; Ferri, C.; Casadei, V.; Grimaldi, L.M. Increased plasma levels of interleukin-1, interleukin-6 and alpha-1-antichymotrypsin in patients with Alzheimer's disease: Peripheral inflammation or signals from the brain? *J. Neuroimmunol.* **2000**, *103*, 97–102. [CrossRef]
71. De Felice, F.G.; Ferreira, S.T. Inflammation, defective insulin signaling, and mitochondrial dysfunction as common molecular denominators connecting type 2 diabetes to Alzheimer disease. *Diabetes* **2014**, *63*, 2262–2272. [CrossRef] [PubMed]
72. Spielman, L.J.; Little, J.P.; Klegeris, A. Inflammation and insulin/IGF-1 resistance as the possible link between obesity and neurodegeneration. *J. Neuroimmunol.* **2014**, *273*, 8–21. [CrossRef] [PubMed]
73. Innamorato, N.G.; Lastres-Becker, I.; Cuadrado, A. Role of microglial redox balance in modulation of neuroinflammation. *Curr. Opin. Neurol.* **2009**, *22*, 308–314. [CrossRef] [PubMed]
74. Kierdorf, K.; Prinz, M. Factors regulating microglia activation. *Front. Cell Neurosci.* **2013**, *7*, 44. [CrossRef] [PubMed]
75. Rojo, A.I.; McBean, G.; Cindric, M.; Egea, J.; Lopez, M.G.; Rada, P.; Zarkovic, N.; Cuadrado, A. Redox control of microglial function: Molecular mechanisms and functional significance. *Antioxid Redox Signal* **2014**, *21*, 1766–1801. [CrossRef]
76. Dheen, S.T.; Kaur, C.; Ling, E.A. Microglial activation and its implications in the brain diseases. *Curr. Med. Chem.* **2007**, *14*, 1189–1197. [CrossRef]
77. Franco, R.; Vargas, M.R. Redox Biology in Neurological Function, Dysfunction, and Aging. *Antioxid Redox Signal* **2018**, *28*, 1583–1586. [CrossRef]
78. Handy, D.E.; Loscalzo, J. Redox regulation of mitochondrial function. *Antioxid Redox Signal* **2012**, *16*, 1323–1367. [CrossRef]

79. Rossi, S.; Zanier, E.R.; Mauri, I.; Columbo, A.; Stocchetti, N. Brain temperature, body core temperature, and intracranial pressure in acute cerebral damage. *J. Neurol. Neurosurg. Psychiatry* **2001**, *71*, 448–454. [CrossRef]
80. Belanger, M.; Allaman, I.; Magistretti, P.J. Brain energy metabolism: Focus on astrocyte-neuron metabolic cooperation. *Cell Metab.* **2011**, *14*, 724–738. [CrossRef]
81. Rose, J.; Brian, C.; Woods, J.; Pappa, A.; Panayiotidis, M.I.; Powers, R.; Franco, R. Mitochondrial dysfunction in glial cells: Implications for neuronal homeostasis and survival. *Toxicology* **2017**, *391*, 109–115. [CrossRef] [PubMed]
82. Herrero-Mendez, A.; Almeida, A.; Fernandez, E.; Maestre, C.; Moncada, S.; Bolanos, J.P. The bioenergetic and antioxidant status of neurons is controlled by continuous degradation of a key glycolytic enzyme by APC/C-Cdh1. *Nat. Cell Biol.* **2009**, *11*, 747–752. [CrossRef] [PubMed]
83. Van Horssen, J.; van Schaik, P.; Witte, M. Inflammation and mitochondrial dysfunction: A vicious circle in neurodegenerative disorders? *Neurosci. Lett.* **2019**, *710*, 132931. [CrossRef] [PubMed]
84. Gibson, G.E.; Zhang, H.; Sheu, K.F.; Bogdanovich, N.; Lindsay, J.G.; Lannfelt, L.; Vestling, M.; Cowburn, R.F. Alpha-ketoglutarate dehydrogenase in Alzheimer brains bearing the APP670/671 mutation. *Ann. Neurol.* **1998**, *44*, 676–681. [CrossRef]
85. Mastrogiacoma, F.; Lindsay, J.G.; Bettendorff, L.; Rice, J.; Kish, S.J. Brain protein and alpha-ketoglutarate dehydrogenase complex activity in Alzheimer's disease. *Ann. Neurol.* **1996**, *39*, 592–598. [CrossRef]
86. Nijland, P.G.; Molenaar, R.J.; van der Pol, S.M.; van der Valk, P.; van Noorden, C.J.; de Vries, H.E.; van Horssen, J. Differential expression of glucose-metabolizing enzymes in multiple sclerosis lesions. *Acta Neuropathol. Commun.* **2015**, *3*, 79. [CrossRef]
87. Nagra, R.M.; Becher, B.; Tourtellotte, W.W.; Antel, J.P.; Gold, D.; Paladino, T.; Smith, R.A.; Nelson, J.R.; Reynolds, W.F. Immunohistochemical and genetic evidence of myeloperoxidase involvement in multiple sclerosis. *J. Neuroimmunol.* **1997**, *78*, 97–107. [CrossRef]
88. Reynolds, W.F.; Rhees, J.; Maciejewski, D.; Paladino, T.; Sieburg, H.; Maki, R.A.; Masliah, E. Myeloperoxidase polymorphism is associated with gender specific risk for Alzheimer's disease. *Exp. Neurol.* **1999**, *155*, 31–41. [CrossRef]
89. Shi, Q.; Xu, H.; Yu, H.; Zhang, N.; Ye, Y.; Estevez, A.G.; Deng, H.; Gibson, G.E. Inactivation and reactivation of the mitochondrial alpha-ketoglutarate dehydrogenase complex. *J. Biol. Chem.* **2011**, *286*, 17640–17648. [CrossRef]
90. Lunnon, K.; Ibrahim, Z.; Proitsi, P.; Lourdusamy, A.; Newhouse, S.; Sattlecker, M.; Furney, S.; Saleem, M.; Soininen, H.; Kloszewska, I.; et al. Mitochondrial dysfunction and immune activation are detectable in early Alzheimer's disease blood. *J. Alzheimers Dis.* **2012**, *30*, 685–710. [CrossRef]
91. Doll, D.N.; Rellick, S.L.; Barr, T.L.; Ren, X.; Simpkins, J.W. Rapid mitochondrial dysfunction mediates TNF-alpha-induced neurotoxicity. *J. Neurochem.* **2015**, *132*, 443–451. [CrossRef] [PubMed]
92. Kastl, L.; Sauer, S.W.; Ruppert, T.; Beissbarth, T.; Becker, M.S.; Suss, D.; Krammer, P.H.; Gulow, K. TNF-alpha mediates mitochondrial uncoupling and enhances ROS-dependent cell migration via NF-kappaB activation in liver cells. *FEBS Lett.* **2014**, *588*, 175–183. [CrossRef] [PubMed]
93. Lee, I.; Huttemann, M. Energy crisis: The role of oxidative phosphorylation in acute inflammation and sepsis. *Biochim. Biophys. Acta* **2014**, *1842*, 1579–1586. [CrossRef] [PubMed]
94. Samavati, L.; Lee, I.; Mathes, I.; Lottspeich, F.; Huttemann, M. Tumor necrosis factor alpha inhibits oxidative phosphorylation through tyrosine phosphorylation at subunit I of cytochrome c oxidase. *J. Biol. Chem.* **2008**, *283*, 21134–21144. [CrossRef]
95. Suliman, H.B.; Welty-Wolf, K.E.; Carraway, M.; Tatro, L.; Piantadosi, C.A. Lipopolysaccharide induces oxidative cardiac mitochondrial damage and biogenesis. *Cardiovasc. Res.* **2004**, *64*, 279–288. [CrossRef]
96. Moe, G.W.; Marin-Garcia, J.; Konig, A.; Goldenthal, M.; Lu, X.; Feng, Q. In vivo TNF-alpha inhibition ameliorates cardiac mitochondrial dysfunction, oxidative stress, and apoptosis in experimental heart failure. *Am. J. Physiol. Heart Circ. Physiol.* **2004**, *287*, H1813–H1820. [CrossRef]
97. Venters, H.D.; Dantzer, R.; Kelley, K.W. A new concept in neurodegeneration: TNFalpha is a silencer of survival signals. *Trends Neurosci.* **2000**, *23*, 175–180. [CrossRef]
98. Prajapati, P.; Sripada, L.; Singh, K.; Bhatelia, K.; Singh, R.; Singh, R. TNF-alpha regulates miRNA targeting mitochondrial complex-I and induces cell death in dopaminergic cells. *Biochim. Biophys. Acta* **2015**, *1852*, 451–461. [CrossRef]

99. Palomer, X.; Alvarez-Guardia, D.; Rodriguez-Calvo, R.; Coll, T.; Laguna, J.C.; Davidson, M.M.; Chan, T.O.; Feldman, A.M.; Vazquez-Carrera, M. TNF-alpha reduces PGC-1alpha expression through NF-kappaB and p38 MAPK leading to increased glucose oxidation in a human cardiac cell model. *Cardiovasc. Res.* **2009**, *81*, 703–712. [CrossRef]
100. Hahn, W.S.; Kuzmicic, J.; Burrill, J.S.; Donoghue, M.A.; Foncea, R.; Jensen, M.D.; Lavandero, S.; Arriaga, E.A.; Bernlohr, D.A. Proinflammatory cytokines differentially regulate adipocyte mitochondrial metabolism, oxidative stress, and dynamics. *Am. J. Physiol. Endocrinol. Metab.* **2014**, *306*, E1033–E1045. [CrossRef]
101. Motori, E.; Puyal, J.; Toni, N.; Ghanem, A.; Angeloni, C.; Malaguti, M.; Cantelli-Forti, G.; Berninger, B.; Conzelmann, K.K.; Gotz, M.; et al. Inflammation-induced alteration of astrocyte mitochondrial dynamics requires autophagy for mitochondrial network maintenance. *Cell Metab.* **2013**, *18*, 844–859. [CrossRef] [PubMed]
102. Yuan, J.; Amin, P.; Ofengeim, D. Necroptosis and RIPK1-mediated neuroinflammation in CNS diseases. *Nat. Rev. Neurosci.* **2019**, *20*, 19–33. [CrossRef] [PubMed]
103. Daniels, B.P.; Snyder, A.G.; Olsen, T.M.; Orozco, S.; Oguin, T.H., 3rd; Tait, S.W.G.; Martinez, J.; Gale, M., Jr.; Loo, Y.M.; Oberst, A. RIPK3 Restricts Viral Pathogenesis via Cell Death-Independent Neuroinflammation. *Cell* **2017**, *169*, 301–313. [CrossRef] [PubMed]
104. Ito, Y.; Ofengeim, D.; Najafov, A.; Das, S.; Saberi, S.; Li, Y.; Hitomi, J.; Zhu, H.; Chen, H.; Mayo, L.; et al. RIPK1 mediates axonal degeneration by promoting inflammation and necroptosis in ALS. *Science* **2016**, *353*, 603–608. [CrossRef] [PubMed]
105. Zhang, S.; Tang, M.B.; Luo, H.Y.; Shi, C.H.; Xu, Y.M. Necroptosis in neurodegenerative diseases: A potential therapeutic target. *Cell Death Dis.* **2017**, *8*, e2905. [CrossRef] [PubMed]
106. Ofengeim, D.; Ito, Y.; Najafov, A.; Zhang, Y.; Shan, B.; DeWitt, J.P.; Ye, J.; Zhang, X.; Chang, A.; Vakifahmetoglu-Norberg, H.; et al. Activation of necroptosis in multiple sclerosis. *Cell Rep.* **2015**, *10*, 1836–1849. [CrossRef]
107. Iliev, A.I.; Stringaris, A.K.; Nau, R.; Neumann, H. Neuronal injury mediated via stimulation of microglial toll-like receptor-9 (TLR9). *FASEB J.* **2004**, *18*, 412–414. [CrossRef]
108. Ajmone-Cat, M.A.; Bernardo, A.; Greco, A.; Minghetti, L. Non-Steroidal Anti-Inflammatory Drugs and Brain Inflammation: Effects on Microglial Functions. *Pharmaceuticals* **2010**, *3*, 1949–1965. [CrossRef]
109. Koch, J.C.; Tatenhorst, L.; Roser, A.E.; Saal, K.A.; Tonges, L.; Lingor, P. ROCK inhibition in models of neurodegeneration and its potential for clinical translation. *Pharmacol. Ther.* **2018**, *189*, 1–21. [CrossRef]
110. Yu, Y.; Shen, Q.; Lai, Y.; Park, S.Y.; Ou, X.; Lin, D.; Jin, M.; Zhang, W. Anti-inflammatory Effects of Curcumin in Microglial Cells. *Front. Pharmacol.* **2018**, *9*, 386. [CrossRef]
111. Gan, P.; Zhang, L.; Chen, Y.; Zhang, Y.; Zhang, F.; Zhou, X.; Zhang, X.; Gao, B.; Zhen, X.; Zhang, J.; et al. Anti-inflammatory effects of glaucocalyxin B in microglia cells. *J. Pharmacol. Sci.* **2015**, *128*, 35–46. [CrossRef] [PubMed]
112. Qureshi, M.; Al-Suhaimi, E.A.; Wahid, F.; Shehzad, O.; Shehzad, A. Therapeutic potential of curcumin for multiple sclerosis. *Neurol. Sci.* **2018**, *39*, 207–214. [CrossRef] [PubMed]
113. Ullah, F.; Liang, A.; Rangel, A.; Gyengesi, E.; Niedermayer, G.; Munch, G. High bioavailability curcumin: An anti-inflammatory and neurosupportive bioactive nutrient for neurodegenerative diseases characterized by chronic neuroinflammation. *Arch. Toxicol.* **2017**, *91*, 1623–1634. [CrossRef] [PubMed]
114. Jun-Long, H.; Yi, L.; Bao-Lian, Z.; Jia-Si, L.; Ning, Z.; Zhou-Heng, Y.; Xue-Jun, S.; Wen-Wu, L. Necroptosis Signaling Pathways in Stroke: From Mechanisms to Therapies. *Curr. Neuropharmacol.* **2018**, *16*, 1327–1339. [CrossRef] [PubMed]
115. Shao, B.Z.; Cao, Q.; Liu, C. Targeting NLRP3 Inflammasome in the Treatment of CNS Diseases. *Front. Mol. Neurosci.* **2018**, *11*, 320. [CrossRef]
116. Korniluk, A.; Koper, O.; Kemona, H.; Dymicka-Piekarska, V. From inflammation to cancer. *Ir. J. Med. Sci.* **2017**, *186*, 57–62. [CrossRef]
117. Multhoff, G.; Molls, M.; Radons, J. Chronic inflammation in cancer development. *Front. Immunol.* **2011**, *2*, 98. [CrossRef] [PubMed]
118. Hussain, S.P.; Harris, C.C. Inflammation and cancer: An ancient link with novel potentials. *Int. J. Cancer* **2007**, *121*, 2373–2380. [CrossRef] [PubMed]
119. Colotta, F.; Allavena, P.; Sica, A.; Garlanda, C.; Mantovani, A. Cancer-related inflammation, the seventh hallmark of cancer: Links to genetic instability. *Carcinogenesis* **2009**, *30*, 1073–1081. [CrossRef] [PubMed]

120. Hanahan, D.; Weinberg, R.A. The hallmarks of cancer. *Cell* **2000**, *100*, 57–70. [CrossRef]
121. Coussens, L.M.; Werb, Z. Inflammation and cancer. *Nature* **2002**, *420*, 860–867. [CrossRef] [PubMed]
122. Vringer, E.; Tait, S.W.G. Mitochondria and Inflammation: Cell Death Heats Up. *Front. Cell Dev. Biol.* **2019**, *7*, 100. [CrossRef] [PubMed]
123. Lee, N.; Kim, D. Cancer Metabolism: Fueling More than Just Growth. *Mol. Cells* **2016**, *39*, 847–854. [CrossRef] [PubMed]
124. Lopez-Armada, M.J.; Riveiro-Naveira, R.R.; Vaamonde-Garcia, C.; Valcarcel-Ares, M.N. Mitochondrial dysfunction and the inflammatory response. *Mitochondrion* **2013**, *13*, 106–118. [CrossRef] [PubMed]
125. Maximo, V.; Botelho, T.; Capela, J.; Soares, P.; Lima, J.; Taveira, A.; Amaro, T.; Barbosa, A.P.; Preto, A.; Harach, H.R.; et al. Somatic and germline mutation in GRIM-19, a dual function gene involved in mitochondrial metabolism and cell death, is linked to mitochondrion-rich (Hurthle cell) tumours of the thyroid. *Br. J. Cancer* **2005**, *92*, 1892–1898. [CrossRef] [PubMed]
126. Putignani, L.; Raffa, S.; Pescosolido, R.; Aimati, L.; Signore, F.; Torrisi, M.R.; Grammatico, P. Alteration of expression levels of the oxidative phosphorylation system (OXPHOS) in breast cancer cell mitochondria. *Breast Cancer Res. Treat.* **2008**, *110*, 439–452. [CrossRef]
127. Bonora, E.; Porcelli, A.M.; Gasparre, G.; Biondi, A.; Ghelli, A.; Carelli, V.; Baracca, A.; Tallini, G.; Martinuzzi, A.; Lenaz, G.; et al. Defective oxidative phosphorylation in thyroid oncocytic carcinoma is associated with pathogenic mitochondrial DNA mutations affecting complexes I and III. *Cancer Res.* **2006**, *66*, 6087–6096. [CrossRef]
128. Stankov, K.; Biondi, A.; D'Aurelio, M.; Gasparre, G.; Falasca, A.; Romeo, G.; Lenaz, G. Mitochondrial activities of a cell line derived from thyroid Hurthle cell tumors. *Thyroid* **2006**, *16*, 325–331. [CrossRef]
129. Simonnet, H.; Alazard, N.; Pfeiffer, K.; Gallou, C.; Beroud, C.; Demont, J.; Bouvier, R.; Schagger, H.; Godinot, C. Low mitochondrial respiratory chain content correlates with tumor aggressiveness in renal cell carcinoma. *Carcinogenesis* **2002**, *23*, 759–768. [CrossRef]
130. Modica-Napolitano, J.S.; Singh, K.K. Mitochondrial dysfunction in cancer. *Mitochondrion* **2004**, *4*, 755–762. [CrossRef]
131. Chandel, N.S.; Maltepe, E.; Goldwasser, E.; Mathieu, C.E.; Simon, M.C.; Schumacker, P.T. Mitochondrial reactive oxygen species trigger hypoxia-induced transcription. *Proc. Natl. Acad. Sci. USA* **1998**, *95*, 11715–11720. [CrossRef] [PubMed]
132. King, A.; Selak, M.A.; Gottlieb, E. Succinate dehydrogenase and fumarate hydratase: Linking mitochondrial dysfunction and cancer. *Oncogene* **2006**, *25*, 4675–4682. [CrossRef] [PubMed]
133. Hold, G.L.; El-Omar, E.M. Genetic aspects of inflammation and cancer. *Biochem. J.* **2008**, *410*, 225–235. [CrossRef] [PubMed]
134. Lewis, C.A.; Parker, S.J.; Fiske, B.P.; McCloskey, D.; Gui, D.Y.; Green, C.R.; Vokes, N.I.; Feist, A.M.; Vander Heiden, M.G.; Metallo, C.M. Tracing compartmentalized NADPH metabolism in the cytosol and mitochondria of mammalian cells. *Mol. Cell* **2014**, *55*, 253–263. [CrossRef]
135. Khansari, N.; Shakiba, Y.; Mahmoudi, M. Chronic inflammation and oxidative stress as a major cause of age-related diseases and cancer. *Recent Pat. Inflamm. Allergy Drug Discov.* **2009**, *3*, 73–80. [CrossRef]
136. Segal, A.W. How superoxide production by neutrophil leukocytes kills microbes. *Novartis Found. Symp.* **2006**, *279*, 92–98, discussion 98-100, 216-109.
137. Beckman, K.B.; Ames, B.N. Oxidative decay of DNA. *J. Biol. Chem.* **1997**, *272*, 19633–19636. [CrossRef]
138. Trifunovic, A.; Hansson, A.; Wredenberg, A.; Rovio, A.T.; Dufour, E.; Khvorostov, I.; Spelbrink, J.N.; Wibom, R.; Jacobs, H.T.; Larsson, N.G. Somatic mtDNA mutations cause aging phenotypes without affecting reactive oxygen species production. *Proc. Natl. Acad. Sci. USA* **2005**, *102*, 17993–17998. [CrossRef]
139. Villanueva, T. Metabolism: The mitochondria that wag the dog. *Nat. Rev. Cancer* **2011**, *11*, 155. [CrossRef]
140. Tan, A.S.; Baty, J.W.; Dong, L.F.; Bezawork-Geleta, A.; Endaya, B.; Goodwin, J.; Bajzikova, M.; Kovarova, J.; Peterka, M.; Yan, B.; et al. Mitochondrial genome acquisition restores respiratory function and tumorigenic potential of cancer cells without mitochondrial DNA. *Cell Metab.* **2015**, *21*, 81–94. [CrossRef]
141. Berridge, M.V.; Dong, L.; Neuzil, J. Mitochondrial DNA in Tumor Initiation, Progression, and Metastasis: Role of Horizontal mtDNA Transfer. *Cancer Res.* **2015**, *75*, 3203–3208. [CrossRef]

142. Torralba, D.; Baixauli, F.; Villarroya-Beltri, C.; Fernandez-Delgado, I.; Latorre-Pellicer, A.; Acin-Perez, R.; Martin-Cofreces, N.B.; Jaso-Tamame, A.L.; Iborra, S.; Jorge, I.; et al. Priming of dendritic cells by DNA-containing extracellular vesicles from activated T cells through antigen-driven contacts. *Nat. Commun.* **2018**, *9*, 2658. [CrossRef]
143. Liu, S.; Feng, M.; Guan, W. Mitochondrial DNA sensing by STING signaling participates in inflammation, cancer and beyond. *Int. J. Cancer* **2016**, *139*, 736–741. [CrossRef]
144. Bononi, A.; Bonora, M.; Marchi, S.; Missiroli, S.; Poletti, F.; Giorgi, C.; Pandolfi, P.P.; Pinton, P. Identification of PTEN at the ER and MAMs and its regulation of Ca(2+) signaling and apoptosis in a protein phosphatase-dependent manner. *Cell Death Differ.* **2013**, *20*, 1631–1643. [CrossRef]
145. Giorgi, C.; Bonora, M.; Sorrentino, G.; Missiroli, S.; Poletti, F.; Suski, J.M.; Galindo Ramirez, F.; Rizzuto, R.; Di Virgilio, F.; Zito, E.; et al. p53 at the endoplasmic reticulum regulates apoptosis in a Ca2+-dependent manner. *Proc. Natl. Acad. Sci. USA* **2015**, *112*, 1779–1784. [CrossRef]
146. Kuchay, S.; Giorgi, C.; Simoneschi, D.; Pagan, J.; Missiroli, S.; Saraf, A.; Florens, L.; Washburn, M.P.; Collazo-Lorduy, A.; Castillo-Martin, M.; et al. PTEN counteracts FBXL2 to promote IP3R3- and Ca(2+)-mediated apoptosis limiting tumour growth. *Nature* **2017**, *546*, 554–558. [CrossRef]
147. Missiroli, S.; Bonora, M.; Patergnani, S.; Poletti, F.; Perrone, M.; Gafa, R.; Magri, E.; Raimondi, A.; Lanza, G.; Tacchetti, C.; et al. PML at Mitochondria-Associated Membranes Is Critical for the Repression of Autophagy and Cancer Development. *Cell Rep.* **2016**, *16*, 2415–2427. [CrossRef]
148. Yin, Y.; Choi, S.C.; Xu, Z.; Perry, D.J.; Seay, H.; Croker, B.P.; Sobel, E.S.; Brusko, T.M.; Morel, L. Normalization of CD4+ T cell metabolism reverses lupus. *Sci. Transl. Med.* **2015**, *7*. [CrossRef]
149. Andrejeva, G.; Rathmell, J.C. Similarities and Distinctions of Cancer and Immune Metabolism in Inflammation and Tumors. *Cell Metab.* **2017**, *26*, 49–70. [CrossRef]
150. Chen, Y.; Wen, H.; Zhou, C.; Su, Q.; Lin, Y.; Xie, Y.; Huang, Y.; Qiu, Q.; Lin, J.; Huang, X.; et al. TNF-alpha derived from M2 tumor-associated macrophages promotes epithelial-mesenchymal transition and cancer stemness through the Wnt/beta-catenin pathway in SMMC-7721 hepatocellular carcinoma cells. *Exp. Cell Res.* **2019**, *378*, 41–50. [CrossRef]
151. Berod, L.; Friedrich, C.; Nandan, A.; Freitag, J.; Hagemann, S.; Harmrolfs, K.; Sandouk, A.; Hesse, C.; Castro, C.N.; Bahre, H.; et al. De novo fatty acid synthesis controls the fate between regulatory T and T helper 17 cells. *Nat. Med.* **2014**, *20*, 1327–1333. [CrossRef] [PubMed]
152. Neagu, M.; Constantin, C.; Popescu, I.D.; Zipeto, D.; Tzanakakis, G.; Nikitovic, D.; Fenga, C.; Stratakis, C.A.; Spandidos, D.A.; Tsatsakis, A.M. Inflammation and Metabolism in Cancer Cell-Mitochondria Key Player. *Front. Oncol.* **2019**, *9*, 348. [CrossRef] [PubMed]
153. Li, X.; Fang, P.; Mai, J.; Choi, E.T.; Wang, H.; Yang, X.F. Targeting mitochondrial reactive oxygen species as novel therapy for inflammatory diseases and cancers. *J. Hematol. Oncol.* **2013**, *6*, 19. [CrossRef] [PubMed]
154. Christofk, H.R.; Vander Heiden, M.G.; Harris, M.H.; Ramanathan, A.; Gerszten, R.E.; Wei, R.; Fleming, M.D.; Schreiber, S.L.; Cantley, L.C. The M2 splice isoform of pyruvate kinase is important for cancer metabolism and tumour growth. *Nature* **2008**, *452*, 230–233. [CrossRef] [PubMed]
155. Anastasiou, D.; Poulogiannis, G.; Asara, J.M.; Boxer, M.B.; Jiang, J.K.; Shen, M.; Bellinger, G.; Sasaki, A.T.; Locasale, J.W.; Auld, D.S.; et al. Inhibition of pyruvate kinase M2 by reactive oxygen species contributes to cellular antioxidant responses. *Science* **2011**, *334*, 1278–1283. [CrossRef]
156. Hahn, T.; Polanczyk, M.J.; Borodovsky, A.; Ramanathapuram, L.V.; Akporiaye, E.T.; Ralph, S.J. Use of anti-cancer drugs, mitocans, to enhance the immune responses against tumors. *Curr. Pharm. Biotechnol.* **2013**, *14*, 357–376. [CrossRef]
157. Gillies, R.J.; Gatenby, R.A. Metabolism and its sequelae in cancer evolution and therapy. *Cancer J.* **2015**, *21*, 88–96. [CrossRef]
158. Hartman, M.L.; Czyz, M. Pro-apoptotic activity of BH3-only proteins and BH3 mimetics: From theory to potential cancer therapy. *Anticancer Agents Med. Chem.* **2012**, *12*, 966–981. [CrossRef]
159. Manole, E.; Ceafalan, L.C.; Popescu, B.O.; Dumitru, C.; Bastian, A.E. Myokines as Possible Therapeutic Targets in Cancer Cachexia. *J. Immunol. Res.* **2018**, *2018*, 8260742. [CrossRef]
160. Roberts, A.W.; Seymour, J.F.; Brown, J.R.; Wierda, W.G.; Kipps, T.J.; Khaw, S.L.; Carney, D.A.; He, S.Z.; Huang, D.C.; Xiong, H.; et al. Substantial susceptibility of chronic lymphocytic leukemia to BCL2 inhibition: Results of a phase I study of navitoclax in patients with relapsed or refractory disease. *J. Clin. Oncol.* **2012**, *30*, 488–496. [CrossRef]

161. Selivanov, V.A.; Votyakova, T.V.; Pivtoraiko, V.N.; Zeak, J.; Sukhomlin, T.; Trucco, M.; Roca, J.; Cascante, M. Reactive oxygen species production by forward and reverse electron fluxes in the mitochondrial respiratory chain. *PLoS Comput. Biol.* **2011**, *7*, e1001115. [CrossRef]
162. Egawa, Y.; Saigo, C.; Kito, Y.; Moriki, T.; Takeuchi, T. Therapeutic potential of CPI-613 for targeting tumorous mitochondrial energy metabolism and inhibiting autophagy in clear cell sarcoma. *PLoS ONE* **2018**, *13*, e0198940. [CrossRef]
163. Lycan, T.W.; Pardee, T.S.; Petty, W.J.; Bonomi, M.; Alistar, A.; Lamar, Z.S.; Isom, S.; Chan, M.D.; Miller, A.A.; Ruiz, J. A Phase II Clinical Trial of CPI-613 in Patients with Relapsed or Refractory Small Cell Lung Carcinoma. *PLoS ONE* **2016**, *11*, e0164244. [CrossRef]
164. Alistar, A.; Morris, B.B.; Desnoyer, R.; Klepin, H.D.; Hosseinzadeh, K.; Clark, C.; Cameron, A.; Leyendecker, J.; D'Agostino, R., Jr.; Topaloglu, U.; et al. Safety and tolerability of the first-in-class agent CPI-613 in combination with modified FOLFIRINOX in patients with metastatic pancreatic cancer: A single-centre, open-label, dose-escalation, phase 1 trial. *Lancet Oncol.* **2017**, *18*, 770–778. [CrossRef]
165. Conroy, T.; Desseigne, F.; Ychou, M.; Bouche, O.; Guimbaud, R.; Becouarn, Y.; Adenis, A.; Raoul, J.L.; Gourgou-Bourgade, S.; de la Fouchardiere, C.; et al. FOLFIRINOX versus gemcitabine for metastatic pancreatic cancer. *New Engl. J. Med.* **2011**, *364*, 1817–1825. [CrossRef]
166. Wang, F.; Ogasawara, M.A.; Huang, P. Small mitochondria-targeting molecules as anti-cancer agents. *Mol. Asp. Med.* **2010**, *31*, 75–92. [CrossRef]
167. Young, K.E.; Flaherty, S.; Woodman, K.M.; Sharma-Walia, N.; Reynolds, J.M. Fatty acid synthase regulates the pathogenicity of Th17 cells. *J. Leukoc. Biol.* **2017**, *102*, 1229–1235. [CrossRef]
168. Engin, A.B.; Engin, A.; Gonul, I.I. The effect of adipocyte-macrophage crosstalk in obesity-related breast cancer. *J. Mol. Endocrinol.* **2019**, *62*, R201–R222. [CrossRef]
169. Sabharwal, S.S.; Schumacker, P.T. Mitochondrial ROS in cancer: Initiators, amplifiers or an Achilles' heel? *Nat. Rev. Cancer* **2014**, *14*, 709–721. [CrossRef]
170. Rimessi, A.; Bezzerri, V.; Patergnani, S.; Marchi, S.; Cabrini, G.; Pinton, P. Mitochondrial Ca2+-dependent NLRP3 activation exacerbates the Pseudomonas aeruginosa-driven inflammatory response in cystic fibrosis. *Nat. Commun.* **2015**, *6*, 6201. [CrossRef]
171. Palty, R.; Silverman, W.F.; Hershfinkel, M.; Caporale, T.; Sensi, S.L.; Parnis, J.; Nolte, C.; Fishman, D.; Shoshan-Barmatz, V.; Herrmann, S.; et al. NCLX is an essential component of mitochondrial Na+/Ca2+ exchange. *Proc. Natl. Acad. Sci. USA* **2010**, *107*, 436–441. [CrossRef] [PubMed]
172. Missiroli, S.; Patergnani, S.; Caroccia, N.; Pedriali, G.; Perrone, M.; Previati, M.; Wieckowski, M.R.; Giorgi, C. Mitochondria-associated membranes (MAMs) and inflammation. *Cell Death Dis.* **2018**, *9*, 329. [CrossRef] [PubMed]

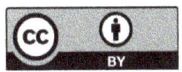

© 2020 by the authors. Licensee MDPI, Basel, Switzerland. This article is an open access article distributed under the terms and conditions of the Creative Commons Attribution (CC BY) license (http://creativecommons.org/licenses/by/4.0/).

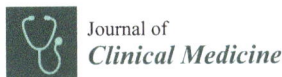 

Review

# Rescue of TCA Cycle Dysfunction for Cancer Therapy

Jubert Marquez [1,†], Jessa Flores [2,†], Amy Hyein Kim [1], Bayalagmaa Nyamaa [2,3], Anh Thi Tuyet Nguyen [2], Nammi Park [4] and Jin Han [1,2,4,*]

1. Department of Health Science and Technology, College of Medicine, Inje University, Busan 47392, Korea; jcuevas.marquez@gmail.com (J.M.); amyhikim@gmail.com (A.H.K.)
2. Department of Physiology, College of Medicine, Inje University, Busan 47392, Korea; jeflores1@up.edu.ph (J.F.); n_bayalgaa@yahoo.com (B.N.); nguyenthituyetanh_t57@hus.edu.vn (A.T.T.N.)
3. Department of Hematology, Mongolian National University of Medical Sciences, Ulaanbaatar 14210, Mongolia
4. Cardiovascular and Metabolic Disease Center, Paik Hospital, Inje University, Busan 47392, Korea; nammi780314@gmail.com
* Correspondence: phyhanj@inje.ac.kr; Tel.: +8251-890-8748
† Authors contributed equally.

Received: 10 November 2019; Accepted: 4 December 2019; Published: 6 December 2019

**Abstract:** Mitochondrion, a maternally hereditary, subcellular organelle, is the site of the tricarboxylic acid (TCA) cycle, electron transport chain (ETC), and oxidative phosphorylation (OXPHOS)—the basic processes of ATP production. Mitochondrial function plays a pivotal role in the development and pathology of different cancers. Disruption in its activity, like mutations in its TCA cycle enzymes, leads to physiological imbalances and metabolic shifts of the cell, which contributes to the progression of cancer. In this review, we explored the different significant mutations in the mitochondrial enzymes participating in the TCA cycle and the diseases, especially cancer types, that these malfunctions are closely associated with. In addition, this paper also discussed the different therapeutic approaches which are currently being developed to address these diseases caused by mitochondrial enzyme malfunction.

**Keywords:** mitochondria; TCA; cancer; IDH; SDH; FH; MDH; CRISPR/Cas9; miRNA

## 1. Introduction

Mitochondrion is a maternally hereditary, subcellular organelle which plays a role in bioenergetics, biosynthesis, and cell signaling [1]. The human mitochondrial proteome is composed of a subset of ~20,000 distinct mammalian proteins which are localized in the said organelle. Thirteen of these proteins are encoded by mitochondrial DNA (mtDNA) and the rest are encoded by nuclear DNA (nDNA) [2]. Mutations in these mitochondrial protein genes are notably implicated in diseases such as cancer and diabetes, as well as a plethora of other genetic diseases [3]. Mitochondria have a double lipid membrane with various types of membrane proteins which are divided into four divisions: The intermembrane space (IMS), outer mitochondrial membrane (OMM), inner mitochondrial membrane (IMM), which has a highly particular structure to create cristae of large surface area for ATP production, and the mitochondrial matrix [4]. The mitochondria play a key role in ATP production and circulation based on the availability of energy from calories and oxygen, along with the demands for cellular maintenance and reproduction [3]. Carbon sources from glycolysis, fatty acids, and glutamine are utilized to produce ATP. Carbon sources entering the tricarboxylic acid (TCA) cycle in the mitochondrial matrix produce NADH and FADH$_2$, which transfer their electrons to the electron transport chain (ETC) located in the IMM [5]. In the ETC system, the electrons transferred from NADH/FADH$_2$ to oxygen induce an oxidation-reduction reaction at each step, and energy from the oxidized electron is utilized to pump protons from the mitochondrial matrix into the intermembrane space through complex I

(NADH dehydrogenase), complex III (CoQH2-cytochrome c reductase), and complex IV (cytochrome c oxidase) [6]. The proton gradient is harnessed to drive the switch of ADP to ATP by complex V (ATP synthase), during which concurrently pumped protons return to the matrix. In the matrix, lipids are oxidized by β-oxidation as a breakdown of fatty chains to produce acetyl-CoA [7].

Energy production during the metabolic process has recently been in the spotlight due to its capability to generate signaling molecules for various cellular responses. Recent technological developments have further supported long-withstanding hypotheses regarding the key role of aberrant energy production and metabolism in disease models (Figure 1). Therefore, in this review, we discussed the metabolic differences in normal and disease models, and highlighted TCA enzymes and proteins critical in further understanding disease progression along with how we can harness the knowledge regarding these enzymes and proteins in order to address diseases, especially in cancer.

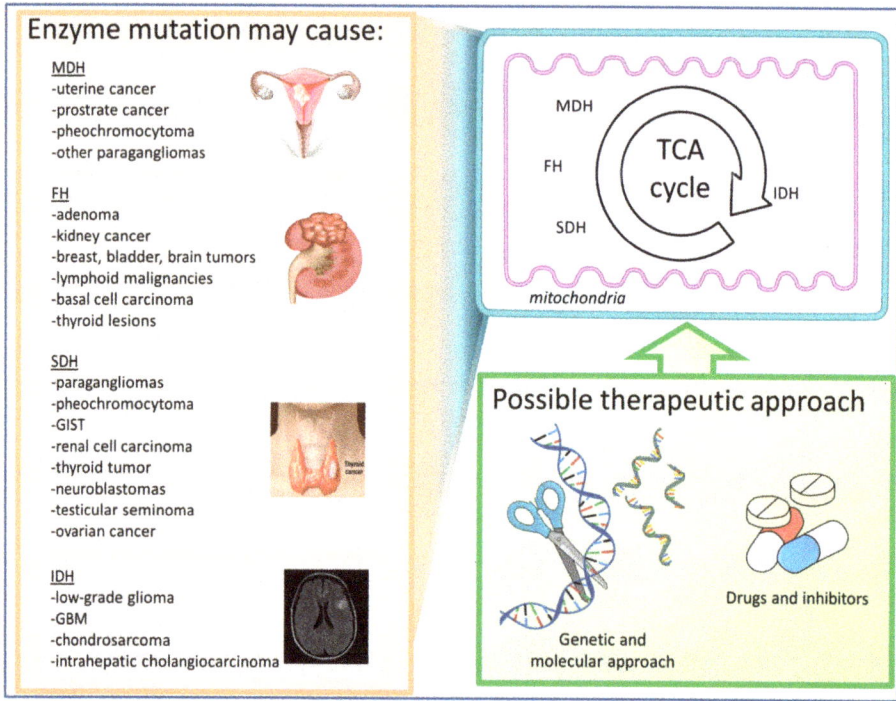

**Figure 1.** Mutations in the tricarboxylic acid (TCA) cycle enzymes may result in various kinds of cancers. These diseases may possibly be treated through pharmacological and genetic therapeutic approaches. IDH, isocitrate dehydrogenase; SDH, succinate dehydrogenase; FH, fumarate hydratase; MDH, malate dehydrogenase.

## 2. The TCA Cycle: In Sickness and in Health

The TCA cycle unifies the carbohydrate, lipid, and protein metabolism pathways. In a healthy, normal cell, glycolysis is responsible for the oxidation of the glucose molecule into pyruvate to produce ATP, which is then decarboxylated into acetyl-CoA as it enters the mitochondria, allowing it to enter the TCA cycle. However, each body part exhibits strikingly different metabolic profiles. For example, in the human brain, with the exception of prolonged fasting states, glucose is the main source of energy [8]. Muscles, on the other hand, have a vast reservoir of glycogen that can easily be converted into glucose 6-phosphate [9]. The liver, which is controlled by both neuronal and hormonal systems, provides energy for organs, such as the brain and muscle, in addition to extrahepatic tissues. The liver can produce glucose by breaking down its stored glycogen and through gluconeogenesis. However, in the fasting state, ketone bodies' conversion from fatty acids is facilitated through mitochondrial β-oxidation and ketogenesis [10,11].

TCA intermediates also play important roles in pathways in which they leave the cycle to be converted into glucose, fatty acids, or non-essential amino acids. Once removed, these intermediates need to be replaced to allow continued function and cycle, known as anaplerosis [12]. In heart and skeletal tissues, anaplerosis maintains steady-state concentrations of TCA intermediates [13]. Cancer cells, on the other hand, transport glucose-derived pyruvate into the mitochondria, where it is used as an anaplerotic substrate to replace TCA intermediates used for biosynthesis [14]. Inadequate amounts of glutamine or suppressed glutaminase forces the cancer cells to depend on glucose carbon flux through pyruvate carboxylase to keep oxaloacetate production and continue downstream TCA cycle activity [15]. In cases like non-small-cell lung carcinoma and glioblastoma, they more frequently rely on pyruvate anaplerosis to maintain TCA cycle flux.

In comparison to the organs previously mentioned, there is an immense demand for energy in mammalian hearts due to its continuous and incessant beating. Central to energy transduction in the heart, the mitochondria generate more than 95% of the ATP used by the heart. In a normal heart, fatty acyl-coenzyme A (CoA) and pyruvate fuel the mitochondria. The entry of long-chain acyl-CoA into the mitochondria is rate-limited by carnitine-palmitoyl transferase-1 (CPT1), while pyruvate dehydrogenase (PDH) reaction regulates pyruvate oxidation. Substrates, such as lactate, ketone bodies, and amino acids, freely enter the mitochondria for oxidation [16].

## 3. TCA Enzymes: The Future to Understanding The Complexities of Diseases

Diseases of the TCA cycle constitute a group of rare human diseases that affect core mitochondrial metabolism [17]. The deficiency of enzymes involving the TCA cycle was detected in order to obtain crucial roles in several human diseases.

Emerging evidences suggest that cancer is mitochondrial in nature [18,19]. Warburg originally observed and postulated that excess lactate production by tumors in the presence of oxygen is a sign of mitochondrial dysfunction, eventually giving rise to the idea of aerobic glycolysis or the 'Warburg effect' [20]. Recent studies proved that the dysfunction observed by Warburg is merely an altered state of the mitochondria and is a part of a bigger picture in cancer bioenergetics [21–23]. The majority of cancer cells generate most of their ATP through the mitochondria. Few tumors bear TCA enzymes mutations, such as isocitrate dehydrogenase (IDH), succinate dehydrogenase (SDH), fumarate hydratase (FH), and malate dehydrogenase (MDH) [24]. Their mutations are also involved directly or indirectly, which comprises the activation of a hypoxic cellular response and high levels of ROS often found in cancer cells [25].

### 3.1. Isocitrate Dehydrogenase

Isocitrate dehydrogenase (IDH) is mainly known for its role in catalyzing the oxidative decarboxylation of isocitrate, resulting in 2-oxoglutarate ($α$-KG) and $CO_2$ (Figure 2). IDH exists in three isoforms: IDH1 is present in the cytoplasm and peroxisomes, while IDH2 and IDH3 are located in the mitochondrial matrix. IDH1/2 isoforms were also identified to mediate the reverse reductive carboxylation of $α$-KG to isocitrate, which oxidizes NADPH to NADP+. Meanwhile, IDH3 only facilitates the irreversible, NAD-dependent conversion of isocitrate to $α$-KG [26,27]. ODH3 mutation of IDH1/2 is found in low-grade glioma and secondary glioblastoma (GBM), chondrosarcoma, intrahepatic cholangiocarcinomas, hematologic malignancies, premalignant diseases, and rare inherited metabolism disorders [28]. In a clinical study, IDH1 and IDH2 mutations were observed in 16%–17% of patients with AML, in around 20% of angioimmunoblastic T-cell lymphomas (AITL) with worse prognosis [29], and in some low-frequency cancer malignancies [30–33]. Mutations in the gene-encoding the said enzymes cause increased production of R-2-hydroxyglutarate (R-2HG), an oncogenic factor promoting leukemogenesis (Figure 3) [34,35]. R-2HG produced by mutant IDH in low-grade glioma was shown to activate the mammalian target of rapamycin (mTOR) signaling pathway, which is important for cell growth and metabolism [36]. Moreover, inhibition of the IDH2/R140Q somatic mutant inhibitor induces differentiation of the human erythroleukemic cell line (HEL) and human primary AML cells [37]. Furthermore, mutant IDH induces hypermethylation of *MIRNA148A*, a tumor-suppressive miRNA in glioma CpG island methylator phenotype (G-CIMP) [38].

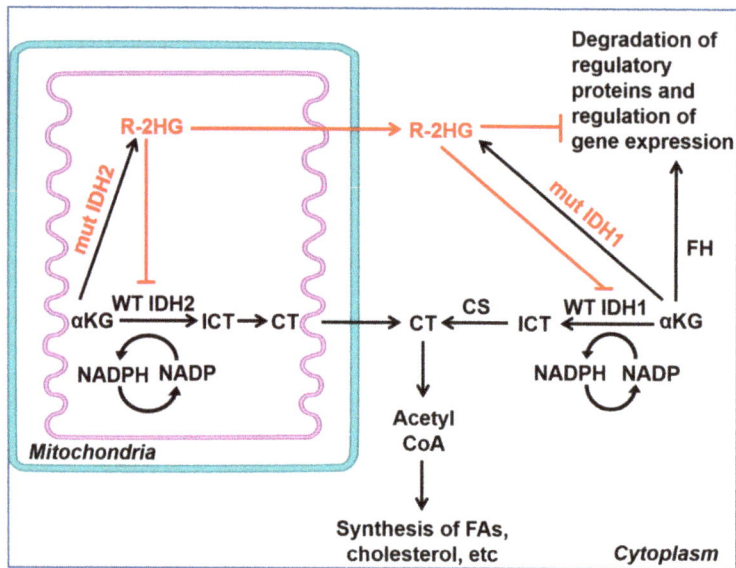

**Figure 2.** Schematic presentation of the difference in cellular pathways of wild-type and mutated IDH1/2 enzymes during reverse reductive carboxylation reaction. IDH1/2 enzymes catalyzes both the forward and reverse conversion of isocitrate to αKG. Mutations in IDH1/2 cause elevated levels of R-2HG (D-2HG), which is a pro-oncogenic factor. αKG, α-ketoglutarate; ICT, isocitrate; CT, citrate; CS, citrate synthase; FH, fumarate hydratase; FAs, fatty acids. Adapted from Al-Khallaf H. (2017) [26].

The most common IDH mutation found in cancer is the substitution of a single arginine in the catalytic site of the enzyme, R132 in IDH1 and R140 or R172 in IDH2, which results in a gain of function. Alterations in R132 in IDH1 and either R172 or R140 in IDH2 represent the majority of IDH mutations identified in cancers [39]. IDH1/R132 and IDH2/R172 are commonly found in gliomas, cholangiocarcinomas, and chondrosarcomas, with a higher frequency of IDH1/R132 mutation occurring in these cancers (58%–90%, 40%–50%, and 50%–60% respectively) compared to IDH2/R172 (3%–5%, 5%–10%, and 10%). These mutations are also found at relatively lower frequencies in AML. Meanwhile, IDH2/R140 is the most common mutation found in AML (30%–50%). However, IDH2/R140, unlike IDH1/R132 and IDH2/R172 mutations, is not found in gliomas, cholangiocarcinomas, and chondrosarcomas [40]. IDH2/R140Q is the most common mutation (75%–80%) and confers a favorable or insignificant impact on overall survival [41–45]. However, IDH2/R172K mutation is found in 20% of the cases, with a lower complete remission rate, higher relapse rate, and lower overall survival [46,47]. Three variants that occur in exon 4 were discovered upon IDH2 gene screening: c.543+45G>A, c. 389 A>T, p. Lys120Met and c.414 T>C, and p.Thr138Thr. These gene variants were found in two independent patients classified under French and Tunisian familial cases which, despite ethnic differences, were similarly diagnosed with non-Hodgkin lymphoma [48]. Melissa Carbonneau et al. found that the molecular mechanism underlying the oncogenic activity of mutant IDH1/2 involved mTOR signaling via KDM4A inhibition, an αKG-dependent enzyme [35].

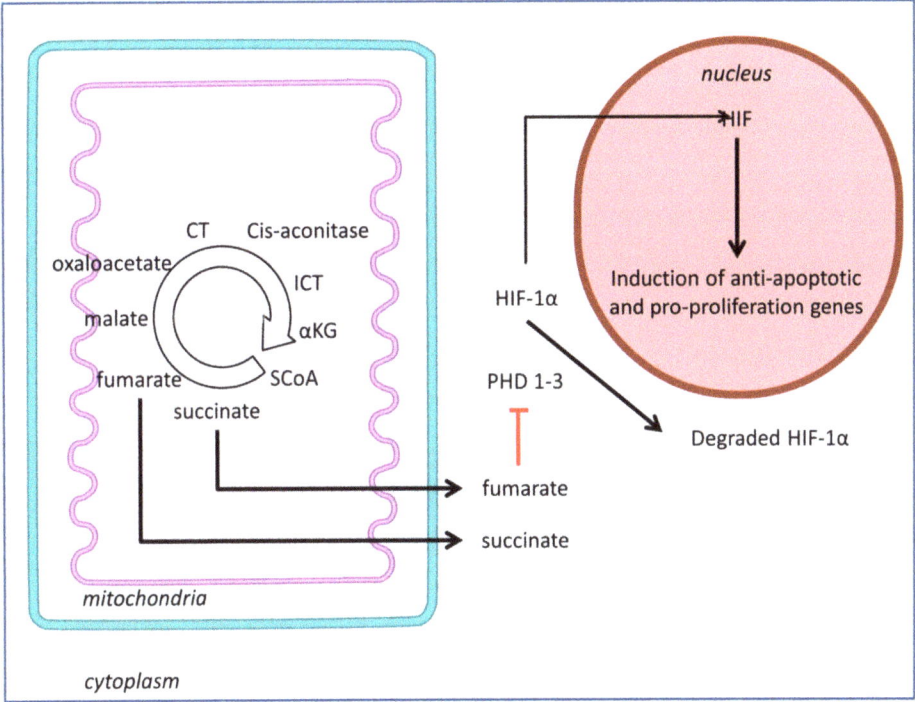

**Figure 3.** Schematic diagram of tumorigenesis in succinate dehydrogenase (SDH) and fumarate hydratase (FH). SDH and FH deficiency causes accumulation of succinate and fumarate, respectively, inside the mitochondria. These will be subsequently transported into the cytosol. High levels of succinate and fumarate can inhibit prolyl hydroxylases (PDH1-3), which plays a role in the degradation of HIF-1α under normoxic conditions. HIF-1α, when stabilized, induces transcription of nuclear genes involved in tumor suppression. αKG, α-ketoglutarate; ICT, isocitrate; CT, citrate; SCoA, Succinyl-coA; HIF, hypoxia-inducible factor Adapted from Zanssen S, Schon EA (2005) [49] and Shuch, B., Linehan, W.M., & Srinivasan, R. (2013) [50].

### 3.2. Succinate Dehydrogenase

Succinate dehydrogenase (SDH) is an enzyme bound to the inner mitochondrial membrane, where it oxidizes succinate to fumarate, and is classified as a tumor suppressor [51]. The SDH complex consists of four subunits (SDHA, SDHB, SDHC, and SDHD), and a deficiency of this enzyme is known to activate tumor formation through dysregulation of HIF activity [52]. HIF, which is a transcription factor, can activate anti-apoptotic and pro-proliferation genes, leading to tumor formation of cancer cells (Figure 3). In addition, deficiency of the enzyme can cause accumulation of the metabolite, succinate. Succinate was shown to exert pro-inflammatory effects through the generation of mtROS [53]. The SDH complex gene-associated cancers include paragangliomas, pheochromocytomas, gastrointestinal stromal tumors (GIST), SDH-deficient renal cell carcinoma [54,55], thyroid tumors, neuroblastomas, testicular seminoma, and ovarian cancer [56].

The SDHA gene is responsible for encoding SDH enzyme major catalytic subunit, possessing a covalently attached flavin adenine dinucleotide (FAD) prosthetic group which can bind with substrates, such as fumarate and succinate, and also with physiological regulators, such as oxaloacetate and ATP. Inactivation of SDHA has been shown to promote neurodegenerative diseases like Leigh syndrome, which is an early-onset encephalopathy [57–59], as well as late-onset optic atrophy, ataxia, and myopathy [60]. In addition, a missense mutation in SDHA was shown to cause a multisystemic failure, leading to neonatal death [61]. Meanwhile, in SDH-deficient GISTs, despite the presence of other SDH subunit gene germline mutations, *SDHA* is the most prevalent among the four [62].

SDHB is an enzyme that catalyzes succinate oxidation. SDHB mutations normally lead to extra-adrenal paragangliomas (PGLs), which are usually characterized by highly aggressive tumors, poor prognosis, and early-age onset (~30 years) [63,64]. To a lesser extent, it may also impose risks of adrenal pheochromocytoma (PCC) and head and neck paragangliomas (HNPGLs) [63–66]. In addition, renal cell carcinoma and T-cell acute leukemia are also associated with SDHB mutations [67,68]. In the study of Fishbein et al., the authors collected and screened data of 173 PGLs/PCCs patients from The Cancer Genome Atlas. *SDHB* appeared to be the most common germline mutation (9%) and exhibited the highest number of copy number alteration (57%) [69].

SDHC mutations were initially implicated with HNPGLs alone. However, recent rare cases of adrenal PCCs and extra-adrenal PGLs were observed to be related to SDHC mutation as well [70–72]. Clinically, features of SDHC-associated cases are similar to symptoms of sporadic HNPGLs [73]. In addition, somatic *SDHC* mutations were also detected in 5% of sporadic thyroid cancer cases in a cohort study [74].

SDHD mutations are usually related to multifocal HNPGLs and sometimes to adrenal PCCs and extra-adrenal PGLs, which are usually benign. Metastatic HNPGLs have been described within SDHD mutation carriers with 0%–10% prevalence [70,75]. In the study of Marc Bennedbaek et al., the authors identified 18 different germline variants of SDH in the Danish PGL and PCC patients, wherein 12 were likely pathogenic/pathogenic [76]. Furthermore, PGL/PCC syndrome has also been associated with mutations in SDH assembly factor 2 (SDHAF2) [77,78], which is required for the flavination of SDH [79]. Meanwhile, in sporadic thyroid cancers, about 6% of patients showed germline mutation of *SDHB* or *SDHD* [74].

3.3. Fumarate Hydratase

Fumarate hydratase (FH) is responsible for the hydration/dehydration of fumarate to malate, an integral process in cellular respiration and energy production. Similarly to succinate, an increase in fumarate inhibits prolyl hydroxylases, which are responsible for the regulation of HIF-1α degradation. Fumarate upregulation may also cause post-translational modification and inactivation of Kelch-like ECH-associated protein 1 (KEAP1). KEAP1 is a substrate adapter protein for the E3 ubiquitin ligase complex which targets nuclear factor erythroid 2-related factor (NRF2) [80]. NRF2, on the other hand, is a regulator of cellular antioxidant defense [81]. Fumarate have also been proved to bind with glutathione to form the oncometabolite succinate glutathione (GSF), which can act as an alternative substrate to glutathione reductase, thus decreasing NADPH levels and enhancing mt ROS and HIF-1 activation. The aforementioned binding can also cause a further increase in oxidative stress due to the depletion of the antioxidant molecules in the system. Furthermore, in the study by Tyrakis et al., increased fumarate due to the deficiency of FH caused the impairment of the respiratory chain complex 2 via the succination of members of Fe-S cluster biogenesis proteins, which are important for the activity of mitochondrial enzymes [82].

Fumarase gene germline mutation is connected to multiple cutaneous and uterine leiomyomas (MCUL) and hereditary leiomyomatosis and renal cell cancer (HLRCC) [83,84]. Meanwhile, in a study where tissue samples from leiomyosarcoma and uterine leiomyoma patients were analyzed, no somatic mutations in the *fumarate* gene was detected, implying that the somatic mutation in gene-encoding the said enzyme does not play a major role in the development of sporadic leiomyosarcomas or uterine leiomyomas [85]. On the other hand, in the cohort study of PGLs conducted by Letouzé et al., *FH* somatic mutation was detected in the only sample of hypermethylated PGL that did not possess SDHx mutation [86].

An estimated 90% (76%–100%) of families were found to have clinically suggestive HLRCC with predisposed early onset, aggressive form of type 2 papillary renal cell carcinoma [87,88]. FH mutation in kidney cancer has been shown to induce an increase in glucose uptake, glycolytic rate, and contribution of glucose to the pentose phosphate pathway [89]. In another study in clear cell renal cancer, a mutation in FH led to the accumulation of HIF-2α, a promotor renal carcinogenesis [90]. However, Tong. W.H. et al. showed that FH mutations in kidney cancer are associated with a reduction in the activity of the metabolic sensor, AMP-activated protein kinase (AMPK), which leads to increased synthesis of fatty acids and proteins to support ongoing cellular anabolism [91]

### 3.4. Malate Dehydrogenase

Malate dehydrogenase is responsible for the reversible oxidation of malate to oxaloacetate through NAD+ to NADH reduction in the ETC, a critical step in the cellular respiration of cells. However, the role of MDH is not only limited to the ETC, as it also plays important roles in metabolic pathways, including glyoxylate bypass, amino acid synthesis, glucogenesis, and oxidation/reduction balance [92].

The ubiquity of MDH is related to its numerous isoforms, which have different areas of subcellular localization and co-enzyme specificity. In eukaryotic cells, there are two main isoenzymes: The mitochondrial and the cytoplasmic malate dehydrogenase. Mitochondrial malate dehydrogenase (MDH2) is critical in the citric acid cycle, as it catalyzes the reaction of malate to oxaloacetate. The other, cytosolic malate dehydrogenase (MDH1), is a key participant in the malate/aspartate shuttle and catalyzes the conversion of oxaloacetate (OAA) to malate, making transport possible. A third isoenzyme, albeit a minor one, was found in the yeast glyoxysomes, where it catalyzes the malate production from glyoxylate. For comparison, the prokaryotic *Escherichia coli* has only one form and is highly similar in sequence identity and tertiary structure to that of MDH2 [92,93].

Online databases, such as MalaCards, have listed diseases associated with MDH1 to include tetanus neonatorum and x-linked sideroblastic anemia with ataxia. However, a cross-reference has only presented predictability of disease occurrence, and no published literature or data can support the claim. Mutations in the MDH2 gene are related to several cancers, including uterine cancer, prostate cancer, pheochromocytoma, and other paragangliomas. MDH2 is a possible target in cancer therapeutics due to its effect on ATP production and drug sensitivity during knockdown. MDH2 was observed to be overexpressed in doxorubicin-resistant uterine cancer cells and prostate cancer cells and may contribute to drug resistance in disease models [94,95]. Its overexpression could supply more energy for P-glycoprotein in order to flush the chemotherapeutic drugs out, which may account for the shorter periods of relapse-free survival by patients with overexpressed MDH2 after chemotherapy. It is also likely that through the JNK pathway, MDH2 is able to lend docetaxel resistance in prostate cancer cells.

Recently, there has been a lot of interest in the use of potent inhibitors, such as visnagin, which holds potential cardioprotective and anticancer benefits. Researches regarding the inhibition of MDH2 as the only mechanism underlying the visnagin-induced cardioprotection are still in their early stages and require further evaluation.

Extensive research about MDH and its role in cancer is still needed, especially in the clinical aspect. In one recent study, DNA samples from 830 patients with PCCs/PGLs negative for the main PGL driver genes were analyzed. MDH2 variants of unknown significance were interpreted using an algorithm based on 20 computational predictions, enzymatic and immunofluorescence assays, and/or molecular dynamic simulation approach. The researchers identified five MDH2 variants with potential involvement in pathogenicity. Three of these variants were missense mutations and the two remaining ones were an in-frame deletion and a splice-site variant, respectively. All of the mutations were germline and are associated with noradrenergic PCCs/PGLs [96].

## 4. Future Direction of Metabolic Strategies in Combating Diseases Caused by TCA Malfunction

Although common methods such as radiotherapy and chemotherapy exert effectiveness in most patients, they sometimes pose more risks, leading to the development of cardiovascular diseases and eventual progression to heart failure. Any disruption or inefficiency in the metabolic homeostasis can undoubtedly contribute to cardiac pathologies. Such disruptions could stem from factors such as, but not limited to, the inadequate delivery of oxygen and substrates, decreased amounts of high-energy phosphate and the PCR/ATP ratio, and inefficient energy transfer or feedback [97].

When addressing cancer therapeutics, the effects of these strategies should also be considered, since focusing on targets such as enzymes can also prove to be detrimental to the physiological functions of normal cells and tissues. Metabolic inhibitors should minimally, if not entirely, interfere with the patient's immune system [98]. Nevertheless, new technology has uncovered more novel target pathways that pose less unwanted side effects to the patient.

### 4.1. Inhibitors and Drugs

Multiple preclinical studies have shown IDH as the recent target with the most potential for cancer drugs (Table 1). Preliminary trials indicate the selective inhibitory strength of AG-120 and AG-221 compounds in IDH1 and IDH2 mutant enzymes, respectively, by inhibiting mutant IDH activity and 2-HG accumulation, an oncometabolite [99,100]. AG-120 and another mutant IDH inhibitor, Novartis-530, were found to be the most biochemically potent inhibitors among all nine inhibitors tested in a comparative study [101]. In the same study, both proved to cause the highest reduction of 2-HG levels in six different cancer cell lines with IDH mutation (HT1080 fibrosarcoma, SNU1079, and RBE cholangiocarcinoma, JJ012 chondrosarcoma, U87 glioblastoma, and THP-1 AML). AG-221, on the other hand, significantly improved survival in an IDH2-mutant AML primary xenograft mouse model. Meanwhile, in preliminary phase I clinical trials in patients with advanced hematologic malignancies, the objective response rate ranged from 31% to 40%, with durable responses (>1 year) observed [102]. In addition, AG-881, a brain-penetrant dual IDH1/2 mutant inhibitor, is currently in phase I trial against solid tumors [101].

**Table 1.** Drugs and inhibitors and their respective TCA or TCA-related enzyme targets.

| Drug/Inhibitor | Target | Role of Target | Action of Drug to Target | Sample Type | Reference |
|---|---|---|---|---|---|
| AG-120 (Ivosidenib) | IDH1 | Catalyze conversion of isocitrate to α-ketoglutarate | inhibit | Clinical trial: glioma, adcanced hematologic malignancy | [87,88] |
| AG-221 | IDH2 | Catalyze conversion of isocitrate to α-ketoglutarate | inhibit | Clinical trial: acute myeloid leukemia and myelodysplastic syndrome patients | [86] |
| Novartis-530 | IDH1 | Catalyze conversion of isocitrate to α-ketoglutarate | inhibit | Cancer cell lines with somatic IDH1 mutation | [88] |
| FX 11 | LDH-A | Forward and reverse conversion of pyruvate to lactate | inhibit | human lymphoma and pancreatic cancer xenografts | [91] |
| Dichloroacetate (DCA) | PDK | Phosphorylation and inhibition of PDC | inhibit | Human lung carcinoma cell | [95,96] |

Inhibition of LDH-A, which facilitates pyruvate conversion to lactate, diminished MYC-driven tumors in xenograft models. In NSCLC mouse models, LDH-A inhibition caused the regression of established tumors without associated toxicity [103,104]. In addition, the genetic ablation of LDH-A has been observed to delay the progression of myeloid leukemia [105]. However, the impact of LDH-A on the adaptive immune system is yet to be explored. Lactate exhibited inhibitory action against cytotoxic T cells. Thus, blocking LDH-A activity may synergize with other immuno-inhibitors to improve host inflammatory T cell activity, which will eventually lead to the targeted tumor cells [106].

Meanwhile, in another clinical trial, dichloroacetate (DCA) was used in patients with lactic acidosis caused by rare inborn errors of mitochondrial metabolism. This small molecule targets pyruvate dehydrogenase kinase (PDK), an enzyme increased in different cancers due to increased activation of hypoxiainducible factor (HIF). PDK negatively regulates the pyruvate dehydrogenase complex (PDH) and blocks the oxidative decarboxylation of pyruvate to acetylCoA, which is important in leading pyruvate into the TCA cycle and away from lactate production [107]. Therefore, PDK inhibition by DCA causes the activation of PDH, enhanced pyruvate to acetyl CoA conversion, and decreased lactate production. More importantly, DCA is well-tolerated by patients even at doses that can affect the mitochondrial membrane potential [108,109].

### 4.2. Novel Approaches to TCA Targeting

However, due to the probable unwanted side effects of drug inhibitors, researchers have turned to revolutionary techniques, such as targeting microRNA (miRNA) and the use of CRISPR/Cas9 to address cancer therapy. Considering current cancer treatment regimens employing DNA-damaging drugs and/or radiation, these new approaches were conceived to be less genotoxic and cause less undesired DNA lesions in cells. This approach also outweighs the ethical limitations of mitochondrial replacement therapy. Here, we concisely discuss miRNA targeting and CRISPR/Cas9 system, both of which are promising candidates in addressing cancer therapies.

### 4.3. miRNA Targeting

MicroRNAs were recently brought to the spotlight due to their key roles in cancer cell metabolism, as multiple pieces of evidence have shown miRNA dysregulation in several types of cancer [113]. MicroRNAs are small, highly evolutionarily conserved, single-stranded, non-coding RNA molecules involved in the regulation of various gene expression. Their regulatory functions are performed through the assembly of RNA-induced silencing complex (RISC), which targets the 3' untranslated region (UTR) of their respective mRNA [114]. The miRNA serves as a guide for the RISC by base-pairing with the target mRNA, and the level of complementarity between the guide and the target determines the mechanism of silencing: (1) Cleavage of target mRNA with subsequent degradation or (2) translation inhibition [115].

miRNAs can regulate the TCA cycle both directly and indirectly. miRNAs can downregulate subunits of pyruvate dehydrogenase (PDH), the enzyme responsible for the process that bridges glycolysis and TCA cycle—the conversion of pyruvate to acetyl CoA [116]. For example, miR-26a can inhibit the PDH protein X component (PDHX) [110], while miR-146b-5p and miR-370 can downregulate the PDHB subunit [111,112]. On the other hand, glutamine provides a major source of energy for proliferating cancer cells, and glutamine intermediates can be converted to $\alpha$-KG. miR-137 targets ASC family transporter 2 (ASCT2), a glutamine transporter upregulated in different kinds of cancer. This downregulation of the transporter decreases the level of glutamine metabolism and affects cell survival in colorectal carcinoma, glioblastoma, prostate, and pancreatic cancers [117]. Glutamine metabolism suppression is increasingly being considered as a possible anticancer strategy. Glutaminase inhibitor CB-839 is currently undergoing a phase one clinical trial. CB-839 obstructs glutamine during the glutamate conversion process and changes the pathways of several downstream processes, such as the TCA cycle, glutathione production, and amino acid synthesis [118]. Epigallocatechin gallate (EGCG) reduced tumor growth in preclinical studies by interrupting the anaplerotic use of glutamine in the TCA cycle and is currently undergoing early phase one clinical trials [119].

In addition, miRNAs also play a pivotal role in regulating IDH. miR-183 has been shown to suppress IDH2, which causes a decrease of $\alpha$-KG levels and a subsequent increase in aerobic glycolysis in glioma cells [120]. Meanwhile, in solid cancer tumors that rely heavily on lipid oxidation for energy source, IDH1, a cytoplasmic isoform of IDH, serves as an important contributor to lipid synthesis. This contribution can be traced back to the role of IDH in converting $\alpha$-KG to isocitrate, which is subsequently converted to citrate, a precursor for the formation of monounsaturated fatty acids. miR-181a, which targets IDH1, causes a decrease of expression of genes related to lipid synthesis and increases the expression of genes involved in $\beta$-oxidation, which subsequently reduces lipid accumulation [121]. Moreover, miR-181a has also shown to sensitize A549 lung cancer cells to cancer drugs by stimulating Bax oligomerization and the activation of proapoptotic caspases [122]. The increased expression of the aforementioned miRNA was also found to increase the sensitivity of mature T cells to peptide antigens.

Hence, inhibiting miR-181a in immature T cells not only reduces its sensitivity, but also impairs the positive and negative selection function of immune cells [123].

To take advantage of the significant role of miRNAs as post-transcriptional regulators, several miRNA-based gene therapies were developed for use against cancers. One strategy is to import exogenous tumor suppressor miRNAs, which can either inhibit the tumor cell proliferation or induce apoptosis. These exogenous miRNAs are chemically synthesized mimics of endogenous miRNAs, which are usually downregulated in tumors. These miRNA mimics can be delivered through plasmid DNA or viral vectors. Another strategy is to inhibit the function of oncogenic miRNAs using antisense oligonucleotide. In this strategy, the antagonistic oligonucleotide is complementary to the sequence of the endogenous miRNA and is chemically modified to increase its affinity with the target miRNA. This causes it to be trapped in a configuration that will either result in the inability of RISC processing or degradation of the miRNA itself [124].

The use of miRNA-based gene therapy against cancer is very promising (Table 2). With the advancement of genetic technology, it is highly possible that more miRNA targeting TCA enzymes will be discovered and studied. However, despite its strong logical rationale, there are still problems regarding its logistics and efficiency. miRNA-based therapies specific to TCA cycle enzymes need to be studied further in order to establish its use for TCA enzyme-related cancers.

Table 2. miRNAs and their respective TCA or TCA-related enzyme targets.

| miRNA Name | Target | Role of Target | Action of miRNA to Target | Sample Type | Reference |
|---|---|---|---|---|---|
| miR-26a | PDHX | Catalyzes conversion of pyruvate to acetyl coA | inhibit | Colorectal cancer cell lines | [110] |
| miR-146b-5p | PDHB | Conversion of glucose-derived pyruvate to acetyl coA | inhibit | Human colorectal cancer tissue samples, colorectal cancer cell lines | [111] |
| miR-370 | PDHB | Conversion of glucose-derived pyruvate to acetyl coA | inhibit | Human melanoma tissue samples, human melanoma cell line | [112] |
| miR-137 | ASCT2 | Transport of glutamine | inhibit | Human neuroblastoma cell line | [107] |
| miR-183 | IDH2 | Catalyze conversion of isocitrate to α-ketoglutarate | inhibit | Glioblastoma cell lines | [108] |
| miR-181a | IDH1 | Catalyze conversion of isocitrate to α-ketoglutarate | inhibit | Tail-tip fibroblast, mouse embryonic fibroblast | [109] |
| | | | | Human lung cancer cell line, human colon cancer cell line, human cervical cancer cell line | [110] |
| | | | | Mouse T-cells | [111] |

### 4.4. CRISPR/Cas9 System

Clustered regularly interspaced short palindromic repeats (CRISPR) and CRISPR-associated protein 9, also known as the CRISPR/Cas9 system, was recently found as a potential therapy for cancer due to its gene-editing capability. This was discovered in prokaryotes, which possess CRISPR segments of DNA with short repetitions of base sequences. These sequences are interrupted by spacer sequences, which are remnants of viral or bacteriophage genetic codes, and thus enable recording of DNA sequences that the bacteria have been exposed to [125]. This then strengthens the immune function of the progeny by helping them to detect and to destroy bacteriophages once they attempt to invade the bacteria again. The spacer sequences were transcribed to RNA (crRNA), which recognizes the foreign DNA sequence. The Cas nucleases, on the other hand, mediate DNA cleavage [126]. For use in therapy, the spacer sequences can be genetically modified to recognize mutations in the DNA or predefined sites in the cellular genome and to facilitate cleavage.

Recently, a group of researchers, with the use of this gene-editing tool, designed sgRNAs for 88% of reported cancer mutations [127]. The team envisions this approach as potentially transferable to primary patient samples and for use as a therapeutic approach for personalized treatment. For example, the delivery of Cas9 and mutation-specific sgRNAs into tumor cells byoncolytic viruses could be an efficient technique for targeted therapy. Also, since specific ssgRNAs can be administered together, this strategy could be useful for combination therapy where more than two cancer mutations are targeted at the same time. However, because the method is still in its early stages, the repair mechanism after Cas9-mediated DNA cleavage is limited, resulting in sgRNA-resistant clones or off-target cleavage. In one study, this technique was also used to disrupt the CTCF motif in *IDH* gene in IDH wild-type gliomaspheres. The CTCF insulator protein is an important transcription factor in creating chromatin loops and boundaries that partition topological genome domains. Hypermethylation and/or disruption of binding sites of this transcription factor leads to loss of insulation between topological domains and aberrant gene activation. The aforementioned CRISPR-mediated disruption of the CTCF binding site caused an upregulation of PDGFRA, a prominent glioma oncogene, and increased cell proliferation [128].

In addition to the aforementioned limitations of the approach, several obstacles need to be surpassed in order to effectively use this system, such as possibilities of incomplete editing, inaccurate editing, and off-target mutations [129]. Such inaccuracy of the system may cause inactivation of essential genes, activation of pro-oncotic genes, or rearrangement of chromosomes. The therapy may also impose the risk of causing genetic mosaicism if it fails to affect all cells uniformly. A recent study showed that the genome editing capability of the system is affected by the tumor suppressor p53 [130]. p53 binds to DNA and can stimulate the transcription and activity of p21. p21 will, in turn, interact with cell division-stimulating protein (cdk2), hindering cell division. The CRISPR/Cas9 system has lower efficiency in p53 wild-type cells compared to that of knockout cells. Aside from increasing the efficiency of the CRISPR/Cas9 system, the inhibition of p53 can also decrease the selective advantage of pre-existing p53-deficient/mutant clones, a common characteristic of cancer cells. However, the inhibition of the said tumor suppressor will also increase the risk of cell vulnerability to chromosomal rearrangements and tumorigenic mutations [130].

The CRISPR/Cas9 system is a potentially promising cure for cancer. However, as it is still in its early stages, further research and improvements are needed to ensure its safety. Improving the balance of efficient DNA editing and suppression of potential tumorigenic effects is also important. Considering the ease of its use, its application to other TCA enzymes opens another area for medical research.

## 5. Conclusions

Understanding the mechanisms involving mitochondria is important to further develop strategies in treating mitochondria-associated diseases and dysfunction. The majority of studies to date have focused more on OXPHOS, which is another process that occurs in the mitochondrion and connects the mitochrondion to cancer physiology. However, the TCA cycle is also now being recognized as a key player in certain cancers which involve enzyme dysfunction. This review presented different studies regarding these mitochondrial TCA enzymes and cited diseases where they play a pivotal role. In addition, we also discussed available and prospective treatments, such as the drugs mentioned in the previous section. Last, this review was able to explore two novel approaches which are both promising strategies for cancer treatment: CRISPR/Cas9 and microRNA. However, both strategies require further research to ensure their specificity and efficiency.

**Author Contributions:** Conceptualization of this review paper was done by J.M. and J.H.; writing and the original draft was by J.M., J.F., B.N., A.T.T.N., N.P., J.H.; review, and editing by J.M., A.H.K., N.P., and J.H.; visualization by J.F.; supervised byN.P., J.H.; and funding acquisition, J.H.

**Funding:** This work was supported by the Priority Research Centers Program (2010-0020224). This work was also supported by the National Research Foundation of Korea (NRF) grant funded by the Korean government (MSIT) (2018R1A2A3074998).

**Conflicts of Interest:** The authors declare no conflict of interest.

## References

1. Vyas, S.; Zaganjor, E.; Haigis, M.C. Mitochondria and Cancer. *Cell* **2016**, *166*, 555–566. [CrossRef] [PubMed]
2. Calvo, S.E.; Mootha, V.K. The mitochondrial proteome and human disease. *Annu. Rev. Genom. Hum. Genet.* **2010**, *11*, 25–44. [CrossRef] [PubMed]
3. Taylor, R.W.; Turnbull, D.M. Mitochondrial DNA mutations in human disease. *Nat. Rev. Genet.* **2005**, *6*, 389–402. [CrossRef] [PubMed]
4. Lu, P.; Bruno, B.J.; Rabenau, M.; Lim, C.S. Delivery of drugs and macromolecules to the mitochondria for cancer therapy. *J. Control. Release* **2016**, *240*, 38–51. [CrossRef] [PubMed]
5. Yang, Y.; Karakhanova, S.; Hartwig, W.; D'Haese, J.G.; Philippov, P.P.; Werner, J.; Bazhin, A.V. Mitochondria and Mitochondrial ROS in Cancer: Novel Targets for Anticancer Therapy. *J. Cell. Physiol.* **2016**, *231*, 2570–2581. [CrossRef] [PubMed]
6. Beutner, G.; Alavian, K.N.; Jonas, E.A.; Porter, G.A., Jr. The Mitochondrial Permeability Transition Pore and ATP Synthase. *Handb. Exp. Pharmacol.* **2016**. [CrossRef]
7. Rogers, G.W.; Nadanaciva, S.; Swiss, R.; Divakaruni, A.S.; Will, Y. Assessment of fatty acid beta oxidation in cells and isolated mitochondria. *Curr. Protoc. Toxicol.* **2014**, *60*, 25.3.1–25.3.19. [CrossRef]
8. Mergenthaler, P.; Lindauer, U.; Dienel, G.A.; Meisel, A. Sugar for the brain: The role of glucose in physiological and pathological brain function. *Trends Neurosci.* **2013**, *36*, 587–597. [CrossRef]
9. Jensen, J.; Rustad, P.I.; Kolnes, A.J.; Lai, Y.C. The role of skeletal muscle glycogen breakdown for regulation of insulin sensitivity by exercise. *Front. Physiol.* **2011**, *2*, 112. [CrossRef]
10. Rui, L. Energy metabolism in the liver. *Compr. Physiol.* **2014**, *4*, 177–197. [CrossRef]
11. Nguyen, P.; Leray, V.; Diez, M.; Serisier, S.; Le Bloc'h, J.; Siliart, B.; Dumon, H. Liver lipid metabolism. *J. Anim. Physiol. Anim. Nutr.* **2008**, *92*, 272–283. [CrossRef] [PubMed]
12. Owen, O.E.; Kalhan, S.C.; Hanson, R.W. The key role of anaplerosis and cataplerosis for citric acid cycle function. *J. Biol. Chem.* **2002**, *277*, 30409–30412. [CrossRef] [PubMed]
13. Gibala, M.J.; Young, M.E.; Taegtmeyer, H. Anaplerosis of the citric acid cycle: Role in energy metabolism of heart and skeletal muscle. *Acta Physiol. Scand.* **2000**, *168*, 657–665. [CrossRef] [PubMed]
14. Ahn, C.S.; Metallo, C.M. Mitochondria as biosynthetic factories for cancer proliferation. *Cancer Metab.* **2015**, *3*, 1. [CrossRef] [PubMed]
15. Cheng, T.; Sudderth, J.; Yang, C.; Mullen, A.R.; Jin, E.S.; Mates, J.M.; DeBerardinis, R.J. Pyruvate carboxylase is required for glutamine-independent growth of tumor cells. *Proc. Natl. Acad. Sci. USA* **2011**, *108*, 8674–8679. [CrossRef] [PubMed]
16. Kolwicz, S.C., Jr.; Purohit, S.; Tian, R. Cardiac metabolism and its interactions with contraction, growth, and survival of cardiomyocytes. *Circ. Res.* **2013**, *113*, 603–616. [CrossRef] [PubMed]
17. Smith, A.C.; Robinson, A.J. A metabolic model of the mitochondrion and its use in modelling diseases of the tricarboxylic acid cycle. *BMC Syst. Biol.* **2011**, *5*, 102. [CrossRef]
18. Seyfried, T.N.; Flores, R.E.; Poff, A.M.; D'Agostino, D.P. Cancer as a metabolic disease: Implications for novel therapeutics. *Carcinogenesis* **2014**, *35*, 515–527. [CrossRef]
19. Seyfried, T.N. Cancer as a mitochondrial metabolic disease. *Front. Cell Dev. Biol.* **2015**, *3*, 43. [CrossRef]
20. Warburg, O. On the origin of cancer cells. *Science* **1956**, *123*, 309–314. [CrossRef]
21. Pavlova, N.N.; Thompson, C.B. The Emerging Hallmarks of Cancer Metabolism. *Cell Metab.* **2016**, *23*, 27–47. [CrossRef] [PubMed]
22. Courtnay, R.; Ngo, D.C.; Malik, N.; Ververis, K.; Tortorella, S.M.; Karagiannis, T.C. Cancer metabolism and the Warburg effect: The role of HIF-1 and PI3K. *Mol. Biol. Rep.* **2015**, *42*, 841–851. [CrossRef] [PubMed]
23. Payne, S.R.; Kemp, C.J. Tumor suppressor genetics. *Carcinogenesis* **2005**, *26*, 2031–2045. [CrossRef] [PubMed]
24. Chen, J.Q.; Russo, J. Dysregulation of glucose transport, glycolysis, TCA cycle and glutaminolysis by oncogenes and tumor suppressors in cancer cells. *Biochim. Biophys. Acta* **2012**, *1826*, 370–384. [CrossRef] [PubMed]
25. Laurenti, G.; Tennant, D.A. Isocitrate dehydrogenase (IDH), succinate dehydrogenase (SDH), fumarate hydratase (FH): Three players for one phenotype in cancer? *Biochem. Soc. Trans.* **2016**, *44*, 1111–1116. [CrossRef]

26. Al-Khallaf, H. Isocitrate dehydrogenases in physiology and cancer: Biochemical and molecular insight. *Cell Biosci.* **2017**, *7*, 37. [CrossRef]
27. Stoddard, B.L.; Dean, A.; Koshland, D.E., Jr. Structure of isocitrate dehydrogenase with isocitrate, nicotinamide adenine dinucleotide phosphate, and calcium at 2.5-A resolution: A pseudo-Michaelis ternary complex. *Biochemistry* **1993**, *32*, 9310–9316. [CrossRef]
28. Mondesir, J.; Willekens, C.; Touat, M.; de Botton, S. IDH1 and IDH2 mutations as novel therapeutic targets: Current perspectives. *J. Blood Med.* **2016**, *7*, 171–180. [CrossRef]
29. Cairns, R.A.; Iqbal, J.; Lemonnier, F.; Kucuk, C.; de Leval, L.; Jais, J.P.; Parrens, M.; Martin, A.; Xerri, L.; Brousset, P.; et al. IDH2 mutations are frequent in angioimmunoblastic T-cell lymphoma. *Blood* **2012**, *119*, 1901–1903. [CrossRef]
30. Kang, M.R.; Kim, M.S.; Oh, J.E.; Kim, Y.R.; Song, S.Y.; Seo, S.I.; Lee, J.Y.; Yoo, N.J.; Lee, S.H. Mutational analysis of IDH1 codon 132 in glioblastomas and other common cancers. *Int. J. Cancer* **2009**, *125*, 353–355. [CrossRef]
31. Yen, K.E.; Bittinger, M.A.; Su, S.M.; Fantin, V.R. Cancer-associated IDH mutations: Biomarker and therapeutic opportunities. *Oncogene* **2010**, *29*, 6409–6417. [CrossRef]
32. Abbas, S.; Lugthart, S.; Kavelaars, F.G.; Schelen, A.; Koenders, J.E.; Zeilemaker, A.; van Putten, W.J.; Rijneveld, A.W.; Lowenberg, B.; Valk, P.J. Acquired mutations in the genes encoding IDH1 and IDH2 both are recurrent aberrations in acute myeloid leukemia: Prevalence and prognostic value. *Blood* **2010**, *116*, 2122–2126. [CrossRef] [PubMed]
33. Paschka, P.; Schlenk, R.F.; Gaidzik, V.I.; Habdank, M.; Kronke, J.; Bullinger, L.; Spath, D.; Kayser, S.; Zucknick, M.; Gotze, K.; et al. IDH1 and IDH2 mutations are frequent genetic alterations in acute myeloid leukemia and confer adverse prognosis in cytogenetically normal acute myeloid leukemia with NPM1 mutation without FLT3 internal tandem duplication. *J. Clin. Oncol.* **2010**, *28*, 3636–3643. [CrossRef] [PubMed]
34. Xu, W.; Yang, H.; Liu, Y.; Yang, Y.; Wang, P.; Kim, S.H.; Ito, S.; Yang, C.; Xiao, M.T.; Liu, L.X.; et al. Oncometabolite 2-hydroxyglutarate is a competitive inhibitor of alpha-ketoglutarate-dependent dioxygenases. *Cancer Cell* **2011**, *19*, 17–30. [CrossRef] [PubMed]
35. Carbonneau, M.; Gagné, L.M.; Lalonde, M.E.; Germain, M.A.; Motorina, A.; Guiot, M.C.; Secco, B.; Vincent, E.E.; Tumber, A.; Hulea, L.; et al. The oncometabolite 2-hydroxyglutarate activates the mTOR signalling pathway. *Nat. Commun.* **2016**, *7*, 12700. [CrossRef]
36. Populo, H.; Lopes, J.M.; Soares, P. The mTOR signalling pathway in human cancer. *Int. J. Mol. Sci.* **2012**, *13*, 1886–1918. [CrossRef]
37. Whetstine, J.R.; Nottke, A.; Lan, F.; Huarte, M.; Smolikov, S.; Chen, Z.; Spooner, E.; Li, E.; Zhang, G.; Colaiacovo, M.; et al. Reversal of histone lysine trimethylation by the JMJD2 family of histone demethylases. *Cell* **2006**, *125*, 467–481. [CrossRef]
38. Li, T.; Cox, C.D.; Ozer, B.H.; Nguyen, N.T.; Nguyen, H.N.; Lai, T.J.; Li, S.; Liu, F.; Kornblum, H.I.; Liau, L.M.; et al. D-2-Hydroxyglutarate Is Necessary and Sufficient for Isocitrate Dehydrogenase 1 Mutant-Induced MIR148A Promoter Methylation. *Mol. Cancer Res.* **2018**, *16*, 947–960. [CrossRef]
39. Dang, L.; White, D.W.; Gross, S.; Bennett, B.D.; Bittinger, M.A.; Driggers, E.M.; Fantin, V.R.; Jang, H.G.; Jin, S.; Keenan, M.C.; et al. Cancer-associated IDH1 mutations produce 2-hydroxyglutarate. *Nature* **2009**, *462*, 739–744. [CrossRef]
40. Losman, J.A.; Kaelin, W.G., Jr. What a difference a hydroxyl makes: Mutant IDH, (R)-2-hydroxyglutarate, and cancer. *Genes Dev.* **2013**, *27*, 836–852. [CrossRef]
41. Mardis, E.R.; Ding, L.; Dooling, D.J.; Larson, D.E.; McLellan, M.D.; Chen, K.; Koboldt, D.C.; Fulton, R.S.; Delehaunty, K.D.; McGrath, S.D.; et al. Recurring mutations found by sequencing an acute myeloid leukemia genome. *N. Engl. J. Med.* **2009**, *361*, 1058–1066. [CrossRef] [PubMed]
42. Im, A.P.; Sehgal, A.R.; Carroll, M.P.; Smith, B.D.; Tefferi, A.; Johnson, D.E.; Boyiadzis, M. DNMT3A and IDH mutations in acute myeloid leukemia and other myeloid malignancies: Associations with prognosis and potential treatment strategies. *Leukemia* **2014**, *28*, 1774–1783. [CrossRef] [PubMed]
43. Molenaar, R.J.; Thota, S.; Nagata, Y.; Patel, B.; Clemente, M.; Przychodzen, B.; Hirsh, C.; Viny, A.D.; Hosano, N.; Bleeker, F.E.; et al. Clinical and biological implications of ancestral and non-ancestral IDH1 and IDH2 mutations in myeloid neoplasms. *Leukemia* **2015**, *29*, 2134–2142. [CrossRef] [PubMed]

44. Patel, J.P.; Gonen, M.; Figueroa, M.E.; Fernandez, H.; Sun, Z.; Racevskis, J.; Van Vlierberghe, P.; Dolgalev, I.; Thomas, S.; Aminova, O.; et al. Prognostic relevance of integrated genetic profiling in acute myeloid leukemia. *N. Engl. J. Med.* **2012**, *366*, 1079–1089. [CrossRef] [PubMed]
45. Abdel-Wahab, O.; Patel, J.; Levine, R.L. Clinical implications of novel mutations in epigenetic modifiers in AML. *Hematol. Oncol. Clin. N. Am.* **2011**, *25*, 1119–1133. [CrossRef] [PubMed]
46. Boissel, N.; Nibourel, O.; Renneville, A.; Huchette, P.; Dombret, H.; Preudhomme, C. Differential prognosis impact of IDH2 mutations in cytogenetically normal acute myeloid leukemia. *Blood* **2011**, *117*, 3696–3697. [CrossRef]
47. Green, C.L.; Evans, C.M.; Zhao, L.; Hills, R.K.; Burnett, A.K.; Linch, D.C.; Gale, R.E. The prognostic significance of IDH2 mutations in AML depends on the location of the mutation. *Blood* **2011**, *118*, 409–412. [CrossRef]
48. Hamadou, W.S.; Bourdon, V.; Letard, S.; Brenet, F.; Laarif, S.; Besbes, S.; Paci, A.; David, M.; Penard-Lacronique, V.; Youssef, Y.B.; et al. Familial hematological malignancies: New IDH2 mutation. *Ann. Hematol.* **2016**. [CrossRef]
49. Zanssen, S.; Schon, E.A. Mitochondrial DNA mutations in cancer. *PLoS Med.* **2005**, *2*, e401. [CrossRef]
50. Shuch, B.; Linehan, W.M.; Srinivasan, R. Aerobic glycolysis: A novel target in kidney cancer. *Expert Rev. Anticancer Ther.* **2013**, *13*, 711–719. [CrossRef]
51. Baysal, B.E.; Ferrell, R.E.; Willett-Brozick, J.E.; Lawrence, E.C.; Myssiorek, D.; Bosch, A.; van der Mey, A.; Taschner, P.E.; Rubinstein, W.S.; Myers, E.N.; et al. Mutations in SDHD, a mitochondrial complex II gene, in hereditary paraganglioma. *Science* **2000**, *287*, 848–851. [CrossRef] [PubMed]
52. Selak, M.A.; Armour, S.M.; MacKenzie, E.D.; Boulahbel, H.; Watson, D.G.; Mansfield, K.D.; Pan, Y.; Simon, M.C.; Thompson, C.B.; Gottlieb, E. Succinate links TCA cycle dysfunction to oncogenesis by inhibiting HIF-alpha prolyl hydroxylase. *Cancer Cell* **2005**, *7*, 77–85. [CrossRef] [PubMed]
53. Ryan, D.G.; Murphy, M.P.; Frezza, C.; Prag, H.A.; Chouchani, E.T.; O'Neill, L.A.; Mills, E.L. Coupling Krebs cycle metabolites to signalling in immunity and cancer. *Nat. Metab.* **2019**, *1*, 16–33. [CrossRef] [PubMed]
54. Niemann, S.; Muller, U. Mutations in SDHC cause autosomal dominant paraganglioma, type 3. *Nat. Genet.* **2000**, *26*, 268–270. [CrossRef]
55. Astuti, D.; Latif, F.; Dallol, A.; Dahia, P.L.; Douglas, F.; George, E.; Skoldberg, F.; Husebye, E.S.; Eng, C.; Maher, E.R. Gene mutations in the succinate dehydrogenase subunit SDHB cause susceptibility to familial pheochromocytoma and to familial paraganglioma. *Am. J. Hum. Genet.* **2001**, *69*, 49–54. [CrossRef]
56. Bardella, C.; Pollard, P.J.; Tomlinson, I. SDH mutations in cancer. *Biochim. Biophys. Acta* **2011**, *1807*, 1432–1443. [CrossRef]
57. Bourgeron, T.; Rustin, P.; Chretien, D.; Birch-Machin, M.; Bourgeois, M.; Viegas-Pequignot, E.; Munnich, A.; Rotig, A. Mutation of a nuclear succinate dehydrogenase gene results in mitochondrial respiratory chain deficiency. *Nat. Genet.* **1995**, *11*, 144–149. [CrossRef]
58. Parfait, B.; Chretien, D.; Rotig, A.; Marsac, C.; Munnich, A.; Rustin, P. Compound heterozygous mutations in the flavoprotein gene of the respiratory chain complex II in a patient with Leigh syndrome. *Hum. Genet.* **2000**, *106*, 236–243. [CrossRef]
59. Horvath, R.; Abicht, A.; Holinski-Feder, E.; Laner, A.; Gempel, K.; Prokisch, H.; Lochmuller, H.; Klopstock, T.; Jaksch, M. Leigh syndrome caused by mutations in the flavoprotein (Fp) subunit of succinate dehydrogenase (SDHA). *J. Neurol. Neurosurg. Psychiatry* **2006**, *77*, 74–76. [CrossRef]
60. Birch-Machin, M.A.; Taylor, R.W.; Cochran, B.; Ackrell, B.A.; Turnbull, D.M. Late-onset optic atrophy, ataxia, and myopathy associated with a mutation of a complex II gene. *Ann. Neurol.* **2000**, *48*, 330–335. [CrossRef]
61. Van Coster, R.; Seneca, S.; Smet, J.; Van Hecke, R.; Gerlo, E.; Devreese, B.; Van Beeumen, J.; Leroy, J.G.; De Meirleir, L.; Lissens, W. Homozygous Gly555Glu mutation in the nuclear-encoded 70 kDa flavoprotein gene causes instability of the respiratory chain complex II. *Am. J. Med. Genet. A* **2003**, *120*, 13–18. [CrossRef] [PubMed]
62. Lin, G.; Doyle, L.A. An update on the application of newly described immunohistochemical markers in soft tissue pathology. *Arch. Pathol. Lab. Med.* **2015**, *139*, 106–121. [CrossRef] [PubMed]
63. Neumann, H.P.; Pawlu, C.; Peczkowska, M.; Bausch, B.; McWhinney, S.R.; Muresan, M.; Buchta, M.; Franke, G.; Klisch, J.; Bley, T.A.; et al. Distinct clinical features of paraganglioma syndromes associated with SDHB and SDHD gene mutations. *JAMA* **2004**, *292*, 943–951. [CrossRef] [PubMed]

64. Timmers, H.J.; Kozupa, A.; Eisenhofer, G.; Raygada, M.; Adams, K.T.; Solis, D.; Lenders, J.W.; Pacak, K. Clinical presentations, biochemical phenotypes, and genotype-phenotype correlations in patients with succinate dehydrogenase subunit B-associated pheochromocytomas and paragangliomas. *J. Clin. Endocrinol. Metab.* **2007**, *92*, 779–786. [CrossRef] [PubMed]
65. Benn, D.E.; Gimenez-Roqueplo, A.P.; Reilly, J.R.; Bertherat, J.; Burgess, J.; Byth, K.; Croxson, M.; Dahia, P.L.; Elston, M.; Gimm, O.; et al. Clinical presentation and penetrance of pheochromocytoma/paraganglioma syndromes. *J. Clin. Endocrinol. Metab.* **2006**, *91*, 827–836. [CrossRef] [PubMed]
66. Young, A.L.; Baysal, B.E.; Deb, A.; Young, W.F., Jr. Familial malignant catecholamine-secreting paraganglioma with prolonged survival associated with mutation in the succinate dehydrogenase B gene. *J. Clin. Endocrinol. Metab.* **2002**, *87*, 4101–4105. [CrossRef]
67. Vanharanta, S.; Buchta, M.; McWhinney, S.R.; Virta, S.K.; Peczkowska, M.; Morrison, C.D.; Lehtonen, R.; Januszewicz, A.; Jarvinen, H.; Juhola, M.; et al. Early-onset renal cell carcinoma as a novel extraparaganglial component of SDHB-associated heritable paraganglioma. *Am. J. Hum. Genet.* **2004**, *74*, 153–159. [CrossRef]
68. Baysal, B.E. A recurrent stop-codon mutation in succinate dehydrogenase subunit B gene in normal peripheral blood and childhood T-cell acute leukemia. *PLoS ONE* **2007**, *2*, e436. [CrossRef]
69. Fishbein, L.; Leshchiner, I.; Walter, V.; Danilova, L.; Robertson, A.G.; Johnson, A.R.; Lichtenberg, T.M.; Murray, B.A.; Ghayee, H.K.; Else, T.; et al. Comprehensive Molecular Characterization of Pheochromocytoma and Paraganglioma. *Cancer Cell* **2017**, *31*, 181–193. [CrossRef]
70. Burnichon, N.; Rohmer, V.; Amar, L.; Herman, P.; Leboulleux, S.; Darrouzet, V.; Niccoli, P.; Gaillard, D.; Chabrier, G.; Chabolle, F.; et al. The succinate dehydrogenase genetic testing in a large prospective series of patients with paragangliomas. *J. Clin. Endocrinol. Metab.* **2009**, *94*, 2817–2827. [CrossRef]
71. Mannelli, M.; Ercolino, T.; Giache, V.; Simi, L.; Cirami, C.; Parenti, G. Genetic screening for pheochromocytoma: Should SDHC gene analysis be included? *J. Med. Genet.* **2007**, *44*, 586–587. [CrossRef] [PubMed]
72. Mannelli, M.; Castellano, M.; Schiavi, F.; Filetti, S.; Giacche, M.; Mori, L.; Pignataro, V.; Bernini, G.; Giache, V.; Bacca, A.; et al. Clinically guided genetic screening in a large cohort of italian patients with pheochromocytomas and/or functional or nonfunctional paragangliomas. *J. Clin. Endocrinol. Metab.* **2009**, *94*, 1541–1547. [CrossRef] [PubMed]
73. Schiavi, F.; Boedeker, C.C.; Bausch, B.; Peczkowska, M.; Gomez, C.F.; Strassburg, T.; Pawlu, C.; Buchta, M.; Salzmann, M.; Hoffmann, M.M.; et al. Predictors and prevalence of paraganglioma syndrome associated with mutations of the SDHC gene. *JAMA* **2005**, *294*, 2057–2063. [CrossRef] [PubMed]
74. Ni, Y.; Seballos, S.; Ganapathi, S.; Gurin, D.; Fletcher, B.; Ngeow, J.; Nagy, R.; Kloos, R.T.; Ringel, M.D.; LaFramboise, T.; et al. Germline and somatic SDHx alterations in apparently sporadic differentiated thyroid cancer. *Endocr. Relat. Cancer* **2015**, *22*, 121–130. [CrossRef] [PubMed]
75. Ricketts, C.J.; Forman, J.R.; Rattenberry, E.; Bradshaw, N.; Lalloo, F.; Izatt, L.; Cole, T.R.; Armstrong, R.; Kumar, V.K.; Morrison, P.J.; et al. Tumor risks and genotype-phenotype-proteotype analysis in 358 patients with germline mutations in SDHB and SDHD. *Hum. Mutat.* **2010**, *31*, 41–51. [CrossRef] [PubMed]
76. Bennedbaek, M.; Rossing, M.; Rasmussen, A.K.; Gerdes, A.M.; Skytte, A.B.; Jensen, U.B.; Nielsen, F.C.; Hansen, T.V. Identification of eight novel SDHB, SDHC, SDHD germline variants in Danish pheochromocytoma/paraganglioma patients. *Hered. Cancer Clin. Pract.* **2016**, *14*, 13. [CrossRef] [PubMed]
77. Burnichon, N.; Briere, J.J.; Libe, R.; Vescovo, L.; Riviere, J.; Tissier, F.; Jouanno, E.; Jeunemaitre, X.; Benit, P.; Tzagoloff, A.; et al. SDHA is a tumor suppressor gene causing paraganglioma. *Hum. Mol. Genet.* **2010**, *19*, 3011–3020. [CrossRef]
78. Bayley, J.P.; Kunst, H.P.; Cascon, A.; Sampietro, M.L.; Gaal, J.; Korpershoek, E.; Hinojar-Gutierrez, A.; Timmers, H.J.; Hoefsloot, L.H.; Hermsen, M.A.; et al. SDHAF2 mutations in familial and sporadic paraganglioma and phaeochromocytoma. *Lancet Oncol.* **2010**, *11*, 366–372. [CrossRef]
79. Hao, H.X.; Khalimonchuk, O.; Schraders, M.; Dephoure, N.; Bayley, J.P.; Kunst, H.; Devilee, P.; Cremers, C.W.; Schiffman, J.D.; Bentz, B.G.; et al. SDH5, a gene required for flavination of succinate dehydrogenase, is mutated in paraganglioma. *Science* **2009**, *325*, 1139–1142. [CrossRef]
80. Zhang, D.D.; Hannink, M. Distinct cysteine residues in Keap1 are required for Keap1-dependent ubiquitination of Nrf2 and for stabilization of Nrf2 by chemopreventive agents and oxidative stress. *Mol. Cell. Biol.* **2003**, *23*, 8137–8151. [CrossRef]
81. Ma, Q. Role of nrf2 in oxidative stress and toxicity. *Annu. Rev. Pharmacol. Toxicol.* **2013**, *53*, 401–426. [CrossRef] [PubMed]

82. Tyrakis, P.A.; Yurkovich, M.E.; Sciacovelli, M.; Papachristou, E.K.; Bridges, H.R.; Gaude, E.; Schreiner, A.; D'Santos, C.; Hirst, J.; Hernandez-Fernaud, J.; et al. Fumarate Hydratase Loss Causes Combined Respiratory Chain Defects. *Cell Rep.* **2017**, *21*, 1036–1047. [CrossRef] [PubMed]
83. Launonen, V.; Vierimaa, O.; Kiuru, M.; Isola, J.; Roth, S.; Pukkala, E.; Sistonen, P.; Herva, R.; Aaltonen, L.A. Inherited susceptibility to uterine leiomyomas and renal cell cancer. *Proc. Natl. Acad. Sci. USA* **2001**, *98*, 3387–3392. [CrossRef] [PubMed]
84. Tomlinson, I.P.; Alam, N.A.; Rowan, A.J.; Barclay, E.; Jaeger, E.E.; Kelsell, D.; Leigh, I.; Gorman, P.; Lamlum, H.; Rahman, S.; et al. Germline mutations in FH predispose to dominantly inherited uterine fibroids, skin leiomyomata and papillary renal cell cancer. *Nat. Genet.* **2002**, *30*, 406–410. [CrossRef]
85. Barker, K.T.; Bevan, S.; Wang, R.; Lu, Y.J.; Flanagan, A.M.; Bridge, J.A.; Fisher, C.; Finlayson, C.J.; Shipley, J.; Houlston, R.S. Low frequency of somatic mutations in the FH/multiple cutaneous leiomyomatosis gene in sporadic leiomyosarcomas and uterine leiomyomas. *Br. J. Cancer* **2002**, *87*, 446–448. [CrossRef]
86. Letouze, E.; Martinelli, C.; Loriot, C.; Burnichon, N.; Abermil, N.; Ottolenghi, C.; Janin, M.; Menara, M.; Nguyen, A.T.; Benit, P.; et al. SDH mutations establish a hypermethylator phenotype in paraganglioma. *Cancer Cell* **2013**, *23*, 739–752. [CrossRef]
87. Smit, D.L.; Mensenkamp, A.R.; Badeloe, S.; Breuning, M.H.; Simon, M.E.; van Spaendonck, K.Y.; Aalfs, C.M.; Post, J.G.; Shanley, S.; Krapels, I.P.; et al. Hereditary leiomyomatosis and renal cell cancer in families referred for fumarate hydratase germline mutation analysis. *Clin. Genet.* **2011**, *79*, 49–59. [CrossRef]
88. Schmidt, L.S.; Linehan, W.M. Hereditary leiomyomatosis and renal cell carcinoma. *Int. J. Nephrol. Renovasc. Dis.* **2014**, *7*, 253–260. [CrossRef]
89. Zhao, S.; Lin, Y.; Xu, W.; Jiang, W.; Zha, Z.; Wang, P.; Yu, W.; Li, Z.; Gong, L.; Peng, Y.; et al. Glioma-derived mutations in IDH1 dominantly inhibit IDH1 catalytic activity and induce HIF-1alpha. *Science* **2009**, *324*, 261–265. [CrossRef]
90. Sudarshan, S.; Shanmugasundaram, K.; Naylor, S.L.; Lin, S.; Livi, C.B.; O'Neill, C.F.; Parekh, D.J.; Yeh, I.T.; Sun, L.Z.; Block, K. Reduced expression of fumarate hydratase in clear cell renal cancer mediates HIF-2alpha accumulation and promotes migration and invasion. *PLoS ONE* **2011**, *6*, e21037. [CrossRef]
91. Tong, W.H.; Sourbier, C.; Kovtunovych, G.; Jeong, S.Y.; Vira, M.; Ghosh, M.; Romero, V.V.; Sougrat, R.; Vaulont, S.; Viollet, B.; et al. The glycolytic shift in fumarate-hydratase-deficient kidney cancer lowers AMPK levels, increases anabolic propensities and lowers cellular iron levels. *Cancer Cell* **2011**, *20*, 315–327. [CrossRef] [PubMed]
92. Musrati, R.A.; Kollarova, M.; Mernik, N.; Mikulasova, D. Malate dehydrogenase: Distribution, function and properties. *Gen. Physiol. Biophys.* **1998**, *17*, 193–210. [PubMed]
93. Minarik, P.; Tomaskova, N.; Kollarova, M.; Antalik, M. Malate dehydrogenases–structure and function. *Gen. Physiol. Biophys.* **2002**, *21*, 257–265. [PubMed]
94. Lo, Y.W.; Lin, S.T.; Chang, S.J.; Chan, C.H.; Lyu, K.W.; Chang, J.F.; May, E.W.; Lin, D.Y.; Chou, H.C.; Chan, H.L. Mitochondrial proteomics with siRNA knockdown to reveal ACAT1 and MDH2 in the development of doxorubicin-resistant uterine cancer. *J. Cell. Mol. Med.* **2015**, *19*, 744–759. [CrossRef]
95. Liu, Q.; Harvey, C.T.; Geng, H.; Xue, C.; Chen, V.; Beer, T.M.; Qian, D.Z. Malate dehydrogenase 2 confers docetaxel resistance via regulations of JNK signaling and oxidative metabolism. *Prostate* **2013**, *73*, 1028–1037. [CrossRef]
96. Calsina, B.; Curras-Freixes, M.; Buffet, A.; Pons, T.; Contreras, L.; Leton, R.; Comino-Mendez, I.; Remacha, L.; Calatayud, M.; Obispo, B.; et al. Role of MDH2 pathogenic variant in pheochromocytoma and paraganglioma patients. *Genet. Med.* **2018**, *20*, 1652–1662. [CrossRef]
97. Ventura-Clapier, R.; Garnier, A.; Veksler, V. Energy metabolism in heart failure. *J. Physiol.* **2004**, *555*, 1–13. [CrossRef]
98. Erez, A.; DeBerardinis, R.J. Metabolic dysregulation in monogenic disorders and cancer—Finding method in madness. *Nat. Rev. Cancer* **2015**, *15*, 440–448. [CrossRef]
99. Chen, J.; Yang, J.; Cao, P. The Evolving Landscape in the Development of Isocitrate Dehydrogenase Mutant Inhibitors. *Mini Rev. Med. Chem.* **2016**, *16*, 1344–1358. [CrossRef]
100. Caino, M.C.; Altieri, D.C. Molecular Pathways: Mitochondrial Reprogramming in Tumor Progression and Therapy. *Clin. Cancer Res.* **2016**, *22*, 540–545. [CrossRef]

101. Urban, D.J.; Martinez, N.J.; Davis, M.I.; Brimacombe, K.R.; Cheff, D.M.; Lee, T.D.; Henderson, M.J.; Titus, S.A.; Pragani, R.; Rohde, J.M.; et al. Assessing inhibitors of mutant isocitrate dehydrogenase using a suite of pre-clinical discovery assays. *Sci. Rep.* **2017**, *7*, 12758. [CrossRef] [PubMed]
102. Fujii, T.; Khawaja, M.R.; DiNardo, C.D.; Atkins, J.T.; Janku, F. Targeting isocitrate dehydrogenase (IDH) in cancer. *Discov. Med.* **2016**, *21*, 373–380. [PubMed]
103. Fantin, V.R.; St-Pierre, J.; Leder, P. Attenuation of LDH-A expression uncovers a link between glycolysis, mitochondrial physiology, and tumor maintenance. *Cancer Cell* **2006**, *9*, 425–434. [CrossRef]
104. Le, A.; Cooper, C.R.; Gouw, A.M.; Dinavahi, R.; Maitra, A.; Deck, L.M.; Royer, R.E.; Vander Jagt, D.L.; Semenza, G.L.; Dang, C.V. Inhibition of lactate dehydrogenase A induces oxidative stress and inhibits tumor progression. *Proc. Natl. Acad. Sci. USA* **2010**, *107*, 2037–2042. [CrossRef]
105. DeBerardinis, R.J.; Chandel, N.S. Fundamentals of cancer metabolism. *Sci. Adv.* **2016**, *2*, e1600200. [CrossRef] [PubMed]
106. Haas, R.; Smith, J.; Rocher-Ros, V.; Nadkarni, S.; Montero-Melendez, T.; D'Acquisto, F.; Bland, E.J.; Bombardieri, M.; Pitzalis, C.; Perretti, M.; et al. Lactate Regulates Metabolic and Pro-inflammatory Circuits in Control of T Cell Migration and Effector Functions. *PLoS Biol.* **2015**, *13*, e1002202. [CrossRef] [PubMed]
107. Bonnet, S.; Archer, S.L.; Allalunis-Turner, J.; Haromy, A.; Beaulieu, C.; Thompson, R.; Lee, C.T.; Lopaschuk, G.D.; Puttagunta, L.; Bonnet, S.; et al. A mitochondria-K+ channel axis is suppressed in cancer and its normalization promotes apoptosis and inhibits cancer growth. *Cancer Cell* **2007**, *11*, 37–51. [CrossRef]
108. Michelakis, E.D.; Sutendra, G.; Dromparis, P.; Webster, L.; Haromy, A.; Niven, E.; Maguire, C.; Gammer, T.L.; Mackey, J.R.; Fulton, D.; et al. Metabolic modulation of glioblastoma with dichloroacetate. *Sci. Transl. Med.* **2010**, *2*, 31ra34. [CrossRef]
109. Vander Heiden, M.G. Targeting cancer metabolism: A therapeutic window opens. *Nat. Rev. Drug Discov.* **2011**, *10*, 671–684. [CrossRef]
110. Chen, B.; Liu, Y.; Jin, X.; Lu, W.; Liu, J.; Xia, Z.; Yuan, Q.; Zhao, X.; Xu, N.; Liang, S. MicroRNA-26a regulates glucose metabolism by direct targeting PDHX in colorectal cancer cells. *BMC Cancer* **2014**, *14*, 443. [CrossRef]
111. Zhu, Y.; Wu, G.; Yan, W.; Zhan, H.; Sun, P. miR-146b-5p regulates cell growth, invasion, and metabolism by targeting PDHB in colorectal cancer. *Am. J. Cancer Res.* **2017**, *7*, 1136–1150. [PubMed]
112. Wei, S.; Ma, W. MiR-370 functions as oncogene in melanoma by direct targeting pyruvate dehydrogenase B. *Biomed. Pharmacother.* **2017**, *90*, 278–286. [CrossRef]
113. Peng, Y.; Croce, C.M. The role of MicroRNAs in human cancer. *Signal Transduct. Target. Ther.* **2016**, *1*, 15004. [CrossRef] [PubMed]
114. Macfarlane, L.A.; Murphy, P.R. MicroRNA: Biogenesis, Function and Role in Cancer. *Curr. Genom.* **2010**, *11*, 537–561. [CrossRef] [PubMed]
115. Bartel, D.P. MicroRNAs: Genomics, biogenesis, mechanism, and function. *Cell* **2004**, *116*, 281–297. [CrossRef]
116. Subramaniam, S.; Jeet, V.; Clements, J.A.; Gunter, J.H.; Batra, J. Emergence of MicroRNAs as Key Players in Cancer Cell Metabolism. *Clin. Chem.* **2019**. [CrossRef] [PubMed]
117. Dong, J.; Xiao, D.; Zhao, Z.; Ren, P.; Li, C.; Hu, Y.; Shi, J.; Su, H.; Wang, L.; Liu, H.; et al. Epigenetic silencing of microRNA-137 enhances ASCT2 expression and tumor glutamine metabolism. *Oncogenesis* **2017**, *6*, e356. [CrossRef]
118. Anderson, N.M.; Mucka, P.; Kern, J.G.; Feng, H. The emerging role and targetability of the TCA cycle in cancer metabolism. *Protein Cell* **2018**, *9*, 216–237. [CrossRef]
119. Choi, Y.K.; Park, K.G. Targeting Glutamine Metabolism for Cancer Treatment. *Biomol. Ther.* **2018**, *26*, 19–28. [CrossRef]
120. Tanaka, H.; Sasayama, T.; Tanaka, K.; Nakamizo, S.; Nishihara, M.; Mizukawa, K.; Kohta, M.; Koyama, J.; Miyake, S.; Taniguchi, M.; et al. MicroRNA-183 upregulates HIF-1alpha by targeting isocitrate dehydrogenase 2 (IDH2) in glioma cells. *J. Neurooncol.* **2013**, *111*, 273–283. [CrossRef]
121. Chu, B.; Wu, T.; Miao, L.; Mei, Y.; Wu, M. MiR-181a regulates lipid metabolism via IDH1. *Sci. Rep.* **2015**, *5*, 8801. [CrossRef] [PubMed]
122. Galluzzi, L.; Morselli, E.; Vitale, I.; Kepp, O.; Senovilla, L.; Criollo, A.; Servant, N.; Paccard, C.; Hupe, P.; Robert, T.; et al. miR-181a and miR-630 regulate cisplatin-induced cancer cell death. *Cancer Res.* **2010**, *70*, 1793–1803. [CrossRef] [PubMed]

123. Li, Q.J.; Chau, J.; Ebert, P.J.; Sylvester, G.; Min, H.; Liu, G.; Braich, R.; Manoharan, M.; Soutschek, J.; Skare, P.; et al. miR-181a is an intrinsic modulator of T cell sensitivity and selection. *Cell* **2007**, *129*, 147–161. [CrossRef] [PubMed]
124. Bader, A.G.; Brown, D.; Winkler, M. The promise of microRNA replacement therapy. *Cancer Res.* **2010**, *70*, 7027–7030. [CrossRef]
125. Hsu, P.D.; Lander, E.S.; Zhang, F. Development and applications of CRISPR-Cas9 for genome engineering. *Cell* **2014**, *157*, 1262–1278. [CrossRef]
126. Doudna, J.A.; Charpentier, E. Genome editing. The new frontier of genome engineering with CRISPR-Cas9. *Science* **2014**, *346*, 1258096. [CrossRef]
127. Gebler, C.; Lohoff, T.; Paszkowski-Rogacz, M.; Mircetic, J.; Chakraborty, D.; Camgoz, A.; Hamann, M.V.; Theis, M.; Thiede, C.; Buchholz, F. Inactivation of Cancer Mutations Utilizing CRISPR/Cas9. *J. Natl. Cancer Inst.* **2017**, *109*. [CrossRef]
128. Flavahan, W.A.; Drier, Y.; Liau, B.B.; Gillespie, S.M.; Venteicher, A.S.; Stemmer-Rachamimov, A.O.; Suva, M.L.; Bernstein, B.E. Insulator dysfunction and oncogene activation in IDH mutant gliomas. *Nature* **2016**, *529*, 110–114. [CrossRef]
129. Fogleman, S.; Santana, C.; Bishop, C.; Miller, A.; Capco, D.G. CRISPR/Cas9 and mitochondrial gene replacement therapy: Promising techniques and ethical considerations. *Am. J. Stem Cells* **2016**, *5*, 39–52.
130. Haapaniemi, E.; Botla, S.; Persson, J.; Schmierer, B.; Taipale, J. CRISPR-Cas9 genome editing induces a p53-mediated DNA damage response. *Nat. Med.* **2018**, *24*, 927–930. [CrossRef]

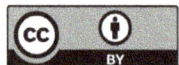

© 2019 by the authors. Licensee MDPI, Basel, Switzerland. This article is an open access article distributed under the terms and conditions of the Creative Commons Attribution (CC BY) license (http://creativecommons.org/licenses/by/4.0/).

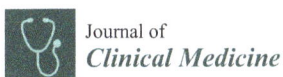

*Review*

# The Rise of Mitochondria in Peripheral Arterial Disease Physiopathology: Experimental and Clinical Data

Mégane Pizzimenti [1,2], Marianne Riou [1,2], Anne-Laure Charles [1], Samy Talha [1,2], Alain Meyer [1,2], Emmanuel Andres [3], Nabil Chakfé [1,4], Anne Lejay [1,4] and Bernard Geny [1,2,*]

1. Unistra, Translational Medicine Federation of Strasbourg (FMTS), Faculty of Medicine, Team 3072 «Mitochondria, Oxidative Stress and Muscle Protection», 11 Rue Humann, 67000 Strasbourg, France; megane.pizzimenti@hotmail.fr (M.P.); marianne.riou@chru-strasbourg.fr (M.R.); anne.laure.charles@outlook.fr (A.-L.C.); samy.talha@chru-strasbourg.fr (S.T.); alain.meyer1@chru-strasbourg.fr (A.M.); nabil.chakfe@chru-strasbourg.fr (N.C.); anne.lejay@chru-strasbourg.fr (A.L.)
2. Physiology and Functional Exploration Service, University Hospital of Strasbourg, 1 Place de l'Hôpital, 67091 Strasbourg CEDEX, France
3. Internal Medicine, Diabete and Metabolic Diseases Service, University Hospital of Strasbourg, 1 Place de l'Hôpital, 67091 Strasbourg CEDEX, France; emmanuel.andres@chru-strasbourg.fr
4. Vascular Surgery and Kidney Transplantation Service, University Hospital of Strasbourg, 1 Place de l'Hôpital, 67091 Strasbourg CEDEX, France
* Correspondence: bernard.geny@chru-strasbourg.fr

Received: 10 November 2019; Accepted: 29 November 2019; Published: 2 December 2019

**Abstract:** Peripheral arterial disease (PAD) is a frequent and serious condition, potentially life-threatening and leading to lower-limb amputation. Its pathophysiology is generally related to ischemia-reperfusion cycles, secondary to reduction or interruption of the arterial blood flow followed by reperfusion episodes that are necessary but also—per se—deleterious. Skeletal muscles alterations significantly participate in PAD injuries, and interestingly, muscle mitochondrial dysfunctions have been demonstrated to be key events and to have a prognosis value. Decreased oxidative capacity due to mitochondrial respiratory chain impairment is associated with increased release of reactive oxygen species and reduction of calcium retention capacity leading thus to enhanced apoptosis. Therefore, targeting mitochondria might be a promising therapeutic approach in PAD.

**Keywords:** peripheral arterial disease; ischemia-reperfusion; mitochondria; oxidative stress; reactive oxygen species; antioxidant; calcium retention capacity; apoptosis

---

## 1. Introduction

Peripheral arterial diseases (PAD) is a major concern for public healthcare, affecting more than 200 million individual worldwide [1,2]. Its prevalence varies from 3% to 10%, but can reach up to 20% in the elderly population [3].

PAD is defined by a narrowing of the peripheral arterial vasculature. It mostly affects lower limbs, leading to overall functional disability and reduced quality of life. Initially asymptomatic, PAD progressively compromises lower limb vascularization, leading to obstruction of the vessels by atheroma. PAD includes all stages of the disease, from asymptomatic with abolition of distal pulses, to intermittent claudication or critical limb threatening ischemia (CLTI) characterized by rest pain and/or ulcers. PAD is also often associated with cognitive dysfunction characterized by reduced performance in nonverbal reasoning, reduced verbal fluency, and decreased information processing speed [4]. Thus, PAD is a serious condition threatening both limb (risk of amputation) and vital prognosis of the patients. Indeed, despite recent therapeutic progress, morbidity and mortality rates remain incompressible around 20% and 15% five years after a diagnosis of symptomatic or asymptomatic PAD [5]. On average, the life expectancy of claudicating patients is reduced by 10 years, with a majority of death attributable to cardiovascular causes.

The treatment of PAD is mainly based on revascularization of the ischemic limb [6]. Nevertheless, this surgical procedure is not always possible, notably when the vascular state is too precarious or when the local evolution is too advanced. It appears therefore important to better understand PAD pathophysiology to offer optimal patient care. Indeed, insufficient oxygen supply was long presumed to be the main and sole cause for PAD symptoms. However, recent advances in understanding PAD physiopathology identified mitochondria as a key element in the deleterious process of PAD [7,8].

Thus, skeletal muscles alterations significantly participate in PAD injuries, modulating its prognosis, and this review aims to describe muscle mitochondrial dysfunctions. Particularly, we will analyze data focused on mitochondrial respiratory chain respiration, on reactive oxygen species release and on mitochondrial calcium retention capacity which decrease is associated with enhanced apoptosis (Figure 1).

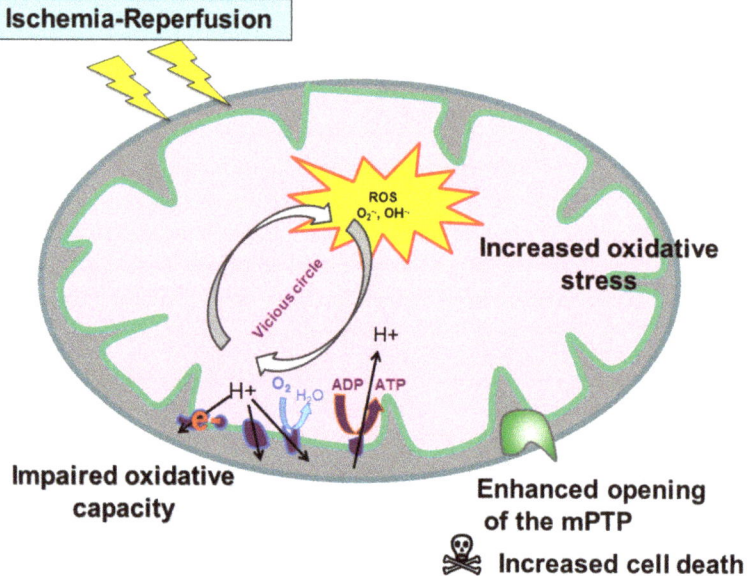

**Figure 1.** Mitochondrial dysfunction during peripheral arterial disease (PAD). mPTP: mitochondrial permeability transition pore.

## 2. Mitochondrial Function under Normal and Pathological Conditions

### 2.1. Normal Condition

Life requires energy, and this energy is stored in adenosine triphosphate (ATP) molecules, that are produced in the mitochondria by oxidative phosphorylation and assessed through mitochondrial respiration determination. Specifically, the oxidation of nutrients through the Krebs cycle provides reduced coenzymes (the reduced form of nicotinamide adenine dinucleotide (NADH)) and to a lesser extent flavin adenine dinucleotide ($FADH_2$), which are electron donors. This flow of electrons is supported by different redox reactions provided by the four complexes of the mitochondrial respiratory chain, up to the reduction of molecular oxygen in water. The respiratory complexes use the energy generated by this electron transfer to allow an active translocation of protons from the matrix to the inter-membrane mitochondrial space. This expulsion of protons results in the generation of a concentration gradient and a mitochondrial membrane potential across the inner membrane. ATP synthases use the transmembrane protonmotive force as a source of energy to drive a mechanical rotary mechanism leading to the chemical synthesis of ATP from ADP and Pi. The $F_1F_0$ ATP synthase enzymes allow proton flux and ATP synthesis through a and c subunits of the $F_0$ domain. The maintenance of this electrochemical gradient, also called protomotive force, is an essential element for the energetic role of the mitochondria [9–11].

Mitochondrial respiration generates free radicals derived from oxygen, the reactive oxygen species (ROS). A free radical is a chemical species containing an unpaired electron. Extremely unstable, this compound can react with more stable molecules to match its electron. It can then pull out an electron and behave as an oxidant, usually leading to the formation of new radicals in the chain and causing significant cell damage. Main ROS comprise superoxide anion, the hydroxyl radical and the highly reactive compound hydrogen peroxide ($H_2O_2$). Detoxification systems exist, enzymatic (superoxide dismutase, catalase, glutathione peroxidase) or not (vitamins and trace elements).

Nevertheless, when the radical production remains contained below a certain threshold, the ROS activate defenses pathways involving the development of cellular antioxidants and mitochondrial biogenesis. Also named mitohormesis, these mechanisms constitute one of the therapeutic targets that can limit the lesions linked to repeated cycles of ischemia-reperfusion in PAD [12].

## 2.2. Ischemic Condition

During ischemia, ATP is generated by anaerobic glycolysis, leading to glycogen storage depletion, anaerobic metabolism activation and local lactic acidosis. The resulting depletion of ATP reduces the function of membrane pumps and causes cellular edema. Indeed, the cell tends to correct the acidosis by expelling the H+ ions via the Na+/H+ exchanger, thus saturating the cytoplasm with Na + ions and causing an osmotic shift to the cytoplasm. Cell edema is aggravated by Na+/K+ ATP-dependent exchanger dysfunction due to lack of ATP, which also leads to Na+ accumulation in the cytoplasm. Acidosis also activates mediators, such as phospholipaseA2, that metabolize membrane phospholipids to arachidonic acid, a precursor of inflammatory mediators such as leukotrienes and prostaglandins. Ischemia will also initiate conversion of xanthine dehydrogenase to xanthine oxidase [13].

Reperfusion is able to prevent the irreversible damages of ischemia. Nevertheless, this process also generates lesions that aggravate the pre-existing tissue damages. At the cellular level, reoxygenation interrupts the lesions induced by ischemia, but causes reperfusion injury. During the first few minutes of reperfusion, the rapid correction of acidosis increases the cytosolic $Ca^{2+}$, thus promoting the opening of the mitochondrial permeability transition pore [14]. This opening causes a sudden change in the mitochondrial membrane permeability, resulting in energy collapse incompatible with cell survival and inducing the release of pro-apoptotic factors from the inter-membrane mitochondrial space to the cytosol, leading to cell death. It is the intrinsic mitochondrial apoptosis pathway.

In parallel, reperfusion generates massive oxidative stress since xanthine oxidase and succinate, produced during ischemia, catalyzes the formation of uric acid from hypoxanthine and of ubiquinol, respectively, accompanied by the formation of large amounts of free radicals. Very interestingly, Chouchani et al. demonstrated a conserved metabolic response of tissues to ischemia-reperfusion (IR) revealing that reducing ischemia-induced succinate increase and its oxidation after reperfusion might be an important therapeutic during IR settings. [15–17].

The ROS thus produced exceed the cellular antioxidant defenses creating a vicious circle. Production of free radicals will cause a dysfunction of the mitochondrial respiratory chain, which in turn generate more ROS. Such ROS overproduction leads to several deleterious effects: lipid peroxidation, protein oxidation and DNA mutations, but also to the opening of the mitochondrial permeability transition pore.

## 3. Mitochondrial Oxidative Capacities in PAD

### 3.1. Experimental Data

Impairments in mitochondrial respiration were observed in both claudicating and CLTI experimental models. Indeed, significant reduction in mitochondrial complexes I, II and IV activities was found in muscles of rats submitted to hindlimb ischemia-reperfusion compared to contralateral muscles [18–21]. Similarly, mouse models of CLTI presented decreased activities of the complexes I, III and IV in ischemic muscles compared with controls [22].

The respiratory impairments were shown to be strain-, muscle-, age- and disease- specific. Indeed, mitochondrial respiration was affected by hindlimb ischemia-reperfusion in limb muscles of BALB/c mice, but not of C57BL/6 mice [23]. Secondly, ischemia-reperfusion injury was shown to affect more severely the respiration in glycolytic muscles than in oxidative ones [24]. Furthermore, the impairments in mitochondrial respiration observed in young mice were greater in older animals submitted to ischemia-reperfusion injury [25]. Lastly, the decline in mitochondrial oxidative capacity was more severe in diabetic rats compared to non-diabetic animals (Table 1) [26].

**Table 1.** Mitochondrial oxidative capacity and peripheral arterial disease in selected experimental studies.

| Animals | Study Design Ischemia-Reperfusion Duration | Outcomes Measured | Main Results | Reference |
|---|---|---|---|---|
| Mice, n = 25 young (23 ± 1 weeks) and old (84 ± 1 weeks) | Unilateral tourniquet I: 2 h/R: 2 h | Skeletal muscle mitochondrial capacity (by oxygraphy) | Impaired mitochondrial respiration in young PAD mice compared with sham ($V_{ADP}$ 33.0 ± 2.4 for the contralateral limb versus 18.4 ± 3.8 for the ischemic limb, $p < 0.01$). Enhanced impairment in old PAD mice ($V_{ADP}$ 5.9 ± 2.7 pmol/s/mg wet weight, $p < 0.001$). | Paradis et al., 2019, Antioxidants [25]. |
| Rats, n = 36 diabetic and non-diabetic | Aortic banding I: 3 h/R: 2 h | Skeletal muscle mitochondrial capacity (by oxygraphy) | Significant decline in mitochondrial respiration after ischemia-reperfusion injury in diabetic rats compared to non-diabetic ($p < 0.05$). | Pottecher et al., 2018, Front Physiol [26]. |
| Mice, n = 69 BALB/c (ischemia susceptible) and C57BL/6 (ischemia protected) | Aortic banding I and R: duration not specified | Skeletal muscle mitochondrial capacity (by western blot and oxygraphy) | Skeletal muscle mitochondrial impairments in BALB/c limb muscle but not in C57BL/6 ($p < 0.01$). | Schmidt et al., 2017, J Vasc Surg [23]. |
| Mice, n = 22 | Aortic banding I: 3 h/R: 2 h | Skeletal muscle mitochondrial capacity (by oxygraphy) | Decreased mitochondrial respiration in glycolytic versus oxidative muscles. | Charles et al., 2017, Front Physiol [24]. |
| Rats, n = 12 Old 71-73 weeks | Unilateral tourniquet I: 3 h/R: 2 h | Skeletal muscle mitochondrial capacity (by oxygraphy) | Reduced mitochondrial complexes I, II and IV activities in PAD muscles compared with contralateral ones ($V_{MAX}$ 7.34 ± 1.5 versus 2.87 ± 1.22 µmol $O_2$/min/g dry weight for PAD muscles, $p < 0.05$). | Pottecher et al., 2016, Fundam Clin Pharmacol [18]. |
| Rats n = 28 | Aortic banding I: 3 h/R: 2 h | Skeletal muscle mitochondrial capacity (by oxygraphy) | IR reduced V(max) (−21.2%, 6.6 ± 1 versus 5.2 ± 1 µmol $O_2$/min/g dry weight, $p = 0.001$), V(succ) (−22.2%, $p = 0.032$), and V(TMPD) (−22.4%, $p = 0.033$). | Mansour et al., 2012, J Vasc Surg [21]. |
| Rats, n = 22 | Unilateral tourniquet I: 5 h R: 5 min | Skeletal muscle mitochondrial capacity (by oxygraphy) | Reduced mitochondrial complexes I, II and IV activities in PAD rats compared with sham ($V_{MAX}$ 4.4 ± 0.4 versus 8.7 ± 0.5 µmol $O_2$/min/g dry weight, $p < 0.001$). | Thaveau et al., 2010, Fundam Clin Pharmacol [19]. |

Table 1. Cont.

| Animals | Study Design Ischemia-Reperfusion Duration | Outcomes Measured | Main Results | Reference |
|---|---|---|---|---|
| Mice, n = 48 | CLTI Sequential left femoral and iliac ligations R: week 12 | Skeletal muscle mitochondrial capacity (by oxygraphy) | Reduced activity of complexes I (by 34%), III (by 45%) and IV (by 42%) in ischemic muscles compared with controls ($p < 0.05$). | Pipinos et al., 2008, Am J Physiol Regul Integr Comp Physiol [22]. |
| Rats, n = 20 | Unilateral tourniquet I: 5 h | Respiration of isolated mitochondria (by polarographic analysis) | Inhibition of the mitochondrial respiratory chain | Brandão et al., J Surg Res. 2003 [20]. |

CLTI: critical limb threatening ischemia; I: ischemia; PAD: peripheral arterial disease; R: reperfusion. TMPD, N, N, N', N'-tetramethyl-p-phenylenediamine dihydrochloride.

## 3.2. Clinical Data

Oxygraphy measurements in PAD patients revealed significantly altered respiratory activity, notably of complexes I, III and IV, and of the acceptor control ratio [27–30]. Interestingly, more recent studies reported no difference in the mitochondrial respiration rate between PAD patients and healthy controls, despite alterations in $O_2$ delivery, tissue-reoxygenation and ATP synthesis rate during exercise [31,32]. These conflicting findings could be explained by disparities in disease severity. Indeed, the alterations in mitochondrial oxidative capacity may have been the result of factors associated with higher morbidity in PAD, such as sarcopenia [33–35].

Mitochondrial energy metabolism was shown to decrease in PAD patients compared to controls [36, 37]. In contrast, Hou et al. found similar mitochondrial ATP production rate in both PAD patients and healthy controls [38]. Again, such differences might be explained by differences in disease severity or morbidity factors rate.

It is important to note that patients suffering from both PAD and type II diabetes (DT2) are more susceptible to reduced O2 consumption and mitochondrial oxidative phosphorylation compared to patients with PAD alone or to controls (Table 2) [39,40].

Table 2. Mitochondrial oxidative capacities and peripheral arterial disease in clinical studies.

| Population | Number Studied (Symptomatic/Controls) | Outcomes Measured | Main Results | Reference |
|---|---|---|---|---|
| Early stage PAD | 10/11 | $O_2$ delivery, tissue oxygenation and Vmax (by high-resolution respirometry). Skeletal muscle mitochondrial capacity (by oxygraphy) | PAD patients exhibited significantly lower $O_2$ delivery ($p < 0.05$), tissue-reoxygenation ($58 \pm 3$ % for controls versus $44 \pm 3$ % for PAD patients, $p < 0.05$) and Vmax ($p < 0.05$) during exercise, compared with healthy controls. No differences were found in the mitochondrial respiration rate. | Hart et al., 2018, Am J Physiol Heart Circ Physiol [31]. |
| Claudicant PAD | 10/12 | Skeletal muscle mitochondrial capacity (by oxygraphy) | No differences were found in the mitochondrial respiration rate between PAD patients and healthy controls. | Hart et al., 2018, Exp Physiol [32]. |
| Claudicant PAD; claudicant PAD + DT2 | 15 (PAD)/15 (PAD + DT2)/10 (controls) | Skeletal muscle mitochondrial capacity (by oxygraphy) | Significant reduction in oxygen consumption in the PAD+DT2 group compared with the PAD group or the control group ($p < 0.05$). No differences were found in the mitochondrial respiration rate between PAD patients and healthy controls. | Lindegaard et al., 2017, Int Angiol [39]. |

Table 2. Cont.

| Population | Number Studied (Symptomatic/Controls) | Outcomes Measured | Main Results | Reference |
| --- | --- | --- | --- | --- |
| Patients with low ABI | 82 (ABI of 0.90 to 1.10)/281 (ABI of 1.11 to 1.40) | Phosphocreatine recovery (by phosphorus-31 magnetic resonance spectroscopy) | Significantly lower muscle mitochondrial energy production in patients with lower ABI, compared with those with higher ABI (20.8 ms$^{-1}$ for higher ABI versus 19.3 ms$^{-1}$ for lower ABI, $p = 0.015$). | AlGhatrif et al., 2017, J Am Heart Assoc [36]. |
| PAD (no stage specified) | 30/30 | Skeletal muscle mitochondrial capacity (by oxygraphy) | PAD subjects presented significantly lower respiratory activity compared with controls ($p < 0.05$). | Koutakis et al., 2015, J Histochem Cytochem [27]. |
| Claudicant PAD + neuropathy + DT2 | 7/14 | Phosphocreatine recovery (by phosphorus-31 magnetic resonance spectroscopy) | Reduced mitochondrial oxidative phosphorylation in DT2 patients with lower extremity complications (neuropathy and PAD) ($p < 0.05$). | Tecilazich et al., 2013, J Vasc Surg [40]. |
| Claudicant PAD; CLI | 25/16 | Skeletal muscle mitochondrial capacity (by spectrophotometry) | Decreased activity of complexes I, III and IV in PAD muscle compared to control ($p < 0.05$). | Pipinos et al., 2006, Free Radic Biol Med [28]. |
| Claudicant PAD; CLI | 9/9 | Skeletal muscle mitochondrial capacity (by oxygraphy) | Significantly lower respiratory rates, and lower acceptor control ratio ($2.90 \pm 0.20$ for controls versus $1.41 \pm 0.10$ for PAD) in patients with PAD compared with controls ($p < 0.05$). | Pipinos et al., 2003, J Vasc Surg [29]. |
| Claudicant PAD | 7/11 | ATP synthesis (by luminometer) | Similar mitochondrial ATP production rate were in PAD patients and healthy controls. | Hou et al., 2002, Clin Physiol Funct Imaging [38]. |
| Claudicant PAD | 17/9 | Skeletal muscle mitochondrial capacity (by spectrophotometry) | Significant reduction in NADH dehydrogenase and ubiquinol-cytochrome c oxidoreductase activity by 27% and 38%, respectively, in PAD compared with controls ($p < 0.05$). | Brass et al., 2001, Am J Physiol Heart Circ Physiol [30]. |
| Claudicant PAD | 12/14 | Phosphocreatine and ADP recovery (by phosphorus-31 magnetic resonance spectroscopy) | Defective phosphocreatine ($44 \pm 3$ s for controls versus $137 \pm 41$ s for PAD) and ADP recovery ($29 \pm 2$ s versus $60 \pm 10$ s for PAD) in PAD compared with controls ($p < 0.05$). | Pipinos et al., 2000, J Vasc Surg [37]. |

ABI: ankle brachial index; CLTI: critical limb threatening ischemia; DT2: type II diabetes; PAD: peripheral arterial disease.

## 4. Reactive Oxygen Species Production, Proteins, Lipids and DNA Alterations and Impaired Antioxidant Defense, in PAD

The interaction between mitochondria and oxidative stress in skeletal muscle is modulated by repeated cycles of ischemia-reperfusion in the context of PAD. The vascular damages create an imbalance between oxygen supply and demand during efforts, generating a situation of ischemia; followed by a situation of reperfusion when the patient is at rest. Repetition of ischemia and reperfusion cycles are deleterious for skeletal muscle and lead to myopathy and to remote organ damage [7,28,41].

### 4.1. Experimental Data

ROS production was found increased in both animal models of PAD (acute ischemia-reperfusion and CLTI) as compared to controls, using either measurements of 1) free radical species by electron paramagnetic resonance spectroscopy, 2) dihydroethidium (DHE) by epifluorescence microscopy or 3) $H_2O_2$ by Amplex Red peroxide assay [24,42,43]. Interestingly, ROS production was greater in PAD animals presenting with hypercholesterolemia or diabetes [26,44]. These evidences suggest an association between PAD comorbidity factors and enhanced mitochondrial dysfunction.

Furthermore, deleterious effects of oxidative stress were also observed in ischemic skeletal muscles, as highlighted by higher levels of oxidative stress markers (superoxide dismutase [45], protein carbonyls and 4-hydroxy-2-nonenanal protein (HNE) adducts) [22], and elevated DNA alterations [46].

Finally, antioxidant defenses have been shown to be impaired by ischemia-reperfusion. Indeed, alterations in the expression of superoxide dismutase 1 and 2 (SOD1 and SOD2), catalase and manganese superoxide dismutase (MnSOD) were observed in ischemic muscles compared with controls (Table 3) [22,45,47].

**Table 3.** Reactive oxygen species production during peripheral arterial disease in experimental studies.

| Animals | Study Design Ischemia-Reperfusion Duration | Outcomes Measured | Main Results | Reference |
|---|---|---|---|---|
| Mice, n = 7 ApoE-/- versus ApoE+/+ | CLTI Sequential right femoral and iliac ligations. R: day 40 | Free radical measurement (by electron paramagnetic resonance spectroscopy) | Enhanced ROS production in muscles of ApoE-/- (+63.6%) and ApoE+/+ (+41.4%) mice compared with contralateral muscles. | Lejay et al., 2019, Eur J Vasc Endovasc Surg [44]. |
| Rats, n = 36 diabetic versus non-diabetic | Aortic banding I: 3 h/R: 2 h | DHE measures of ROS (by epifluorescence microscopy) | Increase in normalized DHE fluorescence in diabetic PAD compared to diabetic controls ($p < 0.001$). | Pottecher et al., 2018, Front Physiol [26]. |
| Mice, n = 20 | CLTI Left femoral ligation. R: day 21 | mtDNA damage quantification (by quantitative PCR) | Increase in mtDNA damages in ischemic muscles of PAD mice compared with sham ($p < 0.05$). | Miura et al., 2017, Int J Mol Sci [46]. |
| Mice, n = 20 | CLTI Sequential right femoral and iliac ligations. R: day 30 | Antioxidant quantification (by quantitative PCR) | Significant decrease in mRNA expression of the antioxidant enzymes SOD1 ($0.39 \pm 0.10$ for sham limb versus $0.10 \pm 0.06$ for ischemic limb), SOD2 ($0.32 \pm 0.16$ versus $0.11 \pm 0.07$) and catalase ($0.38 \pm 0.04$ versus $0.22 \pm 0.11$) in ischemic muscles compared with control ones ($p < 0.05$). | Lejay et al., 2017, Front Physiol [47]. |
| Mice, n = 22 | Aortic banding I: 3 h/R: 2 h | Free radical measurement (by electron paramagnetic resonance spectroscopy) | Ischemia-reperfusion injury increased ROS production in ischemic muscles compared to no ischemic contralateral ($+79.15 \pm 28.72\%$, $p = 0.04$). | Charles et al., 2017, Front Physiol [24]. |
| Mice, n = 6 | CLTI Right femoral ligation. R: day 10 | $H_2O_2$ measurement (by Amplex Red assay) | Significant increase in $H_2O_2$ level in ischemic muscles compared with sham ones ($p < 0.05$). | Kwon et al., 2016, Int J Pharm [43]. |
| Mice, n = 28 | CLTI Sequential right femoral and iliac ligations. R: day 30. | Free radical measurement (by electron paramagnetic resonance spectroscopy) DHE measures of ROS (by epifluorescence microscopy) | CLI induced a significant increase in ROS production in ischemic muscles compared with controls. DHE staining was higher in ischemic muscles ($p < 0.01$). | Lejay et al., 2015, Eur J Vasc Endovasc Surg [42]. |
| Rats, n = 35 | Aortic banding I: 2 h/R: 10 min and 2 h | DHE staining (by epifluorescence microscopy) | ROS increased significantly after ischemia alone ($+324 \pm 66\%$, $p = 0.038$), normalized after 10 min of reperfusion, and increased again at 2 h of reperfusion ($+349.2 \pm 67\%$, $p = 0.024$). Oxidative stress preceded skeletal muscle mitochondrial dysfunction. | Guillot et al., 2014, J Vasc Surg [48]. |
| Mice, n = 18 | Unilateral tourniquet I: 3 h/R: 4 h | Superoxide anion production measurement (by luminometer); Quantification of MnSOD (by Western blot) | Increased superoxide production and decreased activity of the mitochondria-targeted SOD isoform) in the ischemia-reperfusion group. | Tran et al., 2011, Eur J Pharmacol [45]. |
| Mice, n = 48 | CLTI Sequential left femoral and iliac ligations R: week 12 | Protein carbonyls, HNE adducts and MnSOD expression quantification (by reverse phase protein lysate microarray) | Significantly higher expression of protein carbonyls, HNE adducts and MnSOD in ischemic muscles compared with controls ($p < 0.05$). | Pipinos et al., 2008, Am J Physiol Regul Integr Comp Physiol [22]. |

CLTI: critical limb threatening ischemia; DHE: dihydroethidium; dw: dry weight; HNE: 4-hydroxy-2-nonenal; I: ischemia; MnSOD: manganese superoxide dismutase; mtDNA: mitochondrial DNA; PAD: peripheral arterial disease; PCR: polymerase chain reaction; R: reperfusion; ROS: reactive oxygen species; SOD: superoxide dismutase.

## 4.2. Clinical Data

Similar to the findings on experimental models, PAD patients displayed increased mitochondria-derived ROS production characterized by elevated levels of free radical species [32].

Moreover, oxidative damages were also observed in patients suffering from PAD, as reported by higher levels of oxidative stress markers (protein carbonyl groups, HNE-protein adducts and lipid hydroperoxides), and elevated DNA alterations [28,49–53].

Lastly, evidence of reduced antioxidant defenses has been shown in PAD patients, notably with altered activities of the antioxidant enzymes SOD, catalase and glutathione peroxidase (Table 4) [28].

**Table 4.** Reactive oxygen species production during peripheral arterial disease in clinical studies.

| Population | Number Studied (Symptomatic/Controls) | Outcomes Measured | Main Results | Reference |
|---|---|---|---|---|
| Claudicant PAD | 10/34 | Mitochondrial DNA copy number (by quantitative PCR) | Significant association between disease severity and increased mitochondrial DNA copy number ($p < 0.05$). | McDermott et al., 2018, Vasc Med [49]. |
| Claudicant PAD | 10/12 | Free radical measurement (by electron paramagnetic resonance spectroscopy) | Significant increase in mitochondria-derived ROS production in PAD ($1.0 \pm 0.36$ AU/mg tissue for controls versus $4.3 \pm 1.0$ AU/mg tissue for PAD, $p < 0.05$). | Hart et al., 2018, Exp Physiol [32]. |
| Claudicant PAD; CLTI | 28 claudicants/25 CLTI/25 controls | Carbonyl groups quantification (by quantitative fluorescence microscopy) | Observation of a 25% increase in carbonyl groups (markers of oxidative damage) in myofibers of all PAD patients compared with controls ($p < 0.05$). | Koutakis et al., 2014, Redox Biol [50]. |
| Claudicant PAD; CLTI | 34/21 | Carbonyl groups and HNE adducts quantification (by quantitative fluorescence microscopy) | Significant increase in carbonyl groups (30%, $p < 0.0001$) and HNE adducts (40%, $p < 0.0001$) in PAD myofibers compared to controls. | Weiss et al., 2013, J Transl Med [51]. |
| Claudicant PAD; CLTI | 16/10 | Lipid hydroperoxides measurement (by ferrous oxidation/xylenol orange technique); Protein carbonyls measurments (using an Enzyme Immuno-Assay kit); HNE detection (by western blot); Antioxidant activity (by spectrophotometry) | Higher levels of lipid hydroperoxides ($12.45 \pm 0.74$ mmol/g wet weight for controls versus $20.32 \pm 1.02$ for PAD), protein carbonyls ($0.22 \pm 0.02$ nmol/mg for controls versus $0.35 \pm 0.04$) and HNE ($191.2 \pm 7.17$ total binding versus $226.4 \pm 10.4$) was found in PAD patients compared to controls ($p < 0.05$). Significant decrease in SOD activity, and increase in catalase and glutathione peroxidase activities. | Pipinos et al., 2006, Free Radic Biol Med [28]. |
| Claudicant PAD | 9 claudicants | Quantification of mitochondrial DNA injury (by PCR) | Substantial injury to mitochondrial DNA in PAD patients occurring bilaterally in patients with unilateral PAD. | Brass et al., 2000, Vasc Med [52]. |
| Claudicant PAD | 8/10 | Quantification of mitochondrial DNA injury (by PCR) | Accumulation of 4977-bp mitochondrial deletion frequency in patients with PAD compared with controls ($0.05 \pm 0.01$ % for controls versus $0.43 \pm 0.28$ % for the less-affected limb versus $0.88 \pm 0.53$ % for the worse-affected limb, $p < 0.05$). | Bhat et al., 1999, Circulation [53]. |

CLTI: critical limb threatening ischemia; HNE: 4-hydroxy-2-nonenal; mtDNA: mitochondrial DNA; PAD: peripheral arterial disease; PCR: polymerase chain reaction; SOD: superoxide dismutase.

## 5. Mitochondrial Implication in Apoptosis during PAD

### 5.1. Experimental Data

Rodent models of PAD displayed elevated protein expression of the apoptotic factors cleaved-caspase 3, cleaved-poly (ADP-robose) polymerase (PARD) and mitochondrial and cytosolic Bcl2-associated X (Bax), and reduced protein expression of the anti-apoptotic factor Bcl-2, compared with controls [21,54,55]. Furthermore, a decrease in mitochondrial calcium retention capacity was observed in ischemic limbs compared with contralateral ones (Table 5) [25,44,47,56,57].

**Table 5.** Mitochondrial implication in apoptosis during peripheral arterial disease in experimental studies.

| Animals | Study Design Ischemia-Reperfusion Duration | Outcomes Measured | Main Results | Reference |
|---|---|---|---|---|
| Mice, n = 7 ApoE-/- versus ApoE+/+ | CLTI Sequential right femoral and iliac ligations. | Calcium retention capacity (by spectrofluometry) | Impairment in calcium retention capacity in ischemic muscles of ApoE-/- and ApoE+/+ mice compared with contralateral muscles ($p = 0.001$). | Lejay et al., 2019, Eur J Vasc Endovasc Surg [44]. |
| Mice, n = 25 young (23 weeks) versus aged (84 weeks) C57Bl6J | Unilateral tourniquet I: 2 h/R: 2 h | Calcium retention capacity (by spectrofluometry) | Significant reduction in calcium retention capacity in young (-60.9 ± 7.3%) and aged (-60.9 ± 4.6%) mice compared with sham ones ($p < 0.001$). | Paradis et al., 2019, Antioxidants [25]. |
| Rats, n = 12 | CLTI Left femoral ligation. R: day 14 | Protein expression of indicators of apoptosis (by Western blot) | Higher expression of proteins cleaved-caspase 3, cleaved-PARP and mitochondrial Bax in CLTI muscles compared with sham ones ($p < 0.05$). | Hsu et al., 2019, Am J Transl Res [54]. |
| Mice, n = 16 | Unilateral tourniquet I: 2 h/R: 2 h | Calcium retention capacity (by spectrofluometry) | Decrease in calcium retention capacity in ischemic limbs compared with contralateral ones (-61.1 ± 6.8%, $p < 0.01$). | Tetsi et al., 2019. Antioxidants [56]. |
| Mice, n = 20 | CLTI Sequential right femoral and iliac ligations. R: day 30. | Calcium retention capacity (by spectrofluometry) | Significant reduction of calcium retention capacity in ischemic limbs compared with contralateral ones ($p < 0.001$). | Lejay et al., 2018, Eur J Vasc Endovasc Surg [57]. |
| Mice, n = 20 | CLTI Sequential right femoral and iliac ligations. | Calcium retention capacity (by spectrofluometry) | Lower calcium retention capacity in ischemic limbs compared with controls ($p < 0.001$). | Lejay et al., 2017, Front Physiol [47]. |
| Rats, n = 16 | CLTI Right femoral ligation. R: day 14 | Protein expression of indicators of apoptosis and anti-apoptotic factor (by Western blot) | Higher expression of the proteins cleaved-caspase 3, cleaved-PARP and cytosolic Bax in CLTI muscles compared with sham ones ($p < 0.001$). Lower expression of the anti-apoptotic marker Bcl-2 in CLTI muscles compared with sham ones ($p < 0.001$). | Sheu et al., 2015, J Transl Med [55]. |
| Rats n = 28 | Aortic banding I: 3 h/R: 2 h | Quantification of gene expression (by quantitative PCR) | IR increased Bax (63.4%, $p = 0.020$) and Bax/Bcl-2 ratio (+84.6%, $p = 0.029$). SODs and GPx messenger RNA were not modified, but glutathione tended to be decreased after IR. | Mansour et al., 2012, J Vasc Surg [21]. |

CLTI: critical limb threatening ischemia; I: ischemia; IR: ischemia-reperfusion; PAD: peripheral arterial disease; R: reperfusion.

## 5.2. Clinical Data

Human investigations also showed a clear implication of apoptosis in PAD pathophysiology. Indeed, PAD patients displayed elevated levels of genes mediating apoptosis [58], increased DNA fragmentation and caspase-3 activity [59]. Additionally, multiple studies reported higher levels of apoptotic cells in different cell types, notably endothelial cells and lymphocytes [60,61]. Interestingly, another study reported similar levels of endothelial apoptosis in both PAD and control groups. This result is likely due to disparities in patient's selection, with patients presenting with lower associated risk factors (Table 6) [62].

**Table 6.** Mitochondrial implication in apoptosis during peripheral arterial disease in clinical studies.

| Population | Number Studied (Symptomatic/Controls) | Outcomes Measured | Main Results | Reference |
|---|---|---|---|---|
| Claudicant PAD | 130/36 | Caspase activity measurement (by caspase Assay) | No difference observed in apoptosis between the PAD and the control group ($p = 0.463$). | Gardner et al., 2014, Angiology [62]. |
| Claudicant PAD | 156/16 | Caspase activity measurement (by caspase Assay) | Higher percentage of endothelial cell apoptosis in the PAD group compared with the control group (+164%, $p < 0.001$). | Gardner et al., 2014, Int J Vasc Med [60]. |
| Claudicant PAD | 19/18 | Quantification of gene expression (by quantitative PCR) | Upregulation in genes mediating apoptosis: *BCL-2, G0S2, KLF6, PTP4A1* and *CFLAR*. | Masud et al., 2012, J Clin Bioinforma [58]. |
| Claudicant PAD | 10/10 | Detection and quantification of apoptosis (by fluorescence microscopy) | Higher percentage of late apoptotic lymphocytes (by 33%) in the PAD patients compared with healthy controls. | Skórkowska-Telichowska et al., 2009, Clin Invest Med [61]. |
| Claudicant PAD | 26/28 | Apoptosis detection (by TUNEL Assay); Caspase activity measurement (by caspase Assay) | The fraction of TUNEL-positive nuclei was greater in PAD patients compared with controls ($1.53\% \pm 0.96$ for controls *versus* $3.83\% \pm 2.6$ for PAD, $p < 0.001$). Caspase-3 activity was increased in PAD group compared with control group ($0.22 \pm 0.05$ units mg$^{-1}$ soluble protein *versus* $0.39 \pm 0.09$ for PAD, $p < 0.001$). | Mitchell et al., 2007, Vasc Med [59]. |

PAD: peripheral arterial disease; PCR: polymerase chain reaction.

## 6. Conclusions

In summary, PAD is a public health issue even when poorly symptomatic [63], and mitochondria are importantly involved in its pathophysiology. Not only because mitochondrial alterations reduce the energy available for cell function, but also because mitochondria participate in the increased ROS production (and therefore to a greater oxidative stress) and in the enhanced opening of the mitochondrial permeability pore which favor the intrinsic pathway of cell apoptosis. These data account for the fact that skeletal muscle mitochondrial function might be considered as a prognostic factor in the setting of PAD in humans. On the other hand, if ROS production remains contained below a certain threshold, mitohormesis and stimulation of the antioxidant defenses can be protective supporting that mitochondrial function modulation might be a therapeutic target. Thus, further studies focused on mitochondria are warranted to optimize the care of patients presenting with PAD.

**Author Contributions:** Conceptualization, M.R., A.-L.C., A.L., and B.G.; methodology, M.P., M.R., A.-L.C., A.L., and B.G.; validation, M.P., M.R., A.-L.C., S.T., A.M., E.A., N.C., A.L., and B.G.; writing—original draft preparation, M.P., A.L., and B.G. writing—review and editing, M.P., N.C. A.L. and B.G.; supervision, A.L. and B.G.

**Funding:** This research received no external funding.

**Conflicts of Interest:** The authors declare no conflict of interest.

## References

1. Criqui, M.H.; Aboyans, V. Epidemiology of peripheral artery disease. *Circ. Res.* **2015**, *116*, 1509–1526. [CrossRef]
2. Duff, S.; Mafilios, M.S.; Bhounsule, P.; Hasegawa, J.T. The burden of critical limb ischemia: A review of recent literature. *Vasc. Health. Risk. Manag.* **2019**, *15*, 187–208. [CrossRef] [PubMed]
3. Dua, A.; Lee, C.J. Epidemiology of Peripheral Arterial Disease and Critical Limb Ischemia. *Tech. Vasc. Interv. Radiol.* **2016**, *19*, 91–95. [CrossRef] [PubMed]
4. Leardini-Tristao, M.; Charles, A.L.; Lejay, A.; Pizzimenti, M.; Meyer, A.; Estato, V.; Tibiriçá, E.; Andres, E.; Geny, B. Beneficial Effect of Exercise on Cognitive Function during Peripheral Arterial Disease: Potential Involvement of Myokines and Microglial Anti-Inflammatory Phenotype Enhancement. *J. Clin. Med.* **2019**, *8*, 653. [CrossRef] [PubMed]

5. Aboyans, V.; Ricco, J.B.; Bartelink, M.L.E.L.; Björck, M.; Brodmann, M.; Cohnert, T.; Collet, J.P.; Czerny, M.; De Carlo, M.; Debus, S.; et al. Editor's Choice—2017 ESC Guidelines on the Diagnosis and Treatment of Peripheral Arterial Diseases, in collaboration with the European Society for Vascular Surgery (ESVS). *Eur. J. Vasc. Endovasc. Surg.* **2018**, *55*, 305–368. [CrossRef]
6. Conte, M.S.; Bradbury, A.W.; Kolh, P.; White, J.V.; Dick, F.; Fitridge, R.; Mills, J.L.; Ricco, J.B.; Suresh, K.R.; Murad, M.H.; et al. Global Vascular Guidelines on the Management of Chronic Limb-Threatening Ischemia. *Eur. J. Vasc. Endovasc. Surg.* **2019**, *58*, S1–S109.e33. [CrossRef]
7. Paradis, S.; Charles, A.L.; Meyer, A.; Lejay, A.; Scholey, J.W.; Chakfé, N.; Zoll, J.; Geny, B. Chronology of mitochondrial and cellular events during skeletal muscle ischemia-reperfusion. *Am. J. Physiol.-Cell Physiol.* **2016**, *310*, C968–C982. [CrossRef]
8. Koutakis, P.; Ismaeel, A.; Farmer, P.; Purcell, S.; Smith, R.S.; Eidson, J.L.; Bohannon, W.T. Oxidative stress and antioxidant treatment in patients with peripheral artery disease. *Physiol. Rep.* **2018**, *6*, e13650. [CrossRef]
9. Walker, J.E. ATP Synthesis by Rotary Catalysis (Nobel lecture). *Angew. Chem. Int. Edit.* **1998**, *37*, 2308–2319. [CrossRef]
10. Walker, J.E.; Dickson, V.K. The peripheral stalk of the mitochondrial ATP synthase. *Biochim. Biophys. Acta (BBA)—Bioenerg.* **2006**, *1757*, 286–296. [CrossRef]
11. Walker, J.E. The ATP synthase: The understood, the uncertain and the unknown. *Biochem. Soc. Trans.* **2013**, *41*, 1–16. [CrossRef] [PubMed]
12. Lejay, A.; Meyer, A.; Schlagowski, A.I.; Charles, A.L.; Singh, F.; Bouitbir, J.; Pottecher, J.; Chakfé, N.; Zoll, J.; Geny, B. Mitochondria: Mitochondrial participation in ischemia-reperfusion injury in skeletal muscle. *Int. J. Biochem. Cell Biol.* **2014**, *50*, 101–105. [CrossRef] [PubMed]
13. Makris, K.I.; Nella, A.A.; Zhu, Z.; Swanson, S.A.; Casale, G.P.; Gutti, T.L.; Judge, A.R.; Pipinos, I.I. Mitochondriopathy of peripheral arterial disease. *Vascular* **2007**, *15*, 336–343. [CrossRef]
14. Bernardi, P. The mitochondrial permeability transition pore: A mystery solved? *Front. Physiol.* **2013**, *4*, 95. [CrossRef] [PubMed]
15. Chouchani, E.T.; Pell, V.R.; James, A.M.; Work, L.M.; Saeb-Parsy, K.; Frezza, C.; Krieg, T.; Murphy, M.P. A Unifying Mechanism for Mitochondrial Superoxide Production during Ischemia-Reperfusion Injury. *Cell Metab.* **2016**, *23*, 254–263. [CrossRef]
16. Chouchani, E.T.; Pell, V.R.; Gaude, E.; Aksentijević, D.; Sundier, S.Y.; Robb, E.L.; Logan, A.; Nadtochiy, S.M.; Ord, E.N.J.; Smith, A.C.; et al. Ischaemic accumulation of succinate controls reperfusion injury through mitochondrial ROS. *Nature* **2014**, *515*, 431–435. [CrossRef]
17. Chouchani, E.T.; Methner, C.; Nadtochiy, S.M.; Logan, A.; Pell, V.R.; Ding, S.; James, A.M.; Cochemé, H.M.; Reinhold, J.; Lilley, K.S.; et al. Cardioprotection by S-nitrosation of a cysteine switch on mitochondrial complex I. *Nat. Med.* **2013**, *19*, 753–759. [CrossRef]
18. Pottecher, J.; Kindo, M.; Chamaraux-Tran, T.N.; Charles, A.L.; Lejay, A.; Kemmel, V.; Vogel, T.; Chakfe, N.; Zoll, J.; Diemunsch, P.; et al. Skeletal muscle ischemia-reperfusion injury and cyclosporine A in the aging rat. *Fundam. Clin. Pharmacol.* **2016**, *30*, 216–225. [CrossRef]
19. Thaveau, F.; Zoll, J.; Bouitbir, J.; N'guessan, B.; Plobner, P.; Chakfe, N.; Kretz, J.G.; Richard, R.; Piquard, F.; Geny, B. Effect of chronic pre-treatment with angiotensin converting enzyme inhibition on skeletal muscle mitochondrial recovery after ischemia/reperfusion. *Fundam. Clin. Pharmacol.* **2010**, *24*, 333–340. [CrossRef]
20. Brandão, M.L.; Roselino, J.E.S.; Piccinato, C.E.; Cherri, J. Mitochondrial alterations in skeletal muscle submitted to total ischemia. *J. Surg. Res.* **2003**, *110*, 235–240. [CrossRef]
21. Mansour, Z.; Bouitbir, J.; Charles, A.L.; Talha, S.; Kindo, M.; Pottecher, J.; Zoll, J.; Geny, B. Remote and local ischemic preconditioning equivalently protects rat skeletal muscle mitochondrial function during experimental aortic cross-clamping. *J. Vasc. Surg.* **2012**, *55*, 497–505. [CrossRef] [PubMed]
22. Pipinos, I.I.; Swanson, S.A.; Zhu, Z.; Nella, A.A.; Weiss, D.J.; Gutti, T.L.; McComb, R.D.; Baxter, B.T.; Lynch, T.G.; Casale, G.P. Chronically ischemic mouse skeletal muscle exhibits myopathy in association with mitochondrial dysfunction and oxidative damage. *Am. J. Physiol. Regul. Integr. Comp. Physiol.* **2008**, *295*, R290–R296. [CrossRef] [PubMed]
23. Schmidt, C.A.; Ryan, T.E.; Lin, C.T.; Inigo, M.M.R.; Green, T.D.; Brault, J.J.; Spangenburg, E.E.; McClung, J.M. Diminished force production and mitochondrial respiratory deficits are strain-dependent myopathies of subacute limb ischemia. *J. Vasc. Surg.* **2017**, *65*, 1504–1514.e11. [CrossRef] [PubMed]

24. Charles, A.L.; Guilbert, A.S.; Guillot, M.; Talha, S.; Lejay, A.; Meyer, A.; Kindo, M.; Wolff, V.; Bouitbir, J.; Zoll, J.; et al. Muscles Susceptibility to Ischemia-Reperfusion Injuries Depends on Fiber Type Specific Antioxidant Level. *Front. Physiol.* **2017**, *8*, 52. [CrossRef]

25. Paradis, S.; Charles, A.L.; Georg, I.; Goupilleau, F.; Meyer, A.; Kindo, M.; Laverny, G.; Metzger, D.; Geny, B. Aging Exacerbates Ischemia-Reperfusion-Induced Mitochondrial Respiration Impairment in Skeletal Muscle. *Antioxidants (Basel)* **2019**, *8*, 168. [CrossRef]

26. Pottecher, J.; Adamopoulos, C.; Lejay, A.; Bouitbir, J.; Charles, A.L.; Meyer, A.; Singer, M.; Wolff, V.; Diemunsch, P.; Laverny, G.; et al. Diabetes Worsens Skeletal Muscle Mitochondrial Function, Oxidative Stress, and Apoptosis After Lower-Limb Ischemia-Reperfusion: Implication of the RISK and SAFE Pathways? *Front. Physiol.* **2018**, *9*, 579. [CrossRef]

27. Koutakis, P.; Miserlis, D.; Myers, S.A.; Kim, J.K.S.; Zhu, Z.; Papoutsi, E.; Swanson, S.A.; Haynatzki, G.; Ha, D.M.; Carpenter, L.A.; et al. Abnormal accumulation of desmin in gastrocnemius myofibers of patients with peripheral artery disease: Associations with altered myofiber morphology and density, mitochondrial dysfunction and impaired limb function. *J. Histochem. Cytochem.* **2015**, *63*, 256–269. [CrossRef]

28. Pipinos, I.I.; Judge, A.R.; Zhu, Z.; Selsby, J.T.; Swanson, S.A.; Johanning, J.M.; Baxter, B.T.; Lynch, T.G.; Dodd, S.L. Mitochondrial defects and oxidative damage in patients with peripheral arterial disease. *Free Radic. Biol. Med.* **2006**, *41*, 262–269. [CrossRef]

29. Pipinos, I.I.; Sharov, V.G.; Shepard, A.D.; Anagnostopoulos, P.V.; Katsamouris, A.; Todor, A.; Filis, K.A.; Sabbah, H.N. Abnormal mitochondrial respiration in skeletal muscle in patients with peripheral arterial disease. *J. Vasc. Surg.* **2003**, *38*, 827–832. [CrossRef]

30. Brass, E.P.; Hiatt, W.R.; Gardner, A.W.; Hoppel, C.L. Decreased NADH dehydrogenase and ubiquinol-cytochrome c oxidoreductase in peripheral arterial disease. *Am. J. Physiol. Heart Circ. Physiol.* **2001**, *280*, H603–H609. [CrossRef]

31. Hart, C.R.; Layec, G.; Trinity, J.D.; Le Fur, Y.; Gifford, J.R.; Clifton, H.L.; Richardson, R.S. Oxygen availability and skeletal muscle oxidative capacity in patients with peripheral artery disease: Implications from in vivo and in vitro assessments. *Am. J. Physiol. Heart Circ. Physiol.* **2018**, *315*, H897–H909. [CrossRef] [PubMed]

32. Hart, C.R.; Layec, G.; Trinity, J.D.; Kwon, O.S.; Zhao, J.; Reese, V.R.; Gifford, J.R.; Richardson, R.S. Increased skeletal muscle mitochondrial free radical production in peripheral arterial disease despite preserved mitochondrial respiratory capacity. *Exp. Physiol.* **2018**, *103*, 838–850. [CrossRef]

33. Morisaki, K.; Furuyama, T.; Matsubara, Y.; Inoue, K.; Kurose, S.; Yoshino, S.; Nakayama, K.; Yamashita, S.; Yoshiya, K.; Yoshiga, R.; et al. External validation of CLI Frailty Index and assessment of predictive value of modified CLI Frailty Index for patients with critical limb ischemia undergoing infrainguinal revascularization. *Vascular* **2019**, 1708538119836005. [CrossRef] [PubMed]

34. Taniguchi, R.; Deguchi, J.; Hashimoto, T.; Sato, O. Sarcopenia as a Possible Negative Predictor of Limb Salvage in Patients with Chronic Limb-Threatening Ischemia. *Ann. Vasc. Dis.* **2019**, *12*, 194–199. [CrossRef] [PubMed]

35. Matsubara, Y.; Matsumoto, T.; Aoyagi, Y.; Tanaka, S.; Okadome, J.; Morisaki, K.; Shirabe, K.; Maehara, Y. Sarcopenia is a prognostic factor for overall survival in patients with critical limb ischemia. *J. Vasc. Surg.* **2015**, *61*, 945–950. [CrossRef] [PubMed]

36. AlGhatrif, M.; Zane, A.; Oberdier, M.; Canepa, M.; Studenski, S.; Simonsick, E.; Spencer, R.G.; Fishbein, K.; Reiter, D.; Lakatta, E.G.; et al. Lower Mitochondrial Energy Production of the Thigh Muscles in Patients with Low-Normal Ankle-Brachial Index. *J. Am. Heart Assoc* **2017**, *6*. [CrossRef] [PubMed]

37. Pipinos, I.I.; Shepard, A.D.; Anagnostopoulos, P.V.; Katsamouris, A.; Boska, M.D. Phosphorus 31 nuclear magnetic resonance spectroscopy suggests a mitochondrial defect in claudicating skeletal muscle. *J. Vasc. Surg.* **2000**, *31*, 944–952. [CrossRef] [PubMed]

38. Hou, X.Y.; Green, S.; Askew, C.D.; Barker, G.; Green, A.; Walker, P.J. Skeletal muscle mitochondrial ATP production rate and walking performance in peripheral arterial disease. *Clin. Physiol. Funct. Imaging* **2002**, *22*, 226–232. [CrossRef]

39. Lindegaard, B.P.; Bækgaard, N.; Quistorff, B. Mitochondrial dysfunction in calf muscles of patients with combined peripheral arterial disease and diabetes type 2. *Int. Angiol.* **2017**, *36*, 482–495.

40. Tecilazich, F.; Dinh, T.; Lyons, T.E.; Guest, J.; Villafuerte, R.A.; Sampanis, C.; Gnardellis, C.; Zuo, C.S.; Veves, A. Postexercise phosphocreatine recovery, an index of mitochondrial oxidative phosphorylation, is reduced in diabetic patients with lower extremity complications. *J. Vasc. Surg.* **2013**, *57*, 997–1005. [CrossRef]

41. Zorov, D.B.; Juhaszova, M.; Sollott, S.J. Mitochondrial ROS-induced ROS release: An update and review. *Biochim. Biophys. Acta.* **2006**, *1757*, 509–517. [CrossRef] [PubMed]
42. Lejay, A.; Choquet, P.; Thaveau, F.; Singh, F.; Schlagowski, A.; Charles, A.L.; Laverny, G.; Metzger, D.; Zoll, J.; Chakfe, N.; et al. A new murine model of sustainable and durable chronic critical limb ischemia fairly mimicking human pathology. *Eur. J. Vasc. Endovasc. Surg.* **2015**, *49*, 205–212. [CrossRef] [PubMed]
43. Kwon, B.; Kang, C.; Kim, J.; Yoo, D.; Cho, B.R.; Kang, P.M.; Lee, D. $H_2O_2$-responsive antioxidant polymeric nanoparticles as therapeutic agents for peripheral arterial disease. *Int. J. Pharm.* **2016**, *511*, 1022–1032. [CrossRef] [PubMed]
44. Lejay, A.; Charles, A.L.; Georg, I.; Goupilleau, F.; Delay, C.; Talha, S.; Thaveau, F.; Chakfe, N.; Geny, B. Critical limb ischemia exacerbates mitochondrial dysfunction in ApoE-/- mice compared to ApoE+/+ mice, but N-acetyl cysteine still confers protection. *Eur. J. Vasc. Endovasc. Surg.* **2019**, *58*, 576–582. [CrossRef]
45. Tran, T.P.; Tu, H.; Pipinos, I.I.; Muelleman, R.L.; Albadawi, H.; Li, Y.L. Tourniquet-induced acute ischemia-reperfusion injury in mouse skeletal muscles: Involvement of superoxide. *Eur. J. Pharmacol.* **2011**, *650*, 328–334. [CrossRef]
46. Miura, S.; Saitoh, S.; Kokubun, T.; Owada, T.; Yamauchi, H.; Machii, H.; Takeishi, Y. Mitochondrial-Targeted Antioxidant Maintains Blood Flow, Mitochondrial Function, and Redox Balance in Old Mice Following Prolonged Limb Ischemia. *Int. J. Mol. Sci.* **2017**, *18*, 1897. [CrossRef]
47. Lejay, A.; Laverny, G.; Paradis, S.; Schlagowski, A.I.; Charles, A.L.; Singh, F.; Zoll, J.; Thaveau, F.; Lonsdorfer, E.; Dufour, S.; et al. Moderate Exercise Allows for shorter Recovery Time in Critical Limb Ischemia. *Front. Physiol.* **2017**, *8*, 523. [CrossRef]
48. Guillot, M.; Charles, A.L.; Chamaraux-Tran, T.N.; Bouitbir, J.; Meyer, A.; Zoll, J.; Schneider, F.; Geny, B. Oxidative stress precedes skeletal muscle mitochondrial dysfunction during experimental aortic cross-clamping but is not associated with early lung, heart, brain, liver, or kidney mitochondrial impairment. *J. Vasc. Surg.* **2014**, *60*, 1043–1051.e5. [CrossRef]
49. McDermott, M.M.; Peterson, C.A.; Sufit, R.; Ferrucci, L.; Guralnik, J.M.; Kibbe, M.R.; Polonsky, T.S.; Tian, L.; Criqui, M.H.; Zhao, L.; et al. Peripheral artery disease, calf skeletal muscle mitochondrial DNA copy number, and functional performance. *Vasc. Med.* **2018**, *23*, 340–348. [CrossRef]
50. Koutakis, P.; Weiss, D.J.; Miserlis, D.; Shostrom, V.K.; Papoutsi, E.; Ha, D.M.; Carpenter, L.A.; McComb, R.D.; Casale, G.P.; Pipinos, I.I. Oxidative damage in the gastrocnemius of patients with peripheral artery disease is myofiber type selective. *Redox. Biol.* **2014**, *2*, 921–928. [CrossRef]
51. Weiss, D.J.; Casale, G.P.; Koutakis, P.; Nella, A.A.; Swanson, S.A.; Zhu, Z.; Miserlis, D.; Johanning, J.M.; Pipinos, I.I. Oxidative damage and myofiber degeneration in the gastrocnemius of patients with peripheral arterial disease. *J. Transl. Med.* **2013**, *11*, 230. [CrossRef] [PubMed]
52. Brass, E.P.; Wang, H.; Hiatt, W.R. Multiple skeletal muscle mitochondrial DNA deletions in patients with unilateral peripheral arterial disease. *Vasc. Med.* **2000**, *5*, 225–230. [CrossRef] [PubMed]
53. Bhat, H.K.; Hiatt, W.R.; Hoppel, C.L.; Brass, E.P. Skeletal muscle mitochondrial DNA injury in patients with unilateral peripheral arterial disease. *Circulation* **1999**, *99*, 807–812. [CrossRef] [PubMed]
54. Hsu, S.L.; Yin, T.C.; Shao, P.L.; Chen, K.H.; Wu, R.W.; Chen, C.C.; Lin, P.Y.; Chung, S.Y.; Sheu, J.J.; Sung, P.H.; et al. Hyperbaric oxygen facilitates the effect of endothelial progenitor cell therapy on improving outcome of rat critical limb ischemia. *Am. J. Transl. Res.* **2019**, *11*, 1948–1964.
55. Sheu, J.J.; Lee, F.Y.; Wallace, C.G.; Tsai, T.H.; Leu, S.; Chen, Y.L.; Chai, H.T.; Lu, H.I.; Sun, C.K.; Yip, H.K. Administered circulating microparticles derived from lung cancer patients markedly improved angiogenesis, blood flow and ischemic recovery in rat critical limb ischemia. *J. Transl. Med.* **2015**, *13*. [CrossRef]
56. Tetsi, L.; Charles, A.L.; Georg, I.; Goupilleau, F.; Lejay, A.; Talha, S.; Maumy-Bertrand, M.; Lugnier, C.; Geny, B. Effect of the Phosphodiesterase 5 Inhibitor Sildenafil on Ischemia-Reperfusion-Induced Muscle Mitochondrial Dysfunction and Oxidative Stress. *Antioxidants (Basel)* **2019**, *8*, 93. [CrossRef]
57. Lejay, A.; Paradis, S.; Lambert, A.; Charles, A.L.; Talha, S.; Enache, I.; Thaveau, F.; Chakfe, N.; Geny, B. N-Acetyl Cysteine Restores Limb Function, Improves Mitochondrial Respiration, and Reduces Oxidative Stress in a Murine Model of Critical Limb Ischaemia. *Eur. J. Vasc. Endovasc. Surg.* **2018**, *56*, 730–738. [CrossRef]
58. Masud, R.; Shameer, K.; Dhar, A.; Ding, K.; Kullo, I.J. Gene expression profiling of peripheral blood mononuclear cells in the setting of peripheral arterial disease. *J. Clin. Bioinforma.* **2012**, *2*, 6. [CrossRef]

59. Mitchell, R.G.; Duscha, B.D.; Robbins, J.L.; Redfern, S.I.; Chung, J.; Bensimhon, D.R.; Kraus, W.E.; Hiatt, W.R.; Regensteiner, J.G.; Annex, B.H. Increased levels of apoptosis in gastrocnemius skeletal muscle in patients with peripheral arterial disease. *Vasc. Med.* **2007**, *12*, 285–290. [CrossRef]
60. Gardner, A.W.; Parker, D.E.; Montgomery, P.S.; Sosnowska, D.; Casanegra, A.I.; Ungvari, Z.; Csiszar, A.; Sonntag, W.E. Greater Endothelial Apoptosis and Oxidative Stress in Patients with Peripheral Artery Disease. *Int. J. Vasc. Med.* **2014**, *2014*. [CrossRef]
61. Skórkowska-Telichowska, K.; Adamiec, R.; Tuchendler, D.; Gasiorowski, K. Susceptibility to apoptosis of lymphocytes from patients with peripheral arterial disease. *Clin. Investig. Med.* **2009**, *32*, E345–E351. [CrossRef] [PubMed]
62. Gardner, A.W.; Parker, D.E.; Montgomery, P.S.; Sosnowska, D.; Casanegra, A.I.; Esponda, O.L.; Ungvari, Z.; Csiszar, A.; Sonntag, W.E. Impaired vascular endothelial growth factor A and inflammation in patients with peripheral artery disease. *Angiology* **2014**, *65*, 683–690. [CrossRef] [PubMed]
63. Alves-Cabratosa, L.; Garcia-Gil, M.; Comas-Cufí, M.; Blanch, J.; Ponjoan, A.; Martí-Lluch, R.; Elosua-Bayes, M.; Parramon, D.; Camós, L.; Ramos, R. Role of Low Ankle-Brachial Index in Cardiovascular and Mortality Risk Compared with Major Risk Conditions. *J. Clin. Med.* **2019**, *8*, 870. [CrossRef] [PubMed]

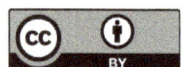

© 2019 by the authors. Licensee MDPI, Basel, Switzerland. This article is an open access article distributed under the terms and conditions of the Creative Commons Attribution (CC BY) license (http://creativecommons.org/licenses/by/4.0/).

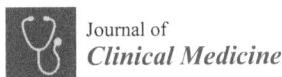

*Review*

# An Intriguing Involvement of Mitochondria in Cystic Fibrosis

**Maria Favia [1,2,*], Lidia de Bari [1], Antonella Bobba [1] and Anna Atlante [1,*]**

[1] Istituto di Biomembrane, Bioenergetica e Biotecnologie Molecolari—CNR, Via G. Amendola 122/O, 70126 Bari, Italy; l.debari@ibiom.cnr.it (L.d.B.); a.bobba@ibiom.cnr.it (A.B.)
[2] Dipartimento di Bioscienze, Biotecnologie e Biofarmaceutica, Università di Bari, Via E. Orabona 4, 70126 Bari, Italy
* Correspondence: mariafavia@hotmail.com (M.F.); a.atlante@ibiom.cnr.it (A.A.)

Received: 14 October 2019; Accepted: 4 November 2019; Published: 6 November 2019

**Abstract:** Cystic fibrosis (CF) occurs when the cystic fibrosis transmembrane conductance regulator (CFTR) protein is not synthetized and folded correctly. The CFTR protein helps to maintain the balance of salt and water on many body surfaces, such as the lung surface. When the protein is not working correctly, chloride becomes trapped in cells, then water cannot hydrate the cellular surface and the mucus covering the cells becomes thick and sticky. Furthermore, a defective CFTR appears to produce a redox imbalance in epithelial cells and extracellular fluids and to cause an abnormal generation of reactive oxygen species: as a consequence, oxidative stress has been implicated as a causative factor in the aetiology of the process. Moreover, massive evidences show that defective CFTR gives rise to extracellular GSH level decrease and elevated glucose concentrations in airway surface liquid (ASL), thus encouraging lung infection by pathogens in the CF advancement. Recent research in progress aims to rediscover a possible role of mitochondria in CF. Here the latest new and recent studies on mitochondrial bioenergetics are collected. Surprisingly, they have enabled us to ascertain that mitochondria have a leading role in opposing the high ASL glucose level as well as oxidative stress in CF.

**Keywords:** cystic fibrosis; cystic fibrosis transmembrane conductance regulator; mitochondria; bioenergetics; oxidative stress; glucose; airway surface liquid

## 1. Introduction

"The powerhouse of the cell" is surely the first memorable phrase in biology concerning mitochondria. Although this is still true, an explosion of new information about mitochondria reveals that their importance extends well beyond their time-honoured function as the "powerhouse of the cell", essential for life.

In recent years, a large body of research has established that mitochondria are not simply static, passively producing adenosine 5'-triphosphate (ATP) for fuel, but that they sense and respond to changing cellular environments and stresses. This is the reason the research on mitochondria is feverish worldwide: an increasing number of studies place mitochondrion at the heart of cell life as well as mitochondrial dysfunction at the heart of disease, thus opening new frontiers in health and disease.

Since the 1980s, with the beginnings of molecular biology and the detection of pathogenic defects of mitochondrial DNA, it has been found that a large number of mitochondrial disorders were underlying of pathogenesis of common human diseases. This is not surprising considering that mitochondria—establishing a dynamic network intimately combined with other cellular and extracellular compartments—influence the physiology and regulate communication between cells and tissues.

Moreover, considering that mitochondrial functions respond to a number of genetic, metabolic, neuroendocrine signals, it follows that mitochondrial defects contribute to the development of various diseases by altering complex cellular and physiological functions. In fact, it is now ascertained that many seemingly disconnected diseases have tangled roots in dysfunctional mitochondria. At the same time, it is also true that modern research has also endowed us with the knowledge on how to optimize their function, which is of critical importance to our health and longevity.

Reflecting on the fact that mitochondria have received increasing attention, especially in recent decades, we argue that their increasing relevance to modern medicine [1,2], is attributable to the convergence of key signalling pathways and biological processes onto the mitochondrion. Moreover, since mitochondria have an enormous potential to influence health, the optimizing of their metabolism could really to be the focus of an effective therapeutic treatment. Consequently, it is no wonder that mitochondria failure risks the collapse of most crucial cellular functions: this is the reason for which mitochondrial dysfunction is strictly connected to the aging phenomenon and numerous human diseases. It happens that biomedical scientists frequently 'fortuitously' encounter mitochondria during the natural development of their research program, as well as recent studies have brought to light unsuspected pathophysiological mechanisms involving this organelle. However, it is not yet clear whether mitochondrial dysfunction is a trigger for or a consequence of disease. For example, no one would have suspected, mitochondrial involvement in cystic fibrosis (CF) progression, an inherited disease characterized by alterations in the cystic fibrosis transmembrane conductance regulator (CFTR) protein, which plays a role in regulating hydrosaline balance on many surfaces in the body.

At the beginning of the research about the direct involvement of mitochondria in CF, a consideration is worthy of note: it is a question of building a cathedral in a desert. At the moment, the small steps that research is making in this direction are almost invisible and surely researchers, who are now laying the foundations to promote it, will not reap the benefits. However, every step will have great importance for who will outline the molecular mechanisms responsible for the implication of these cellular organelles in CF in the future. Discovering the invisible traces of the thousands of metabolic reactions in which mitochondrial enzymes are involved, can reveal the secrets of the CF cell and find the points of attack on which to act to obtain therapeutic responses.

That's why the authors of this Review embarked on this venture: to collect all the data—at the moment very few—available on the involvement of mitochondria in CF to understand how to proceed with exploration of mechanism underlying regulation of mitochondrial function with the last hope of glimpsing viable paths for future therapies.

## 2. Cystic Fibrosis: News on the Disease

CF is the most common and severe multisystem genetic disease among Caucasians and is estimated to affect about 36000 individuals in the European Union [3], and approximately 80,000 people in the world [4], with an incidence of 1 in 2500 Caucasians [5,6].

CF is caused by a defective gene *cftr* [7] that encodes for a protein called CFTR. The CFTR is a cAMP-regulated anion ($Cl^-$) channel. Playing crucial roles in both absorption and secretion [8,9], it is found primarily in wet epithelia, consistent with the symptoms that define CF. Besides being directly involved in the transport of chloride, it participates in the transport of other ions, as sodium and bicarbonate, so controlling salt and water transport across epithelial cell membranes of many tissues [10]. Indeed, CFTR protein is expressed in various epithelial cells lining many organs including the lung, pancreas, liver, the digestive and reproductive tracts [8,9,11,12]. However, CFTR protein is also present in non-epithelial cells from blood, brain, heart, liver, kidney and other tissues [13–19]. Additionally, CFTR is transcribed in the central, peripheral, and enteric nervous systems [20]. Although many organs are affected in CF, the most severe pathological consequences are lung-associated. For this reason the paper will be focused on the cell affected by CF in airways.

*2.1. CFTR Protein*

2.1.1. Domain Structure of CFTR

The CFTR protein belongs to the superfamily of ABC (ATP Binding Cassette) transporters proteins that have a characteristic modular structure consisting of two hydrophobic transmembrane domain, usually made of six membrane-spanning α-helices, and two cytosolic nucleotide-binding domains (NBD1 and NBD2) [21]. In addition, CFTR is unique among ABC transporters to have a regulatory (R) domain that links two homologous halves [22]. CFTR activation requires both ATP binding to the interface between NBD1 and NBD2 and protein kinase A (PKA)-mediated phosphorylation of the R domain [23–26].

CFTR activity (i.e., channel opening and closing) is controlled both by phosphorylation and dephosphorylation processes, via protein kinases and phosphatases, and by cellular ATP levels. It is also known that CFTR functional expression is regulated by interactions of CFTR protein with several proteins [27–32] in order to form a macromolecular complex.

2.1.2. CFTR Synthesis and Trafficking

In order to ensure that its functioning on the apical membrane is optimal, CFTR protein must be synthesized, folded, and transported in a correct manner. For this to happen, it must be subjected to a stringent quality control which removes any misfolded protein that could fail to function properly [33]. The normal biogenesis of CFTR starts with the translation of the CFTR protein in the rough endoplasmic reticulum (ER). Simultaneously a glycan (sugar molecule) is attached to a nitrogen atom of the protein in a process called N-linked glycosylation. Several proteins, as the chaperones, are involved in the correct folding of CFTR [4,34,35].

An important cytosolic chaperone, calnexin [36], interacting with the immature form of CFTR in ER, favours its proper folding. After folding in the ER, the CFTR is submitted to the ER-associated degradation process, involving the ubiquitin proteasome system [33]. Now, the aberrantly folded CFTR proteins undergo polyubiquitylation, removed from the ER membrane and degraded by a proteasome in the cytoplasm [37], whereas the correctly folded CFTR protein is sent to the Golgi by the coat protein complex II (COPII). Thanks to COPII, CFTR protein maintains the right structure, conformation, and protein-protein interactions. Next, within the Golgi, CFTR assumes its mature form and it is moved to the apical membrane via clathrin-coated vesicles [38]. In the plasma membrane, CFTR has a half-life of about 12–24 h; then it is internalized by clathrin-coated endosomes and either sent back to the plasma membrane or degraded within lysosomes [33].

2.1.3. CFTR Function in Physiological Conditions

In the lung, CFTR protein is expressed on the apical membrane of the cells lining the airways where it functions as a regulated chloride ion channel to maintain the balance of salt and water on lung surface. In fact, through an ATP-ase activity, requiring the use of an ATP molecule, CFTR protein favours the passage of chloride (but also of other electrolytes, such as sodium) from the inside to the outside of cells, with consequent secretion of water [39].

In addition, CFTR has been implicated in the secretion of bicarbonate, necessary for the bactericidal activity of the fluid that wets the airways, and also in the glutathione (GSH) efflux from cells [39], then implicating a role for CFTR in the control of oxidative stress in the airways [40]. Moreover, of note is the fact that CFTR protein regulates the activity of other chloride and sodium channels at the cell surface epithelium [39]. The balance between these transport functions is thought to lead to an optimal airway surface liquid (ASL) volume to promote ciliary clearance of mucus and bacteria (see Figures 1 and 2).

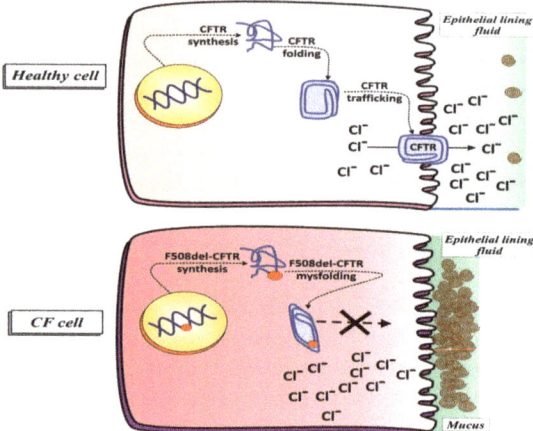

**Figure 1.** CFTR activity in the cell. In a *HEALTHY CELL*, a correct insertion of normal CFTR on the membrane allows for the ion movement across airway epithelium; in a *CF CELL*, transport Cl⁻ ions does not occur due to the mutated-CFTR channel protein (F508del-) inability for reaching the plasma membrane.

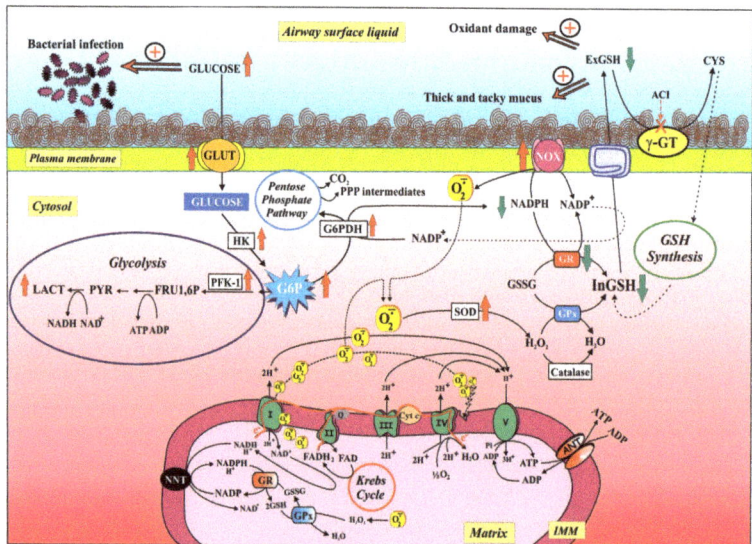

**Figure 2.** An overview of both the GSH turnover and the principal glucose related metabolic pathways: modulation of ROS and glucose levels in airway surface liquid and fight oxidative stress in cystic fibrosis cells. *Main abbreviations:* ACI, Acivicin; ANT, adenine nucleotide translocator; CYS; Cysteine; CI, Complex I or NADH-ubiquinone oxidoreductase; II, Complex II or succinate-ubiquinone oxidoreductase; III, Complex III or ubiquinone–cytochrome-c oxidoreductase; IV, Complex IV or cytochrome-c oxidase; V, Complex V or FoF1 ATP synthase; GLUT, Glucose Transporter/s; G6P, Glucose-6-phosphate; G6PDH, glucose-6-phosphate dehydrogenase; exGSH, extracellular GSH; inGSH, intracellular GSH; GPx, glutathione peroxidase; GR, glutathione reductase; GSSG, oxidized glutathione; γGT, γ-glutamyltransferase; HK, Hexokinase; $H_2O_2$, hydrogen peroxide; IMS, intermembrane mitochondrial space; MIM, mitochondrial inner membrane; NOX, NAD(P)H oxidases; $O_2^{-\bullet}$, Superoxide anion; OMM, outer mitochondrial membrane; PPP, pentose phosphate pathway; ROS, reactive oxygen species; SOD, Superoxide dismutase.

### 2.1.4. CFTR Function in Pathological Conditions (Cystic Fibrosis)

In CF, the gene mutation determines the production of a defective CFTR protein or even prevents its synthesis, with disruption of ion transport and the consequence that the secretions are poor in water, therefore dense and not very flowing, thus preventing effective ciliary activity [41]. In fact, mutated CFTR is not able to maintain the proper chloride levels, leading to an increase in intracellular chloride levels and a decrease in extracellular ones (see Figure 1). In particular, in CF the impairment of chloride transport is coupled with an increased sodium absorption by the airway epithelial cells, followed by an excessive movement of water into the airway epithelial cells. This represents a key step in the pathogenesis of CF lung disease, i.e., airway surface liquid dehydration, leading to thick and sticky mucus formation [39], ineffective mucociliary clearance [42] and exaggerated inflammation in response to infection. Chronic inflammation of the lung, as a consequence of persistent bacterial infections by several opportunistic pathogens, represents the main cause of morbidity and mortality in patients affected by CF [43]. Moreover an increase in anionic polyelectrolytes, including DNA derived from bacteria and lysed inflammatory cells, contributes to thicken the mucus [42].

In addition to the epithelial cell defects, a growing body of evidence has emerged indicating that neutrophils and macrophages, being central to the infectious and pulmonary pathology, account for the majority of CF mortality [44]. The intrinsic effect of CFTR deficiency in neutrophils and macrophages appears to be an inability to effectively kill bacteria [45]. Recent works prove that autophagy, a process clearing pathogens and dysfunctional protein aggregates within macrophages, is impaired in CF patients and CF mice, as their macrophages exhibit limited autophagy activity. This is the reason for which the study of microRNAs (Mirs), and other noncoding RNAs offers new therapeutic targets, with the aim to elucidate the role of Mirs in dysregulated autophagy-related genes in CF macrophages, and then target them to restore this host-defense function and improve CFTR channel function [46]. Furthermore, CF neutrophils are deficient in chlorination of bacterial components due to a limited chloride supply to the phagolysosomal compartment. About this, CFTR channel expression in neutrophils and its dysfunction affect neutrophil chlorination of phagocytosed bacteria [47].

Of note, these particular aspects of the disease, besides to have a clinical value because a cause-and-effect relationship has been established between ion transport and gene expression in CF immune cells, also transform the way we look at CF, which is now classified as an immune deficiency disorder [44,48].

### 2.1.5. Classes of Mutations

To date, more than 2000 mutations of the *cftr* gene have been described (Cystic Fibrosis Mutation Database; www.genet.sickkids.on.ca), although the most frequent mutation causing CF disease is the deletion of three base pairs in both copies of the gene that causes the loss of phenylalanine residue at position 508 of the CFTR protein (F508del) [49]. Different mutations prompt varying effects on CFTR function, resulting in diverse phenotypes of the disease.

Mutations known to affect the CFTR protein have been divided into classes (I to VI). The mutations belonging to classes I, II and III most alter the fate of the protein, not allowing any production (class I) or producing a very defective protein (class II and III); those of class IV allow the synthesis of a defective protein but capable of carrying out its function, even if in reduced measure; those of class V lead to a reduced amount of functional CFTR protein. Lastly, class VI mutations reduce CFTR stability, causing to accelerated channel removal from the plasma membrane [37].

#### F508del CFTR

Nearly 70–90% of the CF patients carry the allele F508, where phenylalanine at position 508 (F508del CFTR) in the NBD1 domain of the protein is lost leading to misfolding of the protein causing the most severe defect, that is the mistrafficking of CFTR protein that remains trapped in the endoplasmic reticulum and is subsequently degraded, before reaching the membrane.

However, in some CF airway cells a negligible expression of F508del CFTR can be detected at the cell surface due to the fact that ER retention is not complete [50,51]. Furthermore, the F508del-mutation reduces its apical membrane half-life [52] by accelerating its endocytic retrieval from the plasma membrane and its consequent degradation [53].

## 2.2. Clinical Trials in Cystic Fibrosis

### 2.2.1. Treatments of CF Symptoms

Quality of life as well as survival are affected by this disease. Although life expectancy has improved [54,55], current treatments for CF are neither preventive nor curative. In fact, since its recognition CF has been treated symptomatically.

One of the most common treatments is the inhalation of osmotic agents which, assuring an increase in mucociliary clearance [56], leads to better lung function within CF patients [57].

Another common treatment for CF patients is the inhalation of an enzyme deoxyribonuclease I that cleaves DNA in order to reduce the viscosity of the mucus [56,58]. Another treatment helping to slow the progression of CF disease is the chest physiotherapy [59].

Furthermore, since there are a wide variety of bacterial infections that can take hold in CF patients' lungs, there is also a large amount of antibiotic treatments focus on the controlling pulmonary infections. Lastly, lung transplantation is a complex, high-risk, potentially life-saving therapy for the end-stage of CF [60].

### 2.2.2. Latest Breakthrough Therapies

Daily, expensive drug-based options for treating the downstream effects of the CFTR gene defect, having the potential to improve survival and quality of life in patients with CF, are the major areas of focus of clinical trials.

In fact, the findings that restoration of small amounts of functional CFTR protein (20–30% of normal levels) [61] can greatly ameliorate the disease severity, have prompted researchers to identify modulator molecules able to rescue the CFTR defect thus restoring its folding, trafficking, and insertion into the plasma membrane (correctors) and/or improving its regulated function once its insertion on the surface (potentiators). Correctors are small molecules designed to increase the availability of CFTR protein at the apical membrane of epithelial cells and stay there longer (see Figure 1). Two F508del-CFTR corrector molecules, VX-809 and 4,6,4'-trimethylangelicin (TMA), were used in our studies in order to improve mitochondrial impairments, associated with the $\Delta$F508 mutation (see below, Section 5.2.1) [61,62].

However, the combined use of corrector and potentiator may work on residual function allowing more chloride to flow through cell epithelium and reduce the symptoms of CF.

To these molecules acting as modulators, others recently are added: the amplifiers. They are CFTR modulators that improve translation of CFTR mRNA to increase CFTR protein production. However, amplifiers are not yet available.

Other alternative approaches have been proposed, such as inhibiting ENaC activity [63] or activating an alternative chloride channel [64].

Lastly, since CF is a recessive genetic disorder, the addition of a single copy of the properly functioning CFTR gene into affected CF airway cells could represent the only rational and feasible way to prevent or treat CF airway disease for all CFTR mutation classes [65].

## 3. Lung: Information and Facts

The primary function of the respiratory system is to exchange oxygen and carbon dioxide. The inhaled oxygen enters the lungs and reaches alveoli and the bloodstream, by which it is transferred to all the tissues and organs of the body. Besides the skin, the lung is the only organ that is in direct contact with the external environment. As a consequence, it is constantly exposed to inhaled microbes, allergens and particulate material, which must be cleared without inducing inflammation, so as to maintain homeostasis. Airway epithelium, functioning as a physical barrier against external environmental insults, protects the lungs. Therefore, structurally and/or functionally damage to the epithelium may contribute to inflammation establishment and to alteration of repairing process following an injury.

*3.1. Lung: A Metabolically Active Organ*

Although the lung is often not considered a metabolically active organ, biochemical studies demonstrated that glucose utilization in lung [66] surpasses that of many other organs, including the heart, kidney, and brain. As for most tissues, glucose represents the primary source of energy also for the lung. In fact, glucose oxidation has been estimated to be 40–50 µmol/(h·g) of dry lung weight, which is a value equal to or greater than most other metabolically active organs [67,68].

The first step in glucose metabolism consists in its phosphorylation by hexokinase (HK) that occurs inside the cell. This process has the double advantage of trapping glucose inside the cell and providing a transmembrane concentration gradient to uptake more glucose (see below, Section 3.4).

In the cell, glucose metabolism involves four pathways: Krebs cycle and oxidative phosphorylation (OXPHOS) occurring in the mitochondria, and glycolysis and pentose phosphate pathway (PPP), which take place in the cytoplasm. Glycolysis and the Krebs cycle provide reducing equivalents for OXPHOS and finally produce ATP and NADH, while PPP, of which glucose-6-phosphate dehydrogenase (G6PDH) is the first and rate-limiting enzyme [66] and NADPH is the main product, mainly plays an important role in the fight against oxidative stress. Therefore, G6P is at the nexus of the PPP oxidative arm, glycogen synthesis—via conversion to glucose-1-phosphate—and glycolysis. The predominant fate of G6P depends on the cell type and metabolic demand.

In the lung, mitochondria preferably use substrates derived from glucose, such as pyruvate, for the production of oxidative energy, however, other energy sources are also used, including fatty acids, intermediates of the Krebs cycle, glycerol-3-phosphate and glutamate [69]. With classical teaching, pyruvate is metabolized in mitochondria under aerobic conditions. However, it is interesting to note that pyruvate conversion—by one additional cytosolic enzymatic reaction—to lactate in the cytoplasm appears to be largely independent of oxygen concentration, as levels have been shown to increase only marginally when alveolar $PO_2$ levels are significantly reduced [61]. This suggests that the lung may have evolved to use aerobic glycolysis as a means of minimizing local oxygen consumption, thus improving overall supply of oxygen delivery to other tissues.

Furthermore, it has been proposed that lactate production could serve as an energy source for lung cells, particularly, for those that have not adequate access to nutrients in the pulmonary circulation. This is not surprising if we consider the existence of monocarboxylate transporters and lactate dehydrogenase LDH isoforms in mitochondria in different healthy tissues as previously reported [70] and supported by the MitoCarta list [71].

If true, then the healthy lung would have used a strategy often attributed to cancer cells, in which lactate secretion by the primary tumour cell is important to support the activities of other cells (e.g., stromal cells) in the tumour microenvironment [72]. Moreover, lung mitochondria also have a unique and advantageous metabolic adaptation to aerobic OXPHOS, since the lung possesses its own isoform of the complex IV of the electron transport chain (ETC), cytochrome c oxidase (COX subunit IV-2), present in all lung cells, more oxygen sensitive, thus making the pulmonary COX more two-fold active (oxygen-binding) than COX in other tissues [73].

*3.2. Lung Redox Homeostasis*

As commonly indicated, molecular oxygen is a prerequisite for the life of all aerobic organisms and is essential for its many roles in human physiology. However, it is known that high concentrations of oxygen or its metabolites, i.e., reactive oxygen species (ROS), are able to cause cellular lesions and contribute to the pathogenesis of the disease. In particular, the lung is exposed to several thousand litres of air per day that carry a very large number of compounds with oxidative potential, including air pollution, pollen, and particulate matter. Although bigger particles are efficiently cleared by the nose and upper airways, fine particles can easily access the lower airways and promote greater airway oxidation and inflammation [74,75]. In order to effectively regulate the biological actions of exogenous and endogenous ROS, various enzymatic and non-enzymatic antioxidant defence systems are present in all types of lung cells to provide adequate protection against their harmful effects.

An increase in ROS production or a reduction in the ability to eliminate ROS can destroy redox homeostasis, leading to an overall increase in intracellular ROS levels or oxidative stress. Prolonged activity of cells at abnormal levels of ROS causes genetic mutations, which make them well adapted to oxidative stress. Thus, the cells that survive intrinsic oxidative stress mobilize a series of adaptive mechanisms, which activate ROS-scavenging systems to combat oxidative stress [76].

In this regard, it is important to reflect on what is meant by oxidative stress. Oxidative stress is considered as an imbalance between pro- and antioxidant species, which results in molecular and cellular damage. This definition lends itself to the idea that in reality there is a particular balance and that deviations from it can affect homeostasis and potentially cause or worsen the disease. Therefore, many studies, albeit with disappointing results, have been focused on restoring this "balance" through the use of antioxidants. A problem that should not be underestimated is the difficulty the researcher encounters in distinguishing when, in a given pathological process, oxidative stress is a guiding factor or simply an epiphenomenon.

Acute and chronic lung diseases are thought to be associated with an increase in oxidative stress, evidenced by greater irreversible oxidative changes in proteins or DNA, mitochondrial dysfunction and altered expression or activity of NOX (NAD(P)H oxidases) enzymes and antioxidant enzyme systems. However, it is right to consider that, besides these presumed damaging effects of NOX-derived ROS, NOX-family enzymes participate in other cell functions such as cell proliferation, differentiation, etc. [77,78].

The most accepted hypothesis is that in CF the excessive production of ROS (probably by neutrophils activated during infection cycles) overloads the antioxidant defences and oxidises the components of the lung cell membrane, thus contributing to lung dysfunction, following repeated episodes of infection. In particular, it has been observed that patients with severely impaired pulmonary function had significantly elevated plasma concentrations of lipid hydroperoxides [79,80], suggesting that lipid peroxidation is closely associated with the decrease in pulmonary function seen in CF. In addition, markers of oxidative stress were present in many CF patients, even though they had normal concentrations of circulating antioxidants, thus suggesting that normal levels of antioxidant defences are insufficient to protect against the oxidative stress. As a result, cumulative oxidative lung damage contributes to the progressive decrease in pulmonary function observed in these patients [81].

### 3.3. Airways Surface Liquid: Characteristics and Functions

The common feature of chronic airway diseases in humans is mucociliary dysfunction.

Briefly, mucociliary clearance is an important primary innate defence mechanism that protects the lungs from deleterious effects of inhaled pollutants, allergens, and pathogens. The mucociliary apparatus consists of three functional compartments, namely, the cilia, a protective layer of mucus, and an ASL layer, which work in concert to remove inhaled particles from the lung.

In this context, we will only report information about ASL that is pertinent to what will be discussed later in the paper.

The ASL, initially recognized for its property of reducing the surface tension facilitating alveolar compliance, is now appreciated as a first line of defence against inhaled chemical agents and pathogens [82]. The importance of ASL for the healthy function of the epithelium mainly concerns the correct function of the cilia, which would be unable to beat if ASL was absent, as well as mucociliary transport would be absent. As a consequence, various defensive mechanisms in the airway mucosa would be defective. Therefore, everything related to the ASL, i.e., the volume, pH, ionic and nutrient content is important in regulating antimicrobial activity, ciliary function and mucociliary transport of the airway. In particular, the water content of ASL is controlled by the regulation of ionic transport mediated by chloride channels (CFTR and a calcium-activated [alternative] chloride channel) and the epithelial sodium channel ENaC [43,83]. In detail, airway epithelia absorb $Na^+$ through ENaC and secrete $Cl^-$ through the CFTR anion channel. This balance maintains adequate hydration of superficial airway fluid to permit an effective elimination of the mucus, required to conserve sterility of the lung.

As evidence of the functional importance of these channels, we can consider that a series of human pathologies, including CF [84], chronic bronchitis [85], chronic obstructive pulmonary disease (COPD) [86], and pulmonary edema [87], are associated with the impairment of epithelial ionic transports.

Indeed, in normal airways, CFTR and the ENaC are perfectly functioning [88]. The combination of $Cl^-$ secretion and reduced $Na^+$ reabsorption favours a healthy ASL ion composition and depth, which enables effective ciliary function for appropriate mucociliary clearance [88].

In chronic airway diseases, such as CF, i.e., when CFTR is absent or dysfunctional and ENaC is no longer regulated, hyperabsorption of $Na^+$ and an increased driving force for fluid reabsorption [88] occurs. Furthermore, the ASL depth is reduced, the mucosal glands are hypertrophic and excess mucus is secreted [88]. The excessive production of viscous mucus impairs mucociliary clearance, resulting in airflow obstruction and bacterial colonization of the lungs [88].

*3.4. Glucose Movement Across the Airway Epithelium*

Another task of the ASL is to maintain differential glucose concentration. Glucose is exclusively supplied to the airways by circulating blood, and reaches the basolateral side of epithelial cells, where it can be absorbed. Levels of glucose in the lungs are tightly regulated and are up to 12 times lower in the lung ASL than in circulating levels (differential glucose concentrations between the ASL [~0.4 mM] and the blood/interstitium [5–6 mM]) [89,90].

The glucose concentration in ASL is kept low—an important condition to protect the lung from infections—both by the action of facilitative glucose transporter/s (GLUT/s) and by its subsequent metabolism occurring in lung epithelial cells [91].

Consistently, Bearham et al. [90] hypothesised that movement of glucose in the airway largely depends on its intracellular concentration, which is regulated by the activity of hexokinase. Low intracellular glucose preserves a driving force for glucose to enter the cell. However, if intracellular glucose concentrations rise to the same or higher values of glucose present in ASL, this would favor luminal efflux of glucose.

Since an increase of glucose in the ASL has been associated with an increase in respiratory tract infections in airway disease [92], the knowledge of the dynamics underlying glucose movement across the airway epithelium is fundamental. Recently Bearham et al. [90] showed that inhibition of apical GLUT uptake with Cytochalasin B increased apical glucose accumulation, indicating that without the contribution of GLUT-mediated absorption, glucose levels in ASL are likely to increase further in response to proinflammatory mediators. To confirm this, the clinical observations show that, in humans, airway inflammation is associated with increased ASL glucose concentrations [92]. Therefore, maintaining a low level of ASL glucose is essential for preserving airway sterility.

To confirm that the low concentration of glucose in ASL is a key element in lung defence against infection, a study conducted on patients in intensive care showed that patients with high ASL glucose concentrations were more likely to acquire respiratory infections—particularly with methicillin-resistant *Staphylococcus aureus*, which uses glucose as a growth substrate—compared to those with normal ASL glucose concentrations [93]. Consistently, diabetic patients with and without chronic lung disease are at increased risk of respiratory infection.

However, to date, it has not yet established how the human airway epithelium is able to regulate the concentration of glucose in ASL. Since in healthy subjects, in which blood glucose increase was induced experimentally, glucose concentration in ASL increased [94,95], it appears that glucose moves through the epithelium along the concentration gradient by paracellular diffusion. When the experimental hyperglycemia is reversed, the ASL glucose concentration decreased, suggesting that glucose is removed from the ASL by absorption by cells against a transepithelial glucose concentration gradient since the ASL glucose always remained lower than the concentrations of blood glucose [94,95]. Consistently, it has been observed by [96] that CF-related diabetes is associated with a more rapid decline in lung function. Many evidences indicate that diabetes and hyperglycemia, even in non-CF patients, are associated with reduced lung function compared to control non-diabetic subjects [97]. In addition, high blood glucose concentrations, particularly in CF patients, have been associated with elevated airway glucose levels and an increased risk of bacterial infections [for review see [96]]. Moreover, hyperglycemia may disrupt the benefits of CFTR correctors on airway repair.

## 4. Mitochondria

### 4.1. Mitochondria: A Short Brief and Essential Presentation

Although mitochondria are far more than just power suppliers—having them main roles in apoptosis, calcium homeostasis and oxygen sensing [98–100]—they remain famous for producing ATP via OXPHOS.

The mitochondrion, a semi-autonomous organelle with an own maternally inherited genome as well as the full apparatus for transcription/translational processes [101], is enclosed within outer and inner membranes that identify the two compartments of intermembrane space (IMS) and matrix. The inner membrane (IMM), which protrudes into the matrix with the cristae, harbours the OXPHOS enzyme complexes, which altogether form ETC or respiratory chain (Figure 3). In the matrix, the enzymatic reactions of the tricarboxylic acid cycle (TCA) produce NADH and FADH$_2$ which act as electron-carriers to the respiratory chain complexes, thus inducing oxygen consumption. As a result, the oxidation of food-derived, high-energy molecules, which starts into the cytoplasm and culminates with electron flow along the ETC and oxygen consumption, allowed the chemical energy being trapped into a trans-membrane electrochemical potential ($\Delta\Psi$) [102]. Any defect in the energy flow will alter mitochondrial homeostasis and induce pathological conditions.

The ETC consists of four protein machines (I–IV), which through sequential redox reactions undergo conformational changes to pump protons from the matrix into the IMS. In details, nutrients (e.g., glucose, fatty acids and aminoacids) are degraded to small metabolites (e.g., pyruvate, acetyl-CoA, oxaloacetate, 2-oxoglutarate) which are oxidized by the enzymes of the TCA cycle where electrons, made available in the decarboxylation reactions, are transferred to NAD$^+$ producing NADH.

Complex I (mtCx-I), i.e., NADH:ubiquinone oxidoreductase, also known as Nicotinamide adenine dinucleotide (NADH) dehydrogenase—a sophisticated microscale pump consisting of 45 core subunits, whose biogenesis requires an army of assembly factors [103,104]—thereafter oxidizes NADH and induces the release of electrons that flow through ubiquinone Q to generate ubiquinol. The ubiquinone Q can further receive electrons from other sources, i.e., Complex II (succinate dehydrogenase), electron transfer flavoprotein oxidoreductase, dihydroorotate dehydrogenase, and FAD-linked glycerol-3-phosphate dehydrogenase [105]. Electrons then proceed through cytochrome $c$ and Complex III up to Complex IV where the terminal electron acceptor, i.e., O$_2$, is reduced to H$_2$O (see Figure 3). This flow of electrons along the respiratory complexes is an energetically favourable process sustained by the difference in the redox potentials of NADH (Eo' = $-340$ mV) and O$_2$ (Eo'= $+810$ mV). According to Peter Mitchell's chemiosmotic theory, the electron flow is coupled to the pumping of protons through Complexes I, III, and IV into the intermembrane space and the released energy is temporary stored in the so-called protonmotive force. This energy reservoir allows ATP to be synthesized from ADP and free phosphate when protons move down this gradient at the level of the F$_1$F$_O$-ATP synthase. The newly synthesized ATP can be translocated into the cytosol through the adenine nucleotide translocase (ANT) (Figure 3).

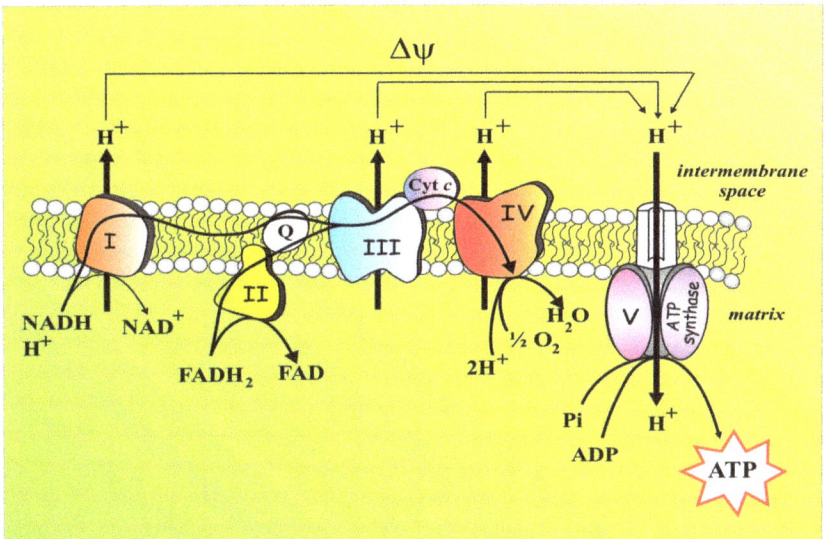

**Figure 3.** A schematic representation of the mitochondrial respiratory chain. Main abbreviations: ANT, adenine nucleotide translocator; I, Complex I or NADH-ubiquinone oxidoreductase; II, Complex II or succinate-ubiquinone oxidoreductase; III, Complex III or ubiquinone–cytochrome-c oxidoreductase; IV, Complex IV or cytochrome-c oxidase; V, Complex V or FoF1 ATP synthase; ΔΨ, Mitochondrial membrane potential.

The ΔΨ, generated at the IMM level, not only provide cell with newly synthetized ATP, but it is a crucial feature of healthy mitochondria [106], being the driving force for other mitochondrial processes, such as mitochondrial protein imports [107] or the key factor that underlies any changes of mitochondrial behaviours in response to mitochondrial dysfunction. In addition, the mitochondrial matrix is central to metabolism, as OXPHOS, the citric acid cycle, fatty acid oxidation, the urea cycle and the biosynthesis of iron sulphur centres and can take place there.

A consequence of mitochondrial respiration is the generation of unpaired electrons. Molecular oxygen can be reduced to $H_2O$ by only one electron at a time, but it may happen that spurious electrons, mainly originating from complex I and III, reduce $O_2$ to produce superoxide anion ($O_2^{-\bullet}$) [108]. $O_2^{-\bullet}$ is an highly ROS that is quickly dismutated to $H_2O_2$, a signalling molecules still belonging to ROS, which is endowed with a longer half-life and increased capacity to cross biological membranes.

In addition to being the main source of ROS, mitochondria also contain the cell's antioxidant defences [109]—such as superoxide dismutase, peroxidases and catalase, and small molecules such as GSH—to curb the damaging effects of ROS, thus protecting the cell. This makes mitochondrion a central player in cellular redox homeostasis. It follows that subtle changes in respiratory chain capacity, substrate supply, GSH levels and membrane potential could determine conditions predisposing towards diseases as well as in genetic disorders.

*4.2. Mitochondria, An Essential Part of the Redox Balance*

It is undisputed that mitochondria, playing a central role in the regulation of cellular bioenergetics, respond to changes in the environment caused by hormones, nutrients, partial oxygen pressure, oxygen amendments and others [110] and are essential for cell viability. It follows that the mitochondrial redox control affects the redox balance of the entire cell [111] that in turn affects all cell metabolism, as we will see below. The cytosolic redox state strictly depends on the reduced/oxidized ratio of specific cofactors—$NADH/NAD^+$, $NADPH/NADP^+$ and glutathione (GSH)/glutathione disulfide

(GSSG)—which are involved in maintaining cell homeostasis and counteracting oxidative stress. The ratio of these redox/active cofactors is greatly influenced by the energy status of the cell, i.e., availability of energy substrates and ATP, as well as by any alteration in physiological conditions.

About the NADH/NAD$^+$ pair, under basal condition, the oxidized form, i.e., NAD$^+$, prevails over the reduced one [112] and as such it is used in the glycolysis within the glyceraldehyde-3-phosphate dehydrogenase reaction which leads to the production of 1,3-diphospho-D-glycerate and NAD(P)H. Thus, the reduced state of this cofactor is closely linked to the pathways that contribute to the synthesis of ATP, i.e., glycolysis and OXPHOS. Indeed, full oxidation of glucose to $CO_2$, occurring first during glycolysis and then in the citric acid cycle, has the effect of reduce the electron acceptor NAD$^+$ to NADH. Due to the continued demand of NAD$^+$, it is regenerated by oxidation of NADH. Cytosolic NADH can be directly oxidized to NAD$^+$ in the last glycolytic reaction which converts pyruvate to lactate, otherwise its electrons can cross the mitochondrial membrane via enzymatic shuttles. Into the matrix, NADH can directly transfers electrons to mtCx-I of the ETC.

In contrast, the redox pair NADPH/NADP$^+$ is in a more reduced state [112] to provide electrons in particular for reductive biosynthesis. It is in fact known that NADPH acts as an electron donor in anabolic as well as antioxidative reactions, such as the reduction of GSSG to the active antioxidant GSH [113,114]. The replenishment of NADPH, which is necessary to maintain a sustainable NADPH/NADP$^+$ ratio, is mainly achieved via NADPH-regenerating enzymes [112]. The activity of these enzymes, which include two enzymes of the oxidative part of the PPP, i.e., G6PDH and 6-phosphogluconate dehydrogenase, the cytosolic NADP$^+$-dependent isocitrate dehydrogenase (ICDH) and the cytosolic malic enzyme (ME), is strictly dependent on cell metabolic state.

As far as the cytosolic isoforms of ICDH and ME are concerned, they can produce NADPH when the metabolic state of the cell allow the withdrawals of isocitrate and malate from citric acid cycle, thus contributing to the synthesis of fatty acids and cholesterol by supplying NADPH. Conversely, during acute oxidative stress, the increase in demand for NADPH is guaranteed mainly by G6PDH, a PPP enzyme, whose complete deficiency is incompatible with life, which utilizes the glucose-6-phosphate continuously produced during the first reaction of glycolysis. Noteworthy with regard to mitochondria, nicotinamide nucleotide transhydrogenase, in a reaction driven by the mitochondrial electrochemical proton gradient, can also produce NADPH from NADP$^+$ by using the NADH derived from TCA cycle as substrate. Consistently, whenever matrix NADH level or mitochondrial membrane potential decrease, due to mitochondrial malfunctioning, also mitochondrial NADPH regeneration will be impaired, leading to oxidative stress [115].

Furthermore, NADPH can be produced by other mitochondrial dehydrogenases, such as mitochondrial isoforms of ICDH and malate dehydrogenase (MDH) [115] and it is also involved in the reaction of the GSH- and thioredoxin-dependent antioxidant enzymes, either cytosolic or mitochondrial, where it participates as an electron donor.

Concerning GSH, it strongly exceeds GSSG levels [116] and constitutes a strong antioxidant protective tool against ROS, mainly in lung. The GSH/GSSG ratio is controlled by several parameters and its value depends not only on the rates of GSH synthesis, GSH oxidation and GSSG reduction, but also on the availability of GSH to participate in other metabolic pathways (cellular processes) and on the export of either GSH or GSSG, outside the cells. In healthy cells, the level of GSH is kept higher than the oxidized form GSSG by glutathione reductase (GR) which constantly removes the GSSG produced in basal conditions. On the other hand, under oxidative stress conditions, an increase in GSSG level occurs since reduced glutathione is oxidized via chemical or enzymatic reaction. In the last case, glutathione peroxidase (GPx) reduces $H_2O_2$ to $H_2O$ by utilizing GSH as an electron donor. GSSG is then reduced back to GSH in the reaction catalysed by GR in the *glutathione cycle*. The capacity to recycle GSH makes this cycle crucial to the cellular antioxidant defence mechanism and prevents depletion of thiols. Besides to the glutathione cycle, the GSH/GSSG ratio is also influenced by the effective availability of GSH inside the cell since it that can be exported outside as such in the oxidized form or after conjugation [112].

The picture that emerges highlights that the three cytosolic redox pairs NADH/NAD$^+$, NADPH/NADP$^+$ and GSH/GSSG could to be more crosslinked than supposed. Indeed, NAD kinase catalyses the production of NADP$^+$ from NAD$^+$ but NADP$^+$ can also be hydrolysed to NAD$^+$ [117]. The GSH/GSSG pair is modulated by GR, a NADPH-consuming enzyme, while glucose-6-phopshate is the substrate for both glycolysis and PPP, two metabolic pathways responsible for the production of NADH and NADPH, respectively. Any alterations of one of these redox pairs will produce effect also on the other and, indeed, G6PDH overexpression induces NADPH, NADH and GSH level increase [118] while inhibition of GR reduces GSH but increases both NADH/NAD$^+$ and NADPH/NADP$^+$ ratios [119].

### 4.3. GSH as Tool to Combat Ox Stress (Infections)

Since its role in the CF is dominant, more information about GSH concerning its synthesis and use are necessary.

GSH is normally present at 2–10 mM concentrations inside cells. It is synthesized *de novo* exclusively in cytosol—where γ-glutamylcysteine synthase (γ-GCS) and glutathione synthetase (GS) reside—from its constituent amino acids by two successive ATP-dependent enzymatic steps.

In the first step, cysteine (CYS) and glutamate are linked in a reaction catalysed by the γ-GCS to form γ-glutamylcysteine. This first reaction is the rate-limiting step in the synthesis of GSH and is regulated by CYS availability. About, the antioxidant function of GSH is proper determined by the redox-active thiol (-SH) of CYS that becomes oxidized when GSH reduces target molecules [120]. The completion of GSH synthesis is catalysed by GS, in a reaction in which γ-glutamyl-cysteine is covalently linked to glycine.

Cytosolic GSH is then distributed among the intracellular organelles including the mitochondria, endoplasmic reticulum (ER), and nucleus—which do not possess the enzymatic machinery to perform *de novo* synthesis of GSH—to control compartment-specific needs and functions [120].

Except for the ER, intracellular GSH is mainly found in its reduced form. In particular, although mitochondrial GSH represents about 10% of the total cellular GSH pool, however, based on the volume of the mitochondrial matrix, its concentration is similar to that found in the cytosol: it is estimated to be about 10–14 mM (see [121]).

In addition, γglutamyltransferase (γGT), which is located on the outer surface of the plasma membrane, can degrade extracellular GSH. GCS and γGT constitute part of a system for transport of GSH between organs and for its recycling between the extracellular and intracellular compartments. As a consequence of GSH export by epithelial cells, GSH is found in high concentration in some extracellular fluids, such as the ASL [122]. Normal human ASL contains a high GSH concentration (i.e., 400 μM) that is 140-fold higher than that in the plasma [123]. Extracellular GSH can serve as a scavenger of carbon-centred free radicals produced by lipid peroxidation and hypochlorous acid produced by neutrophils during inflammation. However, it would be wrong to view GSH only or even most importantly in terms of its antioxidant properties when considering its importance in lung defence. Indeed, a second property of reduced glutathione that should not be overlooked is its promotion of mucolysis. Because of its chemistry, GSH, like N-acetylcysteine (NAC), is able to cleave disulphide bonds, which serves to reduce the viscoelasticity of mucus when the GSH system is functioning normally [124].

## 5. Mitochondria in CF: What Is Known?

To date, the involvement of mitochondria in CF has never been investigated in detail.

The paucity of information is mainly due to the fact that after the primordial suspicion that the mutated protein responsible for the disease was of mitochondrial origin, the researchers did not anymore take into account the hypothetical involvement of mitochondria, centering the main research essentially on the protein encoded by the mutated *cftr* gene (see [125]).

Here we review all the studies concerning the involvement of mitochondria in CF, with particular attention to the more recent ones on the altered mitochondrial function. We believe this effort a necessary starting point to obtain a clear and fruitful overall picture that could help to properly address future studies aimed to clarify the molecular mechanisms of mitochondrial dysfunction in CF.

*5.1. What Was Already Known about Mitochondria in CF?*

That mitochondrial defects could somehow related to CF pathogenesis was first hypothesised in 1979 when mtCx-I impairments was reported [125]. In this study, Shapiro and collaborators sustained that in CF cells oxygen consumption increased and the mtCx-I inhibition by rotenone (ROT) was more effective than in normal cells [125]. Furthemore, treatment with ouabain, an inhibitor of the $Na^+$-$K^+$-exchanging ATPase, was able to reverse the increase in mitochondrial oxygen consumption, thus suggesting that an increase in $Na^+K^+$ATPase activity also occurred to fulfil the energy demands by CF cells [126]. Consistently, about a 50% increase in oxygen consumption was described in epithelial cells derived from nasal polyps in CF patients with respect to control samples. As a consequence, for the increased oxygen consumption by CF cells, the mitochondrial production of both superoxide ($O_2^{-\bullet}$) and peroxide ($H_2O_2$) could increase too [127].

NADH dehydrogenase also showed differences in enzyme kinetics with decreased Km and increased pH optima in CF cells [128], suggesting that the CF-mutant gene might be responsible for the observed mtCx-I alterations [129]. Moreover, it has been reported that in CF fibroblast also cytochrome-c oxidase showed an altered kinetics with increased Km at temperature >25 °C [130]. Other mitochondrial abnormalities have been described in F508del-CFTR cells such as fragmentation of the mitochondria network and reduction of mitochondrial $Ca^{2+}$ uptake, both events presumably linked to a primary mitochondrial membrane depolarization [131]. Taken together, these findings pointed out to an involvement of mutated CFTR into the impairment of mitochondrial structure and function.

Afterwards, several studies described other mitochondrial changes in CF [131] to such an extent that it was initially thought that the mutated protein responsible for the disease was a mitochondrial protein. However, when CFTR was cloned and identified as a chloride channel [131], the hypotheses of possible mitochondrial involvement in CF was totally put aside to the point of concentrating the whole study on the mutated protein forgetting that the cell lives thanks to the presence of the mitochondria. Therefore, the subsequent works concerned mainly the CFTR as chloride channel. Only few studies continued to explore mitochondrial involvement in CF. In particular, it was proven that the 2D electrophoretic patterns of mitochondrial proteins was proved to be different in CF patients with respect to controls [132], as well as intracellular pH increased in CF subjects during workload [133].

Besides being a chloride channel, and as such clearly endowed with a transport activity, the CFTR can also indirectly affect gene expression. It has been reported that some CFTR-dependent genes are involved in specific cell pathways—either metabolic or inflammation-related [124]—and two genes in particular, MT-ND4 and CISD1 encoding for mitochondrial proteins, are downregulated in CF cells [131].

In particular, MT-ND4 gene encodes for one of seven subunits of the mtCx-I, the ND4 subunit. It is crucial to the proper assembly and activity of mtCx-I [131,134,135]. As a consequence, the MT-ND4 downregulation detected in CF cells could be responsible for the low efficiency in NADH oxidation. Indeed, as also discussed below (see Section 5.2.1), the activity of mtCx-I decreased in CF cells (see [131,136]) and it should be considered that, as suggested by Cleeter et al. [137], a deficient mtCx-I may increase the level of ROS, which in turn further affects mtCx-I activity. Conversely, inhibition of the OXPHOS system, described by Esposito et al. [138] in the Ant1(tm2Mgr) (-/-) mouse model which is depleted of the heart/muscle isoform of ANT, induced ROS production as well as the expression of manganese superoxide dismutase (Mn-SOD or SOD2) as a compensatory mechanism [131]. These conditions apparently in antithesis indicate that both the origin and the consequences of high ROS levels are not fully understood.

Whenever the antioxidant system fails to balance the increasing ROS, a damage to mtDNA could easily occur which further impairs the OXPHOS system thus inducing a vicious cycle of additional ROS generation [131]. Such findings have been confirmed in human RPE cells by Lian and

Godley [139]. A mitochondrial impairment, due to increasing oxidative stress, has also been described in CFTR-knockout mice where both an oxidative damage to mtDNA and a reduced aconitase activity have been observed [121].

There are several factors that make CF cells more prone to injury by oxidative stress, and an altered GSH/GSSG ratio is the first among them. As already reported (see Section 4.3), GSH is a key antioxidant compound whose availability inside cell is fundamental to sustain a good redox state and the health of cells. In CF, the low CFTR activity has been correlated to a defective GSH transport [140,141] (see above, Section 2.1.3) resulting in an altered extracellular ratio between reduced and oxidized glutathione [131].

Altered GSH level in CF has already been reported in the initial studies done in the 1970s [121]. Consistently, transfection of normal CFTR has been reported to result in increased GSH [114]. Concerning this, Kelly-Aubert et al. [142] reported that the treatment with a membrane permeable analogue of GSH, i.e., GSH monoethylester (GSH-EE), reverted the reduced mtCx-I activity of CF cells, as well as CFTR knockout mice, to healthy values. Likewise, also the $\Delta\Psi$ was restored by GSH-EE. Taking into account that GSH-EE was found to be able to increase the levels of mitochondrial GSH (mGSH) in different experimental models (see [131]), it clearly emerges that the GSH depletion is a predisposing factor to mitochondrial dysfunction in CF cells. Either in liver or in neurodegenerative disorders, such as Parkinson's and Alzheimer's disease, mGSH depletion has been correlated with alterations of the respiratory chain [142] in particular of mtCx-I the more likely among the respiratory complexes to be inactivated by ROS and/or by GSH/GSSG variations [143].

Any attempt for defining the cause–effect relationship between mtCx-I inhibition and GSH depletion, in order to define which mechanism comes first, is still waiting for an answer. What is known is that each mechanism causes an increase of level of ROS, which in turn modify the GSH/GSSG ratio by consuming GSH and lead to mtCx-I inhibition due to oxidative modifications. mtCx-I inhibition and mtGSH depletion are interconnected in a round loop fuelled by ROS elevation.

Notwithstanding GSH treatment, either by inhalation or oral administration of GSH or NAC, has been administered to CF adults and children enrolled in several clinical trials [144], none of them proved to be really effective in reduce sputum elastase activity and IL-8 levels while a short-term administration only slightly improved lung function. Moreover, GSH-EE was able to re-establish suitable levels of mGSH and to correct the cellular damage [145], but it was found to be toxic at high doses probably as a result of the ethanol production occurring when GSH is released [146]. At present, this issue limits its use in vivo.

Next, taking into account what has been reported so far, we will review the recent findings on mitochondrial alterations found in CF cells and their possible pathophysiological consequences.

*5.2. The Latest Findings on Mitochondria in CF*

From the above, one thing is certain: mitochondria have an enormous potential to influence health. This leads us to firmly believe that optimizing the metabolism of mitochondria in those diseases, such as CF, in which mitochondrial function is compromised, can be the focus of effective treatment therapeutic.

The latest studies to which we will refer in this section started about five years ago.

We approached the study of mitochondria in CF taking into account two assumptions: (i) oxidative stress plays a pivotal role in the pathogenesis of CF [131] and (ii) mitochondria play a major role in cellular redox homeostasis [147–149].

Aim of our study has been to find the intertwined relation between F508del-CFTR and mitochondrial bioenergetics, with respect to both oxidative stress and redox imbalance in-order-to describe some features of the complex CF phenotype and detect potential new targets for therapy.

5.2.1. Characterization of Mitochondrial Function in Cells with Impaired CFTR Function

First, the principal goal has been to investigate mitochondrial function, in particular as it regards the steps of OXPHOS and ROS production, in airway cells. In this regard, experiments concerning this research were made using two human bronchial epithelial cell lines: CFBE41o- cells expressing F508del CFTR and respective control, i.e., CFBE41o-cells stably expressing wildtype CFTR. For convenience these cells will be referred to as 'CF cells' and 'control cells' in the text.

We observed that some steps of OXPHOS, such as ADP/ATP exchange via ANT, oxygen consumption, $\Delta\Psi$ generation and both mtCx-I and COX, activities are impaired in airway cells homozygous for the F508 deletion, while both ROS production and mitochondrial membrane lipid peroxidation increased [136] (Figure 2).

In particular, we found a loss of mtCx-I activity with consequent ROS increase. Further, we proved that ROS-mediated damage of the membrane microenvironment was likely responsible for inhibition of COX, whose activity is strongly dependent on the membrane lipid environment (see Figure 2). Importantly, treatment of CF cells with the small molecules VX-809 and 4,6,4'-trimethylangelicin (TMA), which act as 'correctors' for F508del CFTR by increasing the amount of functional CFTR at the cell surface and rescuing the F508del CFTR-dependent chloride secretion [61,62] (see above, Section 2.2.2), significantly improved all the mitochondrial parameters towards values found in the airway cells expressing wildtype CFTR, strongly suggesting that the restorative action provided by the correctors on mitochondrial functions in CF cells is linked to the rescue of chloride channel activity. Unfortunately, we could not currently provide any molecular mechanism underlying how CFTR dysfunction affects parameters of mitochondrial function, nor how corrector-induced increased CFTR cell surface expression is able to repair these mitochondrial dysfunctions.

At the same time, we obtained the same results by using as a model study primary cells, which provide a microenvironment closer to in vivo situations.

These results were valuable because they represented the starting point to address the next research. Indeed, since (i) the mitochondrial dysfunction and ROS generation are intricately related to changes in the glutathione redox system [147]; (ii) a drop of GSH levels is observed in CF cells [81,150], we studied more precisely GSH and GSH-dependent enzymes in order to trace back the link between mitochondrial dysfunction, low GSH levels and defective F508del-CFTR.

In particular, the research was devoted to:

- Detecting the enzyme/s contributing to the upregulation of intracellular ROS production, besides mitochondria [131,136];
- Studying how the balance between the production and neutralization of ROS is maintained in the presence of antioxidant enzymes, measuring the activity of superoxide dismutase (SOD) and catalase;
- Measuring both the GSH-dependent enzyme, i.e., GPx and GR activities, and the GSH levels, either inside or outside the cell;
- Analysing the redox states of the NAD and NADP pyridine nucleotide pools, which play critical roles in defining the activity of energy producing pathways and in both driving oxidative stress and maintaining antioxidant defences, respectively;
- Identify the involvement of CFTR—if any—as part of the GSH cycle.

It is noteworthy that the objective was not to study changes in enzymatic activities and/or metabolite levels, but to understand the interaction dynamics existing between enzymes and levels of metabolites/cofactors.

The findings, i.e., the increased production of ROS is crucial to the progression of CF [131] and, consistently, the high levels of lipid and protein oxidation products found in bronchoalveolar lavage fluid of CF patients [142], prompted us to investigate further the origin of ROS in CF, besides those coming out by mitochondria activity.

5.2.2. Defective CFTR and NOX/GR Activity Imbalance Contribute to ROS Overproduction

Together with mitochondria [136], NOX was the prominent source of ROS, as revealed by the ability of its inhibitor Diphenyliodonium (DPI) to drastically lower $O_2^{-\bullet}$ level in cells. Moreover, that NOX preferentially uses NADPH over NADH as an electron donor turned out to be extremely interesting—if you think that NADPH mainly plays an important role in fighting oxidative stress (see below). This conclusion was strengthened by NADPH oxidase protein overexpression [116]. Consistently, it is largely known that increased oxidative stress and enhanced ROS production [151] may largely originate from enhanced and/or inappropriate NOX activation in chronic diseases of the respiratory tract, such as COPD, asthma, CF, or in various forms of lung cancer.

However, considering that excessive levels of extracellular and intracellular ROS may result from increased ROS production but also from defective cellular antioxidant (AOX) system, the authors—in the same study—showed a 50% decrease of GR activity, probably due to post-translational enzyme modification since GR protein level remained unchanged.

Then, we are dealing with a perturbation of the equilibrium between two enzymes working in opposition, i.e., NOX, requiring NADPH to produce $O_2^{-\bullet}$, and GR, using NADPH to restore GSH levels, with NADPH being probably channelled preferentially towards NOX rather than GR reaction. In order to confirm that really GR and NOX are competing for cytosolic NADPH, it was observed that GR reaction rate increased in CF cells incubated with NOX inhibitor DPI (Figure 2).

Interesting to note that though an increase of SOD activity—but not of catalase and GPx—was found in CF cells, a slight increase of ROS level was detected in the presence of SOD inhibitor, suggesting a negligible action of this enzyme in protecting CF cells against pro-oxidant insults.

Bounteous of information, useful to our research aim, was the study on the modulation of the ratios of the redox-active cofactors NADH/NAD$^+$, NADPH/NADP$^+$ and GSH/GSSG which hit cell metabolism, an unexplored realm in the search for CF.

Under normal conditions—as reported above (see Section 3.2)—the NADH/NAD+ pair is predominately in the oxidised state (see above); in contrast, the redox pairs NADPH/NADP$^+$ and GSH/GSSG are biased towards the reduced state to supply electrons for reductive biosynthesis and antioxidative processes, respectively.

An overturned situation was found in CF: the cytosolic redox state of the NADH/NAD+ pair was inclined to the reduced state, whereas the NADPH/NADP$^+$ pair to the oxidized one's. These results confirmed the reduced mtCx-I activity to oxidise NADH due to low OXPHOS [129] and, in addition, they suggested that the reduced quantity of NADPH, the main cellular reducing equivalent required by many antioxidant defence systems [152,153], could be responsible, totally or in part, for the low intracellular GSH (inGSH) level (see below) and then have a profound effect on ROS levels in CF cells. In this regard, to avoid getting in the experimental details, we invite the reader to read how the experiments were made as well as the strategic procedure adopted in order to understand the mechanism by which CFTR modulates extracellular GSH (exGSH) level in CF airway cells.

Regarding GSH levels, both extra- and intracellular, this issue merits some considerations. Indeed, since exGSH level is low and it depends on its impaired transport across plasma membrane due to deficient CFTR function, this suggests that contrariwise inGSH increased. But, surprisingly—and contrary to expectations—we found a significant decrease in inGSH content in CF cells, in accordance with [154], which was largely prevented by VX-809-treatment (about 100%).

Then, investigating on the inGSH level which depends upon the equilibrium between its consumption and biosynthesis, the latter process being limited by CYS availability [150,155], we guessed that the CYS could have a role in this dynamics. To confirm this, an increase of inGSH (about 50%) was found when CF cells were preincubated with CYS, suggesting that when CYS is available outside the cells, it is used for intracellular GSH synthesis (see [156]) (see Figure 2). The hypothesis that we advanced thanks to the obtained experimental observations was that a low exGSH amount, consequent to the CFTR deficit, can contribute to the decrease of inGSH level due to a reduced CYS regeneration by γGT (see Figure 2). In support to this hypothesis, we found that: (*i*) treating CF cells with Acivicin (ACI), specific γGT inhibitor [157], the inGSH level further decreased, even below that obtained in untreated CF cells, but it recovered up when cells were treated with ACI plus CYS; (*ii*) treating normal cells with CFTR(inh)-172, a specific inhibitor of CFTR channel [158], the inGSH level decreased of about 40% with respect to the inGSH level of untreated cells and it was almost completely restored when CYS was added together with CFTR(inh)-172.

What has been said so far leads to firmly setting salient points: (*i*) in CF cells some steps of OXPHOS are impaired, with both mitochondrial ROS production and membrane lipid peroxidation increase; (*ii*) ROS overproduction is also due to increased NOX activity; (*iii*) the overt oxidative stress condition elicits the loss of cell redox balance—a condition which sees the involvement of GSH in the front row—with deleterious consequences for metabolic regulation.

This should be kept in mind, especially in light of what will be described in the next paragraphs. Starting from the observation that the high ASL GLU concentration in human patients with CF [87] is responsible for the burst of the lung infection by pathogens [159], together with the highly expression of CFTR in the airway epithelium, it is reasonable to think that a CFTR defect leads to changes in the ASL lining the lungs, causing poor clearance of bacteria which ultimately exacerbates inflammation (see [39,160]).

The current model for airway GLU homeostasis assumes that the concentration of GLU in the ASL is the net effect of paracellular diffusion (and, to a lesser extent, the transcellular flux of GLU) from the blood and interstitial fluid across respiratory epithelium into the ASL and removal of GLU from ASL by GLU transporters (GLUTs) and cellular metabolic enzyme/s [161]. In this context, a metabolomic approach had revealed that the levels of glucose and various glycolytic intermediates were significantly reduced in CF cells [148]. Furthermore, increased activity of four glycolytic enzymes in cultured fibroblasts from CF patients was found [162], whereas in 1981, researchers found a G6PDH deficiency in CF [131].

Our new research path aimed to investigate some of the thousands of metabolic reactions (see Section 5.2.3)—those related to glucose metabolism and the production of NADPH—with the ultimate aim to restrict GLU availability in the ASL, action of extreme importance in order to control lung infection by pathogens.

With the term 'cellular metabolism' refers to the complex set of chemical reactions that permit cells, organs, and entire organisms to function and thrive. Although cellular metabolism is often discussed in the context of individual pathways, survival of an organism is ultimately dependent on the integration of all metabolic pathways. In fact, other than glycolysis, no major metabolic pathway functions entirely on its own; for example, the PPP most commonly relies on G6P from glycolysis in order to proceed, and lipid synthesis cannot move forward without input of both NADPH and ATP from at least two other metabolic pathways. While numerous other examples could be highlighted, the major point is that biochemical events in one metabolic pathway cannot be easily understood if discussed only in isolation.

According to a logical assumption, we all were agreed that the extracellular GLU-lowering action exerted by cell membrane transporter/s and cytosolic enzymes was necessary, but perhaps not sufficient. Biochemical approaches have allowed to respond to questions about how G6P is partitioned between glycolytic and PPP and whether the PPP, appropriately controlled, plays a crucial role against oxidative stress in CF cells. Strategic manipulations of both GLU-utilizing pathway enzymes, i.e., Glycolysis and PPP, and mitochondrial function proved useful for understanding how the cells could fight the high load of ASL GLU and ROS in CF.

5.2.3. Modulation of Glucose-Related Metabolic Pathways Helps both Reduce Glucose Level in ASL and Fight Oxidative Stress

Lung epithelial cells are able to oxidize GLU to produce energy (see Section 3.4). The availability of intracellular GLU is under the control of GLUTs that not only control its movement across the lung epithelium, but are also involved in regulating GLU level in ASL. Once inside the cell, GLU is immediately metabolized by cytosolic enzymes (for detail see above, Sections 3.1 and 3.4).

Considering that the metabolic pathways of glycolysis, Krebs cycle and respiratory chain are tightly interconnected, it becomes easy to realize that any alteration in mitochondrial respiration (see [125,136]) or in the processes regulating GLU uptake and utilization, inevitably involve both mitochondrial and cytosolic metabolic pathways, mutually (see Figure 2).

As far as the GLU metabolism in airways cells is concerned, the first step is the uptake across the cell membrane. In this regard, Garnett et al. [92] have demonstrated that in human H441 airway cells the levels of GLU2 and GLUT10 can be modulated by pro-inflammatory stimuli. Consistently, it has recently been demonstrated that not only GLUT activity increases but also the protein level of GLUT1, the most ubiquitously expressed isoform of GLU transporter in humans (see [161]), is upregulated. However, the overall upregulation of GLU transport seems not to be sufficient to prevent the rise of GLU concentration in ASL. This does not exclude a priori the possibility to intervene on a mechanism that could dynamically regulate the ASL GLU level as it increases during inflammation.

In addition to GLUT, also the activity of the two most important glycolytic enzymes, HK and PFK, increased in CF cells, as well as their protein levels although to a lesser extent. Similarly, in fibroblasts from CF patients, the increase in the activity of four glycolytic enzymes was detected [162].

Different was the situation for G6PDH, a key enzyme in regulating the GSH availability and ensuring protection against cellular ROS in healthy cell. Enzymatic activity and protein level of G6PDH decreased in CF cells as compared to control cells. These findings strongly support the close relationship between NADPH and GSH level decrease (see above) and G6PDH decrease in CF cells where ROS level increased [116].

Recently, a deep investigation has been carried out as to whether a relationship exists between the redox state of the cell and the GLU metabolism both inside the cell and in ALS, taking advantage of a set of compounds able to modulate G6P utilization and glycolytic ATP production.

It was found that in the presence of 6-aminonicotinamide (6AN), G6PDH inhibitor, the level of G6P was almost doubled while ROS levels were reduced by a half, thus suggesting that (i) in CF cells G6P is preferentially metabolized through PPP and (ii) PPP-derived NADPH is likely to be the driving force to generate NOX-derived ROS, being the latter an enzyme whose activity overcomes that of GR [116] (see above, Section 5.2.2).

Unexpectedly, G6P and ASL GLU levels were unchanged in CF cells in the presence of CITR, an anti-glycolytic agent that inhibits PFK, thereby largely inhibiting phosphorylation at the substrate level and slowing glycolysis. This singular effect suggests that when PFK is inhibited by CITR, glycolytic flux is 'gated', as confirmed also by the collapse in L-LAC level. In this condition, G6P reaches a sort of 'steady-state' level being able to inhibit HK from one side, so that no further production of G6P occurs, and to be metabolized by G6PDH along PPP on the other side. Thus, in the presence of CITR, the cell is forced to produce more NADPH, also thanks to a more active G6PDH, in a sort of compensatory mechanism for the inhibited activity of glycolysis and the reduced mitochondrial ETC (see above, Section 5.2.1).

Surprisingly, although the NADPH level increased, the ROS level actually decreased in the presence of CITR in CF cells, suggesting that the increase in NADPH level in the presence of CITR was not able to accelerate NOX activity, thus confirming the hypothesis that the point at which the glycolytic flow is blocked—by CITR—is crucial for the regulation of cell redox status in CF. These results agree with the observations that a high NADPH level is required in CF in response to infection [152] as well as in the temptative to counteract the ongoing oxidative stress [125,131,136].

When the activity of mitochondrial respiratory chain is inhibited at level of Complex I and IV, i.e., in the presence of ROT+OLIGO, a low level of G6P but an increase in L-LAC are detected and these results can be easily explained as an extreme tentative of the cell to upregulate the glycolytic enzymes metabolizing G6P to prevent its accumulation, consistent with Glycolytic index (GI) increase.

Interestingly, GI values, per se higher in CF as compared to control cells (3.1 versus 0.8), further increased when CF cells were treated with ROT+OLIGO confirming that when residual mitochondrial activity is inhibited, cell metabolism strictly depends on the anaerobic glycolytic pathway.

We are facing a dizzying situation: the reduction of mitochondrial respiration seems to be advantageous for the reduction of GLU of ASL and also for the reduction of the level of ROS in CF cells.

To disentangle ourselves in this complex matter, with the aim to interpret the metabolic environment of ASL in CF, two models of disease (Alzheimer's disease and cancer) in which cooperation was observed between mitochondria and glycolytic enzymes have intervened [163].

Due to the close co-operation between cytosolic metabolism, i.e., glycolysis, and mitochondria, it is understandable that when glycolysis is inhibited at the level of PFK, the supply of pyruvate to mitochondria will be reduced with consequent reduction in mitochondrial activity. Indeed, in the presence of CITR, i.e., when mitochondria functions are repressed, the general conditions of CF cells seem to be improved both inside as well outside.

Accordingly, in CF cells treated with CITR, and even more with ROT+OLIGO, the ROS level decreased thus suggesting that ROS-dependent mitochondrial metabolism is central to disease as well as a crucial element of the CF phenotype. On the other hand, the findings that both upregulation of glycolytic enzymes and downregulation of G6PDH, occurring in CF cells, did not reduce ASL GLU clearly suggest that mitochondrial activity has a prominent role in CF cells and, thus, only a low efficiency of mitochondria may restrain the progressive impairment of CF cells.

In conclusion, when the mitochondria are quiescent, i.e., when mitochondrial activity is below a certain threshold value—mitochondria dictate the conditions in which the cell is, having a beneficial effect detectable in the lowering of both ROS and ASL GLU levels, responsible of infection by pathogens in CF.

## 6. Conclusion Remarks

As it is clear from the discussion above, mitochondrial functions extend beyond the boundaries of the cell and influence an organism's physiology by regulating communication between cells and tissues. It is therefore not surprising that mitochondrial dysfunction has emerged as a key factor in a myriad of diseases.

Then, the research field aimed at "targeting mitochondria" is active and expanding.

It goes without saying that one of the important objectives of managing patients with mitochondrial disorders is to prevent drugs from being toxic to mitochondrial functions. In fact, drugs can affect many of the different functions within the mitochondria. Drug therapy-induced ETC dysfunction may result from the direct inhibition of one or more of the enzyme complexes or uncoupling of OXPHOS. As the enzyme complexes are susceptible to free radical-induced oxidative damage, drugs that cause oxidative stress may also result in ETC toxicity.

Significant progress has been made over the last several decades in understanding of energy metabolism in the lung. Recent technological advances have enabled researchers to go beyond studying just whole organ metabolism and begin dissecting the metabolic events driving common and unique behaviours in individual cell populations in the lung. Although the pulmonary community has made significant progress, understanding of pulmonary metabolism still lags behind that of many other fields.

In order to deal with these problems, it will need to invest more heavily in the field, including taking advantage of recent forefront technologies with the wish to yield new biological insights and also to identify previously unrecognized biological markers that can aid in the diagnosis, screening, and/or monitoring of respiratory diseases. Understanding the molecular mechanisms regulating the mitochondrial function of lung cells will help to better define phenotypes and clinical manifestations associated with respiratory diseases and to identify potential diagnostic and therapeutic targets.

Regarding CF, what has been described currently is a pure basic research study, but investigating a poorly explored and undoubtedly interesting topic, i.e., the optimizing of the mitochondrial metabolism knowledge, could prove to be valuable in the future, reaching the focus of an effective therapeutic treatment and assisting the CF patient.

As such, we maintain that it would be interesting if mitochondrial functions were studied in other cells, such as macrophages and neutrophils, considering the importance these cells have in the progression of the disease, as briefly described above (Section 2.1.4).

**Author Contributions:** M.F. and A.A. designed the review outline, wrote the sections—i.e., CF and mitochondria, respectively—and the conclusion and reviewed and edited the entire manuscript. L.d.B. critically discussed and contributed to the final version of the manuscript. A.B. contributed to figure development and critically discussed the entire manuscript.

**Acknowledgments:** The authors thank R.L. for constructive criticism of the manuscript and for assisting with English language editing.

**Conflicts of Interest:** The authors declare no conflicts of interest.

## Abbreviations

| | |
|---|---|
| 6AN | 6-aminonicotinamide |
| ABC | ATP Binding Cassette |
| ACI | Acivicin |
| ANT | Adenine nucleotide translocase |
| AOX | Antioxidant system |
| ASL | Airway surface liquid |
| ATP | Adenosine 5′-triphosphate |
| CF | Cystic Fibrosis |
| CFTR | Cystic Fibrosis Transmembrane Conductance Regulator |
| CITR | Citrate |
| COPII | Protein Complex II |
| COX | Mitochondrial Complex IV |
| CYS | Cysteine |
| DPI | Diphenyliodonium |
| $\Delta\Psi$ | Mitochondrial membrane potential |
| ENaC | Epithelial sodium channel |
| ER | Endoplasmic reticulum |
| ETC | Electron transport chain |
| exGSH | Extracellular GSH |
| GI | Glycolytic index |
| GLU | Glucose |
| GLUT | Glucose transporter |
| G6P | Glucose-6-phpsphate |
| G6PDH | Glucose-6-phosphate dehydrogenase |
| GPx | Glutathione peroxidase |
| GR | Glutathione reductase |
| GSH | Reduced glutathione |
| GSSG | Glutathione disulphide |
| CYS | Cysteine |
| γ-GT | γ-glutamyltransferase |
| γ-GCS | γ-glutamylcysteine synthase |
| HK | Hexokinase |
| $H_2O_2$ | Hydrogen peroxide |
| ICDH | Isocitrate dehydrogenase |
| IMS | Intermembrane space |
| inGSH | Intracellular GSH |
| L-LAC | L-lactate |
| MDH | Malate dehydrogenase |
| ME | Malic enzyme |
| mtCx-I | Mitochondrial Complex I |
| mGSH | mitochondrial GSH |
| Mirs | microRNAs |
| NAC | N-acetylcysteine |
| NOX | NAD(P)H oxidases |
| $O_2$ | Molecular oxygen |

| | |
|---|---|
| $O_2^{-\bullet}$ | Superoxide anion radical |
| OLIGO | Oligomycin |
| OXPHOS | Oxidative phosphorylation |
| PFK | Phosphofructokinase |
| PKA | Protein kinase A |
| PPP | Pentose phosphate pathway |
| ROS | Reactive oxygen species |
| ROT | Rotenone |
| SOD | Superoxide dismutase |
| TCA | Tricarboxylic acid cycle |
| TMA | 4,6,4′-trimethylangelicin |

## References

1. McBride, H.M. Open questions: Seeking a holistic approach for mitochondrial research. *BMC Biol.* **2015**, *13*, 8. [CrossRef] [PubMed]
2. Pagliarini, D.J.; Rutter, J. Hallmarks of a new era in mitochondrial biochemistry. *Genes Dev.* **2013**, *27*, 2615–2627. [CrossRef] [PubMed]
3. Elborn, J.S. Cystic fibrosis. *Lancet* **2016**, *388*, 2519–2531. [CrossRef]
4. Riordan, J.R. CFTR and prospects for therapy. *Annu. Rev. Biochem.* **2008**, *77*, 701–726. [CrossRef] [PubMed]
5. Farrel, P.M. The prevalence of cystic fibrosis in the European Union. *J. Cyst. Fibros.* **2008**, *7*, 450–453. [CrossRef]
6. McCormick, J.; Mehta, G.; Olesen, H.V.; Viviani, L.; Macek, M., Jr.; Mehta, A.; European Registry Working Group. Comparative demographics of the European cystic fibrosis population: A cross-sectional database analysis. *Lancet* **2010**, *375*, 1007–1013. [CrossRef]
7. Riordan, J.R.; Rommens, J.M.; Kerem, B.; Alon, N.; Rozmahel, R.; Grzelczak, Z.; Zielenski, J.; Lok, S.; Plavsic, N.; Chou, J.-L.; et al. Identification of the cystic fibrosis gene: Cloning and characterization of complementary DNA. *Science* **1989**, *245*, 1066–1073. [CrossRef]
8. Rowe, S.M.; Miller, S.; Sorscher, E.J. Cystic fibrosis. *N. Engl. J. Med.* **2005**, *352*, 1992–2001. [CrossRef]
9. Chan, H.C.; Ruan, Y.C.; He, Q.; Chen, M.H.; Chen, H.; Xu, W.M.; Chen, W.Y.; Xie, C.; Zhang, X.H.; Zhou, Z. The cystic fibrosis transmembrane conductance regulator in reproductive health and disease. *J. Physiol.* **2009**, *587*, 2187–2195. [CrossRef]
10. Frizzell, R.A.; Hanrahan, J.W. Physiology of epithelian chloride and fluid secretion. *Cold Spring Harb. Perspect. Med.* **2012**, *2*, a009563. [CrossRef]
11. Quinton, P.M. Physiological basis of cystic fibrosis: A historical perspective. *Physiol. Rev.* **1999**, *79*, S3–S22. [CrossRef] [PubMed]
12. O'Sullivan, B.P.; Freedman, S.D. Cystic fibrosis. *Lancet* **2009**, *373*, 1891–1904. [CrossRef]
13. Yoshimura, K.; Nakamura, H.; Trapnell, B.C.; Chu, C.S.; Dalemans, W.; Pavirani, A.; Lecocq, J.P.; Crystal, R.G. Expression of the cystic fibrosis transmembrane conductance regulator gene in cells of non-epithelial origin. *Nucleic Acids Res.* **1991**, *19*, 5417–5423. [CrossRef] [PubMed]
14. Levesque, P.C.; Hart, P.J.; Hume, J.R.; Kenyon, J.L.; Horowitz, B. Expression of cystic fibrosis transmembrane regulator Cl channels in heart. *Circ. Res.* **1992**, *71*, 1002–1007. [CrossRef]
15. Horowitz, B.; Tsung, S.S.; Hart, P.; Levesque, P.C.; Hume, J.R. Alternative splicing of CFTRCl channels inheart. *Am. J. Physiol.* **1993**, *264*, H2214–H2220.
16. Tizzano, E.F.; Chitayat, D.; Buchwald, M. Cell-specific localization of CFTR mRNA shows developmentally regulated expression in human fetal tissues. *Hum. Mol. Genet.* **1993**, *2*, 219–224. [CrossRef]
17. Mulberg, A.E.; Wiedner, E.B.; Bao, X.; Marshall, J.; Jefferson, D.M.; Altschuler, S.M. Cystic fibrosis transmembrane conductance regulator protein expression in brain. *Neuroreport* **1994**, *5*, 1684–1688. [CrossRef]
18. Kulka, M.; Gilchrist, M.; Duszyk, M.; Befus, A.D. Expression and functional characterization of CFTR in mast cells. *J. Leukoc. Biol.* **2002**, *71*, 54–64.
19. Lange, T.; Jungmann, P.; Haberle, J.; Falk, S.; Duebbers, A.; Bruns, R.; Ebner, A.; Hinterdorfer, P.; Oberleithner, H.; Schillers, H. Reduced number of CFTR molecules in erythrocyte plasma membrane of cystic fibrosis patients. *Mol. Membr. Biol.* **2006**, *23*, 317–323. [CrossRef]

20. Swahn, H.; Harris, A. Cell-selective regulation of CFTR gene expression: Relevance to gene editing therapeutics. *Genes* **2019**, *10*, 235. [CrossRef]
21. Schwiebert, E.M.; Benos, D.J.; Egan, M.E.; Stutts, M.J.; Guggino, W.B. CFTR is a conductance regulator as well as a chloride channel. *Physiol. Rev.* **1999**, *79*, S145–S166. [CrossRef] [PubMed]
22. Sheppard, D.N.; Welsh, M.J. Structure and function of the CFTR chloride channel. *Physiol. Rev.* **1999**, *79*, S23–S45. [CrossRef] [PubMed]
23. Cheng, S.H.; Rich, D.P.; Marshall, J.; Gregory, R.J.; Welsh, M.J.; Smith, A.E. Phosphorylation of the R domain by cAMP-dependent protein kinase regulates the CFTR chloride channel. *Cell* **1991**, *66*, 1027–1036. [CrossRef]
24. Berger, A.L.; Ikuma, M.; Welsh, M.J. Normal gating of CFTR requires ATP binding to both nucleotide-binding domains and hydrolysis at the second nucleotide-binding domain. *Proc. Natl. Acad. Sci. USA* **2005**, *102*, 455–460. [CrossRef]
25. Vergani, P.; Lockless, S.W.; Nairn, A.C.; Gadsby, D.C. CFTR channel opening by ATP-driven tight dimerization of its nucleotide-binding domains. *Nature* **2005**, *433*, 876–880. [CrossRef]
26. Csanady, L.; Vergani, P.; Gadsby, D.C. Strict coupling between CFTR's catalytic cycle and gating of its Cl$^-$ ion pore revealed by distributions of open channel burst durations. *Proc. Natl. Acad. Sci. USA* **2010**, *107*, 1241–1246. [CrossRef]
27. Naren, A.P.; Cobb, B.; Li, C.; Roy, K.; Nelson, D.; Heda, G.D.; Liao, J.; Kirk, K.L.; Sorscher, E.J.; Hanrahan, J.; et al. A macromolecular complex of beta 2 adrenergic receptor, CFTR, and ezrin/radixin/moesin-binding phosphoprotein 50 is regulated by PKA. *Proc. Natl. Acad. Sci. USA* **2003**, *100*, 342–346. [CrossRef]
28. Li, C.; Naren, A.P. Macromolecular complexes of cystic fibrosis transmembrane conductance regulator and its interacting partners. *Pharmacol. Ther.* **2005**, *108*, 208–223. [CrossRef]
29. Li, C.; Naren, A.P. Analysis of CFTR interactome in the macromolecular complexes. *Methods Mol. Biol.* **2011**, *741*, 255–270.
30. Zhang, W.; Penmatsa, H.; Ren, A.; Punchihewa, C.; Lemoff, A.; Yan, B.; Fujii, N.; Naren, A.P. Functional regulation of cystic fibrosis transmembrane conductance regulator-containing macromolecular complexes: A small-molecule inhibitor approach. *Biochem. J.* **2011**, *435*, 451–462. [CrossRef]
31. Guerra, L.; Fanelli, T.; Favia, M.; Riccardi, S.M.; Busco, G.; Cardone, R.A.; Carrabino, S.; Weinman, E.J.; Reshkin, S.J.; Conese, M.; et al. Na$^+$/H$^+$ exchanger regulatory factor isoform 1 overexpression modulates cystic fibrosis transmembrane conductance regulator (CFTR) expression and activity in human airway 16HBE14o- cells and rescues DeltaF508 CFTR functional expression in cystic fibrosis cells. *J. Biol. Chem.* **2005**, *280*, 40925–40933. [PubMed]
32. Favia, M.; Guerra, L.; Fanelli, T.; Cardone, R.A.; Monterisi, S.; Di Sole, F.; Castellani, S.; Chen, M.; Seidler, U.; Reshkin, S.J.; et al. Na$^+$/H$^+$ exchanger regulatory factor 1 overexpression-dependent increase of cytoskeleton organization is fundamental in the rescue of F508del cystic fibrosis transmembrane conductance regulator in human airway CFBE41o- cells. *Mol. Biol. Cell* **2010**, *21*, 73–86. [CrossRef] [PubMed]
33. Rogan, M.P.; Stoltz, D.A.; Hornick, D.B. Cystic fibrosis transmembrane conductance regulator intracellular processing, trafficking, and opportunities for mutation-specific treatment. *Chest* **2011**, *139*, 1480–1490. [CrossRef] [PubMed]
34. Yang, Y.; Janich, S.; Cohn, J.A.; Wilson, J.M. The common variant of cystic fibrosis transmembrane conductance regulator is recognized by hsp70 and degraded in a pre-Golgi nonlysosomal compartment. *Proc. Natl. Acad. Sci. USA* **1993**, *90*, 9480–9484. [CrossRef] [PubMed]
35. Cheung, J.C.; Deber, C.M. Misfolding of the cystic fibrosis transmembrane conductance regulator and disease. *Biochemistry* **2008**, *47*, 1465–1473. [CrossRef] [PubMed]
36. Pind, S.; Riordan, J.R.; Williams, D.B. Participation of the endoplasmic reticulum chaperone calnexin (p88, IP90) in the biogenesis of the cystic fibrosis transmembrane conductance regulator. *J. Biol. Chem.* **1994**, *269*, 12784–12788. [PubMed]
37. Turnbull, E.L.; Rosser, M.F.; Cyr, D.M. The role of the UPS in cystic fibrosis. *BMC Biochem.* **2007**, *8*, S11. [CrossRef]
38. Cheng, J.; Wang, H.; Guggino, W.B. Modulation of mature cystic fibrosis transmembrane regulator protein by the PDZ domain protein CAL. *J. Biol. Chem.* **2004**, *279*, 1892–1898. [CrossRef]
39. Saint-Criq, V.; Gray, M.A. Role of CFTR in epithelial physiology. *Cell. Mol. Life Sci.* **2017**, *74*, 93–115. [CrossRef]

40. Kogan, I.; Ramjeesingh, M.; Li, C.; Kidd, J.F.; Wang, Y.; Leslie, E.M.; Cole, S.P.; Bear, C.E. CFTR directly mediates nucleotide-regulated glutathione flux. *EMBO J.* **2003**, *22*, 1981–1989. [CrossRef]
41. Boucher, R.C. Status of gene therapy for cystic fibrosis lung disease. *J. Clin. Investig.* **1999**, *103*, 441–445. [CrossRef] [PubMed]
42. Fahy, J.V.; Dickey, B.F. Airway mucus function and dysfunction. *N. Engl. J. Med.* **2010**, *363*, 2233–2247. [CrossRef] [PubMed]
43. Hull, J. Cystic fibrosis transmembrane conductance regulator dysfunction and its treatment. *J. R. Soc. Med.* **2012**, *105* (Suppl. 2), S2–S8, review. [CrossRef] [PubMed]
44. Zhang, S.; Shrestha, C.L.; Kopp, B.T. Cystic fibrosis transmembrane conductance regulator (CFTR) modulators have differential effects on cystic fibrosis macrophage function. *Sci. Rep.* **2018**, *8*, 17066. [CrossRef]
45. Ratner, D.; Mueller, C. Immune responses in cystic fibrosis: Are they intrinsically defective? *Am. J. Respir. Cell Mol. Biol.* **2012**, *46*, 715–722. [CrossRef]
46. Tazi, M.F.; Dakhlallah, D.A.; Caution, K.; Gerber, M.M.; Chang, S.W.; Khalil, H.; Kopp, B.T.; Ahmed, A.E.; Krause, K.; Davis, I.; et al. Elevated Mirc1/Mir17-92 cluster expression negatively regulates autophagy and CFTR (cystic fibrosis transmembrane conductance regulator) function in CF macrophages. *Autophagy* **2016**, *12*, 2026–2037. [CrossRef]
47. Painter, R.G.; Valentine, V.G.; Lanson, N.A., Jr.; Leidal, K.; Zhang, Q.; Lombard, G.; Thompson, C.; Viswanathan, A.; Nauseef, W.M.; Wang, G.; et al. CFTR expression in human neutrophils and the phagolysosomal chlorination defect in cystic fibrosis. *Biochemistry* **2006**, *45*, 10260–10269. [CrossRef]
48. Bonfield, T.; Chmiel, J.F. Impaired innate immune cells in cystic fibrosis: Is it really a surprise? *J. Cyst. Fibr.* **2017**, *16*, 433–435. [CrossRef]
49. Lukacs, G.L.; Verkman, A.S. CFTR: Folding, misfolding and correcting the ∆F508 conformational defect. *Trends Mol. Med.* **2012**, *18*, 81–91. [CrossRef]
50. Kälin, N.; Claaß, A.; Sommer, M.; Puchelle, E.; Tümmler, B. ∆F508 CFTR protein expression in tissues from patients with cystic fibrosis. *J. Clin. Investig.* **1999**, *103*, 1379–1389. [CrossRef]
51. Bronsveld, I.; Mekus, F.; Bijman, J.; Ballmann, M.; de Jonge, H.R.; Laabs, U.; Halley, D.J.; Ellemunter, H.; Mastella, G.; Thomas, S.; et al. Chloride conductance and genetic background modulate the cystic fibrosis phenotype of ∆F508 homozygous twins and siblings. *J. Clin. Investig.* **2001**, *108*, 1705–1715. [CrossRef] [PubMed]
52. Gentzsch, M.; Choudhury, A.; Chang, X.B.; Pagano, R.E.; Riordan, J.R. Misassembled mutant DeltaF508 CFTR in the distal secretory pathway alters cellular lipid trafficking. *J. Cell Sci.* **2007**, *120*, 447–455. [CrossRef] [PubMed]
53. Swiatecka-Urban, A.; Brown, A.; Moreau-Marquis, S.; Renuka, J.; Coutermarsh, B.; Barnaby, R.; Karlson, K.H.; Flotte, T.R.; Fukuda, M.; Langford, G.M.; et al. The short apical membrane half-life of rescued ∆F508-cystic fibrosis transmembrane conductance regulator (CFTR) results from accelerated endocytosis of ∆F508-CFTR in polarized human airway epithelial cells. *J. Biol. Chem.* **2005**, *280*, 36762–36772. [CrossRef] [PubMed]
54. Castellani, C.; Assael, B.M. Cystic fibrosis: A clinical view. *Cell. Mol. Life Sci.* **2017**, *74*, 129–140. [CrossRef] [PubMed]
55. Burgel, P.-R.; Bellis, G.; Olesen, H.; Viviani, L.; Zolin, A.; Blasi, F.; Elborn, J.S. Future trends in cystic fibrosis demography in 34 European countries. *Eur. Respir. J.* **2015**, *46*, 133–141.
56. MacConnachie, A.M. Dornase-alfa (DNase, Pulmozyme) for cystic fibrosis. *Intensive Crit. Care Nurs.* **1998**, *14*, 101–102. [CrossRef]
57. Reeves, E.P.; Molloy, K.; Pohl, K.; McElvaney, N.G. Hypertonic saline in treatment of pulmonary disease in cystic fibrosis. *Sci. World J.* **2012**, *2012*, 465230. [CrossRef] [PubMed]
58. Suri, R. The use of human deoxyribonuclease (rhDNase) in the management of cystic fibrosis. *BioDrugs* **2005**, *19*, 135–144. [CrossRef]
59. Pisi, G.; Chetta, A. Airway clearance therapy in cystic fibrosis patients. *Acta Biomed.* **2009**, *80*, 102–106.
60. Adler, F.R.; Aurora, P.; Barker, D.H.; Barr, M.L.; Blackwell, L.S.; Bosma, O.H.; Brown, S.; Cox, D.R.; Jensen, J.L.; Kurland, G.; et al. Lung transplantation for cystic fibrosis. *Proc. Am. Thorac. Soc.* **2009**, *6*, 619–633. [CrossRef]
61. Favia, M.; Mancini, M.T.; Bezzerri, V.; Guerra, L.; Laselva, O.; Abbattiscianni, A.C.; Debellis, L.; Reshkin, S.J.; Gambari, R.; Cabrini, G.; et al. Trimethylangelicin promotes the functional rescue of mutant F508del CFTR protein in cystic fibrosis airway cells. *Am. J. Physiol. Lung Cell. Mol. Physiol.* **2014**, *307*, L48–L61. [CrossRef] [PubMed]

62. Van Goor, F.; Hadida, S.; Grootenhuis, P.D.; Burton, B.; Stack, J.H.; Straley, K.S.; Decker, C.J.; Miller, M.; McCartney, J.; Olson, E.R.; et al. Correction of the F508del-CFTR protein processing defect in vitro by the investigational drug VX-809. *Proc. Natl. Acad. Sci. USA* **2011**, *108*, 18843–18848. [CrossRef] [PubMed]
63. Zhao, K.Q.; Xiong, G.; Wilber, M.; Cohen, N.A.; Kreindler, J.L. A role for two-pore $K^+$ channels in modulating $Na^+$ absorption and $Cl^-$ secretion in normal human bronchial epithelial cells. *Am. J. Physiol. Lung Cell. Mol. Physiol.* **2012**, *302*, L4–L12. [CrossRef] [PubMed]
64. Schiffhauer, E.S.; Vij, N.; Kovbasnjuk, O.; Kang, P.W.; Walker, D.; Lee, S.; Zeitlin, P.L. Dual activation of CFTR and CLCN2 by lubiprostone in murine nasal epithelia. *Am. J. Physiol. Lung Cell. Mol. Physiol.* **2013**, *304*, L324–L331. [CrossRef] [PubMed]
65. Griesenbach, U.; Davies, J.C.; Alton, E. Cystic fibrosis gene therapy: A mutation-independent treatment. *Curr. Opin. Pulm. Med.* **2016**, *22*, 602–609. [CrossRef] [PubMed]
66. Liu, G.; Summer, R. Cellular metabolism in lung health and disease. *Annu. Rev. Physiol.* **2019**, *81*, 403–428. [CrossRef]
67. O'Neil, J.J.; Tierney, D.F. Rat lung metabolism: Glucose utilization by isolated perfused lungs and tissue slices. *Am. J. Physiol.* **1974**, *226*, 867–873. [CrossRef]
68. Tierney, D.F. Intermediary metabolism of the lung. *Fed. Proc.* **1974**, *33*, 2232–2237.
69. Mustafa, M.G.; Cross, C.E. Effects of short-term ozone exposure on lung mitochondrial oxidative and energy metabolism. *Arch. Biochem. Biophys.* **1974**, *162*, 585–594. [CrossRef]
70. Hussien, R.; Brooks, G.A. Mitochondrial and plasma membrane lactate transporter and lactate dehydrogenase isoform expression in breast cancer cell lines. *Physiol. Genomics* **2011**, *43*, 255–264. [CrossRef]
71. Pagliarini, D.J.; Calvo, S.E.; Chang, B.; Sheth, S.A.; Vafai, S.B.; Ong, S.E.; Walford, G.A.; Sugiana, C.; Boneh, A.; Chen, W.K.; et al. A mitochondrial protein compendium elucidates complex I disease biology. *Cell* **2008**, *134*, 112–123. [CrossRef] [PubMed]
72. Faubert, B.; Li, K.Y.; Cai, L.; Hensley, C.T.; Kim, J.; Zacharias, L.G.; Yang, C.; Do, Q.N.; Doucette, S.; Burguete, D.; et al. Lactate metabolism in human lung tumors. *Cell* **2017**, *171*, 358–371.e9. [CrossRef] [PubMed]
73. Hüttemann, M.; Lee, I.; Gao, X.; Pecina, P.; Pecinova, A.; Liu, J.; Aras, S.; Sommer, N.; Sanderson, T.H.; Tost, M.; et al. Cytochrome c oxidase subunit 4 isoform 2-knockout mice show reduced enzyme activity, airway hyporeactivity, and lung pathology. *FASEB J.* **2012**, *26*, 3916–3930. [CrossRef] [PubMed]
74. Squadrito, G.L.; Cueto, R.; Dellinger, B.; Pryor, W.A. Quinoid redox cycling as a mechanism for sustained free radical generation by inhaled airborne particulate matter. *Free Radic. Biol. Med.* **2001**, *31*, 1132–1138. [CrossRef]
75. Dellinger, B.; Pryor, W.A.; Cueto, R.; Squadrito, G.L.; Hegde, V.; Deutsch, W.A. Role of free radicals in the toxicity of airborne fine particulate matter. *Chem. Res. Toxicol.* **2001**, *14*, 1371–1377. [CrossRef]
76. Aravamudan, B.; Thompson, M.A.; Pabelick, C.M.; Prakash, Y.S. Mitochondria in lung diseases. *Expert Rev. Respir. Med.* **2013**, *7*, 631–646. [CrossRef]
77. Segal, B.H.; Grimm, M.J.; Khan, A.N.; Han, W.; Blackwell, T.S. Regulation of innate immunity by NADPH oxidase. *Free Radic. Biol. Med.* **2012**, *53*, 72–80. [CrossRef]
78. van der Vliet, A. Nox enzymes in allergic airway inflammation. *Biochim. Biophys. Acta* **2011**, *1810*, 1035–1044. [CrossRef]
79. Brown, R.K.; Kelly, F.J. Evidence of increased oxidative damage in patients with cystic fibrosis. *Pediatr. Res.* **1994**, *36*, 1–7. [CrossRef]
80. Yagi, K. Lipid peroxides and human diseases. *Chem. Phys. Lipids* **1987**, *45*, 337–351. [CrossRef]
81. Galli, F.; Battistoni, A.; Gambari, R.; Pompella, A.; Bragonzi, A.; Pilolli, F.; Iuliano, L.; Piroddi, M.; Dechecchi, M.C.; Cabrini, G.; et al. Oxidative stress and antioxidant therapy in cystic fibrosis. *Biochim. Biophys. Acta* **2012**, *1822*, 690–713. [CrossRef] [PubMed]
82. Gandhi, V.D.; Vliagoftis, H. Airway epithelium interactions with aeroallergens: Role of secreted cytokines and chemokines in innate immunity. *Front. Immunol.* **2015**, *6*, 147. [CrossRef] [PubMed]
83. Collawn, J.F.; Lazrak, A.; Bebok, Z.; Matalon, S. The CFTR and ENaC debate: How important is ENaC in CF lung disease? *Am. J. Physiol. Lung Cell. Mol. Physiol.* **2012**, *302*, L1141–L1146. [CrossRef] [PubMed]
84. Kunzelmann, K.; Kathöfer, S.; Greger, R. $Na^+$ and $Cl^-$ conductances in airway epithelial cells: Increased $Na^+$ conductance in cystic fibrosis. *Pflugers. Arch* **1995**, *431*, 1–9. [CrossRef] [PubMed]

85. Boucher, R.C. Relationship of airway epithelial ion transport to chronic bronchitis. *Proc. Am. Thorac. Soc.* **2004**, *1*, 66–70. [CrossRef]
86. Zhao, R.; Liang, X.; Zhao, M.; Liu, S.L.; Huang, Y.; Idell, S.; Li, X.; Ji, H.L. Correlation of apical fluid-regulating channel proteins with lung function in human COPD lungs. *PLoS ONE* **2014**, *9*, e109725. [CrossRef]
87. Matthay, M.A.; Folkesson, H.G.; Clerici, C. Lung epithelial fluid transport and the resolution of pulmonary edema. *Physiol. Rev.* **2002**, *82*, 569–600. [CrossRef]
88. Zeitlin, P.L. Cystic fibrosis and estrogens: A perfect storm. *J. Clin. Investig.* **2008**, *118*, 3841–3844. [CrossRef]
89. Rhoades, R.A. Net uptake of glucose, glycerol, and fatty acids by the isolated perfused rat lung. *Am. J. Physiol.* **1974**, *226*, 144–149. [CrossRef]
90. Bearham, J.; Garnett, J.P.; Schroeder, V.; Biggart, M.G.; Baines, D.L. Effective glucose metabolism maintains low intracellular glucose in airway epithelial cells after exposure to hyperglycaemia. *Am. J. Physiol. Cell Physiol.* **2019**. [CrossRef]
91. Kalsi, K.K.; Baker, E.H.; Fraser, O.; Chung, Y.L.; Mace, O.J.; Tarelli, E.; Philips, B.J.; Baines, D.L. Glucose homeostasis across human airway epithelial cell monolayers: Role of diffusion, transport and metabolism. *Pflugers Arch.* **2009**, *457*, 1061–1070. [CrossRef] [PubMed]
92. Garnett, J.P.; Nguyen, T.T.; Moffatt, J.D.; Pelham, E.R.; Kalsi, K.K.; Baker, E.H.; Baines, D.L. Proinflammatory mediators disrupt glucose homeostasis in airway surface liquid. *J. Immunol.* **2012**, *189*, 373–380. [CrossRef] [PubMed]
93. Philips, B.J.; Redman, J.; Brennan, A.; Wood, D.; Holliman, R.; Baines, D.; Baker, E.H. Glucose in bronchial aspirates increases the risk of respiratory MRSA in intubated patients. *Thorax* **2005**, *60*, 761–764. [CrossRef] [PubMed]
94. Baker, E.H.; Clark, N.; Brennan, A.L.; Fisher, D.A.; Gyi, K.M.; Hodson, M.E.; Philips, B.J.; Baines, D.L.; Wood, D.M. Hyperglycemia and cystic fibrosis alter respiratory fluid glucose concentrations estimated by breath condensate analysis. *J. Appl. Physiol.* **1985**, *102*, 1969–1975. [CrossRef]
95. Wood, D.M.; Brennan, A.L.; Philips, B.J.; Baker, E.H. Effect of hyperglycaemia on glucose concentration of human nasal secretions. *Clin. Sci. (Lond.)* **2004**, *106*, 527–533. [CrossRef]
96. Bilodeau, C.; Bardou, O.; Maillé, É.; Berthiaume, Y.; Brochiero, E. Deleterious impact of hyperglycemia on cystic fibrosis airway ion transport and epithelial repair. *J. Cyst. Fibros.* **2016**, *15*, 43–51. [CrossRef]
97. Meo, S.A. Significance of spirometry in diabetic patients. *Int. J. Diabetes Mellit.* **2009**, *2*, 47–50. [CrossRef]
98. Duchen, M.R. Mitochondria in health and disease: Perspectives on a new mitochondrial biology. *Mol. Asp. Med.* **2004**, *25*, 365–451. [CrossRef]
99. Murphy, M.P. How mitochondria produce reactive oxygen species. *Biochem. J.* **2009**, *417*, 1–13. [CrossRef]
100. Murphy, M.P. Mitochondria—A neglected drug target. *Curr. Opin. Investig. Drugs* **2009**, *10*, 1022–1024.
101. Scarpulla, R.C. Transcriptional paradigms in mammalian mitochondrial biogenesis and function. *Physiol. Rev.* **2008**, *88*, 611–638. [CrossRef] [PubMed]
102. Nicholls, D.G.; Fergusson, S.J. *Bioenergetics*; Academic Press: Cambridge, MA, USA, 2013.
103. Diaz, F.; Kotarsky, H.; Fellman, V.; Moraes, C.T. Mitochondrial disorders caused by mutations in respiratory chain assembly factors. *Semin. Fetal Neonatal Med.* **2011**, *16*, 197–204. [CrossRef] [PubMed]
104. Efremov, R.G.; Sazanov, L.A. Respiratory complex I: 'Steam engine' of the cell? *Curr. Opin. Struct. Biol.* **2011**, *21*, 532–540. [CrossRef] [PubMed]
105. Mailloux, R.J.; Jin, X.; Willmore, W.G. Redox regulation of mitochondrial function with emphasis on cysteine oxidation reactions. *Redox Biol.* **2013**, *2*, 123–139. [CrossRef]
106. Mitchell, P. Coupling of phosphorylation to electron and hydrogen transfer by a chemi-osmotic type of mechanism. *Nature* **1961**, *191*, 144–148. [CrossRef]
107. Neupert, W.; Herrmann, J.M. Translocation of proteins into mitochondria. *Annu. Rev. Biochem.* **2007**, *76*, 723–749. [CrossRef]
108. Mailloux, R.J.; Harper, M.E. Uncoupling proteins and the control of mitochondrial reactive oxygen species production. *Free Radic. Biol. Med.* **2011**, *51*, 1106–1115. [CrossRef]
109. Mailloux, R.J. Mitochondrial antioxidants and the maintenance of cellular hydrogen peroxide levels. *Oxid. Med. Cell. Longev.* **2018**, *2018*, 7857251. [CrossRef]
110. Georgieva, E.; Ivanova, D.; Zhelev, Z.; Bakalova, R.; Gulubova, M.; Aoki, I. Mitochondrial dysfunction and redox imbalance as a diagnostic marker of "free radical diseases". *Anticancer Res.* **2017**, *37*, 5373–5381.

111. Apostolova, N.; Victor, V.M. Molecular strategies for targeting antioxidants to mitochondria: Therapeutic implications. *Antioxid. Redox Signal.* **2015**, *22*, 686–729. [CrossRef]
112. Hirrlinger, J.; Dringen, R. The cytosolic redox state of astrocytes: Maintenance, regulation and functional implications for metabolite trafficking. *Brain Res. Rev.* **2010**, *63*, 177–188. [CrossRef] [PubMed]
113. Brown, G.C. Mechanisms of inflammatory neurodegeneration: iNOS and NADPH oxidase. *Biochem. Soc. Trans.* **2007**, *35*, 1119–1121. [CrossRef] [PubMed]
114. Sorce, S.; Krause, K.H. NOX enzymes in the central nervous system: From signaling to disease. *Antioxid. Redox Signal.* **2009**, *11*, 2481–2504. [CrossRef] [PubMed]
115. Handy, D.E.; Loscalzo, J. Redox regulation of mitochondrial function. *Antioxid. Redox Signal.* **2012**, *16*, 1323–1367. [CrossRef] [PubMed]
116. de Bari, L.; Favia, M.; Bobba, A.; Lassandro, R.; Guerra, L.; Atlante, A. Aberrant GSH reductase and NOX activities concur with defective CFTR to pro-oxidative imbalance in cystic fibrosis airways. *J. Bioenerg. Biomembr.* **2018**, *50*, 117–129. [CrossRef]
117. Magni, G.; Orsomando, G.; Raffelli, N.; Ruggieri, S. Enzymology of mammalian NAD metabolism in health and disease. *Front. Biosci.* **2008**, *13*, 6135–6154. [CrossRef]
118. Legan, S.K.; Rebrin, I.; Mockett, R.J.; Radyuk, S.N.; Klichko, V.I.; Sohal, R.S.; Orr, W.C. Overexpression of glucose-6-phosphate dehydrogenase extends the life span of Drosophila melanogaster. *J. Biol. Chem.* **2008**, *283*, 32492–32499. [CrossRef]
119. Zhao, Y.; Seefeldt, T.; Chen, W.; Wang, X.; Matthees, D.; Hu, Y.; Guan, X. Effects of glutathione reductase inhibition on cellular thiol redox state and related systems. *Arch. Biochem. Biophys.* **2009**, *485*, 56–62. [CrossRef]
120. Ribas, V.; García-Ruiz, C.; Fernández-Checa, J.C. Glutathione and mitochondria. *Front. Pharmacol.* **2014**, *5*, 151. [CrossRef]
121. Velsor, L.W.; Kariya, C.; Kachadourian, R.; Day, B.J. Mitochondrial oxidative stress in the lungs of cystic fibrosis transmembrane conductance regulator protein mutant mice. *Am. J. Respir. Cell Mol. Biol.* **2006**, *35*, 579–586. [CrossRef]
122. Forman, H.J.; Zhang, H.; Rinna, A. Glutathione: Overview of its protective roles, measurement, and biosynthesis. *Mol. Asp. Med.* **2009**, *30*, 1–12. [CrossRef] [PubMed]
123. Cantin, A.M.; North, S.L.; Hubbard, R.C.; Crystal, R.G. Normal alveolar epithelial lining fluid contains high levels of glutathione. *J. Appl. Physiol.* **1985**, *63*, 152–157. [CrossRef] [PubMed]
124. Aldini, G.; Altomare, A.; Baron, G.; Vistoli, G.; Carini, M.; Borsani, L.; Sergio, F. N-Acetylcysteine as an antioxidant and disulphide breaking agent: The reasons why. *Free Radic. Res.* **2018**, *52*, 751–762. [CrossRef] [PubMed]
125. Favia, M.; Atlante, A. Mitochondria and cystic fibrosis transmembrane conductance regulator dialogue: Some news. *J. Rare Dis. Res. Treat.* **2016**, *1*, 23–29.
126. Stutts, M.J.; Knowles, M.R.; Gatzy, J.T.; Boucher, R.C. Oxygen consumption and ouabain binding sites in cystic fibrosis nasal epithelium. *Pediatr. Res.* **1986**, *20*, 1316–1320. [CrossRef] [PubMed]
127. Turrens, J.F.; Freeman, B.A.; Levitt, J.G.; Crapo, J.D. The effect of hyperoxia on superoxide production by lung submitochondrial particles. *Arch. Biochem. Biophys.* **1982**, *217*, 401–410. [CrossRef]
128. Awasthi, A.; Prasad, B.; Kumar, J. Altered mitochondrial function and cystic fibrosis. *Hered. Genet. S7* **2015**. [CrossRef]
129. Shapiro, B.L.; Feigal, R.J.; Lam, L.F. Mitochondrial NADH dehydrogenase in cystic fibrosis. *Proc. Nat. Acad. Sci. USA* **1979**, *76*, 2979–2983. [CrossRef] [PubMed]
130. Battino, M.; Rugolo, M.; Romeo, G.; Lenaz, G. Kinetic alterations of cytochrome-c oxidase in cystic fibrosis. *FEBS Lett.* **1986**, *199*, 155–158. [CrossRef]
131. Valdivieso, A.G.; Santa-Coloma, T.A. CFTR activity and mitochondrial function. *Redox Biol.* **2013**, *1*, 190–202. [CrossRef]
132. Picci, L.; Brentagni, L.; Mastella, G.; Scarso, E.; Pizzochero, P.; Mattiazzo, P.; Chiandetti, L.; Anglani, F.; Zacchello, F. 2D-electrophoresis of mitochondrial proteins from cystic fibrosis patients. *Adv. Exp. Med. Biol.* **1991**, *290*, 379–381. [PubMed]
133. de Meer, K.; Jeneson, J.A.; Gulmans, V.A.; van der Laag, J.; Berger, R. Efficiency of oxidative work performance of skeletal muscle in patients with cystic fibrosis. *Thorax* **1995**, *50*, 980–983. [CrossRef] [PubMed]

134. Chomyn, A. Mitochondrial genetic control of assembly and function of complex I in mammalian cells. *J. Bioenerg. Biomembr.* **2001**, *33*, 251–257. [CrossRef] [PubMed]
135. Bai, Y.; Hajek, P.; Chomyn, A.; Chan, E.; Seo, B.B.; Matsuno-Yagi, A.; Yagi, T.; Attardi, G. Lack of complex I activity in human cells carrying a mutation in MtDNA-encoded ND4 subunit is corrected by the Saccharomyces cerevisiae NADH-quinone oxidoreductase (NDI1) gene. *J. Biol. Chem.* **2001**, *276*, 38808–38813. [CrossRef] [PubMed]
136. Atlante, A.; Favia, M.; Bobba, A.; Guerra, L.; Casavola, V.; Reshkin, S.J. Characterization of mitochondrial function in cells with impaired cystic fibrosis transmembrane conductance regulator (CFTR) function. *J. Bioenerg. Biomembr.* **2016**, *48*, 197–210. [CrossRef] [PubMed]
137. Cleeter, M.W.; Cooper, J.M.; Schapira, A.H. Irreversible inhibition of mitochondrial complex I by 1-methyl-4-phenylpyridinium: Evidence for free radical involvement. *J. Neurochem.* **1992**, *58*, 786–789. [CrossRef] [PubMed]
138. Esposito, L.A.; Melov, S.; Panov, A.; Cottrell, B.A.; Wallace, D.C. Mitochondrial disease in mouse results in increased oxidative stress. *Proc. Nat. Acad. Sci. USA* **1999**, *96*, 4820–4825. [CrossRef]
139. Liang, F.Q.; Godley, B.F. Oxidative stress-induced mitochondrial DNA damage in human retinal pigment epithelial cells: A possible mechanism for RPE aging and age-related macular degeneration. *Exp. Eye Res.* **2003**, *76*, 397–403. [CrossRef]
140. Linsdell, P.; Hanrahan, J.W. Glutathione permeability of CFTR. *Am. J. Physiol.* **1998**, *275*, C323–C326. [CrossRef]
141. Gao, L.; Kim, K.J.; Yankaskas, J.R.; Forman, H.J. Abnormal glutathione transport in cystic fibrosis airway epithelia. *Am. J. Physiol. Lung Cell. Mol. Physiol.* **1999**, *277*, L113–L118. [CrossRef]
142. Kelly-Aubert, M.; Trudel, S.; Fritsch, J.; Nguyen-Khoa, T.; Baudouin-Legros, M.; Moriceau, S.; Jeanson, L.; Djouadi, F.; Matar, C.; Conti, M.; et al. GSH monoethyl ester rescues mitochondrial defects in cystic fibrosis models. *Hum. Mol. Genet.* **2011**, *20*, 2745–2759. [CrossRef] [PubMed]
143. Passarelli, C.; Tozzi, G.; Pastore, A.; Bertini, E.; Piemonte, F. GSSG-mediated complex I defect in isolated cardiac mitochondria. *Int. J. Mol. Med.* **2010**, *26*, 95–99. [PubMed]
144. Cantin, A.M. Potential for antioxidant therapy of cystic fibrosis. *Curr. Opin. Pulm. Med.* **2004**, *10*, 531–536. [CrossRef] [PubMed]
145. Anderson, M.F.; Nilsson, M.; Sims, N.R. Glutathione monoethylester prevents mitochondrial glutathione depletion during focal cerebral ischemia. *Neurochem. Int.* **2004**, *44*, 153–159. [CrossRef]
146. Anderson, M.E.; Powrie, F.; Puri, R.N.; Meister, A. Glutathione monoethyl ester: Preparation, uptake by tissues, and conversion to glutathione. *Arch. Biochem. Biophys.* **1985**, *239*, 538–548. [CrossRef]
147. Kang, J.; Pervaiz, S. Mitochondria: Redox metabolism and dysfunction. *Biochem. Res. Int.* **2012**, *2012*, 896751. [CrossRef]
148. Dunn, J.D.; Alvarez, L.A.J.; Zhang, X.; Soldati, T. Reactive oxygen species and mitochondria: A nexus of cellular homeostasis. *Redox Biol.* **2015**, *6*, 472–485. [CrossRef]
149. Willems, P.H.; Rossignol, R.; Dieteren, C.E.; Murphy, M.P.; Koopman, W.J. Redox homeostasis and mitochondrial dynamics. *Cell Metab.* **2015**, *22*, 207–218. [CrossRef]
150. Hudson, V.M. New insights into the pathogenesis of cystic fibrosis: Pivotal role of glutathione system dysfunction and implications for therapy. *Treat. Respir. Med.* **2004**, *3*, 353–363. [CrossRef]
151. van der Vliet, A. NADPH oxidases in lung biology and pathology: Host defense enzymes, and more. *Free Radic. Biol. Med.* **2008**, *44*, 938–955. [CrossRef]
152. Birben, E.; Sahiner, U.M.; Sackesen, C.; Erzurum, S.; Kalayci, O. Oxidative stress and antioxidant defense. *World Allergy Organ. J.* **2012**, *5*, 9–19. [CrossRef] [PubMed]
153. Blacker, T.S.; Duchen, M.R. Investigating mitochondrial redox state using NADH and NADPH autofluorescence. *Free Radic. Biol. Med.* **2016**, *100*, 53–65. [CrossRef] [PubMed]
154. Wetmore, D.R.; Joseloff, E.; Pilewski, J.; Lee, D.P.; Lawton, K.A.; Mitchell, M.W.; Milburn, M.V.; Ryals, J.A.; Guo, L. Metabolomic profiling reveals biochemical pathways and biomarkers associated with pathogenesis in cystic fibrosis cells. *J. Biol. Chem.* **2010**, *285*, 30516–30522. [CrossRef] [PubMed]
155. Hudson, V.M. Rethinking cystic fibrosis pathology: The critical role of abnormal reduced glutathione (GSH) transport caused by CFTR mutation. *Free Radic. Biol. Med.* **2001**, *30*, 1440–1461. [CrossRef]

156. Włodek, P.; Sokołowska, M.; Smoleński, O.; Włodek, L. The γ-glutamyltransferase activity and non-protein sulfhydryl compounds levels in rat kidney of different age groups. *Acta Biochim. Pol.* **2002**, *49*, 501–507. [PubMed]
157. Corti, A.; Franzini, M.; Paolicchi, A.; Pompella, A. Gamma-glutamyltransferase of cancer cells at the crossroads of tumor progression, drug resistance and drug targeting. *Anticancer Res.* **2010**, *30*, 1169–1181.
158. Ma, T.; Thiagarajah, J.R.; Yang, H.; Sonawane, N.D.; Folli, C.; Galietta, L.J.V.; Verkman, A.S. Thiazolidinone CFTR inhibitor identified by high-throughput screening blocks cholera toxin-induced intestinal fluid secretion. *J. Clin. Investig.* **2002**, *110*, 1651–1658. [CrossRef]
159. Pezzulo, A.A.; Gutiérrez, J.; Duschner, K.S.; McConnell, K.S.; Taft, P.J.; Ernst, S.E.; Yahr, T.L.; Rahmouni, K.; Klesney-Tait, J.; Stoltz, D.A.; et al. Glucose depletion in the airway surface liquid is essential for sterility of the airways. *PLoS ONE* **2011**, *6*, e16166. [CrossRef]
160. Tabary, O.; Corvol, H.; Boncoeur, E.; Chadelat, K.; Fitting, C.; Cavaillon, J.M.; Clément, A.; Jacquot, J. Adherence of airway neutrophils and inflammatory response are increased in CF airway epithelial cell neutrophil interactions. *Am. J. Phys. Lung Cell. Mol. Phys.* **2006**, *290*, L588–L596.
161. Favia, M.; de Bari, L.; Lassandro, R.; Atlante, A. Modulation of glucose-related metabolic pathways controls glucose level in airway surface liquid and fight oxidative stress in cystic fibrosis cells. *J. Bioenerg. Biomembr.* **2019**, *51*, 203–218. [CrossRef]
162. Bardon, A.; Ceder, O.; Kollberg, H. Increased activity of four glycolytic enzymes in cultured fibroblasts from cystic fibrosis patients. *Res. Commun. Chem. Pathol. Pharmacol.* **1986**, *51*, 405–408. [PubMed]
163. Atlante, A.; de Bari, L.; Bobba, A.; Amadoro, G. A disease with a sweet tooth: Exploring the Warburg effect in Alzheimer's disease. *Biogerontology* **2017**, *18*, 301–319. [CrossRef] [PubMed]

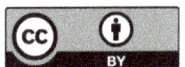

© 2019 by the authors. Licensee MDPI, Basel, Switzerland. This article is an open access article distributed under the terms and conditions of the Creative Commons Attribution (CC BY) license (http://creativecommons.org/licenses/by/4.0/).

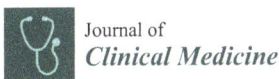 

Article

# Novel Insights into the Role of UBE3A in Regulating Apoptosis and Proliferation

Lilach Simchi [†], Julia Panov [†], Olla Morsy, Yonatan Feuermann and Hanoch Kaphzan *

Laboratory for Neurobiology of Psychiatric Disorders, Sagol Department of Neurobiology, University of Haifa, 199 Aba Khoushy Ave., Mt. Carmel, Haifa 3498838, Israel; simchi.lilach@gmail.com (L.S.); juliapanov.uni@gmail.com (J.P.); aloush223@gmail.com (O.M.); yfeuerman@univ.haifa.ac.il (Y.F.)
* Correspondence: hkaphzan@univ.haifa.ac.il
† Lilach Simchi and Julia Panov contributed equally to this paper.

Received: 5 March 2020; Accepted: 17 May 2020; Published: 22 May 2020

**Abstract:** The *UBE3A* gene codes for a protein with two known functions, a ubiquitin E3-ligase which catalyzes ubiquitin binding to substrate proteins and a steroid hormone receptor coactivator. UBE3A is most famous for its critical role in neuronal functioning. Lack of UBE3A protein expression leads to Angelman syndrome (AS), while its overexpression is associated with autism. In spite of extensive research, our understanding of UBE3A roles is still limited. We investigated the cellular and molecular effects of *Ube3a* deletion in mouse embryonic fibroblasts (MEFs) and Angelman syndrome (AS) mouse model hippocampi. Cell cultures of MEFs exhibited enhanced proliferation together with reduced apoptosis when *Ube3a* was deleted. These findings were supported by transcriptome and proteome analyses. Furthermore, transcriptome analyses revealed alterations in mitochondria-related genes. Moreover, an analysis of adult AS model mice hippocampi also found alterations in the expression of apoptosis- and proliferation-associated genes. Our findings emphasize the role UBE3A plays in regulating proliferation and apoptosis and sheds light into the possible effects UBE3A has on mitochondrial involvement in governing this balance.

**Keywords:** UBE3A; Angelman syndrome; apoptosis; proliferation; mitochondria; bioinformatics; RNA editing

## 1. Introduction

The *UBE3A* gene that encodes for the ubiquitin E3-ligase protein UBE3A is located in the q11–q13 region of chromosome 15 in humans and at 28.65 cm of chromosome 7 in mice. UBE3A possesses five well-characterized functional domains: an HECT domain, E6 binding domain, p53 binding domain, three nuclear receptor interaction domains, and an activation domain [1,2]. So far, UBE3A has been identified to be expressed in the heart, liver, kidney, brain, and possibly other tissues [3,4]. In general, UBE3A has two main functions. First, it can act as a hormone-dependent coactivator for nuclear hormone receptors, such as androgen receptors (AR), estrogen receptors (ER), and some auxiliary regulatory proteins [5]. This function was found mainly in the prostate and mammary glands [1]. Second, UBE3A functions as an E3 ligase from the HECT domain family, catalyzing ubiquitin binding to substrate proteins [6]. As an E3 ligase, UBE3A can bind its substrates either directly, as in the case of p27, progesterone receptor-B (PR-B), Sox9, and HHR23A [7,8], or indirectly via the human papillomavirus E6 protein for p53, BAK, and interleukin-1β [9–11]. Interestingly, the hormone receptor coactivator function is not related to its ubiquitin E3 ligase activity [1,5,12]. Alterations in UBE3A levels are associated with several human diseases, such as cervical cancer, prostate cancer, and breast cancer [13–16]. Yet, the most well-known implication of alteration in UBE3A function is in neurodevelopment, where it plays a critical role. UBE3A loss of activity results in Angelman syndrome (AS) [17], while its overexpression leads to autism [18]. In most cases (65–70%), AS is caused by a small deletion of the maternal copy of chromosome

15 (q11–q13) that includes the *UBE3A* gene. Around birth, the paternal copy of *UBE3A* is imprinted in most brain areas, including the hippocampus, and only the maternal copy is expressed [19,20]. Thus, this maternal deletion leads to a lack of expression of the UBE3A protein in AS patients' brains. In order to understand the consequences of *UBE3A* deletion in Angelman syndrome, a mouse model that carries the maternal deletion of exon 2 of the *Ube3a* gene [21] was generated. This model has been shown to recapitulate most phenotypes seen in AS patients, such as impaired motor function, seizures, and cognitive and hippocampal-dependent long-term memory deficits, making these models an efficient tool for investigating AS [21–23].

To date, previous studies by us and others have suggested that UBE3A may play a role in regulating apoptosis [24] and mitochondrial functioning [25]. Apoptosis is an essential cellular mechanism regulating normal physiological processes in many organs and tissues, including the brain. During development, neuronal-programmed cell death removes neurons that are produced in excess to allow the tissue to sculpt the mature brain [26]. In addition, molecular apoptotic pathways regulate the process of synaptogenesis and synaptic pruning, thus shaping brain connectivity [27–32]. Interestingly, the regulation of dendritic arborization by the apoptotic-related mechanism of caspase-3 activity was specifically found in relation to UBE3A expression [33]. Malfunction in the neuronal connectivity is one of the significant developmental defects that lead to autism spectrum disorders (ASD) in general [34] and Angelman syndrome (AS) in particular [35].

One of the major intersections in regulating the apoptotic response is the mitochondria. Apoptosis usually entails alterations of mitochondrial production of reactive oxygen species (ROS) and the release of cytochrome c, which initiate the post-mitochondrial apoptotic cascade [36,37]. Mitochondrial activity is regulated by two genomes: the mitochondrial genome (mtDNA), which encodes 13 essential oxidative phosphorylation (OXPHOS) components, and the nuclear genome. Nuclear-encoded proteins (~1500 in humans and ~1200 in mice) are synthesized by cytosolic ribosomes and imported into the mitochondria via membrane channels [38].

Several types of neurodevelopmental disorders and diseases, such as autism [39], schizophrenia [40,41], Rett syndrome [42], Down Syndrome [43], and others [44,45], have been associated with apoptosis and mitochondrial dysfunction. In the AS mouse model, the mitochondria in CA1 hippocampal neurons were reported to be smaller, denser, and have altered cristae [46]. These findings, combined with studies that showed higher ROS production in AS neurons [25,47], imply that the mitochondria might be involved in the pathophysiology of AS.

In spite of vast efforts invested in studying UBE3A activity and function, the basic molecular mechanisms governing AS pathology are still unclear. This emphasizes the need to discover the basic molecular pathways governed by this multifunctional protein. For this reason, we chose to investigate the cellular and molecular effects of *Ube3a* deletion in mouse embryonic fibroblasts (MEFs) and in the hippocampi of AS model mice.

## 2. Materials and Methods

### 2.1. MEFs Generation

Mice used were all on a C57BL/6 background. The MEFs from null ($Ube3a^{-/-}$) and wild-type ($Ube3a^{+/+}$) 13.5-day-old embryos were generated by breeding $Ube3a^{+/-}$ mice [21] (Figure S1). For the MEF isolation, embryos from 13.5-day pregnant mice were washed with phosphate-buffered saline (PBS). The head and visceral tissues were removed, and the remaining bodies were washed in fresh PBS and minced using a pair of scissors. MEF cells were isolated using the Primary Mouse Embryonic Fibroblast Isolation Kit (Thermo Fisher Scientific #88279, Rockford, IL, USA) according to the manufacturer's instructions. Cells were collected by centrifugation ($200\times g$ for 5 min at 4 °C) and resuspended in fresh DMEM medium with 15% fetal bovine serum (FBS; Biological Industries #04-127-1A, Beit HaEmek, Israel). Cells ($1 \times 10^6$) were cultured on 100-mm dishes at 37 °C with 5% $CO_2$. In this study, we used MEFs within three to five passages to avoid replicative senescence. Housing, handling, and experimental procedures were performed in accordance with the National Institutes of Health guidelines and were approved by the University of Haifa animal ethics committee.

## 2.2. BrdU Incorporation

MEFs were incubated in DMEM with 15% FBS with a final concentration of 10-μM 5-bromo-2-deoxyuridine (BrdU). After 1 h, the cells were washed with PBS, trypsinized, and washed with PBS again. Immediately after the final wash, the cells were fixed, permeabilized, stained, and analyzed by Fluorescence-activated cell sorting (FACS) according to the manufacturer's instructions (BD Pharmingen™ # 552598, San Jose, CA, USA).

## 2.3. Cell Proliferation Assay

Cells were cultured in 96-well plates (625, 1250, or 2500 cells/well). Cell proliferation assay (XTT-based) (Biological Industries #20-300-1000, Beit HaEmek, Israel) was added to the wells for 2 h to measure cell proliferation according to the manufacturer's instructions. The absorbance was recorded at 475 nm (reference wavelength, 660 nm).

## 2.4. Apoptosis

Apoptosis of MEFs was determined by staining cells with Fluorescein isothiocyanate (FITC)-conjugated annexin-V/PI using a MEBCYTO Apoptosis Kit (MBL #4700, Nagoya, Japan) and analyzed by FACS according to the manufacturer's recommendations.

## 2.5. Caspase 3/7 Activity

Caspase 3/7 activity was measured using the Caspase-Glo® 3/7 Assay kit (Promega # G8091, Madison, WI, USA) following the manufacturer's protocols. Briefly, $1 \times 10^3$ and $5 \times 10^3$ MEFs were seeded in coated 96-well white plates with clear bottoms. After 48 h of incubation in 100-μL culture medium, 100-μL caspase 3/7 substrates were added. Immediately before this assay, the wells were examined under the microscope to confirm no over-confluence and no detached cells. After incubation at 37 °C for 30 min, the luminescence was measured to determine the caspase 3/7 activity. The luminescence signal was normalized to dimethyl sulfoxide (DMSO)-treated cells.

## 2.6. Western Blot Analysis

Western blot analysis was carried out for $Ube3a^{-/-}$ and $Ube3a^{+/+}$ MEFs. The cells were washed with PBS, collected, and homogenized by sonication with an ice-cold lysis buffer containing the following (in mM): 10 HEPES pH 7.5, 150 NaCl, 50 NaF, 1 EDTA, 1 EGTA, 10 Na4P2O7 (EMD Millipore, Billerica, MA, USA), PMSF (Roche, Mannheim, Germany), and protease inhibitor cocktail (Roche, Mannheim, Germany). The samples (15 μg) were loaded on an SDS PAGE 4–20% gradient, followed by a transfer to polyvinylidene difluoride (PVDF; Roche, Mannheim, Germany) membranes and probed with primary antibodies using standard techniques. The primary antibodies and the dilutions for the Western blots were as follows: BAX 1:2000 (α-rabbit; Abcam #ab182733, Cambridge, UK), BCL-2 1:2000 (α-rabbit, Abcam #ab182858, Cambridge, UK), and UBE3A 1:1000 (α-mouse; Sigma-Aldrich #E8655, St. Louis, MO, USA). β-ACTIN 1:40,000 (α-mouse; MP Biomedicals #69100, Irvine, CA, USA) was used as a loading control. Secondary antibodies were used, respectively. The blots were developed and imaged using the Image Quant LAS 4000 system. All signals were normalized by the total protein and quantified using Image Studio Lite Ver 5.2 software.

## 2.7. Live Cell Imaging

$Ube3a^{-/-}$ and $Ube3a^{+/+}$ MEFs were cultured in 12-well plates ($35 \times 10^4$ cells/well). Imaging was started 24 h after seeding. Multilocation imaging was performed inside the incubator scope for the duration of 12 h. Bright-field images were acquired with a frequency of 16 frames every 5 min, for proliferation capacity of the cells was analyzed using software tools (tTt) for single-cell tracking and quantification of the cellular and molecular properties [48].

*2.8. CytoPainter Cell Proliferation Assay*

Staining was performed as recommended by the supplier (Abcam, #ab176736, Cambridge, UK). In brief, cells were incubated with CytoPainter cell proliferation red fluorescence reagent, and the median fluorescence intensity was measured by flow cytometry on BD-FACSCanto II at T0 and 48 h post-labeling. At least 10,000 events were collected in each analysis. Data analysis was performed using FlowJo software (TreeStar, OR, USA).

*2.9. SILAC*

$Ube3a^{-/-}$ and $Ube3a^{+/+}$ MEFs were cultured for 5 passages in SILAC medium (SILAC Protein Quantification Kit, Thermo Fisher Scientific, A33972, Rockford, IL, USA) according to the manufacturer's protocols. After collecting the cells, proteins were extracted from the cell pellets in 9-M urea, 400-mM ammonium bicarbonate, and 10-mM DTT and 2 cycles of sonication. Protein (1 mg) from each sample were mixed heavy (H) with light (L), reduced (60 °C for 30 min), modified with 35-mM iodoacetamide in 400-mM ammonium bicarbonate (in the dark, room temperature for 30 min), and digested in 2-M urea and 90-mM ammonium bicarbonate with modified trypsin (Promega, Madison, USA) at a 1:50 enzyme-to-substrate ratio overnight at 37 °C. Additional second trypsinization was done for 4 h in 1-M urea.

*2.10. Mass Spectrometry Analysis*

The resulting tryptic peptides were desalted using C18 tips (Oasis, Waters, Milford, MA, USA). The proteins were analyzed by LC-MS/MS using a Q Exactive Plus mass spectrometer (Thermo Fisher Scientific, Rockford, IL, USA) fitted with a capillary HPLC (easy nLC 1000, Thermo Fisher Scientific). The peptides were loaded onto a homemade capillary column (25 cm, 75 µm ID) packed with Reprosil C18-Aqua (Dr. Maisch GmbH, Ammerbuch-Entringen, Germany) in solvent A (0.1% formic acid in water). The peptide mixture was resolved with a (5–28%) linear gradient of solvent B (95% acetonitrile with 0.1% formic acid) for 105 min followed by 15 min gradient of 28–95% and 15 min at 95% acetonitrile with 0.1% formic acid in water at flow rates of 0.15 µL/min. Mass spectrometry was performed in a positive mode ($m/z$ 350–1800, resolution 70,000) using repetitively full MS scan followed by high collision-induced dissociation (HCD) at 35 normalized collision energy of the 10 most dominant ions (>1 charge) selected from the first MS scan. A dynamic exclusion list was enabled with an exclusion duration of 20 s. The mass spectrometry data were analyzed using MaxQuant software 1.5.2.8. (www.maxquant.org) for peak picking identification and quantification using the Andromeda search engine, searching against the Mus musculus proteome from the UniProt database with a mass tolerance of 20 ppm for the precursor masses and 20 ppm for the fragment ions. Oxidation of methionine and protein N-terminus acetylation were accepted as variable modifications, and carbamidomethyl on cysteine was accepted as a static modification. Minimal peptide length was set to six amino acids, and a maximum of two miscleavages was allowed. Peptide- and protein-level false discovery rates (FDRs) were filtered to 1% using the target-decoy strategy. Protein tables were filtered to eliminate the identifications from the reverse database, common contaminants, and single peptide identifications. Heavy (H)/light (L) ratios for all peptides belonging to a particular protein species were pooled, providing a ratio for each protein.

*2.11. RNA-Seq Library Preparation of MEFs*

$Ube3a^{-/-}$ and $Ube3a^{+/+}$ cultured for 5 passages, as mentioned above, were used for RNA sequencing. After trypsinization cells were collected, total RNA was isolated using the RNeasy Lipid Tissue Mini Kit, Cat No: 74,804 (QIAGEN) according to the manufacturer's instructions. The isolated RNA concentration and quality were determined by Qubit® quantitation assay using a Qubit® 2.0 fluorometer (Invitrogen

Life Technologies, Carlsbad, CA, USA) and Agilent 4200 TapeStation System (Agilent Technologies, Santa Clara, CA, USA). Samples were prepared for Illumina sequencing using NEB's Ultra RNA Library Prep Kit for Illumina (NEB#7530) (BioLabs Inc., Beverly, MA, USA) according to the manufacturer's protocols. Libraries were sequenced with a 2 × 150 bp PE run on Illumina HiSeq 2500 using a V3 flow cell.

*2.12. Bioinformatics Analysis of MEFs Gene Expression*

RNA-seq fastQ files were filtered and trimmed from adaptors using the Trimmomatic algorithm [49]. The reads were aligned to Mus musculus genome assembly and annotation (gtf) file GRCM38:mm10, https://www.ncbi.nlm.nih.gov/assembly/GCF_000001635.20/, using the Bowtie2 algorithm [50]. Gene expression was estimated in Fragments Per Kilobase of transcript per Million mapped reads (FPKM) counts using the RSEM algorithm [51]. Differential expression was quantified with the DeSeq2 algorithm [52]. Log2 fold change of 1.2 was considered as significant, with a *p*-value of less than 0.01. All bioinformatics analyses were performed on the T-BioInfo Platform (http://tauber-data2.haifa.ac.il:3000/). DAVID Bioinformatics [53,54] and the PANTHER Classification System [55] (http://PANTHERdb.org/) were used to classify the differentially expressed genes into functional groups. To identify proteins that are localized to mitochondria, we used a curated database of mitochondrial localized proteins—the MitoCarta2.0 database [56].

*2.13. Bioinformatics Analysis of Mouse Hippocampi Dataset*

For identifying the effects of apoptosis in the Angelman syndrome model mice [19], we utilized hippocampi RNA-seq data generated by us for recent publication [57]. RNA-seq fastQ files were filtered and trimmed from adaptors using the Trimmomatic algorithm [49]. The reads were aligned to Mus musculus genome assembly and annotation (gtf) file GRCM38:mm10, https://www.ncbi.nlm.nih.gov/assembly/GCF_000001635.20/, using the Bowtie2 algorithm [50], and expression levels were quantified in FPKM counts by the RSEM algorithm [51]. The expression table was transformed into a natural logarithm scale, and all genes with expression levels less than 1 in all samples were filtered out. Only male samples were used for further analysis.

Apoptosis-related genes (121) were extracted based on Hallmark (http://software.broadinstitute.org/gsea/msigdb/cards/HALLMARK_APOPTOSIS.html), Biocarta (genes annotated by GO term GO: 0008632), and KEGG (https://www.genome.jp/kegg-bin/show_pathway?mmu04210). Proliferation-associated genes (56) were identified based on the GO term GO: 008283.

Random forest analysis was performed using the R package "randomForest" [58] together with custom R commands with 10,000 iterations, choosing features most frequently identified as differentiating between wild-type (WT) and AS samples. Linear Discriminant Analysis R package [59] was used to validate that the features that were chosen by iterative random forest procedure indeed separated the WT and the AS groups of samples. Principle component analysis (PCA) was used for visualizing the separation of AS and WT hippocampi based on genes identified by random forest procedure.

*2.14. Bioinformatics Analysis of RNA-Editing Sites in MEFs RNA-Seq Data*

RNA-seq fastQ files were filtered and trimmed from adaptors using the Trimmomatic algorithm [49]. The reads were aligned to Mus musculus genome assembly and annotation file GRCM38:mm10 (https://www.ncbi.nlm.nih.gov/assembly/GCF_000001635.20/) using the Bowtie2 algorithm [50]. First, in each sample separately, we identified statistically significant editing sites utilizing GIREMI algorithm [60]. Genes associated with apoptosis or mitochondrial functioning were chosen in a manner similar to the analysis of gene expression data. DAVID Bioinformatics [53,54] and the PANTHER Classification System [55] were used to classify the edited genes and assign a gene ontology term. To identify proteins that are localized to mitochondria, we used a curated database of mitochondrial-localized proteins—the MitoCarta2.0 database [56].

Next, the differentially edited sites in the $Ube3a^{-/-}$ and $Ube3a^{+/+}$ groups of MEFs were identified by utilizing regression-based analysis on the T-BioInfo Platform. In brief, for each position, the frequency of substitution was calculated. The 95% confidence interval for frequency of editing was calculated via the log-likelihood ratio of binomial distributions that generate the chi-square-distributed statistics (Wilks theorem) [61]. The regression analysis-based calculation of significance of differential editing in every position for many versus many replicates was performed by taking into consideration the confidence intervals for the frequencies of editing in every position for each replicate. The differentially edited sites were determined if a position was covered by at least 10 reads in each sample and the significance of the regression slope was more than 3 standard deviations from the confidence limits. DAVID [53,54] and PANTHER [55] software were used for functional annotation and enrichment analysis of differentially edited genes.

### 2.15. Statistical Analysis

Student's unpaired *t*-test was used for in vitro data analysis. Two-tailed *p*-values of 0.05 or less were considered to be statistically significant. Analysis of variance (ANOVA) or repeated-measures analysis of variance (RM-ANOVA) were performed whenever required. Bonferroni correction was used for post-hoc multiple comparisons.

### 2.16. Data Availability

Fastq files of RNA-seq data from the $Ube3a^{-/-}$ and $Ube3a^{+/+}$ MEFs are available in GEO (PRJNA575629).

## 3. Results

### 3.1. Ube3a Deletion Enhances the Growth Capacity of MEFs

Upon preparation and culturing of the MEFs from $Ube3a^{-/-}$ and $Ube3a^{+/+}$ 13.5-day-old embryos, $Ube3a^{-/-}$ MEFs reached confluency faster than their $Ube3a^{+/+}$ controls. In order to quantify this observation, we determined the growth rate by seeding $0.3 \times 10^6$ cells in tissue culture dishes in DMEM with 15% FBS at day zero ($T_0$). Once the $Ube3a^{-/-}$ cells reached 80 percent confluence, all cultures were trypsinized, counted, and replated in a ratio of $0.3 \times 10^6$ cells per dish. Both at the end of the first and the second passages, the cell numbers of the $Ube3a^{-/-}$ MEFs were higher than those of the $Ube3a^{+/+}$ MEFs ($F_{(2,12)} = 43.61$, $p < 0.0001$ for the interaction of the genotype by time in a two-way RM-ANOVA) (Figure 1A). At the end of the experiment, after the second passage ($P_2$), the final averages of MEF counts were $1.37 \times 10^6$ and $0.56 \times 10^6$ for $Ube3a^{-/-}$ and $Ube3a^{+/+}$, respectively ($t_{(18)} = 12.7$, $p < 0.0001$ post-hoc Bonferroni corrected comparison) (Figure 1A). Furthermore, to evaluate the proliferation capacity at the single-cell level, we labeled the cells with a cell membrane probe (deep red fluorescence—Cytopainter). Since the label is stably inherited by daughter cells through successive cell division, the decline in the mean fluorescence intensity of cells is a proxy for the cell division rate, thus enabling its quantification. The bigger the decline of mean fluorescence intensity, the higher the division rate of cells. We found that, after 48 h, the mean fluorescence intensity of the $Ube3a^{-/-}$ MEFs declined by 3.39-fold, while the fluorescence intensity of $Ube3a^{+/+}$ MEFs declined only by 2.53-fold ($t_{(2)} = 11.05$, $p < 0.01$ post-hoc Bonferroni corrected comparison) (Figure 1B,C). To further substantiate our claim regarding this phenotypic effect of Ube3a deletion, we cultured 1250 $Ube3a^{-/-}$ and $Ube3a^{+/+}$ MEFs and evaluated cell viability after 12, 24, and 48 h using an XTT assay. The cell viability of $Ube3a^{-/-}$ MEFs after 24h was, on average, 1.46-fold higher compared to the $Ube3a^{+/+}$ MEFs ($t_{(16)} = 3.43$, $p < 0.05$ post-hoc Bonferroni corrected comparison) and 1.35 after 48h ($t_{(16)} = 6.47$, $p < 0.0001$ post-hoc Bonferroni corrected comparison and $F_{(3,12)} = 28.20$, $p < 0.0001$ for the interaction of the genotype by time in a two-way RM-ANOVA) (Figure 1D). Performing the same XTT assay using lower and higher cell numbers showed similar results of a differential increase of absorbance along time, leading to the same conclusions (Figure S2). Though an XTT assay is often used as a proxy for measuring cell viability and proliferation [62], it is based on the measurement of the mitochondrial metabolic rate and, therefore, does not necessarily reflect cells numbers. Hence, we decided to further investigate the proliferation capacity in a more dynamic fashion. We plated $0.35 \times 10^5$ $Ube3a^{-/-}$ and $Ube3a^{+/+}$ MEFs in 12-well tissue culture plates and utilized live-cell imaging and tracking software to randomly track 75 cells in a single well for 12 h (Figure 1E,F and Vedios S1 and S2). This time lapse tracking showed that the $Ube3a^{-/-}$ MEFs had a higher percentage of dividing cells compared to the $Ube3a^{+/+}$ MEFs (27.33% versus 9.3%) ($n = 75$ cells per well; $n = 2$ wells per each genotype) ($F_{(1,4)} = 29.11$, $p < 0.001$ for the interaction of the genotype by division in a two-way ANOVA and $t_{(4)} = 4.04$, $p < 0.05$ in a post-hoc Bonferroni corrected comparison).

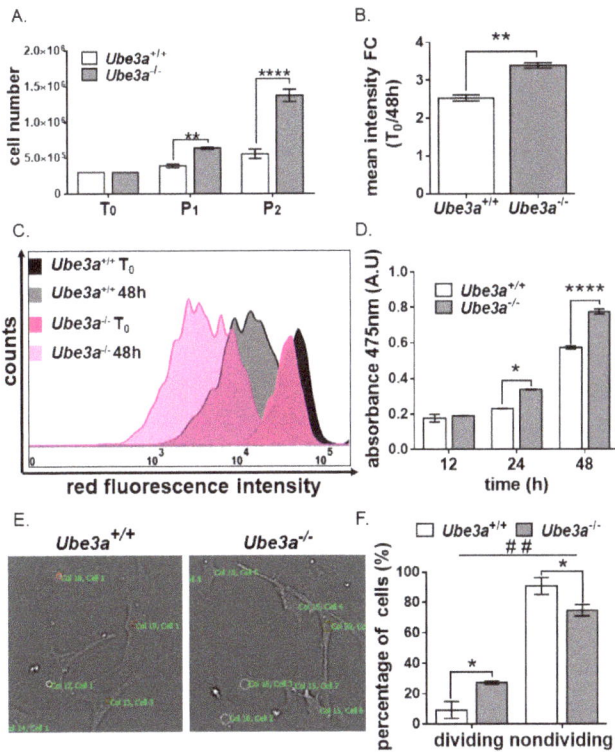

**Figure 1.** Ube3a deletion enhances the growth capacity of mouse embryonic fibroblasts (MEFs). (**A**) Graph showing the comparison in the counts of cells of at different time points: Number of cells seeded at starting point (T$_0$) and two consecutive passages, P$_1$ and P$_2$ ($n = 4$ independent experiments). (**B**) Graph showing the mean intensity signal in $Ube3a^{+/+}$ and $Ube3a^{-/-}$ MEFs at T$_0$ and after 48 h ($n = 3$). (**C**) Representative figure of the fluorescent intensity decline in $Ube3a^{+/+}$ and $Ube3a^{-/-}$ MEFs at T$_0$ and after 48h. (**D**) Graph showing the colorimetric measurements of the cell proliferation XTT assay, displaying differences in the cell viability of $Ube3a^{+/+}$ and $Ube3a^{-/-}$ MEFs at 12 h, 24 h, and 48 h ($n = 3$ per each genotype). (**E**) Representative cell-tracking images of $Ube3a^{+/+}$ and $Ube3a^{-/-}$ MEFs after 12 h. (**F**) Percentage of dividing cells determined by video microscopy-based cell tracking ($n = 75$ cells per well, 2 wells per genotype). The data are presented as the means ± SEM (\* $p < 0.05$, \*\* $p < 0.01$, \*\*\*\* $p < 0.0001$, and ## $p < 0.01$ for interaction of the genotype by division in a two-way ANOVA).

### 3.2. Ube3a Deletion Alters Cell Cycle Progression

Due to the observed enhancement in the growth capacity of $Ube3a^{-/-}$ MEFs, we examined the effects of Ube3a deletion on cell cycle progression. Measuring BrdU incorporation following

1-h incubation showed a difference in the cell-cycle phases between the two genotypes ($F_{(3,16)} = 29.7$, $p < 0.0001$ for the interaction of genotype by the cell-cycle phase in a two-way ANOVA). *Ube3a* deletion increased the percentage of cells found in the S-phase by 1.53-fold and in G0/G1 by 1.24-fold ($t_{(16)} = 3.3$, $p < 0.05$ and $t_{(16)} = 5.9$, $p < 0.0001$, respectively, in a post-hoc Bonferroni corrected comparison). In the G2/M cell population, the significant differences between *Ube3a*$^{-/-}$ and *Ube3a*$^{+/+}$ were also observed ($t_{(16)} = 4.3$, $p < 0.01$ in a post-hoc Bonferroni corrected comparison). The percentage of cells found in the sub-G1 phase was, however, reduced by almost four-fold ($t_{(16)} = 5$, $p < 0.001$ in a post-hoc Bonferroni corrected comparison) (Figure 2).

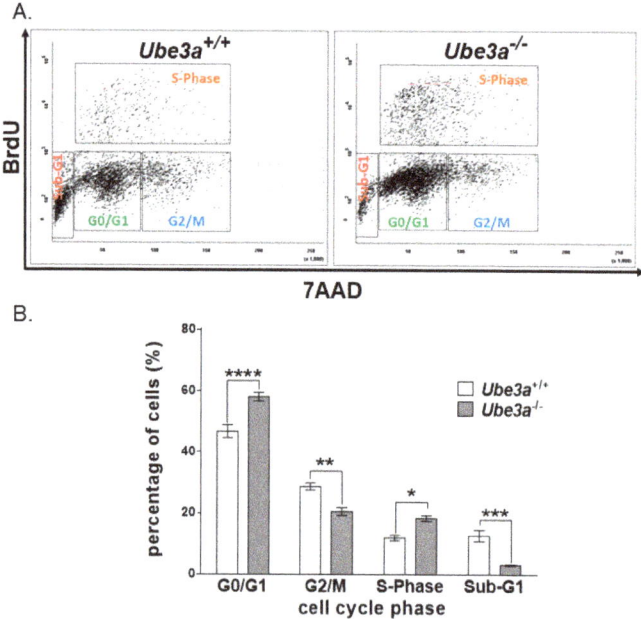

**Figure 2.** *Ube3a* deletion alters cell cycle progression. (**A**) Representative dual-parameter flow cytometry scatter plot showing the cell cycle progression of BrdU versus 7AAD, following 1-h incubation with BrdU in *Ube3a*$^{+/+}$ and *Ube3a*$^{-/-}$ MEFs. (**B**) Graph showing the respective percentages of cells at each cell-cycle stage ($n = 3$ independent experiments). The data are presented as the means ± SEM (* $p < 0.05$, ** $p < 0.01$, *** $p < 0.001$, and **** $p < 0.0001$).

### 3.3. Ube3a Deletion Reduces the Apoptotic Capacity of MEFs

The abovementioned cell cycle status analysis utilized 7-aminoactinomycin D (7-AAD) and BrdU. 7-AAD is usually used to determine the DNA ploidy status [63]. The cell population defined as sub-G1 is characterized by low DNA content, a phenomenon that is usually associated with DNA fragmentation during apoptosis. The fact that the sub-G1 cell population was diminished in the *Ube3a*$^{-/-}$ MEFs led us to suspect that the differences observed in cell counts between the *Ube3a*$^{+/+}$ and *Ube3a*$^{-/-}$ may also arise from the altered mortality rate of these MEFs and not only from enhanced proliferation. For this reason, we evaluated the cellular apoptosis by utilizing the annexin-V/PI assay, which suggested differences in apoptosis/viability ($F_{(2,12)} = 23.13$, $p < 0.0001$ for the interaction of the genotype by apoptosis/viability in a two-way ANOVA). *Ube3a* deletion induced a significant decrease in the percentage of early apoptotic cells: 21.4% versus 12.3% for *Ube3a*$^{+/+}$ and *Ube3a*$^{-/-}$, respectively ($t_{(12)} = 3.2$, $p < 0.05$ post-hoc Bonferroni corrected comparison) (Figure 3A,B). Next, we proceeded to evaluate the pro- and antiapoptosis balance by examining the measure of BAX/BCL2 proteins expression ratio [64].

This ratio between the BAX and BCL-2 protein expression levels was ~40% lower in the $Ube3a^{-/-}$ MEFs than that ratio in the $Ube3a^{+/+}$ MEFs, indicating a balance favoring antiapoptosis (Figure 3C and Figure S3). To further validate the decreased apoptosis in the absence of $Ube3a$, we measured caspase 3/7 enzymatic activity levels in $Ube3a^{-/-}$ and $Ube3a^{+/+}$ MEFs. Caspase 3/7 enzymatic activity is the final common molecular step of apoptotic pathways and, hence, serves as a proxy for apoptosis. We used a caspase glow assay in two independent series of experiments. Each series comprised three different independent experiments, and for each series, we utilized a different number of cells for the assay. The differences were optimized at 5000 cells, but both experimental series showed a significant decrease in caspase 3/7 activity levels. For the 1000-cell experiments, caspase 3/7 activity levels were reduced by ~28% ($t_{(16)} = 8.6$, $p < 0.0001$ in an unpaired $t$-test). In the 5000-cell experiments, caspase 3/7 activity levels were nearly 50% lower in the $Ube3a^{-/-}$ MEFs compared to the controls ($t_{(8)} = 11.4$, $p < 0.0001$ in an unpaired $t$-test) (Figure 3D). This finding further supports that $Ube3a$ deletion results in reduced apoptosis.

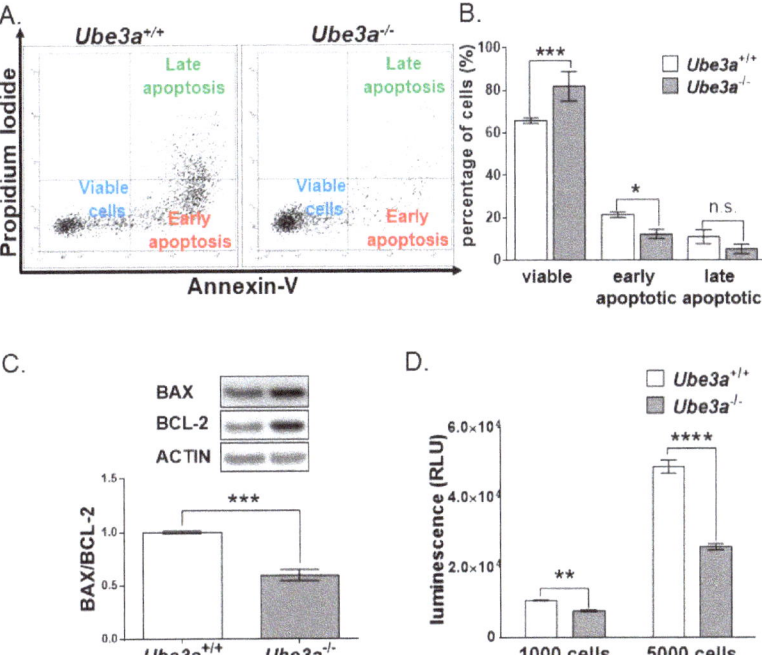

**Figure 3.** $Ube3a$ deletion reduces apoptosis in MEFs. (**A**) Flow cytometry scatter plots for cellular apoptosis analyzed by performing annexin-V/PI double-staining assay in $Ube3a^{+/+}$ and $Ube3a^{-/-}$ MEFs (data represented as an overlay of three experiments). (**B**) The respective cell percentages of viable cells, early apoptotic cells, and late apoptotic cells ($n = 3$ independent experiments). (**C**) Graph depicting BAX to BCL-2 proteins expression ratio in $Ube3a^{+/+}$ and $Ube3a^{-/-}$ MEFs ($n = 4$ per each genotype) (**D**) Graph showing luminescence measurements of the Caspase-Glo 3/7 assay used to determine the activity of caspase 3/7 in $Ube3a^{+/+}$ and $Ube3a^{-/-}$ MEFs utilizing different two series of experiments, each series with a different number of cells ($n = 5$ independent experiments in each series). The data are presented as the means ± SEM (* $p < 0.05$, ** $p < 0.01$, *** $p < 0.001$, and **** $p < 0.0001$, n.s. = non-significant).

### 3.4. Transcriptomic Analyses Support Altered Apoptosis Processes Triggered by Ube3a Deletion

To further study the effects of $Ube3a$ deletion on molecular pathways, we performed polyA RNA sequencing of $Ube3a^{+/+}$ and $Ube3a^{-/-}$ MEF samples. First, we confirmed that our MEFs were correctly labeled as $Ube3a^{+/+}$ and $Ube3a^{-/-}$. We analyzed the alignment of reads on the deleted second exon of the Ube3a gene [21]. This analysis showed a clear difference in alignment between the $Ube3a^{+/+}$ and $Ube3a^{-/-}$ samples. While in $Ube3a^{+/+}$ samples the second exon was enriched by reads, in $Ube3a^{-/-}$ samples, the reads were not aligned to this exon (Figure S4). In addition, to exclude any possibility of a sex effect in our experiment [57], we examined the expression of the Kdm5d and Ddx3y genes. These two genes are highly expressed in males but not in females and, thus, are considered as biomarkers for male samples [65]. All of our $Ube3a^{+/+}$ and $Ube3a^{-/-}$ samples were males (Figure S5).

Differential expression analysis of RNA-seq data yielded 193 differentially expressed genes (Figure 4A). The threshold for a significant difference was set at a 1.2-fold change in average expressions and p-value < 0.01, as calculated by DeSeq2 program [52]. From these, 100 genes were upregulated in $Ube3a^{-/-}$ samples, and 93 were downregulated (Table S1). One of the genes downregulated in the $Ube3a^{-/-}$ samples was the androgen receptor (Ar) (Figure 4B), known to be directly regulated by UBE3A [66]. Enrichment analysis of the dysregulated genes, utilizing PANTHER 14.1 software [55], showed that many significantly enriched gene ontology (GO) terms are related to the cell's fate. The processes of "regulation of cell population proliferation (GO: 0042127)", "regulation of cell death (GO: 0010941)", "regulation of apoptotic process (GO: 0042981)", "regulation of MAPK cascade (GO: 0043408)", "regulation of insulin-like growth factor receptor signaling pathway (GO: 0043567)", and "regulation of the noncanonical Wnt signaling pathway (GO: 2000050)" were significantly enriched in our dataset (Figure 4C). All of these processes are related to cell cycle progression, proliferation, and apoptosis [67–69].

Furthermore, we also observed that the expression of several genes coding for proteins localized to the mitochondria were altered (Dmpk, Abcb6, Bdh1, Bcat1, Fth1, and Acot2) (Table S2).

### 3.5. Dysregulation of RNA Editing Affects Apoptosis-Related Pathways

Recent studies have shown that altered RNA editing may influence apoptotic pathways [70]. For this reason, we performed analyses of mRNA editing in $Ube3a^{-/-}$ and $Ube3a^{+/+}$ MEFs. At first, we examined each sample separately for the editing sites utilizing the GIREMI algorithm [71]. Interestingly, even though the average frequency of editing across the genome in $Ube3a^{-/-}$ MEFs was similar to the frequency of editing in the $Ube3a^{+/+}$ MEFs (Figure 5A), the edited mRNAs were different from the mRNAs edited in the controls (Figure 5B). We found 46 genes uniquely edited in the $Ube3a^{+/+}$ MEFs, while in $Ube3a^{-/-}$ MEFs, 48 different genes were edited (Table S3). From the 46 genes edited in the $Ube3a^{+/+}$ MEFs, 11 genes were either apoptosis-related (Apaf1, Bmp1, Cited2, Crebbp, Fbxw7, Pdcd4, Pim1, and Raf1) or mitochondria-related (Vat1, Mrpl1, and Rhot2) in accordance with GO terms. From the 48 genes edited only in $Ube3a^{-/-}$ MEFs, eight were either apoptosis-related (Btg2, Ccnd2, and Ei24) or mitochondria-related (Adsl, Gpd1, Slc8b1, Spns1, and Car5b) in accordance with their GO terms (Table S3).

Next, utilizing a newly developed approach for identifying differential RNA editing sites in datasets with replicates (see Section 2.14. *Bioinformatics Analysis of RNA-Editing Sites in MEFs RNA-Seq Data*), we found 338 differentially edited nucleotides in 113 genes (Table S4). From these, 206 sites were hyper-edited and 132 were hypo-edited in $Ube3a^{-/-}$ MEFs (Figure 6A,B). Unlike the way we analyzed the results generated by GIREMI, in this type of analysis, the observed edited RNA positions were edited in both $Ube3a^{-/-}$ and $Ube3a^{+/+}$ MEFs. However, the editing frequencies between the groups were significantly different. Enrichment analysis of the differentially edited genes showed that "calcium", "calcium binding", "insulin-like growth factor binding protein", "oxidoreductase", "oxidation-reduction process", and "endoplasmic reticulum" biological processes were significantly enriched (Figure 6C). From the 113 differentially edited genes, 16 genes (14%) were associated with apoptosis according to the GO terms, and 10 genes (9%) were mitochondria-associated (Table S5).

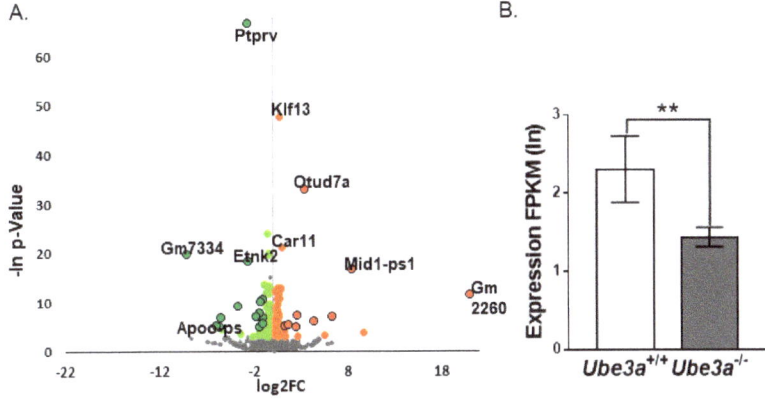

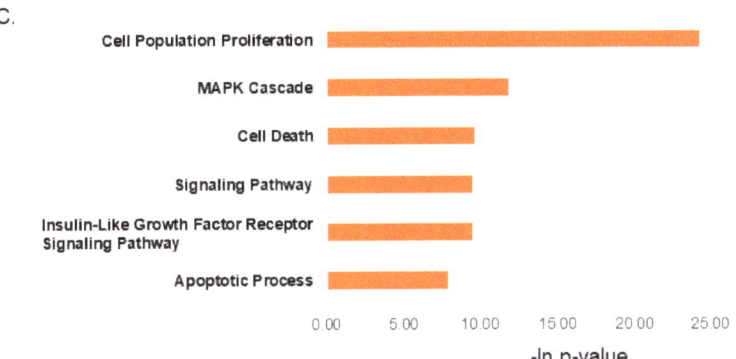

**Figure 4.** RNA-seq analysis reveals differentially expressed genes enriched in apoptotic and proliferative pathways. (**A**) Volcano plots representing the distribution of the gene expression fold changes and $p$-values in $Ube3a^{-/-}$ compared to $Ube3a^{+/+}$ MEFs. A total number of 7365 genes were used for the analysis. Genes with fold changes > 1.5 and $p$-values < 0.01 are indicated in red circles. Genes with fold changes > 1.2 and $p$-values < 0.01 are indicated in orange. Genes with fold changes < 1.5 and $p$-values < 0.01 are indicated in green circles, and genes with fold changes < 0.8 and $p$-values < 0.01 are indicated in light green. Genes with no difference in expression levels are indicated in grey. (**B**) Androgen receptor (Ar) expression profile. Androgen receptor is significantly downregulated (DeSeq2 $p$-value = 0.0053, Fold Change = 0.63) in $Ube3a^{-/-}$ MEFs. (**C**) Enrichment analysis of differentially expressed genes. Topmost significantly enriched biological processes of differentially expressed genes associated with $Ube3a^{-/-}$ samples as analyzed by PANTHER. (** $p < 0.01$).

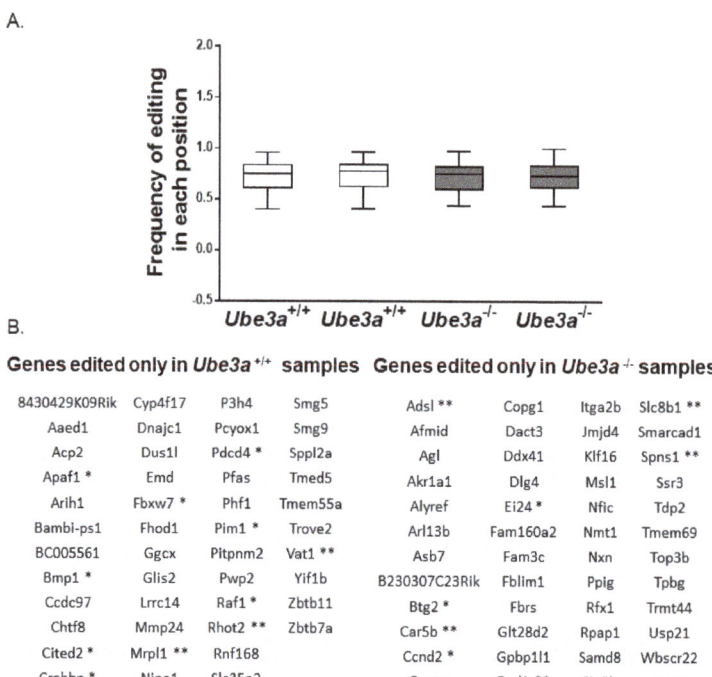

**Figure 5.** Differential RNA editing as determined by the GIREMI algorithm. (**A**) Box plot of RNA editing representing the frequencies of editing across the genome in each sample. The average frequency of RNA editing is not changed in $Ube3a^{-/-}$ compared to $Ube3a^{+/+}$ MEFs. (**B**) Genes uniquely edited in $Ube3a^{+/+}$ and $Ube3a^{-/-}$ MEFs (* signifies apoptosis-associated genes, and ** signifies mitochondria-related genes).

### 3.6. Proteomic Analysis Supports Altered Apoptotic Processes Triggered by Ube3a Deletion

It is known that mRNA expression does not always directly translate to protein abundance [72]. Therefore, in addition to RNA-seq analysis, we also performed a SILAC-based mass spectrometry comparative proteomic analysis (see Methods). The data revealed 30 proteins with at least 20% change in expression, which were replicated in both experiments (Table S6). Interestingly, seventy-three percent (73% = 22 proteins) of these proteins were identified as apoptosis-related based on updated studies (Figure 7A and Table S6). We identified 14 downregulated apoptosis-related proteins and eight upregulated apoptosis-related proteins—out of which, five are known to be involved in antiapoptotic and protective mechanisms: BAG1, FABP5, IL1RN, SERPINB9, and TCIRG1 (Figure 7B and Table S6). One of the most intriguing proteins that we found to be significantly downregulated in $Ube3a^{-/-}$ samples is p16 (CDKN2A). UBE3A has been shown to indirectly regulate p16 expression in non-small cell lung cancer [73].

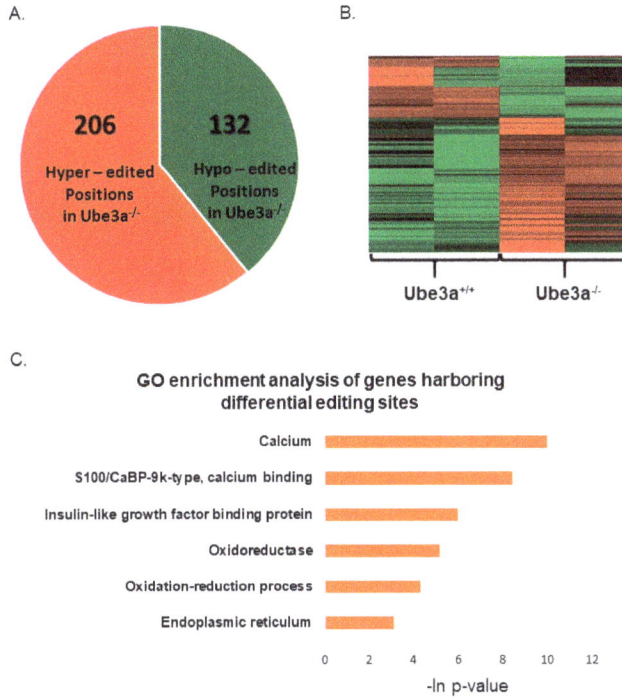

**Figure 6.** Differential RNA editing as determined by regression-based analysis. (**A**) Differentially edited sites in $Ube3a^{-/-}$ MEFs compared to $Ube3a^{+/+}$ MEFs. We identified 206 hyper-edited and 132 hypo-edited sites in $Ube3a^{-/-}$ compared to $Ube3a^{+/+}$ MEFs. (**B**) Heat map for differentially edited genes in $Ube3a^{-/-}$ MEFs. Red represents sites with a higher frequency of editing (hyper-editing), and green represents sites with a lower frequency of editing (hypo-editing) in $Ube3a^{-/-}$ compared to $Ube3a^{+/+}$ MEFs. (**C**) Enrichment analysis of differentially edited genes. Topmost significantly enriched biological processes of differentially edited genes in $Ube3a^{-/-}$ compared to $Ube3a^{+/+}$ MEFs as analyzed by DAVID.

A straightforward way to delineate the effects of differential transcription is to integrate the mRNA expression and their corresponding protein levels. By crossing the transcriptomic and the proteomic datasets, we found 24 proteins/genes significantly dysregulated in a similar direction (the threshold was arbitrarily determined as the protein expression change of more than 15% in at least one of the proteomic experiments and $p < 0.05$ for the mRNA analysis in the $t$-test). Amongst these 24 genes, 13 were upregulated and 11 were downregulated (Table S7). Interestingly, out of these 24 altered genes/proteins, 15 (63%) genes/proteins are apoptosis-related (Tcirg, Lxn, Fhl, Apoo, Pdgfrb, Tpm1, Vps25, Parp3, Copg2, Fam129a (Niban1), Myo5a, Cd151, Ap3s1, Tmx1, and Dscr3).

In addition, we observed many proteins where their expression levels were strongly altered but their mRNA levels were unchanged in $Ube3a^{-/-}$ MEFs. A more stringent threshold of at least 20% change in protein expression levels in both experiments yielded 16 proteins with changed expressions and unchanged mRNA levels. From these, four were upregulated, and 12 were downregulated (Table S8). The four upregulated proteins (P4HA3, FABP5, MVK, and IL1RN) are potential UBE3A substrates. Remarkably, all four proteins are apoptosis-related. Of the 12 downregulated proteins, five (42%) are apoptosis-related (DES, THY1, FTH1, NEK7, and CDKN2A).

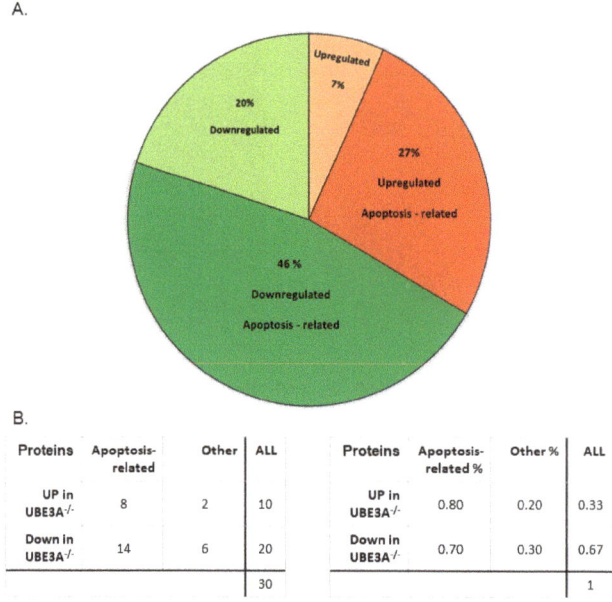

B.

| Proteins | Apoptosis-related | Other | ALL |
|---|---|---|---|
| UP in UBE3A$^{-/-}$ | 8 | 2 | 10 |
| Down in UBE3A$^{-/-}$ | 14 | 6 | 20 |
| | | | 30 |

| Proteins | Apoptosis-related % | Other % | ALL |
|---|---|---|---|
| UP in UBE3A$^{-/-}$ | 0.80 | 0.20 | 0.33 |
| Down in UBE3A$^{-/-}$ | 0.70 | 0.30 | 0.67 |
| | | | 1 |

**Figure 7.** SILAC-based proteomics analysis. (**A**) Pie chart of differentially expressed proteins in $Ube3a^{-/-}$ MEFs. The threshold was set to an at least 20% change in both independent experiments. (**B**) Table of differentially expressed proteins in $Ube3a^{-/-}$ MEFs. From 10 upregulated proteins, we found that 80% ($n = 8$) are associated with apoptosis. From 20 downregulated proteins, 70% ($n = 14$) are associated with apoptosis.

*3.7. Mouse Brain RNA-Seq Data Also Reveals Alterations in Apoptotic Pathways*

Having examined the effect of *Ube3a* deletion in MEFs, we further wanted to investigate the potential role of molecular apoptosis-related pathways in adult AS mice models. For this, we used a random forest approach, utilizing the transcriptome data from the mouse hippocampi we recently produced (see Methods) [57]. Machine-learning methods are progressively being applied to rank ensembles of genes defined by their expression values measured with RNA-seq [74]. Using importance measures generated by the random forest algorithm, we identified groups of 40 apoptosis-related genes and 10 proliferation-related genes that together differentiate between the adult Angelman syndrome model mice and the wild-type (WT) littermates. These genes can identify and differentiate between AS mice from their WT littermates (Table S9) with 100 percent predictability, as was determined by linear discriminant analysis and is demonstrated by a principal component analysis (PCA) plot (Figure 8).

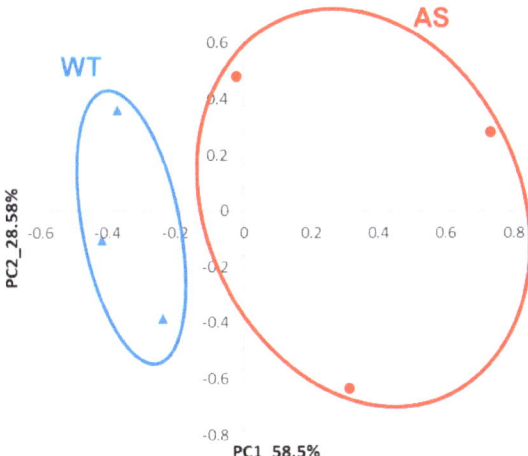

**Figure 8.** Random forest analysis of gene expression data from the hippocampi of Angelman syndrome (AS) model mice and their control littermates identified 40 apoptosis-related and 10 proliferation-related genes as markers of the AS hippocampi. Principal component analysis (PCA) of these 50 genes identified by random forest analysis. First two PCs clearly separate the AS and the wild-type (WT) samples ($n = 3$ per group) as predicted by random forest.

## 4. Discussion

Ubiquitin protein ligase E3A (UBE3A), also known as human papillomavirus E6-associated protein (E6-AP), is one of the E3 ligases in the ubiquitin-proteasome system. Iterations in UBE3A levels, either deletion or overexpression, culminate in severe neurodevelopmental disorders such as Angelman syndrome or autism, respectively. This suggests that cells, especially neurons, are UBE3A dosage-sensitive. For the last few decades, since the discovery of UBE3A as an E3 ligase [10] and the finding of its involvement in Angelman syndrome [75], the biological effects of altered UBE3A have not been completely elucidated.

Around birth, when apoptosis is still an ongoing process in neurons [76], *Ube3a* starts to be imprinted, and mice with maternal deletion do not express the UBE3A protein in neurons. Given the lack of UBE3A protein expression in AS patients [77] and in AS mouse model brains [20] (Figure S6), we utilized $Ube3a^{-/-}$ mouse embryonic fibroblasts (MEFs) to investigate the basic molecular and cellular mechanisms affected by UBE3A. MEFs, in general, have been shown in the past to be a powerful discovery tool for the identification of novel molecular pathways relevant to neurodegenerative disorders [78]. In addition, MEFs lacking UBE3A expression were previously used for the identification of the cellular response to stress and cellular senescence [24,79].

Upon the preparation and culturing of MEFs derived from $Ube3a^{-/-}$ and $Ube3a^{+/+}$ 13.5-day-old male embryos (Figures S1 and S5), we noticed that the $Ube3a^{-/-}$ MEFs exhibited enhanced growth rates when compared to the $Ube3a^{+/+}$ MEFs (Figure 1A). This observation was validated using four different proliferation assays, cell counting, XTT, live cell tracking, and CytoPainter cell proliferation assay (Figure 1B–F).

Further examination of the cell cycle progression showed that *Ube3a* deletion promoted the percentage of cells found in the S-phase, while significantly reducing the percentage of cells in the sub-G1 cell population (Figure 2). The cell population defined as sub-G1 is characterized by their low DNA content, a phenomenon that is usually associated with the DNA fragmentation during apoptosis. The fact that the sub-G1 cell population was reduced in the $Ube3a^{-/-}$ MEFs led us to suspect that the differences observed in cell counts between the $Ube3a^{+/+}$ and $Ube3a^{-/-}$ may also arise from altered mortality rates of these MEFs and not only from enhanced proliferation. However, since cells defined by the Nicoletti assay [80] as the sub-G1 cell population are not necessarily apoptotic cells, we further examined the effects of *Ube3a* deletion in MEFs on apoptosis with other independent techniques. At first, we measured the amount of surface-bound fluorochrome-labeled annexin-V to phosphatidylserine on the plasma membrane outer leaflet, which correlates to apoptosis [81], thus showing that the number of apoptotic cells in the *Ube3a*$^{-/-}$ MEFs was diminished by nearly two-fold (Figure 3A,B). Next, we evaluated the proapoptotic/antiapoptotic balance in the cells by using the proteins expression levels ratio of BAX/BCL2 [64]. The BCL-2 (B-cell lymphoma protein 2) and BAX (Bcl-2-associated X) are cytoplasmic proteins that are responsible for either inhibiting or promoting apoptosis, respectively. BAX interacts with the outer mitochondrial membrane, leading to its perforation, which enables the release of cytochrome-C from the mitochondria. BCL-2 prevents BAX activation, thus inhibiting the successive activation of caspases and, eventually, cell death [82]. Previous studies showed that a low BAX/BCL-2 ratio is typically associated with antiapoptotic properties, while a high BAX/BCL-2 ratio is found in cells that are more sensitive to apoptosis. Furthermore, the BAX/BCL-2 ratio has also been correlated with other factors that induce cell death, such as caspase-3 activation [64]. We show that, in *Ube3a*$^{-/-}$ MEFs, the ratio of BAX/BCL2 was almost two-fold lower (Figure 3C). BAX and BCL2 are representative members of the BCL2 family. However, many more apoptosis-related proteins might be involved in the disruption of apoptosis due to *Ube3a* deletion. Hence, it is important to address the remaining members of this family in future studies under various apoptosis-inducing stimulations. Moreover, when we measured the activity of caspase 3/7 in these cells, the levels of active caspase 3/7 were significantly reduced in the *Ube3a*$^{-/-}$ MEFs (Figure 3D). These findings indicate that *Ube3a* deletion leads to a higher tolerance toward apoptosis, which coincides with the reduction in the sub-G1 cell population in *Ube3a*$^{-/-}$ MEFs. These results also support our hypothesis that the differences in the final cell counts of *Ube3a*$^{-/-}$ and *Ube3a*$^{+/+}$ MEFs (Figure 1A) are not merely attributed to proliferation differences (Figures 1 and 2) but, also, to the differences in the portion of cells undergoing programmed cell death (Figure 3). The involvement of UBE3A in apoptosis is unclear. For example, Zhou et al., who used siRNA to manipulate *Ube3a* expressions, found that, when *Ube3a* was silenced in breast cancer cell lines, the cellular proliferation and invasion were inhibited, while apoptosis was increased [83]. On the other hand, support for our findings can be found in the study conducted by Levav-Cohen et al., who showed that MEFs lacking *Ube3a* have a faster population doubling than WT MEFs, as well as reduced apoptosis [24]. These discrepancies may indicate that the effects of UBE3A are context-dependent, such as cell type or surrounding tissue. Furthermore, while apoptosis is induced by either intrinsic or extrinsic signals, our findings set the stage for future studies in order to delineate the distinct disrupted apoptotic pathways in the absence of *Ube3a*. Future studies should consider addressing each pathway separately under various stimulations.

In order to further study the effects of *Ube3a* deletion on apoptosis mechanisms in MEFs, we utilized transcriptomics and mass-spec SILAC-based proteomics approaches. Most alterations in protein expressions were associated with apoptosis-related proteins (Figure 7A and Table S6), again emphasizing the significance of aberrant apoptosis in *Ube3a*$^{-/-}$ MEFs. Of special interest is the IL1RN protein, which showed the strongest abundance changes. The IL1RN protein is a strong antagonist of Il-1α and Il-1β, which are inducers of apoptosis in general, while Il-1β induces apoptosis specifically in neurons [84,85]. Furthermore, IL1RN was shown to protect neurons by inhibiting apoptosis due to various types of insults [86,87]. Another interesting finding was the reduction of the CDKN2A protein (Table S8). The CDKN2A protein has been implicated in the induction of cellular senescence [88]. Indeed, a previous study of *Ube3a*$^{-/-}$ MEFs has shown impaired senescence in response to stress [24].

Whole transcriptome analyses revealed 193 differentially expressed genes (Figure 4A), most of which belong to the biological processes previously shown to regulate cell growth, cell cycle progression, apoptosis, and cell differentiation [67–69]. Interestingly, one of the genes found to be downregulated by ~40% is the androgen receptor (Ar), whose transcriptional activity is known to be regulated by UBE3A (Figure 4B) [5,89]. This is surprising, because in prostate carcinoma cells,

UBE3A downregulation corresponds with Ar upregulation [13], again showing that UBE3A may act in a cell-type-dependent manner.

Apoptosis, mainly the intrinsic pathway, is governed by the mitochondria. Therefore, we also searched for genes differentially expressed and related to mitochondrial functioning. We found no change in mitochondrially coded genes; however, several nuclear genes coding for proteins localized to the mitochondria were significantly altered (Table S2). Of note, all upregulated genes (Dmpk, Abcb6, and Bdh1) are known to prevent ROS-induced apoptosis or to actively modulate mitochondrial redox activity, thus protecting the cell from apoptosis [90,91]. These findings explain the discrepancy between previously reported elevated ROS activity in AS hippocampi [25] and the antiapoptotic properties of $Ube3a^{-/-}$ MEFs (Figure 3).

In addition to the gene expression analyses, we examined whether UBE3A affects RNA editing. RNA editing is a post-transcriptional modification of the RNA molecules, potentially diversifying the transcriptome and the proteome of the cell [92]. Although the functional roles of the editing are still largely unknown, recent studies found that RNA editing plays an essential role in cancer progression [93] and in neurodevelopmental disorders, such as autism and Prader-Willi syndrome [94,95]. We found dysregulated RNA editing in many genes associated with apoptosis or mitochondrial functioning (Tables S3 and S4). These findings are in-line with recent studies done in cancer cells that report that the ADAR family of proteins implicated in RNA editing are tightly linked with antiapoptotic functions [93,96,97]. It is important to note that, while in cancer studies, changes in RNA editing were associated with altered expressions of the ADAR family of proteins, in our research and in other autism-related studies, like Prader-Willi syndrome and ASD, no differences in the expressions of ADAR proteins were found [94,95]. This again emphasizes the cell-type specificity of these mechanisms.

We found that the mitochondrial-encoded cytochrome-C oxidase 1 gene (Mt-Co1) was differentially edited in the $Ube3a^{-/-}$ MEFs. The Mt-Co1 gene plays a dominant role in the mitochondrial function of oxidative phosphorylation. It is localized to the mitochondrial inner membrane and is an essential component of Complex IV [36]. Mutation in the Mt-Co1 gene leads to elevated reactive oxygen species (ROS) production [98]. This finding is of particular interest, since previously, we showed that the hippocampal CA1 pyramidal cells of AS model mice (which were shown to have smaller and denser mitochondria with abnormal cristae [46]) exhibit elevated ROS levels [25]. In addition, when these AS mice were treated with mitochondria antioxidant, the hippocampal-dependent deficits were rescued [25]. A later in vivo study, using quench-assisted (Quest) MRI, also found elevated ROS levels in AS mice hippocampi [47]. All of the above suggest that the Mt-Co1 editing may play a role in mitochondrial-excessive ROS production.

Taken together, the fact that MEFs have reduced apoptosis in the absence of UBE3A expression suggests that similar deviations might be present in the brains of AS model mice during early development. It was previously shown that reinstating $Ube3a$ in AS mice, immediately after birth, rescued some but not all of AS phenotypes and deficits [99]. Nevertheless, the role of apoptosis-related molecular pathways is not exclusive to early development but is also significant in adult brains. For example, apoptosis is known to be implicated in neurogenesis, which is critical for hippocampal-dependent learning and memory [100,101]. Indeed, AS model mice suffer from severe hippocampal-dependent memory deficits [21,22,25,102]. Remarkably, random forest bioinformatics analysis of transcriptome data derived from the hippocampi of adult Angelman syndrome model mice [57] showed a significant alteration both in apoptotic (for example, Xiap and Casp8) and proliferative (for example, Foxo1 and Pacap) genes between AS model mice and their WT littermates (Figure 8 and Table S9). In addition, several genes found in these analyses are members of the PI3K gene family (Pik3cb, Pik3cd, Pik3r1, and Pik3r3). The PI3K gene family is known to assist cell survival and tumor growth in the case of cancer by inhibiting apoptosis and enhancing the tolerance to low oxygen and nutrient deficiency [103]. Our findings are in-line with earlier reports that UBE3A regulates the PI3K-Akt signaling pathway and, thus, is involved in tumorigenesis [66,104]. The transcriptome analyses we performed provides an additional indication that proliferation and apoptosis are dysregulated not only in MEFs but, also, in mature AS mice hippocampi.

Based on our MEFs and AS mice studies, we suggest that, in the absence of UBE3A expression, the crosstalk between proliferation, apoptosis, and the mitochondrial functioning is disrupted. These findings imply that the fine-tuning of the interaction between the mitochondrial and the proliferation/apoptosis pathways may be of great value when addressing the novel therapeutic approaches for Angelman syndrome patients.

## 5. Conclusions

The herein study indicates that dysregulated levels of UBE3A affects apoptosis and proliferation. Accurate neuronal proliferation during embryonic stages and precise neuronal apoptosis during late embryonic and perinatal stages are required for healthy brain development. This suggests that brains of AS and UBE3A duplication individuals are disrupted at critical early developmental milestones. Hence, later interventions of balancing UBE3A levels might be limited in rescuing some of the phenotypes. The effects of UBE3A dose on apoptosis and proliferation during early brain developmental stages must be further elucidated, so therapeutic strategies beyond correcting UBE3A levels could be considered and investigated.

**Supplementary Materials:** The following are available online at http://www.mdpi.com/2077-0383/9/5/1573/s1. Figure S1: An illustration of $Ube3a^{+/+}$ and $Ube3a^{-/-}$ MEFs generation from E13.5 mouse embryos, Figure S2: XTT assays with different cell numbers at four distinct time points, Figure S3: Western blot analysis of BAX and BCL-2 expression levels in $Ube3a^{+/+}$ and $Ube3a^{-/-}$ MEFs, Figure S4: Alignment of RNA-seq reads on Exon 2 in $Ube3a^{-/-}$ (NULL) and $Ube3a^{+/+}$ (WT) samples, Figure S5: FPKM values of Kdmd5 and Ddx3y genes of individual $Ube3a^{-/-}$ and $Ube3a^{+/+}$ MEFs samples, Figure S6: UBE3A expression levels in MEFs and mice brains. Table S1: Expression table of genes differentially expressed in $Ube3a^{+/+}$ and $Ube3a^{-/-}$ MEFs, Table S2: Expression table of differentially expressed and known to localize to mitochondria (MitoCarta2.0) genes, Table S3: Table with names of genes found as uniquely edited in $Ube3a^{+/+}$ and $Ube3a^{-/-}$ MEFs, Table S4: Table of editing frequencies in genes found as differentially edited in $Ube3a^{+/+}$ and $Ube3a^{-/-}$ MEFs, Table S5: Table of editing frequencies in genes found as differentially edited in $Ube3a^{+/+}$ and $Ube3a^{-/-}$ and that their Gene Ontology term is related to Mitochondrion or Apoptosis, Table S6: Table of differentially expressed proteins, Table S7: Table of expression of up and down regulated proteins and mRNAs Table S8: Table of expression of altered proteins that their mRNAs were found to be unchanged, Table S9: Tables of expression of apoptotic and proliferative genes found as differentiating between WT and AS mice with random forest analysis. Video S1: Representative time-lapse imaging video of $Ube3a^{+/+}$ MEFs over 12 h, Video S2: Representative time-lapse imaging video of $Ube3a^{-/-}$ MEFs over 12 h.

**Author Contributions:** Conceptualization, H.K.; methodology, L.S., J.P, Y.F. and H.K.; validation, L.S., J.P., Y.F. and H.K.; formal analysis, L.S., J.P., Y.F. and H.K.; investigation, L.S., J.P., O.M., Y.F. and H.K.; resources, H.K.; data curation, L.S., J.P., O.M., Y.F. and H.K.; writing—original draft preparation, J.P., L.S., Y.F. and H.K.; writing—review and editing, H.K.; visualization, L.S., J.P., Y.F. and H.K.; supervision, H.K.; project administration, Y.F.; funding acquisition, H.K. All authors have read and agreed to the published version of the manuscript.

**Funding:** Israel Science Foundation (ISF) grant 287/15 and Angelman Syndrome Foundation (ASF)—HK personal grant.

**Acknowledgments:** The Smoler Proteomics Center at the Technion. Tauber Bioinformatics Research Center at the University of Haifa. Center for microscopy and imaging at the University of Haifa.

**Conflicts of Interest:** The authors declare no conflict of interest. The funders had no role in the design of the study; in the collection, analyses, or interpretation of data; in the writing of the manuscript, or in the decision to publish the results.

## References

1. Ramamoorthy, S.; Nawaz, Z. E6-associated protein (E6-AP) is a dual function coactivator of steroid hormone receptors. *Nucl. Recept. Signal.* **2008**, *6*, 6. [CrossRef] [PubMed]
2. Sailer, C.; Offensperger, F.; Julier, A.; Kammer, K.-M.; Walker-Gray, R.; Gold, M.G.; Scheffner, M.; Stengel, F. Structural dynamics of the E6AP/UBE3A-E6-p53 enzyme-substrate complex. *Nat. Commun.* **2018**, *9*, 4441. [CrossRef] [PubMed]

3. Cheng, K.; Li, Y.; Chang, W.-T.; Chen, Z.-C.; Cheng, J.-T.; Tsai, C.-C. Ubiquitin-protein ligase E3a (UBE3A) as a new biomarker of cardiac hypertrophy in cell models. *J. Food Drug Anal.* **2018**, *27*, 355–364. [CrossRef] [PubMed]
4. Gustin, R.M.; Bichell, T.J.V.; Bubser, M.; Daily, J.; Filonova, I.; Mrelashvili, D.; Deutch, A.Y.; Colbran, R.J.; Weeber, E.J.; Haas, K.F. Tissue-specific variation of Ube3a protein expression in rodents and in a mouse model of Angelman syndrome. *Neurobiol. Dis.* **2010**, *39*, 283–291. [CrossRef] [PubMed]
5. Ramamoorthy, S.; Dhananjayan, S.C.; DeMayo, F.J.; Nawaz, Z. Isoform-Specific Degradation of PR-B by E6-AP Is Critical for Normal Mammary Gland Development. *Mol. Endocrinol.* **2010**, *24*, 2099–2113. [CrossRef]
6. Bernassola, F.; Karin, M.; Ciechanover, A.; Melino, G. Review the HECT Family of E3 Ubiquitin Ligases: Multiple Players in Cancer Development. *Cancer Cell* **2008**, *14*, 10–21. [CrossRef]
7. Mishra, A.; Godavarthi, S.K.; Jana, N.R. UBE3A/E6-AP regulates cell proliferation by promoting proteasomal degradation of p27. *Neurobiol. Dis.* **2009**, *36*, 26–34. [CrossRef]
8. Kumar, S.; Talis, A.L.; Howley, P. Identification of HHR23A as a Substrate for E6-associated Protein-mediated Ubiquitination. *J. Biol. Chem.* **1999**, *274*, 18785–18792. [CrossRef]
9. Underbrink, M.P.; Howie, H.L.; Bedard, K.M.; Koop, J.I.; Galloway, D.A. E6 Proteins from Multiple Human Betapapillomavirus Types Degrade Bak and Protect Keratinocytes from Apoptosis after UVB Irradiation. *J. Virol.* **2008**, *82*, 10408–10417. [CrossRef]
10. Scheffner, M.; Huibregtse, J.M.; Vierstra, R.D.; Howley, P. The HPV-16 E6 and E6-AP complex functions as a ubiquitin-protein ligase in the ubiquitination of p53. *Cell* **1993**, *75*, 495–505. [CrossRef]
11. Niebler, M.; Qian, X.; Höfler, D.; Kogosov, V.; Kaewprag, J.; Kaufmann, A.M.; Ly, R.; Böhmer, G.; Zawatzky, R.; Rösl, F.; et al. Post-Translational Control of IL-1β via the Human Papillomavirus Type 16 E6 Oncoprotein: A Novel Mechanism of Innate Immune Escape Mediated by the E3-Ubiquitin Ligase E6-AP and p53. *PLoS Pathog.* **2013**, *9*, e1003536. [CrossRef] [PubMed]
12. Nawaz, Z.; Lonard, D.M.; Dennis, A.P.; Smith, C.L.; O'Malley, B.W. Proteasome-dependent degradation of the human estrogen receptor. *Proc. Natl. Acad. Sci. USA* **1999**, *96*, 1858–1862. [CrossRef] [PubMed]
13. Gao, X.; Mohsin, S.K.; Gatalica, Z.; Fu, G.; Sharma, P.; Nawaz, Z. Decreased Expression of E6-Associated Protein in Breast and Prostate Carcinomas. *Endocrinology* **2005**, *146*, 1707–1712. [CrossRef] [PubMed]
14. Mani, A.; Oh, A.S.; Bowden, E.T.; Lahusen, T.; Lorick, K.L.; Weissman, A.M.; Schlegel, R.; Wellstein, A.; Riegel, A.T. E6AP Mediates Regulated Proteasomal Degradation of the Nuclear Receptor Coactivator Amplified in Breast Cancer 1 in Immortalized Cells. *Cancer Res.* **2006**, *66*, 8680–8686. [CrossRef] [PubMed]
15. Raghu, D.; Paul, P.J.; Gulati, T.; Deb, S.; Khoo, C.; Russo, A.; Gallo, E.; Blandino, G.; Chan, A.-L.; Takano, E.; et al. E6AP promotes prostate cancer by reducing p27 expression. *Oncotarget* **2017**, *8*, 42939–42948. [CrossRef]
16. Shai, A.; Pitot, H.C.; Lambert, P. E6-associated protein is required for human papillomavirus type 16 E6 to cause cervical cancer in mice. *Cancer Res.* **2010**, *70*, 5064–5073. [CrossRef]
17. Sell, G.L.; Margolis, S.S. From UBE3A to Angelman syndrome: A substrate perspective. *Front. Mol. Neurosci.* **2015**, *9*, 75. [CrossRef]
18. Vatsa, N.; Jana, N.R. UBE3A and Its Link with Autism. *Front. Mol. Neurosci.* **2018**, *11*, 448. [CrossRef]
19. Dindot, S.; Antalffy, B.A.; Bhattacharjee, M.B.; Beaudet, A.L. The Angelman syndrome ubiquitin ligase localizes to the synapse and nucleus, and maternal deficiency results in abnormal dendritic spine morphology. *Hum. Mol. Genet.* **2007**, *17*, 111–118. [CrossRef]
20. Kaphzan, H.; Buffington, S.A.; Jung, J.I.; Rasband, M.N.; Klann, E. Alterations in intrinsic membrane properties and the axon initial segment in a mouse model of Angelman syndrome. *J. Neurosci.* **2011**, *31*, 17637–17648. [CrossRef]
21. Jiang, Y.-H.; Armstrong, D.; Albrecht, U.; Atkins, C.; Noebels, J.L.; Eichele, G.; Sweatt, J.D.; Beaudet, A.L. Mutation of the Angelman Ubiquitin Ligase in Mice Causes Increased Cytoplasmic p53 and Deficits of Contextual Learning and Long-Term Potentiation. *Neuron* **1998**, *21*, 799–811. [CrossRef]
22. Kaphzan, H.; Hernandez, P.; Jung, J.I.; Cowansage, K.K.; Deinhardt, K.; Chao, M.V.; Abel, T.; Klann, E. Reversal of impaired hippocampal long-term potentiation and contextual fear memory deficits in Angelman syndrome model mice by ErbB inhibitors. *Biol. Psychiatry* **2012**, *72*, 182–190. [CrossRef] [PubMed]
23. Kaphzan, H.; Buffington, S.A.; Ramaraj, A.B.; Lingrel, J.B.; Rasband, M.N.; Santini, E.; Klann, E. Genetic reduction of the α1 Subunit of Na/K-ATPase corrects multiple hippocampal phenotypes in angelman syndrome. *Cell Rep.* **2013**, *4*, 405–412. [CrossRef] [PubMed]

24. Levav-Cohen, Y.; Wolyniec, K.; Alsheich-Bartok, O.; Chan, A.-L.; Woods, S.J.; Jiang, Y.-H.; Haupt, S.; Haupt, Y. E6AP is required for replicative and oncogene-induced senescence in mouse embryo fibroblasts. *Oncogene* **2011**, *31*, 2199–2209. [CrossRef]
25. Santini, E.; Turner, K.L.; Ramaraj, A.B.; Murphy, M.P.; Klann, E.; Kaphzan, H. Mitochondrial Superoxide Contributes to Hippocampal Synaptic Dysfunction and Memory Deficits in Angelman Syndrome Model Mice. *J. Neurosci.* **2015**, *35*, 16213–16220. [CrossRef]
26. De Zio, D.; Giunta, L.; Corvaro, M.; Ferraro, E.; Cecconi, F. Expanding roles of programmed cell death in mammalian neurodevelopment. *Semin. Cell Dev. Biol.* **2005**, *16*, 281–294. [CrossRef]
27. Lossi, L.; Castagna, C.; Merighi, A. Caspase-3 Mediated Cell Death in the Normal Development of the Mammalian Cerebellum. *Int. J. Mol. Sci.* **2018**, *19*, 3999. [CrossRef]
28. Yamaguchi, Y.; Miura, M. Programmed Cell Death in Neurodevelopment. *Dev. Cell* **2015**, *32*, 478–490. [CrossRef]
29. Thomaidou, D.; Mione, M.C.; Cavanagh, J.F.R.; Parnavelas, J.G. Apoptosis and Its Relation to the Cell Cycle in the Developing Cerebral Cortex. *J. Neurosci.* **1997**, *17*, 1075–1085. [CrossRef]
30. Pozueta, J.; Lefort, R.; Ribe, E.; Troy, C.M.; Arancio, O.; Shelanski, M. Caspase-2 is required for dendritic spine and behavioural alterations in J20 APP transgenic mice. *Nat. Commun.* **2013**, *4*, 1939. [CrossRef]
31. Ertürk, A.; Wang, Y.; Sheng, M. Local Pruning of Dendrites and Spines by Caspase-3-Dependent and Proteasome-Limited Mechanisms. *J. Neurosci.* **2014**, *34*, 1672–1688. [CrossRef] [PubMed]
32. Guo, J.; Ji, Y.; Ding, Y.; Jiang, W.; Sun, Y.; Lu, B.; Nagappan, G. BDNF pro-peptide regulates dendritic spines via caspase-3. *Cell Death Dis.* **2016**, *7*, e2264. [CrossRef] [PubMed]
33. Khatri, N.; Gilbert, J.P.; Huo, Y.; Sharaflari, R.; Nee, M.; Qiao, H.; Man, H.-Y. Faculty Opinions recommendation of The Autism Protein Ube3A/E6AP Remodels Neuronal Dendritic Arborization via Caspase-Dependent Microtubule Destabilization. *J. Neurosci.* **2018**, *38*, 363–378. [CrossRef] [PubMed]
34. Doll, C.A.; Broadie, K. Impaired activity-dependent neural circuit assembly and refinement in autism spectrum disorder genetic models. *Front. Cell. Neurosci.* **2014**, *8*, 1–26. [CrossRef] [PubMed]
35. Scheiffele, P.; Beg, A.A. Angelman syndrome connections. *Nature* **2010**, *468*, 907–908. [CrossRef]
36. Bayır, H.; Kagan, V. Bench-to-bedside review: Mitochondrial injury, oxidative stress and apoptosis—There is nothing more practical than a good theory. *Crit. Care* **2008**, *12*, 206. [CrossRef]
37. Atlante, A.; De Bari, L.; Bobba, A.; Marra, E.; Calissano, P.; Passarella, S. Cytochrome c, released from cerebellar granule cells undergoing apoptosis or excytotoxic death, can generate protonmotive force and drive ATP synthesis in isolated mitochondria. *J. Neurochem.* **2003**, *86*, 591–604. [CrossRef]
38. Stojanovski, D.; Johnston, A.J.; Streimann, I.; Hoogenraad, N.J.; Ryan, M.T. Import of nuclear-encoded proteins into mitochondria. *Exp. Physiol.* **2003**, *88*, 57–64. [CrossRef]
39. Siddiqui, M.F.; Elwell, C.; Johnson, S. Mitochondrial Dysfunction in Autism Spectrum Disorders. *Autism-Open Access* **2016**, *6*, 1–7. [CrossRef]
40. Jarskog, L.F.; Glantz, L.A.; Gilmore, J.H.; Lieberman, J.A. Apoptotic mechanisms in the pathophysiology of schizophrenia. *Prog. Neuro-Psychopharmacol. Biol. Psychiatry* **2005**, *29*, 846–858. [CrossRef]
41. Prabakaran, S.; Swatton, J.E.; Ryan, M.M.; Huffaker, S.J.; Huang, J.T.J.; Griffin, J.L.; Wayland, M.; Freeman, T.; Dudbridge, F.; Lilley, K.S.; et al. Mitochondrial dysfunction in schizophrenia: Evidence for compromised brain metabolism and oxidative stress. *Mol. Psychiatry* **2004**, *9*, 684–697. [CrossRef] [PubMed]
42. Shulyakova, N.; Andreazza, A.C.; Mills, L.R.; Eubanks, J.H. Mitochondrial Dysfunction in the Pathogenesis of Rett Syndrome: Implications for Mitochondria-Targeted Therapies. *Front. Cell. Neurosci.* **2017**, *11*, 185. [CrossRef] [PubMed]
43. Izzo, A.; Mollo, N.; Nitti, M.; Paladino, S.; Cali, G.; Genesio, R.; Bonfiglio, F.; Cicatiello, R.; Barbato, M.; Sarnataro, V.; et al. Mitochondrial dysfunction in down syndrome: Molecular mechanisms and therapeutic targets. *Mol. Med.* **2018**, *24*, 2. [CrossRef] [PubMed]
44. Cagalinec, M.; Liiv, M.; Hodurova, Z.; Hickey, M.; Vaarmann, A.; Mandel, M.; Zeb, A.; Choubey, V.; Kuum, M.; Safiulina, D.; et al. Role of Mitochondrial Dynamics in Neuronal Development: Mechanism for Wolfram Syndrome. *PLoS Biol.* **2016**, *14*, e1002511. [CrossRef]
45. Marazziti, D.; Baroni, S.; Picchetti, M.; Landi, P.; Silvestri, S.; Vatteroni, E.; Catena Dell'Osso, M. Psychiatric disorders and mitochondrial dysfunctions. *Eur. Rev. Med. Pharmacol. Sci.* **2012**, *16*, 270–275.

46. Su, H.; Fan, W.; Coskun, P.E.; Vesa, J.; Gold, J.-A.; Jiang, Y.-H.; Potluri, P.; Procaccio, V.; Acab, A.; Weiss, J.H.; et al. Mitochondrial dysfunction in CA1 hippocampal neurons of the UBE3A deficient mouse model for Angelman syndrome. *Neurosci. Lett.* **2009**, *487*, 129–133. [CrossRef]
47. Berkowitz, B.A.; Lenning, J.; Khetarpal, N.; Tran, C.; Wu, J.Y.; Berri, A.M.; Dernay, K.; Haacke, E.M.; Shafie-Khorassani, F.; Podolsky, R.H.; et al. In vivo imaging of prodromal hippocampus CA1 subfield oxidative stress in models of Alzheimer disease and Angelman syndrome. *FASEB J.* **2017**, *31*, 4179–4186. [CrossRef]
48. Schroeder, T.; Schwarzfischer, M.; Skylaki, S.; SchaubergeriD, B.; Hoppe, P.S.; Loeffler, D.; Kokkaliaris, K.; Hastreiter, S.; Skylaki, E.; Filipczyk, A.; et al. Software tools for single-cell tracking and quantification of cellular and molecular properties. *Nat. Biotechnol.* **2016**, *34*, 703–706. [CrossRef]
49. Bolger, A.M.; Lohse, M.; Usadel, B. Trimmomatic: A flexible trimmer for Illumina sequence data. *Bioinformatics* **2014**, *30*, 2114–2120. [CrossRef]
50. Langmead, B.; Salzberg, S.L. Fast gapped-read alignment with Bowtie 2. *Nat. Methods* **2012**, *9*, 357–359. [CrossRef]
51. Li, B.; Dewey, C.N. RSEM: Accurate transcript quantification from RNA-Seq data with or without a reference genome. *BMC Bioinform.* **2011**, *12*, 323. [CrossRef] [PubMed]
52. Love, M.I.; Huber, W.; Anders, S. Moderated estimation of fold change and dispersion for RNA-seq data with DESeq2. *Genome Biol.* **2014**, *15*, 002832. [CrossRef] [PubMed]
53. Huang, D.W.; Sherman, B.; Tan, Q.; Collins, J.R.; Alvord, W.G.; Roayaei, J.; Stephens, R.M.; Baseler, M.; Lane, H.C.; Lempicki, R. The DAVID Gene Functional Classification Tool: A novel biological module-centric algorithm to functionally analyze large gene lists. *Genome Biol.* **2007**, *8*, R183. [CrossRef] [PubMed]
54. Huang, D.W.; Sherman, B.T.; Lempicki, R.A. Systematic and integrative analysis of large gene lists using DAVID bioinformatics resources. *Nat. Protoc.* **2009**, *4*, 44–57. [CrossRef] [PubMed]
55. Mi, H.; Muruganujan, A.; Huang, X.; Ebert, D.; Mills, C.; Guo, X.; Thomas, P.D. Protocol Update for large-scale genome and gene function analysis with the PANTHER classification system (v.14.0). *Nat. Protoc.* **2019**, *14*, 703–721. [CrossRef] [PubMed]
56. Calvo, S.; Clauser, K.R.; Mootha, V.K. MitoCarta2.0: An updated inventory of mammalian mitochondrial proteins. *Nucleic Acids Res.* **2015**, *44*, D1251–D1257. [CrossRef] [PubMed]
57. Koyavski, L.; Panov, J.; Simchi, L.; Rayi, P.R.; Sharvit, L.; Feuermann, Y.; Kaphzan, H. Sex-Dependent Sensory Phenotypes and Related Transcriptomic Expression Profiles Are Differentially Affected by Angelman Syndrome. *Mol. Neurobiol.* **2019**, *56*, 5998–6016. [CrossRef]
58. Liaw, A.; Wiener, M. Classification and Regression with Random Forest. *R News* **2002**, *2*, 18–22.
59. Venables, W.; Ripley, B. *Modern Applied Statistics with S*, 4th ed.; Springer: New York, NY, USA, 2002; ISBN 0-387-95457-0.
60. Zhang, Q.; Xiao, X. Genome sequence–independent identification of RNA editing sites. *Nat. Methods* **2015**, *12*, 347–350. [CrossRef]
61. Wilks, S.S. The Large-Sample Distribution of the Likelihood Ratio for Testing Composite Hypotheses. *Ann. Math. Stat.* **1938**, *9*, 60–62. [CrossRef]
62. Roehm, N.W.; Rodgers, G.H.; Hatfield, S.M.; Glasebrook, A.L. An improved colorimetric assay for cell proliferation and viability utilizing the tetrazolium salt XTT. *J. Immunol. Methods* **1991**, *142*, 257–265. [CrossRef]
63. Carbonari, M. New use for an old reagent: Cell cycle analysis of DNA content using flow cytometry in formamide treated cells. *Cytom. Part A* **2016**, *89*, 498–503. [CrossRef] [PubMed]
64. Raisova, M.; Hossini, A.M.; Eberle, J.; Riebeling, C.; Wieder, T.; Sturm, I.; Daniel, P.T.; Orfanos, C.E.; Geilen, C.C. The Bax/Bcl-2 ratio determines the susceptibility of human melanoma cells to CD95/Fas-mediated apoptosis. *J. Investig. Dermatol.* **2001**, *117*, 333–340. [CrossRef] [PubMed]
65. Staedtler, F.; Hartmann, N.; Letzkus, M.; Bongiovanni, S.; Scherer, A.; Marc, P.; Johnson, K.J.; Schumacher, M. Robust and tissue-independent gender-specific transcript biomarkers. *Biomarkers* **2013**, *18*, 436–445. [CrossRef] [PubMed]
66. Khan, O.Y.; Fu, G.; Ismail, A.; Srinivasan, S.; Cao, X.; Tu, Y.; Lu, S.; Nawaz, Z. Multifunction Steroid Receptor Coactivator, E6-Associated Protein, Is Involved in Development of the Prostate Gland. *Mol. Endocrinol.* **2006**, *20*, 544–559. [CrossRef]

67. Zhang, W.; Liu, H.T. MAPK signal pathways in the regulation of cell proliferation in mammalian cells. *Cell Res.* **2002**, *12*, 9–18. [CrossRef]
68. Zhang, M.; Liu, J.; Li, M.; Zhang, S.; Lu, Y.; Liang, Y.; Zhao, K.; Li, Y. Insulin-like growth factor 1/insulin-like growth factor 1 receptor signaling protects against cell apoptosis through the PI3K/AKT pathway in glioblastoma cells. *Exp. Ther. Med.* **2018**, *16*, 1477–1482. [CrossRef]
69. Fan, J.; Wei, Q.; Liao, J.; Zou, Y.; Song, D.; Xiong, D.; Ma, C.; Hu, X.; Qu, X.; Chen, L.; et al. Noncanonical Wnt signaling plays an important role in modulating canonical Wnt-regulated stemness, proliferation and terminal differentiation of hepatic progenitors. *Oncotarget* **2017**, *8*, 27105–27119. [CrossRef]
70. Baysal, B.E.; Sharma, S.; Hashemikhabir, S.; Janga, S.C. RNA Editing in Pathogenesis of Cancer. *Cancer Res.* **2017**, *77*, 3733–3739. [CrossRef]
71. Zhang, Q. Analysis of RNA Editing Sites from RNA-Seq Data Using GIREMI. *Methods Mol Biol.* **2018**, *1751*, 101–108. [CrossRef]
72. Liu, Y.; Beyer, A.; Aebersold, R. On the Dependency of Cellular Protein Levels on mRNA Abundance. *Cell* **2016**, *165*, 535–550. [CrossRef]
73. Gamell, C.; Gulati, T.; Levav-Cohen, Y.; Young, R.J.; Do, H.; Pilling, P.; Takano, E.; Watkins, N.; Fox, S.B.; Russell, P.; et al. Reduced abundance of the E3 ubiquitin ligase E6AP contributes to decreased expression of the INK4/ARF locus in non-small cell lung cancer. *Sci. Signal.* **2017**, *10*, eaaf8223. [CrossRef] [PubMed]
74. Wenric, S.; Shemirani, R. Using Supervised Learning Methods for Gene Selection in RNA-Seq Case-Control Studies. *Front. Genet.* **2018**, *9*, 297. [CrossRef] [PubMed]
75. Kishino, T.; Lalande, M.; Wagstaff, J. UBE3A/E6-AP mutations cause Angelman syndrome. *Nat. Genet.* **1997**, *15*, 70–73. [CrossRef] [PubMed]
76. Southwell, D.G.; Paredes, M.F.; Galvao, R.P.; Jones, D.L.; Froemke, R.C.; Sebe, J.Y.; Alfaro-Cervello, C.; Tang, Y.; García-Verdugo, J.M.; Rubenstein, J.L.; et al. Intrinsically determined cell death of developing cortical interneurons. *Nature* **2012**, *491*, 109–113. [CrossRef] [PubMed]
77. Daily, J.; Smith, A.G.; Weeber, E.J. Spatial and temporal silencing of the human maternal UBE3A gene. *Eur. J. Paediatr. Neurol.* **2012**, *16*, 587–591. [CrossRef]
78. Matsui, H.; Gavinio, R.; Asano, T.; Uemura, N.; Ito, H.; Taniguchi, Y.; Kobayashi, Y.; Maki, T.; Shen, J.; Takeda, S.; et al. PINK1 and Parkin complementarily protect dopaminergic neurons in vertebrates. *Hum. Mol. Genet.* **2013**, *22*, 2423–2434. [CrossRef]
79. Wolyniec, K.; Levav-Cohen, Y.; Jiang, Y.-H.; Haupt, S.; Haupt, Y. The E6AP E3 ubiquitin ligase regulates the cellular response to oxidative stress. *Oncogene* **2012**, *32*, 3510–3519. [CrossRef]
80. Nicoletti, I.; Migliorati, G.; Pagliacci, M.; Grignani, F.; Riccardi, C. A rapid and simple method for measuring thymocyte apoptosis by propidium iodide staining and flow cytometry. *J. Immunol. Methods* **1991**, *139*, 271–279. [CrossRef]
81. Vermes, I.; Haanen, C.; Steffens-Nakken, H.; Reutellingsperger, C. A novel assay for apoptosis Flow cytometric detection of phosphatidylserine expression on early apoptotic cells using fluorescein labelled Annexin V. *J. Immunol. Methods* **1995**, *184*, 39–51. [CrossRef]
82. Reed, J.C. Proapoptotic multidomain Bcl-2/Bax-family proteins: Mechanisms, physiological roles, and therapeutic opportunities. *Cell Death Differ.* **2006**, *13*, 1378–1386. [CrossRef] [PubMed]
83. Zhou, X.; Deng, S.; Liu, H.; Liu, Y.; Yang, Z.; Xing, T.; Jing, B.; Zhang, X. Knockdown of ubiquitin protein ligase E3A affects proliferation and invasion, and induces apoptosis of breast cancer cells through regulation of annexin A2. *Mol. Med. Rep.* **2012**, *12*, 1107–1113. [CrossRef] [PubMed]
84. Guadagno, J.; Swan, P.; Shaikh, R.; Cregan, S.P. Microglia-derived IL-1β triggers p53-mediated cell cycle arrest and apoptosis in neural precursor cells. *Cell Death Dis.* **2015**, *6*, e1779. [CrossRef]
85. Shan, H.; Bian, Y.; Shu, Z.; Zhang, L.; Zhu, J.; Ding, J.; Lu, M.; Xiao, M.; Hu, G. Fluoxetine protects against IL-1β-induced neuronal apoptosis via downregulation of p53. *Neuropharmacology* **2016**, *107*, 68–78. [CrossRef] [PubMed]
86. Corbett, G.; Roy, A.; Pahan, K. Gemfibrozil, a lipid-lowering drug, upregulates IL-1 receptor antagonist in mouse cortical neurons: Implications for neuronal self-defense. *J. Immunol.* **2012**, *189*, 1002–1013. [CrossRef] [PubMed]
87. Schizas, N.; Perry, S.; Andersson, B.; Wählby, C.; Kullander, K.; Hailer, N.P. Differential Neuroprotective Effects of Interleukin-1 Receptor Antagonist on Spinal Cord Neurons after Excitotoxic Injury. *Neuroimmunomodulation* **2018**, *24*, 220–230. [CrossRef] [PubMed]

88. Baker, D.J.; Jin, F.; Van Deursen, J. The yin and yang of the Cdkn2a locus in senescence and aging. *Cell Cycle* **2008**, *7*, 2795–2802. [CrossRef]
89. Nawaz, Z.; Lonard, D.M.; Smith, C.L.; Lev-Lehman, E.; Tsai, S.Y.; Tsai, M.-J.; O'Malley, B.W. The Angelman Syndrome-Associated Protein, E6-AP, Is a Coactivator for the Nuclear Hormone Receptor Superfamily. *Mol. Cell. Biol.* **1999**, *19*, 1182–1189. [CrossRef]
90. Pantic, B.; Trevisan, E.; Citta, A.; Rigobello, M.P.; Marin, O.; Bernardi, P.; Salvatori, S.; Rasola, A. Myotonic dystrophy protein kinase (DMPK) prevents ROS-induced cell death by assembling a hexokinase II-Src complex on the mitochondrial surface. *Cell Death Dis.* **2013**, *4*, e858. [CrossRef]
91. Puchalska, P.; Crawford, P. Multi-dimensional Roles of Ketone Bodies in Fuel Metabolism, Signaling, and Therapeutics. *Cell Metab.* **2017**, *25*, 262–284. [CrossRef]
92. Farajollahi, S.; Maas, S. Molecular diversity through RNA editing: A balancing act. *Trends Genet.* **2010**, *26*, 221–230. [CrossRef] [PubMed]
93. Kung, C.-P.; Maggi, L.B.J.; Weber, J.D. The Role of RNA Editing in Cancer Development and Metabolic Disorders. *Front. Endocrinol.* **2018**, *9*, 762. [CrossRef] [PubMed]
94. Tran, S.S.; Jun, H.-I.; Bahn, J.H.; Azghadi, A.; Ramaswami, G.; Van Nostrand, E.L.; Nguyen, T.B.; Hsiao, Y.-H.E.; Lee, C.; Pratt, G.A.; et al. Faculty Opinions recommendation of Widespread RNA editing dysregulation in brains from autistic individuals. *Nat. Neurosci.* **2019**, *22*, 25–36. [CrossRef] [PubMed]
95. Raabe, C.A.; Voss, R.; Kummerfeld, D.-M.; Brosius, J.; Galiveti, C.R.; Wolters, A.; Seggewiss, J.; Huge, A.; Skryabin, B.V.; Rozhdestvensky, T.S. Ectopic expression of Snord115 in choroid plexus interferes with editing but not splicing of 5-Ht2c receptor pre-mRNA in mice. *Sci. Rep.* **2019**, *9*, 4300. [CrossRef] [PubMed]
96. Sakurai, M.; Shiromoto, Y.; Ota, H.; Song, C.; Kossenkov, A.V.; Wickramasinghe, J.; Showe, L.C.; Skordalakes, E.; Tang, H.-Y.; Speicher, D.W.; et al. ADAR1 controls apoptosis of stressed cells by inhibiting Staufen1-mediated mRNA decay. *Nat. Struct. Mol. Biol.* **2017**, *24*, 534–543. [CrossRef] [PubMed]
97. Yang, C.C.; Chen, Y.T.; Chang, Y.F.; Liu, H.; Kuo, Y.P.; Shih, C.T.; Liao, W.C.; Chen, H.W.; Tsai, W.S.; Tan, B.C.M. ADAR1-mediated 3′ UTR editing and expression control of antiapoptosis genes fine-tunes cellular apoptosis response. *Cell Death Dis.* **2017**, *8*, e2833. [CrossRef]
98. Shen, X.; Han, G.; Li, S.; Song, Y.; Shen, H.; Zhai, Y.; Wang, Y.; Zhang, F.; Dong, N.; Li, T.; et al. Association between the T6459C point mutation of the mitochondrial MT-CO1 gene and susceptibility to sepsis among Chinese Han people. *J. Cell. Mol. Med.* **2018**, *22*, 5257–5264. [CrossRef]
99. Silva-Santos, S.; Van Woerden, G.M.; Bruinsma, C.F.; Mientjes, E.; Jolfaei, M.A.; Distel, B.; Kushner, S.A.; Elgersma, Y. Ube3a reinstatement identifies distinct developmental windows in a murine Angelman syndrome model. *J. Clin. Investig.* **2015**, *125*, 2069–2076. [CrossRef]
100. Dupret, D.; Revest, J.-M.; Koehl, M.; Ichas, F.; De Giorgi, F.; Costet, P.; Abrous, N.; Piazza, P.V. Spatial Relational Memory Requires Hippocampal Adult Neurogenesis. *PLoS ONE* **2008**, *3*, e1959. [CrossRef]
101. Dupret, D.; Fabre, A.; Döbrössy, M.D.; Panatier, A.; Rodríguez, J.J.; Lamarque, S.; Lemaire, V.; Oliet, S.H.R.; Piazza, P.-V.; Abrous, N. Spatial learning depends on both the addition and removal of new hippocampal neurons. *PLoS Biol.* **2007**, *5*, e214. [CrossRef]
102. Van Woerden, G.M.; Harris, K.D.; Hojjati, M.R.; Gustin, R.M.; Qiu, S.; Freire, R.D.A.; Jiang, Y.-H.; Elgersma, Y.; Weeber, E.J. Rescue of neurological deficits in a mouse model for Angelman syndrome by reduction of αCaMKII inhibitory phosphorylation. *Nat. Neurosci.* **2007**, *10*, 280–282. [CrossRef] [PubMed]
103. Fruman, D.; Chiu, H.; Hopkins, B.D.; Bagrodia, S.; Cantley, L.C.; Abraham, R.T. The PI3K Pathway in Human Disease. *Cell* **2017**, *170*, 605–635. [CrossRef] [PubMed]
104. Srinivasan, S.; Nawaz, Z. E3 ubiquitin protein ligase, E6-associated protein (E6-AP) regulates PI3K-Akt signaling and prostate cell growth. *Biochim. Biophys. Acta (BBA) Bioenerg.* **2010**, *1809*, 119–127. [CrossRef] [PubMed]

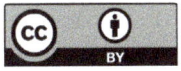

© 2020 by the authors. Licensee MDPI, Basel, Switzerland. This article is an open access article distributed under the terms and conditions of the Creative Commons Attribution (CC BY) license (http://creativecommons.org/licenses/by/4.0/).

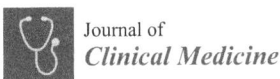 

*Article*

# Mitochondrial Signatures in Circulating Extracellular Vesicles of Older Adults with Parkinson's Disease: Results from the EXosomes in PArkiNson's Disease (EXPAND) Study

Anna Picca [1,2,†], Flora Guerra [3,†], Riccardo Calvani [1,2,*], Federico Marini [4], Alessandra Biancolillo [5], Giovanni Landi [2], Raffaella Beli [3], Francesco Landi [1,2], Roberto Bernabei [1,2], Anna Rita Bentivoglio [2,6], Maria Rita Lo Monaco [2], Cecilia Bucci [3,*] and Emanuele Marzetti [1,2]

[1] Institute of Internal Medicine and Geriatrics, Università Cattolica del Sacro Cuore, 00168 Rome, Italy; anna.picca@guest.policlinicogemelli.it (A.P.); francesco.landi@unicatt.it (F.L.); roberto.bernabei@unicatt.it (R.B.); emanuele.marzetti@policlinicogemelli.it (E.M.)
[2] Fondazione Policlinico Universitario "Agostino Gemelli" IRCCS, 00168 Rome, Italy; giovandi@libero.it (G.L.); annarita.bentivoglio@policlinicogemelli.it (A.R.B.); mariarita.lomonaco@policlinicogemelli.it (M.R.L.M.)
[3] Department of Biological and Environmental Sciences and Technologies, Università del Salento, 73100 Lecce, Italy; guerraflora@gmail.com (F.G.); raffaella.beli@unisalento.it (R.B.)
[4] Department of Chemistry, Sapienza Università di Roma, 00185 Rome, Italy; federico.marini@uniroma1.it
[5] Department of Physical and Chemical Sciences, Università degli Studi dell'Aquila, 67100 L'Aquila, Italy; alessandra.biancolillo@univaq.it
[6] Institute of Neurology, Università Cattolica del Sacro Cuore, 00168 Rome, Italy
* Correspondence: riccardo.calvani@guest.policlinicogemelli.it (R.C.); cecilia.bucci@unisalento.it (C.B.); Tel.: +39-06-3015-5559 (R.C.); +39-08-3229-8900 (C.B.); Fax: +39-06-3051-911 (R.C.); +39-08-3229-8941 (C.B.)
† Equal contribution.

Received: 24 December 2019; Accepted: 9 February 2020; Published: 12 February 2020

**Abstract:** Systemic inflammation and mitochondrial dysfunction are involved in neurodegeneration in Parkinson's disease (PD). Extracellular vesicle (EV) trafficking may link inflammation and mitochondrial dysfunction. In the present study, circulating small EVs (sEVs) from 16 older adults with PD and 12 non-PD controls were purified and characterized. A panel of serum inflammatory biomolecules was measured by multiplex immunoassay. Protein levels of three tetraspanins (CD9, CD63, and CD81) and selected mitochondrial markers (adenosine triphosphate 5A (ATP5A), mitochondrial cytochrome C oxidase subunit I (MTCOI), nicotinamide adenine dinucleotide reduced form (NADH):ubiquinone oxidoreductase subunit B8 (NDUFB8), NADH:ubiquinone oxidoreductase subunit S3 (NDUFS3), succinate dehydrogenase complex iron sulfur subunit B (SDHB), and ubiquinol-cytochrome C reductase core protein 2 (UQCRC2)) were quantified in purified sEVs by immunoblotting. Relative to controls, PD participants showed a greater amount of circulating sEVs. Levels of CD9 and CD63 were lower in the sEV fraction of PD participants, whereas those of CD81 were similar between groups. Lower levels of ATP5A, NDUFS3, and SDHB were detected in sEVs from PD participants. No signal was retrieved for UQCRC2, MTCOI, or NDUFB8 in either participant group. To identify a molecular signature in circulating sEVs in relationship to systemic inflammation, a low level-fused (multi-platform) partial least squares discriminant analysis was applied. The model correctly classified 94.2% ± 6.1% PD participants and 66.7% ± 5.4% controls, and identified seven biomolecules as relevant (CD9, NDUFS3, C-reactive protein, fibroblast growth factor 21, interleukin 9, macrophage inflammatory protein 1β, and tumor necrosis factor alpha). In conclusion, a mitochondrial signature was identified in circulating sEVs from older adults with PD, in association with a specific inflammatory profile. In-depth characterization of sEV trafficking may allow identifying new biomarkers for PD and possible targets for personalized interventions.

**Keywords:** aging; biomarkers; mitophagy; mitochondrial dynamics; mitochondrial quality control; mitochondrial-derived vesicles; exosomes; mitochondrial-lysosomal axis

## 1. Introduction

Parkinson's disease (PD) is the second most common neurodegenerative disease affecting older adults [1]. Among neurodegenerative disorders, PD has shown the fastest growth in prevalence, due to global population aging, greater exposure to environmental risk factors, and longer disease duration [2,3].

Progressive demise of midbrain dopaminergic neurons of the *substantia nigra pars compacta* and dopamine depletion in the *striatum* are pathologic hallmarks of PD, which is characterized clinically by motor (i.e., bradykinesia, postural inability, rigidity, and tremor) and non-motor signs and symptoms (e.g., constipation, depression, sleep disorders, cognitive dysfunction) [4]. Dopaminergic neurotoxicity triggered by aggregation of misfolded α-synuclein is a well-established pathologic trait of PD [5]. However, the molecular events underlying the onset and progression of PD are still debated [5].

Mitochondrial dysfunction is a major factor in the pathogenesis of familial PD [6]. Age-related mitochondrial dyshomeostasis and the ensuing oxidative stress also favor aberrant protein folding and accrual of noxious protein aggregates, including α-synuclein [7]. The co-occurrence of mitochondrial dysfunction and impaired proteostasis during aging is therefore proposed as a mechanism triggering neuronal dysfunction in PD [8]. Remarkably, peripheral changes (e.g., systemic inflammation, metabolic alterations) are thought to precede and contribute to neurodegeneration in PD [9,10]. However, whether and how mitochondrial dysfunction and protein dyshomeostasis in neurons are linked to peripheral processes is currently unknown.

Failing mitochondrial quality control (MQC) processes is acknowledged as a major mechanism underlying mitochondrial dysfunction and loss of mitochondrial DNA (mtDNA) stability during aging and in the setting of neurodegeneration [11,12]. Extracellular vesicles (EVs) are delivery systems through which cells communicate or remove unwanted materials. Among EVs, exosomes originate from endocytic compartments [13]. Exosome precursors, referred to as intraluminal vesicles, are generated from the inward budding of small domains of early endosomal membranes. The accumulation of intraluminal vesicles into endocytic organelles results in the formation of multivesicular bodies (MVBs). MVBs release their cargo—now defined as exosomes—into the extracellular space via fusion with the plasma membrane [13–15]. Here, EV cargo may trigger inflammation [16]. In the setting of failing mitochondrial fidelity pathways, the generation and release of mitochondrial-derived vesicles (MDVs) may act as a further process of MQC orchestrated by mitochondrial–lysosomal crosstalk [17]. Although the release of MDV clears out dysfunctional organelle and avoids the permanence of noxious material within the cell, it may trigger a sterile inflammatory response by binding and activating membrane or cytoplasmic pattern recognition receptors (PRRs) (reviewed in [18]). Indeed, extracellular mtDNA can ignite an inflammatory response through the binding of hypomethylated CpG motifs, similar to those of bacterial DNA, to PRRs. This event could represent a mechanism linking mitochondrial dysfunction to systemic inflammation in PD [19–21]. However, mtDNA might not be the only mitochondrial component displaced into the systemic circulation via EVs to fuel systemic inflammation.

To shed light on the relationship between EV trafficking and inflammation in PD, we purified and characterized the cargo of small EVs (sEVs)/exosomes from the serum of older adults with PD and measured the concentration of a panel of circulating inflammatory biomarkers. Low level-fused (multi-platform) partial least squares discriminant analysis (PLS-DA) was applied to identify the molecular signature related to circulating sEVs and systemic inflammation in PD.

## 2. Materials and Methods

### 2.1. Study Design and Participants

The EXsomes in PArkiNson Disease (EXPAND) study was designed as a case-control investigation aimed at characterizing the cargo of circulating sEVs/exosomes in older adults with PD [21]. The protocol was approved by the Ethics Committee of the Università Cattolica del Sacro Cuore (Rome, Italy) (protocol # 0045298/17). The study was conducted in agreement with legal requirements and international norms (Declaration of Helsinki, 1964).

Participant recruitment was coordinated by the Institute of Neurology at the Università Cattolica del Sacro Cuore, (Rome, Italy) and was carried out at the Fondazione Policlinico Universitario "Agostino Gemelli" IRCCS (Rome, Italy). Analyses were conducted in a convenience sample of 28 participants, 16 cases diagnosed with PD according to the Queen Square Brain Bank criteria [22] under stable dopaminergic therapy for at least 1 month prior to enrolment, and 12 age- and sex-matched controls without any signs of parkinsonism or potential premotor symptoms. As previously detailed [10], drug-induced parkinsonism (dopamine receptor blocker or dopamine-depleting agent) or vascular (arteriosclerotic) parkinsonism, progressive neurological diseases, and cognitive impairment (i.e., Mini Mental State Examination (MMSE) score < 24/30) were considered exclusion criteria for both cases and controls. Prior to enrolment, all participants signed an informed consent form.

### 2.2. Blood Sampling and Serum Separation

Blood samples were collected in the morning by venipuncture of the median cubital vein after overnight fasting, using commercial collection tubes (BD Vacutainer; Becton, Dickinson and Co., Franklin Lakes, NJ, USA). Serum separation was obtained after 30 min of clotting at room temperature and subsequent centrifugation at $1000\times g$ for 15 min at 4 °C. The upper clear fraction (serum) was collected in 0.5-mL aliquots. One aliquot was immediately delivered to the centralized diagnostic laboratory of the Fondazione Policlinico Universitario "Agostino Gemelli" IRCCS for standard blood biochemistry. The remaining aliquots were stored at −80 °C until analysis.

### 2.3. Isolation and Characterization of Small Extracellular Vesicles/Exosomes

#### 2.3.1. Purification of Small Extracellular Vesicles/Exosomes

Purification of sEVs/exosomes was performed as previously described [21]. Briefly, serum samples were diluted with equal volumes of phosphate-buffered saline (PBS) to reduce fluid viscosity and centrifuged at $2000\times g$ at 4 °C for 30 min. Pellets were discarded to remove cell debris, and supernatants were collected and centrifuged at $12,000\times g$ at 4 °C for 45 min to remove apoptotic bodies, mitochondrial fragments, cell debris, and large vesicles (mean size > 200 nm). After discarding pellets, supernatants were ultracentrifuged at $110,000\times g$ at 4 °C for 2 h. Afterwards, pellets were recovered and resuspended in PBS, filtered through a 0.22-μm filter, and further ultracentrifuged at $110,000\times g$ at 4 °C for 70 min to eliminate contaminant proteins. Pellets enriched in purified sEVs/exosomes were resuspended in 100 μL of PBS and proteins were quantified by the Bradford assay [23]. The amount of sEVs was normalized for total serum protein concentration and is shown as percentage of the control group set at 100%. For quality control purposes, sEVs/exosomes from one control and one PD participant were purified through a precipitation method using the miRCURY Exosome Serum/Plasma Kit (Qiagen, Hilden, Germany).

#### 2.3.2. Western Immunoblot Analysis of Small Extracellular Vesicles

The identification of sEV type and the characterization of protein cargo were accomplished by Western immunoblotting, as described elsewhere [24]. Briefly, equal amounts (1.25 μg) of sEV proteins from PD patients and controls were separated by sodium dodecyl sulphate polyacrylamide gel electrophoresis (SDS-PAGE) and subsequently electroblotted onto polyvinylidenefluoride (PVDF)

Immobilon-P membranes (Millipore, Burlington, MA, USA). To determine the type of sEVs, membranes were probed with primary antibodies against CD9, CD63, and CD81 according to the criteria proposed by Kowal et al. [25]. As recommended by the International Society of Extracellular Vesicles [26], the purity of the sEV preparations obtained by ultracentrifugation or precipitation was also ascertained by probing samples for the cytosolic protein flotilin (positive control) and for heterogeneous nuclear ribonucleoprotein A1 (HNRNPA1, negative control).

Small EV protein cargo was characterized using antibodies targeting components of the five complexes of the mitochondrial electron transport chain [adenosine triphosphate 5A (ATP5A; complex V), mitochondrial cytochrome C oxidase subunit I (MTCOI; complex IV), nicotinamide adenine dinucleotide reduced form (NADH):ubiquinone oxidoreductase subunit B8 (NDUFB8; complex I), NADH:ubiquinone oxidoreductase subunit S3 (NDUFS3; complex I), succinate dehydrogenase complex iron sulfur subunit B (SDHB; complex II), and ubiquinol-cytochrome C reductase core protein 2 (UQCRC2; complex III)]. Technical specifications of the primary antibodies used are listed in Table 1. Membranes were incubated overnight and then probed for 1 h at room temperature with anti-mouse peroxidase-conjugated secondary antibodies (1:2000) (Bio-Rad Laboratories, Inc., Hercules, CA, USA). Blots were visualized using the ECL Plus Western blot substrate (Bio-Rad Laboratories) and ECL films (GE Healthcare, Chicago, IL, USA). Images were then acquired with an Epson Perfection V600 Scanner (Epson, Suwa, Japan) and bands were quantified by densitometry using the ImageJ software version 1.5Oi (National Institute of Health, Bethesda, MD, USA).

**Table 1.** Technical specifications of the primary antibodies used for Western immunoblotting.

| Antibody | Manufacturer and Catalog Number | Type | Species | Dilution | Detected Band MW (kDa) |
|---|---|---|---|---|---|
| ATP5A (complex V) MTCOI (complex IV) NDUFB8 (complex I) SDHB (complex II) UQCRC2 (complex III) | Abcam (Cambridge, MA, USA) ab1104413 | Monoclonal | Mouse | 1:250 | 55 40 20 30 48 |
| CD9 | Santa Cruz Biotechnology (Santa Cruz, CA, USA) (sc-13118) | Monoclonal | Mouse | 1:200 | 25 |
| CD63 | Santa Cruz Biotechnology (sc-5275) | Monoclonal | Mouse | 1:200 | 26 |
| CD81 | Santa Cruz Biotechnology (sc-166020) | Monoclonal | Mouse | 1:200 | 25 |
| NDUFS3 (complex I) | Santa Cruz Biotechnology (sc-374283) | Monoclonal | Mouse | 1:200 | 25 |
| Flotilin | Santa Cruz Biotechnology (sc-74566) | Monoclonal | Mouse | 1:200 | 48 |
| HNRNPA1 | Santa Cruz Biotechnology (sc-32301) | Monoclonal | Mouse | 1:1000 | 36 |

*Abbreviations*: ATP5A, adenosine triphosphate 5A; MTCOI, mitochondrial cytochrome C oxidase subunit I; HNRNPA1, heterogeneous nuclear ribonucleoprotein A1; MW, molecular weight; NDUFB8, nicotinamide adenine dinucleotide reduced form (NADH):ubiquinone oxidoreductase subunit B8; NDUFS3, NADH:ubiquinone oxidoreductase subunit S3; SDHB, succinate dehydrogenase complex iron sulfur subunit B; UQCRC2, ubiquinol-cytochrome C reductase core protein 2.

Values of optical density (OD) of immunodetected protein bands were normalized for the amount of sEV total proteins, as determined by the Bradford assay, and related to the control group, whose OD was set at 100%.

## 2.4. Measurement of Serum Concentrations of Inflammatory and Neurotrophic Biomolecules

A biomarker panel was designed on the basis of previous studies by our group in older adult populations [27,28]. Serum samples from PD and control participants were assayed in duplicate for a panel of 27 inflammatory mediators, including cytokines, chemokines, and growth factors using the Bio-Plex Pro Human Cytokine 27-plex Assay kit (#M500KCAF0Y, Bio-Rad Laboratories) on a Bio-Plex System with Luminex xMap Technology (Bio-Rad Laboratories) (Table 2). Data were acquired on Bio-Plex Manager Software 6.1 (Bio-Rad Laboratories) with instrument default settings. Standard curves across all analytes were optimized, outliers were removed, and results were recorded as concentration (pg/mL).

Table 2. Serum inflammatory biomediators assayed by multiplex immunoassay.

| Biomarker Class | Assayed Biomolecules |
|---|---|
| Cytokines | IFNγ, IL1β, IL1Ra, IL2, IL4, IL5, IL6, IL7, IL8, IL9, IL10, IL12, IL13, IL15, IL17, TNF-α |
| Chemokines | CCL5, CCL11, IP-10, MCP-1, MIP-1α, MIP-1β |
| Growth factors | FGF-β, G-CSF, GM-CSF, PDGF-BB |

Abbreviations: CCL, C-C motif chemokine ligand; FGF, fibroblast growth factor; G-CSF, granulocyte colony-stimulating factor; GM-CSF, granulocyte macrophage colony-stimulating factor; IFN, interferon; IL, interleukin; IL1Ra, interleukin 1 receptor agonist; IP: interferon-induced protein; MCP-1: monocyte chemoattractant protein 1; MIP: macrophage inflammatory protein; PDGF-BB, platelet-derived growth factor BB; TNF-α, tumor necrosis factor alpha.

Serum levels of C-reactive protein (CRP), myeloperoxidase (MPO), fibroblast growth factor 21 (FGF21), and brain-derived neurotrophic factor (BDNF) were assayed by commercially available kits on an ELLA automated immunoassay system (Bio-Techne, San Jose, CA, USA) according to the manufacturer's instructions.

## 2.5. Statistical Analysis

Descriptive statistics were run on all data. Differences in demographic, anthropometric, and clinical parameters between PD and control participants were assessed via $t$-test statistics and $\chi^2$ or Fisher's exact tests, for continuous and categorical variables, respectively. All tests were two-sided, with statistical significance set at $p < 0.05$. Descriptive analyses were performed using the GraphPrism 5.03 software (GraphPad Software, Inc., San Diego, CA, USA).

To determine the circulating biomolecule profile of PD and control participants, multivariate analysis was performed through PLS-DA and soft independent modeling of class analogies (SIMCA). Multivariate statistics were conducted using functions written in-house and run under Matlab environment (release R2015b, The Mathworks, Natick, MA, USA).

### 2.5.1. Partial Least Squares Discriminant Analysis

To explore whether it could be possible to classify the PD condition and identify a molecular signature in circulating EVs related to systemic inflammation, a multivariate analytical strategy was enacted [29]. This strategy was based on coupling a classification method (PLS-DA) with extensive validation of both the model performance and the identified biomarkers. PLS-DA operates by building a regression model between the predictors **X** (measured variables) and a dummy binary vector **y** coding for class belonging (in the present study, PD and controls). Regression was carried out through the PLS algorithm, which was based on projecting variables onto a low-dimensional subspace of latent variables (LVs) characterized by being the directions of maximum covariance between the **X** and the **y**, so as to overcome the problems inherent in dealing with a relatively high number of high correlated predictors. Classification was then accomplished by setting a threshold value on the predicted response, so that if the predicted **y** was higher than the threshold, the individual was classified as PD, or otherwise he/she was recognized as a control.

In order to properly validate the results of the classification strategy and to rule out the possibility of chance correlations, the PLS-DA model was validated by repeated double cross-validation (rDCV) and permutation tests [30,31]. In rDCV, two nested cross-validation loops are used to obtain the outcomes of external validation of the model performance (which is accounted for by the external loop) as independent as possible from the model selection stages (which are based on the results of the inner loop). The procedure is repeated a certain number of times (30 in the present study) to avoid the fact that the outcomes may depend on a single data split. Furthermore, to exclude the fact that good results could be due to chance, the values of the three figures of merit (number of misclassifications (NMC), area under the receiver operating characteristic curve (AUROC), and discriminant Q2 (DQ2)), which summarize the double-cross validated classification performances, were compared with their respective distributions under the null hypothesis (which were estimated by a permutation test with 1000 randomizations) [32].

Once the PLS-DA model was built and its predictive ability was tested and validated, model parameters could be inspected to identify potential discriminant biomarkers. Among the possible tools for model interpretation and identification of candidate biomarkers, variable importance in projection (VIP) [33] and rank product (RP) [31] indices were chosen for the present study. VIP scores account for the covariance between the predictors and the response by "apportioning" the variance in the response accounted for by the PLS-DA model to the individual experimental variables. VIP scores were scaled so that a "greater than 1" rule could be used to assess statistical significance. RP, instead, resulted from a model-based ranking of the predictors and accounted for how consistently a variable emerged as relevant in the resampling procedure. RP calculation relied on estimating the discriminant ability of predictors by means of the absolute value of the corresponding PLS-DA regression coefficient. The name RP derives from the fact that, at each iteration of the resampling procedure (in our case, of the rDCV), the absolute values of the PLS-DA regression coefficients are used to rank variables in decreasing order of discriminant ability. The predictor associated with the regression coefficient with the highest absolute value (greatest discriminant power) is given rank 1, the next larger 2, and so on. For each variable, RP is defined as the geometric mean of its ranks in all resampling (rDCV) segments. Predictors with the lowest RPs are identified as potential biomarkers. A more detailed description of PLS-DA and rDCV procedures may be found elsewhere [34].

### 2.5.2. Soft Independent Modeling of Class Analogies

Soft independent modeling of class analogies (SIMCA) falls within the domain of chemometric class modeling techniques, that is, techniques that investigate a single category at a time and test how likely it is for an individual to be part of a specific class or not [35,36]. The model of each category is built by principal component analysis on the class only data, so that, in order to evaluate whether an individual may be considered as coming from that class or not (i.e., be accepted by the class model or not), a distance to the model is defined as

$$d_{ic} = \sqrt{(T^2_{ic,red})^2 + (Q_{ic,red})^2}, \tag{1}$$

where $T^2_{ic,red}$ is the Mahalanobis distance of the $i$th sample from the center of the principal component (PC) space calculated for class $c$, $Q_{ic,red}$ is the orthogonal distance (residual) of the sample from its projection on the PC space of class $c$, and the subscript red indicates that the two statistics are normalized by their respective 95th percentile in order to be made comparable. Accordingly, classification of the unknown samples is achieved by setting a threshold (usually equal to $\sqrt{2}$) to the distance described in Equation (1): if $d_{ic} < \sqrt{2}$, then the individual is accepted by the class model; otherwise he/she is rejected.

## 3. Results

### 3.1. Characteristics of the Study Participants

A total of 28 participants were included in the study—16 older adults with PD and 12 age- and sex-matched controls. Demographic, anthropometric, and clinical characteristics of study participants are presented in Table 3. Age, sex distribution, MMSE score, and number of co-morbid conditions and medications did not differ between groups. Participants with PD had lower body mass index than controls, whereas serum albumin and total serum protein concentrations were comparable between groups.

Table 3. Main characteristics of study participants.

| Characteristic | Controls (n = 12) | PD (n = 16) | p Value |
|---|---|---|---|
| Age (years), mean ± SD | 75.5 ± 4.9 | 74.5 ± 8.4 | 0.6272 |
| Gender (female), n (%) | 5 (42) | 9 (38) | 0.4451 |
| BMI (kg/m$^2$), mean ± SD | 29.2 ± 3.8 | 24.2 ± 3.0 | 0.010 |
| Number of diseases *, mean ± SD | 2.8 ± 2.1 | 3.2 ± 1.6 | 0.4621 |
| Number of medications #, mean ± SD | 2.9 ± 2.0 | 3.4 ± 1.5 | 0.3729 |
| MMSE score, mean ± SD | 27.6 ± 2.4 | 27.4 ± 2.4 | 0.8171 |
| Serum albumin (g/L), mean ± SD | 41.6 ± 7.1 | 40.3 ± 3.9 | 0.5161 |
| Total serum protein (g/L), mean ± SD | 71.8 ± 4.6 | 72.9 ± 4.8 | 0.6541 |
| Disease duration (months), mean ± SD | — | 102.7 ± 69.1 | |
| LEDD (mg), mean ± SD | — | 587.6 ± 223.9 | |

Abbreviations: BMI: body mass index; LEDD: levodopa equivalent daily dose; MMSE: Mini Mental State Examination; PD: Parkinson's disease; SD: standard deviation. * includes hypertension, coronary artery disease, prior stroke, peripheral vascular disease, diabetes, chronic obstructive pulmonary disease, and osteoarthritis. # includes prescription and over-the-counter drugs.

### 3.2. Characterization of Small Extracellular Vesicles in Serum of Participants with and without Parkinson's Disease

#### 3.2.1. Characterization of Small Extracellular Vesicles

The sEV nature of serum preparations obtained by ultracentrifugation or precipitation was ascertained by verifying the presence of three transmembrane proteins (i.e., CD9, CD63, and CD81) and one cytosolic protein (flotilin), and the absence of non-sEV components (i.e., HNRNPA1) [25,26]. As shown in Figure 1, both isolation methods yielded purified sEVs.

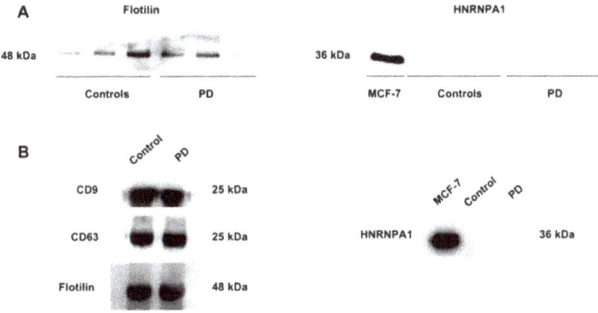

**Figure 1.** Representative blots of preliminary characterization of small extracellular vesicles (sEVs). (**A**) Blots of the cytosolic protein flotilin and ribonucleoprotein (HNRNPA1) as positive and negative markers, respectively, in purified sEVs obtained by ultracentrifugation from controls and participants with Parkinson's disease (PD). MCF-7 cell extract was used as the positive control for the anti-HNRNPA1 antibody. (**B**) Blots of tetraspanins CD9 and CD63, flotilin, and HNRNPA1 in purified sEVs obtained from one control and one PD participant using a commercial precipitation kit.

3.2.2. Quantification of the Amount of Circulating Small Extracellular Vesicles

The total amount of sEVs was significantly greater in PD participants relative to controls ($p < 0.0001$, Figure 2).

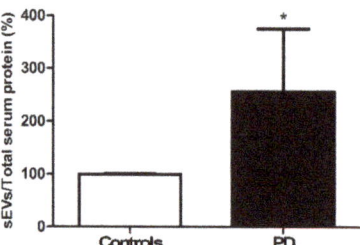

**Figure 2.** Levels of purified small extracellular vesicles (sEVs) in serum of controls ($n = 12$) and participants with Parkinson's disease (PD; $n = 16$). Data were normalized for the amount of total serum protein and are shown as percentage of the control group set at 100%. Bars represent mean values (± standard deviation of the mean). * $p < 0.0001$ vs. controls.

To characterize the population of sEVs in the two participant groups, protein expression levels of tetraspanins CD9, CD63, and CD81 were quantified in purified sEVs (Figure 3). Lower levels of CD9 and CD63 were found in participants with PD relative to controls ($p < 0.0001$, Figure 3A,B), whereas those of CD81 were unvaried between groups ($p = 0.2215$, Figure 3C).

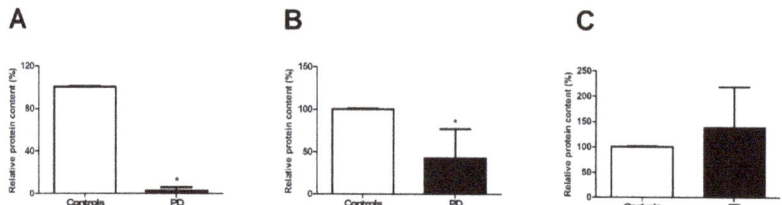

**Figure 3.** Protein expression of (**A**) CD9, (**B**) CD63, and (**C**) CD81 in purified small extracellular vesicles (sEVs) from controls ($n = 12$) and participants with Parkinson's disease (PD; $n = 16$). Data were normalized for the amount of sEV total proteins and are shown as percentage of the control group set at 100%. Bars represent mean values (± standard deviation of the mean). Representative blots are shown in Figure S1. * $p = 0.0001$ vs. controls.

3.2.3. Characterization of the Cargo of Small Extracellular Vesicles

The protein cargo of sEVs was probed for the presence of selected mitochondrial markers [ATP5A (complex V), MTCOI (complex IV), NDUFB8 (complex I), NDUFS3 (complex I), SDHB (complex II), and UQCRC2 (complex III)]. Lower levels of ATP5A, NDUFS3, and SDHB were detected in sEVs from participants with PD compared with controls (Figure 4). No signal was retrieved for UQCRC2, MTCOI, or NDUFB8 in either participant group.

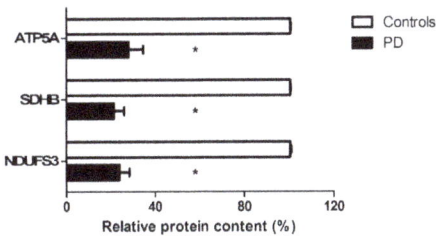

**Figure 4.** Protein expression of adenosine triphosphate 5A (ATP5A), succinate dehydrogenase complex iron sulfur subunit (SDHB), and nicotinamide adenine dinucleotide reduced form (NADH):ubiquinone oxidoreductase subunit S3 (NDUFS3) in purified small extracellular vesicles (sEVs) from controls ($n = 12$) and participants with Parkinson's disease (PD; $n = 16$). Data were normalized for the amount of sEV total proteins and are shown as percentage of the control group set at 100%. Bars represent mean values (± standard deviation of the mean). Representative blots are shown in Figure S1. * $p < 0.0001$ vs. controls.

### 3.3. Identification of a Biomolecular Signature of Parkinson's Disease by Partial Least Squares Discriminant Analysis

Serum levels of 37 biomolecules, including cytokines, chemokines, growth factors, tetraspanins, and mitochondrial markers, were analyzed through PLS-DA models built using a multi-matrix dataset on a low-level data fusion configuration. Prior to PLS-DA analysis, data from the different platforms were autoscaled, followed by normalization of each block by division by its Frobenius' norm. Then, data from the various blocks were concatenated and a PLS-DA model was calculated and validated by rDCV as described in Section 2.5.1. Results are shown in Table 4.

**Table 4.** Discriminant analytes identified by PLS-DA analysis.

|  | Controls ($n = 12$) | PD ($n = 16$) |
|---|---|---|
| CD9 (a.u.) | 1133.4 (2710.4) | 82.3 (53.2) |
| NDUFS3 (a.u.) | 316.6 (881.8) | 96.8 ± 128.0 |
| CRP (mg/L) | 0.5 (0.7) | 1.5 (2.2) |
| FGF21 (pg/mL) | 325.3 (392.0) | 265.5 (151.8) |
| IL9 (pg/mL) | 115.0 (27.1) | 101.8 (3.6) |
| MIP-1β (pg/mL) | 158.6 (97.5) | 184.6 (23.5) |
| TNF-α (pg/mL) | 31.2 (27.4) | 42.2 (10.2) |

Data are shown as median (interquartile range). Grey-shadowed rows correspond to extracellular vesicle-related marker and cargo; white rows correspond to inflammatory mediators. *Abbreviations*: a.u.: arbitrary unit; CRP: C-reactive protein; FGF21: fibroblast growth factor 21; IL9: interleukin 9; MIP-1β: macrophage inflammatory protein 1β; NDUFS3: nicotinamide adenine dinucleotide reduced form (NADH): ubiquinone oxidoreductase subunit S3; PD: Parkinson's disease; PLS-DA: partial least squares discriminant analysis; TNF-α: tumor necrosis factor alpha.

The model correctly classified 94.2% ± 6.1% participants with PD and 66.7% ± 5.4% controls in the outer (external) cross-validation loop, corresponding to a classification ability of 82.4% ± 4.6% in the whole study population. The average AUROC was very close to 1. When compared with their distributions under the null hypothesis, all of the classification figures of merit were statistically significant ($p < 0.0001$).

Among the discriminant analytes identified by the PLS-DA model on the basis of inspection of VIP and RP scores, participants with PD showed lower levels of the sEV marker CD9, the mitochondrial subunit NDUFS3, the metabolic modulator FGF21, and the inflammatory cytokine interleukin 9 (IL9). In addition, participants with PD were characterized by higher serum concentrations of the inflammatory cytokines CRP and tumor necrosis factor alpha (TNF-α), and of the chemokine macrophage inflammatory protein (MIP) 1β (Table 4).

## 3.4. Verification of the Accuracy of Classification by Soft Independent Modeling of Class Analogies

SIMCA was applied to circulating sEV data to obtain a better insight into the characteristics of the PD condition. As described in Section 2.5.2., SIMCA builds and validates individual models for each category of interest and, therefore, allows for evaluation of how likely it is for a sample to belong to any of the modeled classes. Accordingly, SIMCA results are often expressed through two figures of merit (sensitivity and specificity)—the former indicates the percentage of samples from the model class correctly accepted by the model, whereas the latter refers to the percentage of individuals from other categories correctly rejected.

A SIMCA model was built for the PD category and the optimal number of PCs was selected as the one offering the highest efficiency (geometrical average of sensitivity and specificity) in cross-validation. The model is graphically displayed in Figure 5, showing the projection of samples onto the model space described by the variables $T^2_{red}$ and $Q_{red}$ [see also Equation (1)]. A 93.8% sensitivity and 91.7% specificity in calibration, and 87.5% sensitivity and 93.8% specificity in cross-validation were determined.

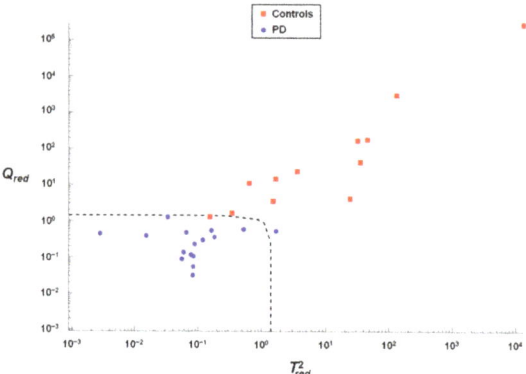

**Figure 5.** Soft independent modeling of class analogies modeling of Parkinson's disease (PD) showing the projection of samples onto the spaces described by the statistical variables $T^2_{red}$ and $Q_{red}$. The dashed line indicates the threshold for acceptance $d = \sqrt{2}$.

## 4. Discussion

Peripheral processes (e.g., inflammation) and neuronal mitochondrial dysfunction contribute to neurodegeneration in PD [37–40]. However, the molecular determinants linking the two processes are underexplored. To help fill this gap in knowledge, we characterized the type and protein cargo of sEVs purified from the serum of elderly people with and without PD.

A greater amount of sEVs (Figure 2) and lower protein content of the two tetraspanins CD9 and CD63 were found in sEVs from participants with PD compared with controls (Figure 3). The protein cargo of sEVs in PD participants was characterized by lower levels of the mitochondrial components ATP5A (complex V), NDUFS3 (complex I), and SDHB (complex II) (Figure 4). The assessment of total protein content of purified sEVs enabled the determination of the overall quantity of the mixed sEV population (Figure 2). On the other hand, the presence of the three tetraspanins CD9, CD63, and CD81 in the purified sEV fraction allowed these vesicles to be identified as endosome-derived exosomes originating from the fusion of MVBs with the plasma membrane [25]. Notably, the identification of mitochondrial signatures indicated the presence of MDVs among sEVs.

MDVs are generated through the selective incorporation of protein cargoes, including outer and inner membranes and matrix content, and may serve as an additional MQC pathway [41]. Indeed, the generation and release of MDVs orchestrated by mitochondrial–lysosomal crosstalk may be triggered as a mechanism to clear out dysfunctional organelles and avoid permanence of noxious material within the cell [17]. Hence, the increased sEV secretion in PD (Figure 2) might have reflected the cell's attempt to dispose dysfunctional mitochondria. In this scenario, the lower secretion of MDVs detected in PD participants (Figure 4) may indicate that the MQC flux was impaired in PD. This finding is in keeping with previous reports showing an association between PD and altered expression of genes encoding proteins involved in mitochondrial homeostasis via quality control mechanisms [e.g., Parkin, phosphatase and tensin homolog (PTEN)-induced putative kinase 1 (PINK1), DJ-1, leucine-rich repeat kinase 2 (LRRK2), ATPase 13A2, vacuolar protein sorting-associated protein 35 (VPS35)) [37,42]. Damaged MDV cargoes may also be delivered to lysosomes for degradation [41]. In support to this hypothesis, alterations of lysosomal function concomitant with impaired mitochondrial biogenesis have been described in Parkin gene (PARK2) mutated fibroblasts from a young patient with PD [38]. These changes were likely sustained by a mitochondrial genetic defect, blocking mitochondrial turnover and triggering premature cellular senescence [38].

Relevant insights into the association of mitochondrial dysfunction with peripheral changes in PD were obtained by integrating mitochondrial and inflammatory markers in the multi-platform PLS-DA analysis, which allowed for the accurate distinguishing of people with PD from controls. Seven biomolecules (i.e., CD9, NDUFS3, CRP, FGF21, IL9, MIP-1β, and TNF-α) were identified as relevant for the discrimination process (Table 4). NDUFS3 is a nuclear-encoded component of mitochondrial complex I, mutations of which are associated with defective complex I activity [43,44]. A large array of clinical conditions, ranging from lethal neonatal diseases to adult-onset neurodegenerative disorders including some forms of PD, show impaired oxidative phosphorylation primarily as a consequence of complex I [45] and III deficiency [46]. In the setting of PD, dysfunction of these mitochondrial subunits together with their insufficient removal via decreased MDV secretion may contribute to protein misfolding via increased oxidative stress [47].

The presence of FGF21 among the discriminant biomolecules in our model is especially remarkable. FGF21, besides being involved in a plethora of metabolic processes [48], has recently been related to dysfunctional MQC in neurons [49]. When mitochondrial dynamics become impaired, neurons activate a multibranched stress response that culminates in the release of FGF21 [49]. The induction of neuron-derived FGF21 has also been detected in brains of mouse models of tauopathy and prion disease [49]. Hence, FGF21 has been attributed a role as mitokine and has been proposed as a candidate marker of brain mitochondrial dysfunction [49].

The identification of a pattern of systemic inflammatory markers in participants with PD (i.e., lower levels of IL9 and higher concentrations of CRP, MIP-1β, and TNF-α) suggests the existence of an inflammatory signature of PD. This view is in keeping with previous reports indicating inflammatory perturbations in both sporadic and familial forms of PD [39,40]. Impairments of innate and adaptive immune response have been described in PD [50]. IL9 is a pleiotropic cytokine with pro-inflammatory and regulatory functions depending on the context in which it is induced and the nature of producing cells. IL9 influences the activity of different cell lines in both the immune and central nervous system (CNS). Notably, Th9 cells/IL9 signaling has been associated with neurodegeneration and autoimmune CNS diseases [51]. However, a neuroprotective role and support in repair functions have also been attributed to IL9 [51,52]. Accordingly, our finding of lower IL9 serum concentrations in PD individuals might suggest that dysregulated IL9 signaling could contribute to impaired neuroprotection/repair capacity in PD [53].

CRP is an acute phase protein commonly measured to monitor disease severity in acute and chronic inflammatory conditions. In advanced age, elevated circulating CRP concentrations independently predict morbidity, functional limitations, and mortality [54]. As such, CRP has been included within the panel of blood-based biomarkers to be implemented in geroscience-guided trials [55]. Noticeably, PD is associated with increased CRP levels in both peripheral blood and the cerebrospinal fluid [56]. Whether elevations in CRP contribute to neurodegeneration or occur as a result of an inflammatory response triggered by PD is presently unclear.

MIP-1β is involved in neurodegeneration by promoting CNS inflammation [57]. Remarkably, circulating MIP-1β levels have been associated with motor symptom severity, depression, and functional status, and have shown to predict their changes over time in a longitudinal study in older people with PD [58]. Finally, TNF-α is a key host defense and inflammatory cytokine that, under certain circumstances, can trigger cell death and tissue degeneration [59]. Our finding of higher serum levels of TNF-α in participants with PD is in line with the possibility that this biomolecule might be implicated in the pathophysiology of PD [60]. Indeed, TNF-α levels increase rapidly in experimental models of PD, and dopaminergic neurons are extremely sensitive to this cytokine [61]. Furthermore, specific polymorphisms in TNF gene characterized by higher TNF-α production are associated with earlier PD onset [62]. Remarkably, the incidence of PD in patients with inflammatory bowel disease was reduced by almost 80% in those exposed to anti-TNF therapy compared with patients who did not receive anti-TNF agents [63].

Albeit proposing novel findings, our study has limitations that need to be discussed. The investigation is associative in nature and cause–effect relationship between candidate mediators and PD pathophysiology cannot be established. Also, despite the fact that participants were carefully characterized, we cannot rule out the possibility that unknown comorbidities may have affected our results. Finally, although a fairly large number of analytes were assayed, it is possible that the inclusion of other biomolecules (e.g., α-synuclein) may provide additional insights into the relationships among sEV trafficking, inflammation, and mitochondrial dysfunction in PD.

Taken as a whole, findings from the present study support the hypothesis that alterations in MQC and release of MDVs may represent an unexplored mechanism through which mitochondrial dysfunction fuels systemic inflammation in PD [19–21]. In-depth characterization of exosomal trafficking may therefore allow identifying new biomarkers for PD and possible targets for interventions.

**Supplementary Materials:** The following is available online at http://www.mdpi.com/2077-0383/9/2/504/s1: Figure S1: Representative blots of biomolecules detected in purified small extracellular vesicles.

**Author Contributions:** Conceptualization, A.P., C.B., E.M., F.G., and R.C.; Data curation, A.P., F.G., and R.B. (Raffaella Beli); Data analysis, A.B. and F.M.; Methodology, A.P., F.G., G.L., M.R.L.M., and R.B. (Raffaella Beli); Writing—original draft preparation, A.P., E.M., M.R.L.M., and R.C.; Writing—review and editing, A.R.B., C.B., F.G., F.L., and R.B. (Raffaella Beli); supervision, A.R.B., F.L., and R.B. (Roberto Bernabei); Funding acquisition, C.B. and R.B. (Roberto Bernabei). All authors have read and agreed to the published version of the manuscript.

**Funding:** This work was supported by Innovative Medicine Initiative-Joint Undertaking (IMI-JU #115621), AIRC (Associazione Italiana per la Ricerca sul Cancro) Investigator grant 2016 #19068 to C.B., Ministero dell'Istruzione, dell'Università e della Ricerca (MIUR) to Consorzio Interuniversitario Biotecnologie (DM 1049, 29/12/2018; CIB N. 112/19 to C.B.), intramural research grants from the Università Cattolica del Sacro Cuore (D3.2 2013 and D3.2 2015), and the nonprofit research foundation "Centro Studi Achille e Linda Lorenzon". Flora Guerra was supported by Fondazione Umberto Veronesi.

**Conflicts of Interest:** The authors declare no conflict of interest. The funders had no role in the design of the study; in the collection, analyses, or interpretation of data; in the writing of the manuscript; or in the decision to publish the results.

## References

1. Brooks, D.J. The early diagnosis of Parkinson's disease. *Ann. Neurol.* **1998**, *44*, S10–S18. [CrossRef] [PubMed]
2. GBD 2016 Parkinson's Disease Collaborators. Global, regional, and national burden of Parkinson's disease, 1990–2016: A systematic analysis for the Global Burden of Disease Study 2016. *Lancet Neurol.* **2018**, *17*, 939–953. [CrossRef]
3. Hou, Y.; Dan, X.; Babbar, M.; Wei, Y.; Hasselbalch, S.G.; Croteau, D.L.; Bohr, V.A. Ageing as a risk factor for neurodegenerative disease. *Nat. Rev. Neurol.* **2019**, *15*, 565–581. [CrossRef] [PubMed]
4. Alexander, G.E. Biology of Parkinson's disease: Pathogenesis and pathophysiology of a multisystem neurodegenerative disorder. *Dialogues Clin. Neurosci.* **2004**, *6*, 259–280.
5. Maiti, P.; Manna, J.; Dunbar, G.L. Current understanding of the molecular mechanisms in Parkinson's disease: Targets for potential treatments. *Transl. Neurodegener.* **2017**, *6*, 28. [CrossRef]

6. Park, J.-S.; Davis, R.L.; Sue, C.M. Mitochondrial dysfunction in Parkinson's disease: New mechanistic insights and therapeutic perspectives. *Curr. Neurol. Neurosci. Rep.* **2018**, *18*, 21. [CrossRef]
7. Melo, T.Q.; Copray, S.J.C.V.M.; Ferrari, M.F.R. Alpha-synuclein toxicity on protein quality control, mitochondria and endoplasmic reticulum. *Neurochem. Res.* **2018**, *43*, 2212–2223. [CrossRef]
8. Cho, B.; Kim, T.; Huh, Y.-J.; Lee, J.; Lee, Y.-I. Amelioration of mitochondrial quality control and proteostasis by natural compounds in parkinson's disease models. *Int. J. Mol. Sci.* **2019**, *20*, 5208. [CrossRef]
9. White, A.J.; Wijeyekoon, R.S.; Scott, K.M.; Gunawardana, N.P.; Hayat, S.; Solim, I.H.; McMahon, H.T.; Barker, R.A.; Williams-Gray, C.H. The peripheral inflammatory response to alpha-synuclein and endotoxin in parkinson's disease. *Front. Neurol.* **2018**, *9*, 946. [CrossRef]
10. Picca, A.; Calvani, R.; Landi, G.; Marini, F.; Biancolillo, A.; Gervasoni, J.; Persichilli, S.; Primiano, A.; Urbani, A.; Bossola, M.; et al. Circulating amino acid signature in older people with Parkinson's disease: A metabolic complement to the EXosomes in PArkiNson Disease (EXPAND) study. *Exp. Gerontol.* **2019**, *128*, 110766. [CrossRef]
11. Picca, A.; Lezza, A.M.S.; Leeuwenburgh, C.; Pesce, V.; Calvani, R.; Landi, F.; Bernabei, R.; Marzetti, E. Fueling inflamm-aging through mitochondrial dysfunction: Mechanisms and molecular targets. *Int. J. Mol. Sci.* **2017**, *18*, 933. [CrossRef] [PubMed]
12. Franco-Iborra, S.; Vila, M.; Perier, C. Mitochondrial quality control in neurodegenerative diseases: Focus on Parkinson's disease and Huntington's disease. *Front. Neurosci.* **2018**, *12*, 342. [CrossRef] [PubMed]
13. Meldolesi, J. Exosomes and ectosomes in intercellular communication. *Curr. Biol.* **2018**, *28*, R435–R444. [CrossRef] [PubMed]
14. Raposo, G.; Stoorvogel, W. Extracellular vesicles: Exosomes, microvesicles, and friends. *J. Cell Biol.* **2013**, *200*, 373–383. [CrossRef]
15. Cocucci, E.; Meldolesi, J. Ectosomes and exosomes: Shedding the confusion between extracellular vesicles. *Trends Cell Biol.* **2015**, *25*, 364–372. [CrossRef]
16. Casella, G.; Colombo, F.; Finardi, A.; Descamps, H.; Ill-Raga, G.; Spinelli, A.; Podini, P.; Bastoni, M.; Martino, G.; Muzio, L.; et al. Extracellular vesicles containing IL-4 modulate neuroinflammation in a mouse model of multiple sclerosis. *Mol. Ther.* **2018**, *26*, 2107–2118. [CrossRef]
17. Picca, A.; Guerra, F.; Calvani, R.; Bucci, C.; Lo Monaco, M.R.; Bentivoglio, A.R.; Coelho-Júnior, H.J.; Landi, F.; Bernabei, R.; Marzetti, E. Mitochondrial dysfunction and aging: Insights from the analysis of extracellular vesicles. *Int. J. Mol. Sci.* **2019**, *20*, 805. [CrossRef]
18. Picca, A.; Lezza, A.M.S.; Leeuwenburgh, C.; Pesce, V.; Calvani, R.; Bossola, M.; Manes-Gravina, E.; Landi, F.; Bernabei, R.; Marzetti, E. Circulating mitochondrial DNA at the crossroads of mitochondrial dysfunction and inflammation during aging and muscle wasting disorders. *Rejuvenat. Res.* **2018**, *21*, 350–359. [CrossRef]
19. Schifferli, J.A. Microvesicles are messengers. *Semin. Immunopathol.* **2011**, *33*, 393–394. [CrossRef]
20. Yoon, Y.J.; Kim, O.Y.; Gho, Y.S. Extracellular vesicles as emerging intercellular communicasomes. *BMB Rep.* **2014**, *47*, 531–539. [CrossRef]
21. Picca, A.; Guerra, F.; Calvani, R.; Bucci, C.; Lo Monaco, M.R.; Bentivoglio, A.R.; Landi, F.; Bernabei, R.; Marzetti, E. Mitochondrial-derived vesicles as candidate biomarkers in Parkinson's disease: Rationale, design and methods of the EXosomes in PArkiNson Disease (EXPAND) study. *Int. J. Mol. Sci.* **2019**, *20*, 2373. [CrossRef] [PubMed]
22. Hughes, A.J.; Daniel, S.E.; Kilford, L.; Lees, A.J. Accuracy of clinical diagnosis of idiopathic Parkinson's disease: A clinico-pathological study of 100 cases. *J. Neurol. Neurosurg. Psychiatry* **1992**, *55*, 181–184. [CrossRef] [PubMed]
23. Théry, C.; Amigorena, S.; Raposo, G.; Clayton, A. Isolation and characterization of exosomes from cell culture supernatants and biological fluids. *Curr. Protoc. Cell Biol.* **2006**, *30*, 3.22.1–3.22.29. [CrossRef] [PubMed]
24. Guerra, F.; Paiano, A.; Migoni, D.; Girolimetti, G.; Perrone, A.M.; De Iaco, P.; Fanizzi, F.P.; Gasparre, G.; Bucci, C. Modulation of RAB7A protein expression determines resistance to cisplatin through late endocytic pathway impairment and extracellular vesicular secretion. *Cancers* **2019**, *11*, 52. [CrossRef] [PubMed]
25. Kowal, J.; Arras, G.; Colombo, M.; Jouve, M.; Morath, J.P.; Primdal-Bengtson, B.; Dingli, F.; Loew, D.; Tkach, M.; Théry, C. Proteomic comparison defines novel markers to characterize heterogeneous populations of extracellular vesicle subtypes. *Proc. Natl. Acad. Sci. USA* **2016**, *113*, E968–E977. [CrossRef]

26. Théry, C.; Witwer, K.W.; Aikawa, E.; Alcaraz, M.J.; Anderson, J.D.; Andriantsitohaina, R.; Antoniou, A.; Arab, T.; Archer, F.; Atkin-Smith, G.K.; et al. Minimal information for studies of extracellular vesicles 2018 (MISEV2018): A position statement of the International Society for Extracellular Vesicles and update of the MISEV2014 guidelines. *J. Extracell. Vesicles* **2018**, *7*, 1535750. [CrossRef]
27. Marzetti, E.; Picca, A.; Marini, F.; Biancolillo, A.; Coelho-Junior, H.J.; Gervasoni, J.; Bossola, M.; Cesari, M.; Onder, G.; Landi, F.; et al. Inflammatory signatures in older persons with physical frailty and sarcopenia: The frailty "cytokinome" at its core. *Exp. Gerontol.* **2019**, *122*, 129–138. [CrossRef]
28. Picca, A.; Ponziani, F.R.; Calvani, R.; Marini, F.; Biancolillo, A.; Coelho-Junior, H.J.; Gervasoni, J.; Primiano, A.; Putignani, L.; Del Chierico, F.; et al. Gut Microbial, Inflammatory and Metabolic Signatures in Older People with Physical Frailty and Sarcopenia: Results from the BIOSPHERE Study. *Nutrients* **2019**, *12*, 65. [CrossRef]
29. Ståhle, L.; Wold, S. Partial least squares analysis with cross-validation for the two-class problem: A Monte Carlo study. *J. Chemom.* **1987**, *1*, 185–196. [CrossRef]
30. Westerhuis, J.A.; Hoefsloot, H.C.J.; Smit, S.; Vis, D.J.; Smilde, A.K.; van Velzen, E.J.J.; van Duijnhoven, J.P.M.; van Dorsten, F.A. Assessment of PLSDA cross validation. *Metabolomics* **2008**, *4*, 81–89. [CrossRef]
31. Smit, S.; van Breemen, M.J.; Hoefsloot, H.C.J.; Smilde, A.K.; Aerts, J.M.F.G.; de Koster, C.G. Assessing the statistical validity of proteomics based biomarkers. *Anal. Chim. Acta* **2007**, *592*, 210–217. [CrossRef] [PubMed]
32. Marzetti, E.; Landi, F.; Marini, F.; Cesari, M.; Buford, T.W.; Manini, T.M.; Onder, G.; Pahor, M.; Bernabei, R.; Leeuwenburgh, C.; et al. Patterns of circulating inflammatory biomarkers in older persons with varying levels of physical performance: A partial least squares-discriminant analysis approach. *Front. Med.* **2014**, *1*, 27. [CrossRef] [PubMed]
33. Wold, S.; Martens, H.; Wold, H. The multivariate calibration problem in chemistry solved by the PLS method. In *Lecture Notes in Mathematics*; Kågström, B., Ruhe, A., Eds.; Springer: Berlin, Germany, 1983; Volume 973, pp. 286–293.
34. Calvani, R.; Picca, A.; Marini, F.; Biancolillo, A.; Gervasoni, J.; Persichilli, S.; Primiano, A.; Coelho-Junior, H.J.; Bossola, M.; Urbani, A.; et al. A Distinct Pattern of Circulating Amino Acids Characterizes Older Persons with Physical Frailty and Sarcopenia: Results from the BIOSPHERE Study. *Nutrients* **2018**, *10*, 1691. [CrossRef] [PubMed]
35. Wold, S. Pattern recognition by means of disjoint principal components models. *Pattern Recognit.* **1976**, *8*, 127–139. [CrossRef]
36. Wold, S.; Sjöström, M. SIMCA: A method for analyzing chemical data in terms of similarity and analogy. *Chemom. Theory Appl.* **1977**, 243–282. [CrossRef]
37. Larsen, S.B.; Hanss, Z.; Krüger, R. The genetic architecture of mitochondrial dysfunction in Parkinson's disease. *Cell Tissue Res.* **2018**, *373*, 21–37. [CrossRef]
38. Guerra, F.; Girolimetti, G.; Beli, R.; Mitruccio, M.; Pacelli, C.; Ferretta, A.; Gasparre, G.; Cocco, T.; Bucci, C. Synergistic effect of mitochondrial and lysosomal dysfunction in Parkinson's disease. *Cells* **2019**, *8*, 452. [CrossRef]
39. Deleidi, M.; Gasser, T. The role of inflammation in sporadic and familial Parkinson's disease. *Cell. Mol. Life Sci.* **2013**, *70*, 4259–4273. [CrossRef]
40. Collins, L.M.; Toulouse, A.; Connor, T.J.; Nolan, Y.M. Contributions of central and systemic inflammation to the pathophysiology of Parkinson's disease. *Neuropharmacology* **2012**, *62*, 2154–2168. [CrossRef]
41. Sugiura, A.; McLelland, G.-L.; Fon, E.A.; McBride, H.M. A new pathway for mitochondrial quality control: Mitochondrial-derived vesicles. *EMBO J.* **2014**, *33*, 2142–2156. [CrossRef]
42. Verstraeten, A.; Theuns, J.; Van Broeckhoven, C. Progress in unraveling the genetic etiology of Parkinson disease in a genomic era. *Trends Genet.* **2015**, *31*, 140–149. [CrossRef] [PubMed]
43. Kirby, D.M.; Salemi, R.; Sugiana, C.; Ohtake, A.; Parry, L.; Bell, K.M.; Kirk, E.P.; Boneh, A.; Taylor, R.W.; Dahl, H.H.M.; et al. NDUFS6 mutations are a novel cause of lethal neonatal mitochondrial complex I deficiency. *J. Clin. Investig.* **2004**, *114*, 837–845. [CrossRef] [PubMed]
44. McFarland, R.; Kirby, D.M.; Fowler, K.J.; Ohtake, A.; Ryan, M.T.; Amor, D.J.; Fletcher, J.M.; Dixon, J.W.; Collins, F.A.; Turnbull, D.M.; et al. De novo mutations in the mitochondrial ND3 gene as a cause of infantile mitochondrial encephalopathy and complex I deficiency. *Ann. Neurol.* **2004**, *55*, 58–64. [CrossRef] [PubMed]
45. Parker, W.D.; Parks, J.K.; Swerdlow, R.H. Complex I deficiency in Parkinson's disease frontal cortex. *Brain Res.* **2008**, *1189*, 215–218. [CrossRef] [PubMed]

46. Amo, T.; Saiki, S.; Sawayama, T.; Sato, S.; Hattori, N. Detailed analysis of mitochondrial respiratory chain defects caused by loss of PINK1. *Neurosci. Lett.* **2014**, *580*, 37–40. [CrossRef]
47. Bouvier-Müller, A.; Ducongé, F. Nucleic acid aptamers for neurodegenerative diseases. *Biochimie* **2018**, *145*, 73–83. [CrossRef]
48. Kharitonenkov, A.; DiMarchi, R. Fibroblast growth factor 21 night watch: Advances and uncertainties in the field. *J. Intern. Med.* **2017**, *281*, 233–246. [CrossRef]
49. Restelli, L.M.; Oettinghaus, B.; Halliday, M.; Agca, C.; Licci, M.; Sironi, L.; Savoia, C.; Hench, J.; Tolnay, M.; Neutzner, A.; et al. Neuronal Mitochondrial Dysfunction activates the integrated stress response to induce fibroblast growth factor 21. *Cell Rep.* **2018**, *24*, 1407–1414. [CrossRef]
50. Kustrimovic, N.; Comi, C.; Magistrelli, L.; Rasini, E.; Legnaro, M.; Bombelli, R.; Aleksic, I.; Blandini, F.; Minafra, B.; Riboldazzi, G.; et al. Parkinson's disease patients have a complex phenotypic and functional Th1 bias: Cross-sectional studies of CD4+ Th1/Th2/T17 and Treg in drug-naïve and drug-treated patients. *J. Neuroinflammat.* **2018**, *15*, 205. [CrossRef]
51. Elyaman, W.; Khoury, S.J. Th9 cells in the pathogenesis of EAE and multiple sclerosis. *Semin. Immunopathol.* **2017**, *39*, 79–87. [CrossRef]
52. Elyaman, W.; Bradshaw, E.M.; Uyttenhove, C.; Dardalhon, V.; Awasthi, A.; Imitola, J.; Bettelli, E.; Oukka, M.; van Snick, J.; Renauld, J.-C.; et al. IL-9 induces differentiation of TH17 cells and enhances function of FoxP3+ natural regulatory T cells. *Proc. Natl. Acad. Sci. USA* **2009**, *106*, 12885–12890. [CrossRef] [PubMed]
53. Schröder, J.B.; Pawlowski, M.; Meyer Zu Hörste, G.; Gross, C.C.; Wiendl, H.; Meuth, S.G.; Ruck, T.; Warnecke, T. Immune cell activation in the cerebrospinal fluid of patients with Parkinson's disease. *Front. Neurol.* **2018**, *9*, 1081. [CrossRef] [PubMed]
54. Chung, H.Y.; Cesari, M.; Anton, S.; Marzetti, E.; Giovannini, S.; Seo, A.Y.; Carter, C.; Yu, B.P.; Leeuwenburgh, C. Molecular inflammation: Underpinnings of aging and age-related diseases. *Ageing Res. Rev.* **2009**, *8*, 18–30. [CrossRef] [PubMed]
55. Justice, J.N.; Ferrucci, L.; Newman, A.B.; Aroda, V.R.; Bahnson, J.L.; Divers, J.; Espeland, M.A.; Marcovina, S.; Pollak, M.N.; Kritchevsky, S.B.; et al. A framework for selection of blood-based biomarkers for geroscience-guided clinical trials: Report from the TAME Biomarkers Workgroup. *GeroScience* **2018**, *40*, 419–436. [CrossRef]
56. Qiu, X.; Xiao, Y.; Wu, J.; Gan, L.; Huang, Y.; Wang, J. C-reactive orotein and risk of Parkinson's disease: A systematic review and meta-analysis. *Front. Neurol.* **2019**, *10*, 384. [CrossRef]
57. Perrin, F.E.; Lacroix, S.; Avilés-Trigueros, M.; David, S. Involvement of monocyte chemoattractant protein-1, macrophage inflammatory protein-1alpha and interleukin-1beta in Wallerian degeneration. *Brain* **2005**, *128*, 854–866. [CrossRef]
58. Ahmadi Rastegar, D.; Ho, N.; Halliday, G.M.; Dzamko, N. Parkinson's progression prediction using machine learning and serum cytokines. *NPJ Park. Dis.* **2019**, *5*, 14. [CrossRef]
59. Probert, L. TNF and its receptors in the CNS: The essential, the desirable and the deleterious effects. *Neuroscience* **2015**, *302*, 2–22. [CrossRef]
60. Montgomery, S.L.; Bowers, W.J. Tumor necrosis factor-alpha and the roles it plays in homeostatic and degenerative processes within the central nervous system. *J. Neuroimmune Pharmacol.* **2012**, *7*, 42–59. [CrossRef]
61. Ferger, B.; Leng, A.; Mura, A.; Hengerer, B.; Feldon, J. Genetic ablation of tumor necrosis factor-alpha (TNF-alpha) and pharmacological inhibition of TNF-synthesis attenuates MPTP toxicity in mouse striatum. *J. Neurochem.* **2004**, *89*, 822–833. [CrossRef]
62. Nishimura, M.; Mizuta, I.; Mizuta, E.; Yamasaki, S.; Ohta, M.; Kaji, R.; Kuno, S. Tumor necrosis factor gene polymorphisms in patients with sporadic Parkinson's disease. *Neurosci. Lett.* **2001**, *311*, 1–4. [CrossRef]
63. Peter, I.; Dubinsky, M.; Bressman, S.; Park, A.; Lu, C.; Chen, N.; Wang, A. Anti-tumor necrosis factor therapy and incidence of Parkinson disease among patients with inflammatory bowel disease. *JAMA Neurol.* **2018**, *75*, 939–946. [CrossRef] [PubMed]

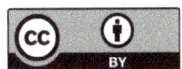

© 2020 by the authors. Licensee MDPI, Basel, Switzerland. This article is an open access article distributed under the terms and conditions of the Creative Commons Attribution (CC BY) license (http://creativecommons.org/licenses/by/4.0/).

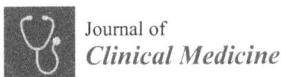 

Article

# Variants in Miro1 Cause Alterations of ER-Mitochondria Contact Sites in Fibroblasts from Parkinson's Disease Patients

Clara Berenguer-Escuder [1,*,†], Dajana Grossmann [1,†], François Massart [1], Paul Antony [1], Lena F. Burbulla [2], Enrico Glaab [1], Sophie Imhoff [3], Joanne Trinh [3], Philip Seibler [3], Anne Grünewald [1,3,‡] and Rejko Krüger [1,4,5,*,‡]

1. Luxembourg Centre for Systems Biomedicine (LCSB), University of Luxembourg, 4367 Belvaux, Luxembourg; dajana.grossmann@uni.lu (D.G.); francois.massart@uni.lu (F.M.); paul.antony@uni.lu (P.A.); enrico.glaab@uni.lu (E.G.); anne.gruenewald@uni.lu (A.G.)
2. Department of Neurology, Northwestern University Feinberg School of Medicine, Chicago, IL 60611, USA; lena.burbulla@northwestern.edu
3. Institute of Neurogenetics, University of Lübeck, 23562 Lübeck, Germany; sophie.imhoff@online.de (S.I.); joanne.trinh@neuro.uni-luebeck.de (J.T.); philip.seibler@neuro.uni-luebeck.de (P.S.)
4. Luxembourg Institute of Health (LIH), 1445 Strassen, Luxembourg
5. Parkinson Research Clinic, Centre Hospitalier de Luxembourg (CHL), 1460 Luxembourg, Luxembourg
* Correspondence: clara.berenguer@uni.lu (C.B.E.); rejko.krueger@uni.lu (R.K.); Tel.: +352-46-66-44-5401 (R.K.)
† These authors contributed equally to the study.
‡ These authors share senior authorship.

Received: 28 October 2019; Accepted: 9 December 2019; Published: 16 December 2019

**Abstract:** Background: Although most cases of Parkinson's disease (PD) are idiopathic with unknown cause, an increasing number of genes and genetic risk factors have been discovered that play a role in PD pathogenesis. Many of the PD-associated proteins are involved in mitochondrial quality control, e.g., PINK1, Parkin, and LRRK2, which were recently identified as regulators of mitochondrial-endoplasmic reticulum (ER) contact sites (MERCs) linking mitochondrial homeostasis to intracellular calcium handling. In this context, Miro1 is increasingly recognized to play a role in PD pathology. Recently, we identified the first PD patients carrying mutations in *RHOT1*, the gene coding for Miro1. Here, we describe two novel *RHOT1* mutations identified in two PD patients and the characterization of the cellular phenotypes. Methods: Using whole exome sequencing we identified two PD patients carrying heterozygous mutations leading to the amino acid exchanges T351A and T610A in Miro1. We analyzed calcium homeostasis and MERCs in detail by live cell imaging and immunocytochemistry in patient-derived fibroblasts. Results: We show that fibroblasts expressing mutant T351A or T610A Miro1 display impaired calcium homeostasis and a reduced amount of MERCs. All fibroblast lines from patients with pathogenic variants in Miro1, revealed alterations of the structure of MERCs. Conclusion: Our data suggest that Miro1 is important for the regulation of the structure and function of MERCs. Moreover, our study supports the role of MERCs in the pathogenesis of PD and further establishes variants in *RHOT1* as rare genetic risk factors for neurodegeneration.

**Keywords:** Parkinson's disease; mitochondria-ER contact sites; Miro1

## 1. Introduction

Parkinson's disease (PD) is a complex neurodegenerative disorder with a largely unknown molecular pathogenesis. Although most PD cases are classified as idiopathic with unknown cause, a growing number of genes and genetic risk factors have been identified, which contribute to the development of PD [1] Many of these genes were found to be involved in common pathways suggesting that, at least in a subgroup of cases, PD might be caused by similar pathological mechanisms. PD-associated mutations in PINK1, Parkin and LRRK2 for example cause impairments of mitochondrial quality control and subsequent mitochondrial dysfunction [2] Mitochondrial-endoplasmic reticulum (ER) contact sites (MERCs) are important connections required for the proper function of mitochondria, i.e., by facilitating the exchange of metabolites, calcium and lipids between both organelles [3,4], thereby maintaining mitochondrial homeostasis. PINK1, Parkin, LRRK2 and α-synuclein (α-syn) were recently found to be involved in the regulation of MERCs. Impaired function of these proteins caused fragmentation of the mitochondrial network, mitochondrial calcium dyshomeostasis and alterations of the amount of MERCs [5–7].

Interestingly, Miro1 plays a central role in a number of molecular and organellar pathways, which are affected in PD. Via its interaction with PINK1, Parkin and LRRK2 [2], Miro1 interferes with mitochondrial quality control and MERCs [5,8,9]. Having access to fibroblasts from PD patients carrying different Miro1 mutations, we explored the role of Miro1 at MERCs in more detail. In this study, we provide further evidence for a role of rare genetic variants in *RHOT1* in PD, now presenting a wider spectrum of Miro1 point mutations in a total of 4 independent patients. In agreement with our previous findings in Miro1-R272Q and Miro1-R450C mutant fibroblasts [10], fibroblasts with the newly identified heterozygous mutations T351A and T610A also display a reduction of MERCs as well as impaired calcium homeostasis. Furthermore, we analyzed the MERC composition in all four Miro1-mutant cultures and found differences in the recruitment of Miro1 protein to MERCs and in the amounts of different types of MERCs compared to control fibroblasts. Our data further establish mutations in *RHOT1* as risk factor for PD and support recent studies implicating dysfunctional MERCs in the pathogenesis of PD.

## 2. Experimental Section

### 2.1. Identification of Miro1-T351A and T610A Mutations

We studied exome data from 86 subjects (62 with PD and 24 controls). The 'convenient patient sample' was comprised of early-onset PD cases. The patients were not known to carry either a pathogenic or likely pathogenic genetic variant in any known PD gene. However, they carried heterozygous variants in Miro1 (T351A and T610A). All patients were examined and diagnosed by movement disorder specialists. The patient harboring the T351A had an age of onset of 60 years and was 65 years old, when the skin biopsy was taken. He suffered from resting tremor, bradykinesia as well as restless legs syndrome. He was treated with a dopamine agonist at the time of examination. The patient with the T610A mutation developed PD at age 40 and was sampled at age 45. He showed signs of bradykinesia, rigidity and a good response to L-DOPA. Moreover, he suffered from depression.

All participants provided informed consent prior to donating a blood sample for genetic analysis and are from Germany or of other European descent. Local ethics approval was obtained from the Research Ethics Board of the University of Lübeck, Germany.

### 2.2. Exome Sequencing

Exome sequencing was performed with Illumina's Nextera Rapid Capture Exome Kit followed by massively parallel sequencing on a NextSeq500 Sequencer (Illumina, San Diego, CA, USA). Raw sequencing reads were converted to fastq format using bcl2fastq software (Illumina). Using an in-house developed pipeline for exome data analysis, the reads were aligned to the human reference genome (GRCh37, hg19 build) with burrows-wheeler algorithm (BWA) software and the mem algorithm. Alignments were converted to binary bam file and variant calling was performed using three different variant callers (GATK HaplotypeCaller, freebayes and samtools). Variants were annotated using Annovar and in-house ad-hoc bioinformatic tools. Exome variants were filtered for (1) minor allele frequency (MAF) <0.01 in Miro-1 (*RHOT1*) in Genome Aggregation Database (GnomAD); (2) functional impact: Non-synonymous, stop-gain, frameshift, and splicing variants; and (3) Phred quality score >220, coverage >20× and variant allele fraction > 40% of called reads. All the selected variants identified in two patients were validated by Sanger sequencing as previously described [11]. Primers with the following sequences were used: for the mutation T351A: (forward: TGTGTTTCTTCAGGATAGAGAC; reverse: GATATCAGCAGCTAATCTTGC); for the mutation T610A: (forward: GGGCCACACTGATAGAATAG; reverse: ACGTAATATATAGCTAGGCAGG).

### 2.3. Fibroblast Cell Culture

Fibroblasts were obtained from the identified two male PD patients. Fibroblasts from three age-matched controls were received from the Neuro-Biobank of the University of Tübingen, Germany. In Lübeck as well as in Tübingen, skin biopsies to establish fibroblast cultures are taken from the arm of the individuals. Cell culture conditions and immortalization of native fibroblasts were explained in our previous study [10].

### 2.4. Western Blot Analysis

Immortalized fibroblasts were lysed in RIPA buffer with 1× complete protease inhibitor (Roche, Mannheim, Germany). Sodium dodecyl sulfate polyacrylamide gel electrophoresis and Western blot analysis was performed using antibodies against Miro1 (Sigma Aldrich, Munich, Germany, WH0055288M1), Tom20 (Santa Cruz Biotechnologies, Dallas, TX, USA, sc-17764), Rab9 (Santa Cruz Biotechnologies, Dallas, TX, USA, sc-74482), and β-Actin (Thermo Scientific, Braunschweig, Germany, MA1-744).

### 2.5. Homology Model of Miro1

Homology models for isoform1 of the human Miro1 protein were built using a crystal structure of sub-domains from this protein in the GMPPCP-bound state with a resolution of 2.5 Å (PDB: 5KSZ) as the main template. Since this template only covers the position of the mutated residue T351, but not the position of the second mutated residue T610, two separate models were built: One high-quality model focusing on the region covered by the template (created using the SWISS-MODEL software [12]), and one lower-quality model covering the entire protein sequence (created using a multi-template approach for protein threading, RaptorX [13]). For all analyses and predictions related to the residue T351, the high-quality model was used, whereas all analyses for residue T610 were conducted using the lower-quality model with complete sequence coverage.

Structure visualizations of the Miro1 isoform1 protein were generated with the software Chimera [14], using the domain annotations from the Uniprot database [15]. Next, the transmembrane regions for the protein were predicted by applying the Constrained Consensus Topology approach (software CCTOP [16] with default parameters). Finally, mutation effects were predicted using the structure-based methods SDM, mCSM [17], DUET [18], and the more sequence-based approaches SIFT [19], Polyphen2 [20] (as implemented in the Variant Effect Predictor software, VEP [21]), and SNAP2 [22].

### 2.6. Live Cell Imaging for Calcium Analysis

The protocol for live cell imaging of cytosolic calcium levels using Fluo4-AM staining and treatment with thapsigargin and Ru360 was described in detail before [10]. Live cell imaging for the analysis of calcium-induced fragmentation using MitoTracker green FM staining and ionomycin treatment was likewise described in detail [10]. The aspect ratio was determined to assess mitochondrial fragmentation. In brief, the aspect ratio is calculated by the minor axis of mitochondria divided by the major axis of mitochondria and indicates mitochondria fragmentation. The smaller the value of the aspect ratio, the smaller the mitochondria, indicating higher fragmentation. Mitochondrial morphology was analyzed using ImageJ software. Images were obtained with a Live cell Microscope

Axiovert 2000 with spinning disc, plan-aprochromate objectives and Hamamatsu camera C11440 (Carl Zeiss Microimaging GmbH, Jena, Germany) in a humidified atmosphere containing 5% $CO_2$ at 37 °C, using a 20× objective for Fluo4-AM or a 40× objective for MitoTracker green, respectively.

### 2.7. Immunocytochemistry for Analysis of MERCs

For quantification and analysis of MERCs, native fibroblasts were fixed in 4% paraformaldehyde for 15 min for subsequent immunocytochemistry. Cells were then labeled with antibodies against protein disulfide-isomerase (PDI) (2446S, dilution 1:1000, secondary antibody: Goat anti-rabbit Alexa Fluor 488; Cell Signaling Technology, Danvers, MA, USA; A-1000, dilution 1:1000; Life Technologies, Carlsbad, CA, USA), Tom20 (sc-17764, dilution 1:500, secondary antibody: Goat anti-mouse Alexa Fluor 647; Santa Cruz Biotechnologies, Dallas, TX, USA; A-21235, dilution 1:1000; Life Technologies, Carlsbad, CA, USA) and Miro1 (Sigma Aldrich, Munich, Germany, WH0055288M1, 1:1000; secondary antibody: Life Technologies, Carlsbad, CA, USA, goat anti-mouse Alexa Fluor 647 1:1000). Data were analyzed using MATLAB. Images were obtained with a Live cell Microscope Axiovert 2000 with spinning disc, plan-aprochromate objectives and Hamamatsu camera C11440 (Carl Zeiss Microimaging GmbH, Jena, Germany), using a 40× objective. Every field consisted of z-stacks of 0.5 µm interval. Data was analyzed using MATLAB. ER area per cell (in pixel) was quantified from the area covered by the PDI signal and mitochondria area per cell (in pixel) was derived from the area covered by Tom20 signal.

### 2.8. Analysis of Miro1 Localization to Different Cellular Compartments

Immortalized fibroblasts were transfected with mito-GFP using TransIT®-2020 transfection reagent (Mirus Bio, Madison, WI, USA, MIR 5400) according to the manufacturer's protocol. At 24 h after transfection, cells were fixed with 4% PFA for 15 min and stained with antibodies against Calnexin (Cell Signaling Technology, Danvers, MA, USA, C5C9, 1:500; secondary antibody: Life Technologies, goat anti-rabbit Alexa Fluor 568, 1:1000) and Miro1 (Sigma Aldrich, Munich, Germany, WH0055288M1, 1:1000; secondary antibody: Life Technologies, Carlsbad, CA, USA, goat anti-mouse Alexa Fluor 647 1:1000). Images were obtained using a Axiovert 2000 Microscope with spinning disc, plan-apochromate objectives and Hamamatsu camera C11440 (Carl Zeiss Microimaging GmbH, Jena, Germany), 63× objective. Image analysis was performed with MATLAB.

### 2.9. Imaging of ER-Mitochondria Contact Sites Using the SPLICS Method

Immortalized fibroblasts were transfected with the SPLICS-short or the SPLICS-long construct [23], respectively, using TransIT®-2020 transfection reagent (Mirus Bio, Madison, WI, USA, MIR 5400). At 12 h after transfection, cells were stained with 0.1 µM MitoTracker deep red FM (Thermo Scientific, Braunschweig, Germany) for 30 min and imaged using a Axiovert 2000 Microscope with spinning disc, plan-apochromate objectives and Hamamatsu camera C11440 (Carl Zeiss Microimaging GmbH, Jena, Germany), 63× objective. Image analysis was performed with MatLab.

### 2.10. Quantification of Co-Localization of Mitochondria and LC3

Immortalized fibroblasts were transiently transfected with mito-DsRed [24] and eGFP-LC3 [25] constructs using TransIT-2020 transfection reagent (Mirus Bio, Madison, WI, USA, MIR 5400). After 24 h, fibroblasts were treated with 25 µM CCCP or 10 nM Bafilomycin A1 for 2 h or 6 h. Co-localization of mitochondria (indicated by mito-DsRed signal) and autophagosomes (indicated by eGFP-LC3 puncta) was considered as mitophagy events.

### 2.11. Analysis of Autophagosome Formation

Immortalized fibroblasts were transfected with mito-dsRed [24] using TransIT-2020 transfection reagent (Mirus Bio, Madison, WI, USA, MIR 5400). After 24 h, autophagosome formation was assessed by staining native fibroblasts with 0.2 mM 18:1 NBD-PS (Sigma Aldrich, Munich, Germany, 810198C) for 30 min at 37 °C. Cells were subsequently starved in medium without FBS for 2 h. Autophagosomes are indicated by 18:1 NBD-PS signal not co-localizing with mitochondria [26].

## 2.12. Statistical Analysis

Statistical significance was determined with GraphPad Prism 8.0 software. Statistical tests and number of replicates are indicated in detail in the figure legend for each experiment. We used nonparametric tests in order to account for the small sample size. All experiments were repeated at least three times (the number of independent biological replicates is indicated by $n$).

## 3. Results

### 3.1. Identification of the Novel Mutations T351A and T610A in the RHOT1 Gene in PD Patients

Recently, we identified the first disease-associated mutations in *RHOT1* in two German PD patients [10]. Here, we describe two additional *RHOT1* mutations found in two male PD patients of German origin. The heterozygous point mutations c.1290A > G and c.2067A > G (NM_001033568) leading to the amino acid exchanges T351A or T610A (NP_001028740), were validated by Sanger sequencing (Figure 1A).

Whole exome sequencing excluded mutations in other known PD genes in these patients. The mutation T351A is located within the second calcium-binding EF-hand domain, while the mutation T610A is located within the C-terminus of Miro1 (Figure 1B). Both affected amino acids are exposed to the cytosol at the surface of the protein (Figure 1C,D).

For the T351A mutation, all effect prediction algorithms consistently estimate a destabilizing effect or, respectively, a "deleterious" or "possibly damaging" effect. For the T610A mutation, different methods estimate different effects, with two approaches (SDM and DUET) predicting a destabilizing effect, and the other methods predicting a stabilizing effect (mCSM), benign or neutral effect (Polyphen2, SNAP2), or a toleration of the mutation (but with low confidence, SIFT; Figure 1E).

The lower confidence and disagreement between the predictions in this case is not surprising, given that the T610 residue was only covered by the lower-quality homology model for Miro1. Both threonine residues in the native structure are highly conserved, and in both cases the mutated residue is smaller and more hydrophobic than the wild-type residue. However, the T351 residue is exposed on the protein surface, whereas only a medium exposure is predicted for the T610 residue (prediction by RaptorX software).

Interestingly, using the further dedicated software tool MutationTaster [27] to assess possible effects on transmembrane domains (TMD), the T610A mutation is predicted to result in the loss of a TMD close to the C-terminal end of the protein structure. Thus, while the T351A mutation is most likely causing a destabilization of the Miro1 protein structure, the T610A mutation may rather only affect the surrounding structural region, possibly including the nearby TMD (Figure 1E).

Western blot analysis revealed that the relative amount of Miro1 protein was not affected in patient-derived mutant fibroblasts compared to control cells (Figure 1F,G). Furthermore, the relative amount of the mitochondrial marker protein Tom20 was comparable between both mutant fibroblasts lines and three control fibroblast lines (Figure 1H,I).

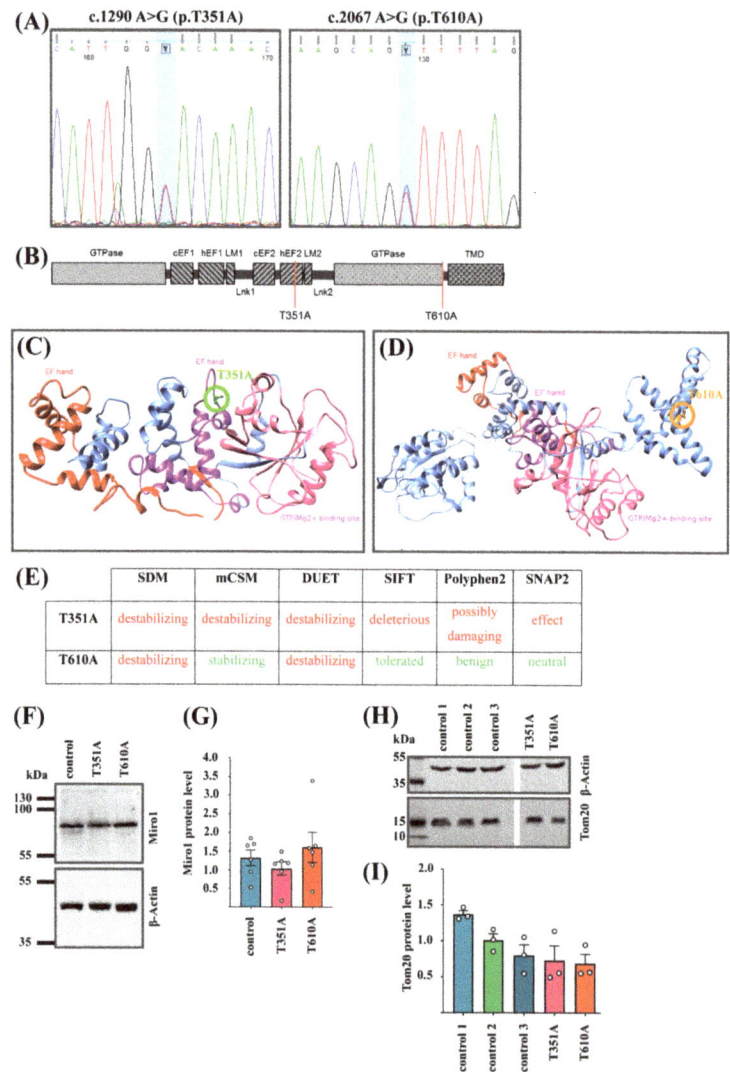

**Figure 1.** (**A**) Sanger sequencing result for the mutations c.1290A > G and c.2067A > G (NM_001033568), leading to the amino acid exchanges T351A or T610A (NP_001028740), respectively. (**B**) Schematic overview of Miro1 protein structure, showing the two newly identified mutations in Miro1: T351A is located within the second EF-hand domain and T610A within the C-terminus. (**C**) Homology model of human Miro1 based on the 3D structure of *Drosophila* Miro. The 3D structure shows both EF-hand domains, the C-terminal GTPase domain and the C-terminus. The amino acid T351 is highlighted with a green circle, (**D**) while the amino acid position T610 is highlighted with an orange circle. (**E**) Overview of the mutation effects on protein stability and functionality as predicted by SDM, mCSB, DUET, SIFT, Polyphen2, and SNAP2. (Red is "destabilizing", "deleterious" or "possibly damaging"; Green is "stabilizing", "tolerated" or "benign". As indicated in the table.) (**F**) Representative Western blot image of Miro1 protein in immortalized fibroblasts with the mutations Miro1-T351A or Miro1-T610A. (**G**) Densitometry of Western blot analysis from (F) for Miro1 protein levels normalized to β-Actin. Data indicated as mean ± SEM ($n = 6$). (**H**) Representative Western blot image of Tom20 protein in immortalized fibroblasts. (**I**) Densitometry of Western blot analysis of Tom20 protein levels normalized to β-Actin. Data indicated as mean ± SEM ($n = 3$).

## 3.2. Increased Calcium Stress is a Shared Phenotype Across Different Miro1 Mutations in PD

Miro1 acts as sensor for cytosolic calcium levels [8,28,29]. Accordingly, we recently showed that patient-derived fibroblasts expressing mutant Miro1 proteins display a decreased capacity to buffer cytosolic calcium after inhibition of ER calcium ATPase by thapsigargin treatment [10]. In the present study, we stained fibroblasts with the cytosolic calcium indicator Fluo4-AM and treated cells during live cell imaging with thapsigargin. In all investigated fibroblast cultures, thapsigargin induced a fast increase of cytosolic calcium levels by inhibition of ER-mediated calcium uptake and depletion of ER calcium stores [30] (Figure 2A). However, calculating the time constant of the exponential decay from the calcium response curve revealed that control cells recover considerably faster from this peak than both Miro1-mutant fibroblasts (Figure 2B).

In order to assess the contribution of mitochondria to the buffering of cytosolic calcium after thapsigargin treatment, we treated fibroblasts in parallel with Ru360, an inhibitor of the mitochondrial calcium uniporter (MCU [28,31,32]). The resulting response curve indicates that blockage of mitochondrial calcium import abolishes the ability of all cell lines to compensate for elevated cytosolic calcium (Figure 2C). This finding suggests that calcium buffering in fibroblasts after thapsigargin treatment is mainly facilitated by mitochondria.

Cytosolic calcium was shown to regulate mitochondrial morphology, with increasing calcium levels causing fragmentation [8]. In the light of this result, we were interested in investigating mitochondrial morphology in response to calcium stress. For this purpose, fibroblasts were stained with MitoTracker green FM and treated with the calcium ionophore ionomycin during live cell imaging. Quantifying the mitochondrial aspect ratios after ionomycin exposure, we observed calcium-mediated mitochondrial fragmentation in all fibroblast lines. By contrast, this fragmentation process was faster and stronger in both Miro1-mutant fibroblast lines compared to controls (Figure 2D,E). These results are in line with our findings in Miro1-R272Q and Miro1-R450C fibroblasts [10], suggesting that all four identified PD-associated Miro1 variants cause a similar calcium phenotype.

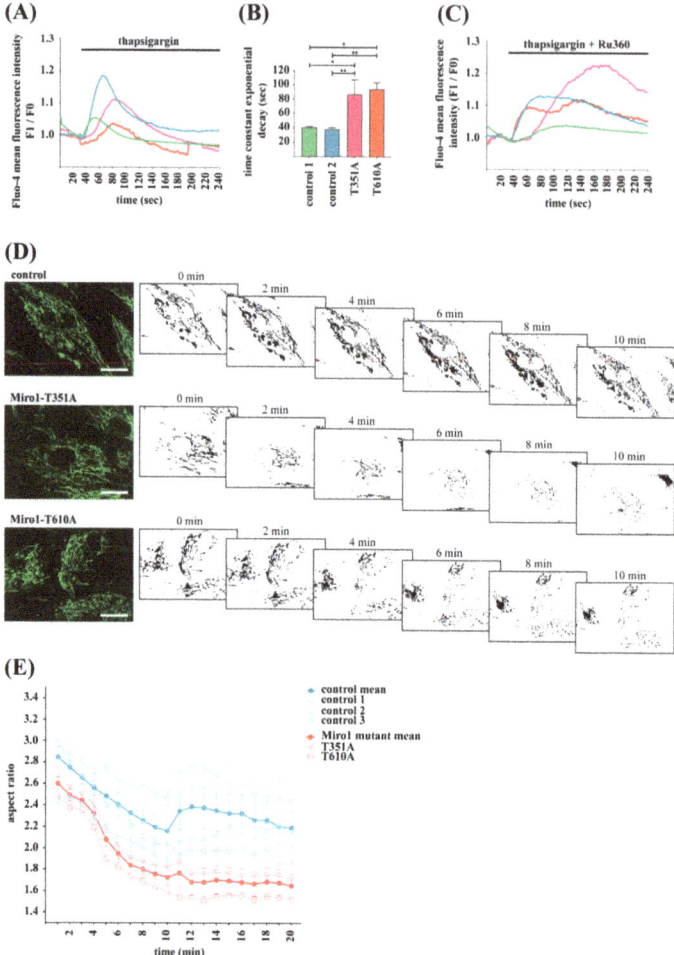

**Figure 2.** (**A**) Immortalized fibroblasts were loaded with the cytosolic calcium indicator Fluo-4 AM for live cell imaging. During imaging, cells were treated with 1 µM thapsigargin in order to inhibit calcium uptake by the SERCA pumps and to deplete endoplasmic reticulum (ER) calcium stores. Imaging was continued for 10 min with a 2 s interval. Images were obtained with a 25× objective. Data indicate the fluorescence signal intensity of Fluo-4 AM expressed as mean fluorescence F1/F0. (**B**) Time constant of the exponential decay calculated from the calcium response curves from (A). The data indicate the time, which is needed to recover from the thapsigargin-induced cytosolic calcium peak shown in (A). Data indicated as mean ± SEM. Significance calculated by Mann-Whitney test ($n = 4$). * $p < 0.05$; **: $p < 0.001$. (**C**) Immortalized fibroblasts were loaded with Fluo-4 AM for live cell imaging and treated with 1 µM thapsigargin and 10 µM Ru360 in order to inhibit calcium buffering by the ER and by the mitochondrial calcium uniporter (MCU). Cells were imaged for 10 min with a 2 sec interval using a 25× objective. Data is expressed as mean Fluo-4 AM fluorescence intensity F1/F0 ($n = 3$). (**D**) Immortalized fibroblasts were stained with MitoTracker green FM for live cell imaging. Images were obtained once per minute using a 40× objective. During imaging, cells were treated with 20 µM ionomycin and mitochondrial morphology was analyzed using ImageJ. Mitochondrial masks from image analysis are shown for all cell lines at different time points. Scale bars indicate 20 µm. (**E**) Analysis of mitochondrial fragmentation in different fibroblast lines, expressed as aspect ratio, from images shown in (D); ($n = 3$–5).

*3.3. Mutations in Miro1 Cause Reduction of MERCs*

Several previous studies showed that cellular calcium buffering depends on MERCs and that their regulation is mediated by Miro1 [5,8]. We stained fixed fibroblasts with antibodies against the ER marker PDI and the mitochondrial marker Tom20 in order to analyze the co-localization of both organelles (Figure 3A). This analysis showed that the amount of MERCs, indicated by the number of co-localization events, was reduced in both Miro1-mutant fibroblast lines, compared to controls (Figure 3B).

Furthermore, quantification of the PDI signal revealed a significantly reduced ER area per cell, which is indicative of ER mass (Figure 3C). When normalized to ER area, the amount of MERCs was not different between controls and mutant fibroblasts (Figure 3D).

We also assessed the mitochondrial mass from the Tom20 signal and found no statistical significant difference between controls and mutants (Figure 3E). The amount of MERCs normalized to mitochondrial area was also significantly reduced in T351A and T610A fibroblasts (Figure 3F). These phenotypes are in line with the observation of reduced MERCs and reduced ER mass in the previously described PD-associated Miro1 mutants R272Q and R450C [10].

*3.4. Reduced Localization of Mutant Miro1 to MERCs*

Since Miro1 is a crucial regulator of MERCs, we were interested to assess whether different mutations in Miro1 have an impact on the proteins localization to MERCs. For this purpose, fibroblasts were first transfected with mito-GFP and afterwards fixed for antibody staining with the ER protein calnexin and Miro1 (Figure 4A). Co-localization analysis showed that Miro1-T351A, but not T610A fibroblasts also present less MERCs without Miro1, compared to control fibroblasts (Figure 4B). Of note, in all fibroblast lines only a subset of MERCs stained positive for Miro1 (Figure 4C), and the mutant T351A and T610A fibroblasts display significantly less MERCs with Miro1 compared to control fibroblasts (Figure 4C).

These results suggest that the observed overall reduction of MERCs in Miro1-mutant fibroblasts is might be driven by a reduction of Miro1-containing MERCs. In line, further image analyses revealed, that all mutant fibroblast lines show a reduction of Miro1 localization to mitochondria and to the ER (Figure 4D).

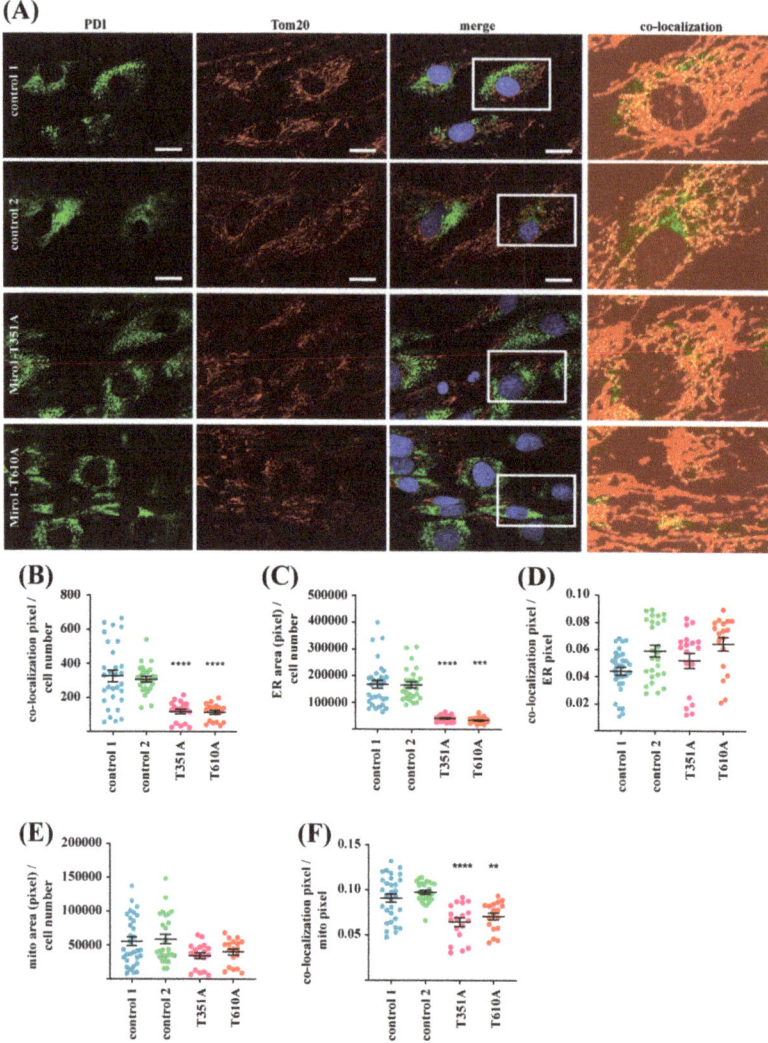

**Figure 3.** (**A**) Native fibroblasts were fixed and stained with antibodies against the ER marker protein protein disulfide-isomerase (PDI) and the mitochondrial marker protein Tom20. Images were obtained using a 63× objectives; scale bars indicate 20 µm. The white boxes in the merged images indicate the magnified regions shown in the co-localization panels. Co-localization of PDI and Tom20 signals was analyzed with MatLab. Co-localization events are highlighted as white dots. (**B**) Quantification of co-localization events of PDI and Tom20 per cell, indicating the amount of mitochondrial-endoplasmic reticulum contact sites (MERCs). (**C**) Quantification of ER area per cell in pixel from the PDI signal. (**D**) Quantification of co-localization events of PDI and Tom20 normalized to PDI-positive ER pixel. (**E**) Quantification of mitochondrial area per cell from the Tom20 signal. (**F**) Quantification of co-localization events of PDI and Tom20 per mitochondrial area. All data indicated as mean ± SEM. Significance calculated using a Kruskal Wallis test ($n = 3$; 25 cells analyzed per fibroblast line per experiment). ** $p < 0.001$; *** $p < 0.0001$; **** $p < 0.00001$.

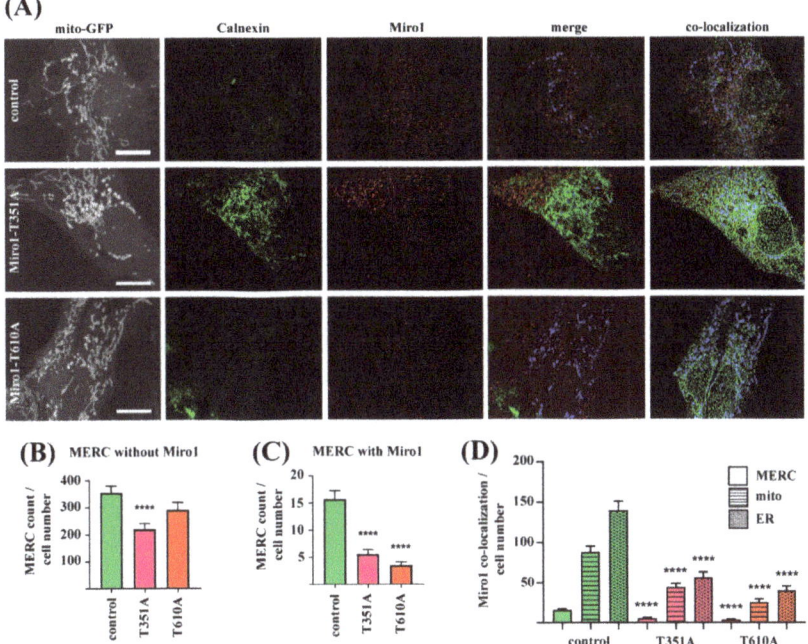

**Figure 4.** (**A**) Immortalized fibroblasts were transfected with mito-GFP and fixed 24 h post-transfection for subsequent labeling with antibodies against Miro1 and the ER marker Calnexin. Images were obtained using a 63× objective; scale bars indicate 20 µm. Co-localization events were analyzed using MatLab. (**B**) Quantification of MERCs without Miro1 and (**C**) MERCs with Miro1 per cell from images shown in (**A**). (**D**) Quantification of co-localization events of Miro1 puncta with MERCs, mitochondria or the ER per cell. All data indicated as mean ± SEM. Significance calculated with Kruskal-Wallis test ($n = 3$; ~20 cells analyzed per fibroblast line per experiment). **** $p < 0.00001$.

### 3.5. Mutations in Miro1 Cause Alterations of MERC Types

To further elucidate the quality of MERCs, we transfected fibroblasts with so-called split-GFP-based contact site sensor (SPLICS) constructs [23]. These constructs express two parts of a split GFP protein in the same plasmid, one part being targeted to the ER and the second part targeted to the mitochondria. As soon as both organelles come in close proximity, the mitochondrial and the ER part of the split GFP align and give a fluorescent signal. While the SPLICS-short construct labels narrow MERCs with a distance between ER and mitochondria of 8–10 nm, the SPLICS-long construct labels wide MERCs with a distance of 40–50 nm between both organelles [33]. Transfected fibroblasts were stained with MitoTracker deep red and live cell imaging showed that the SPLICS signal co-localized with mitochondria (Figure 5A).

Quantification of SPLICS signal per cell revealed that all fibroblasts, controls and mutant lines, have in general more wide MERCs (SPLICS-long) than narrow MERCs (SPLICS-short; Figure 5B,C), a result that fits to previous observations [33]. Both Miro1-mutant fibroblasts display significantly less wide (Figure 5B) and narrow (Figure 5C) MERCs compared to control fibroblasts. These results suggest that mutations in Miro1 cause changes in the structure of MERCs.

Fibroblasts transfected with SPLICS constructs were fixed and stained with an antibody against Miro1 for subsequent quantification of SPLICS signals with Miro1 or without Miro1, respectively. Only the T610A mutant shows a reduction of SPLICS-long signal with Miro1 (Figure 5D), while both mutant fibroblast lines, T351A and T610A, show a significant reduction of SPLICS-long signal without

Miro1 co-localization (Figure 5D). In contrast, both mutant fibroblast lines do not show changes of SPLICS-short signal with Miro1 and a slight reduction of SPLICS-short signal without Miro1 (Figure 5E). These findings support our previous observation that Miro1 mutations cause alterations of the structure of MERCs.

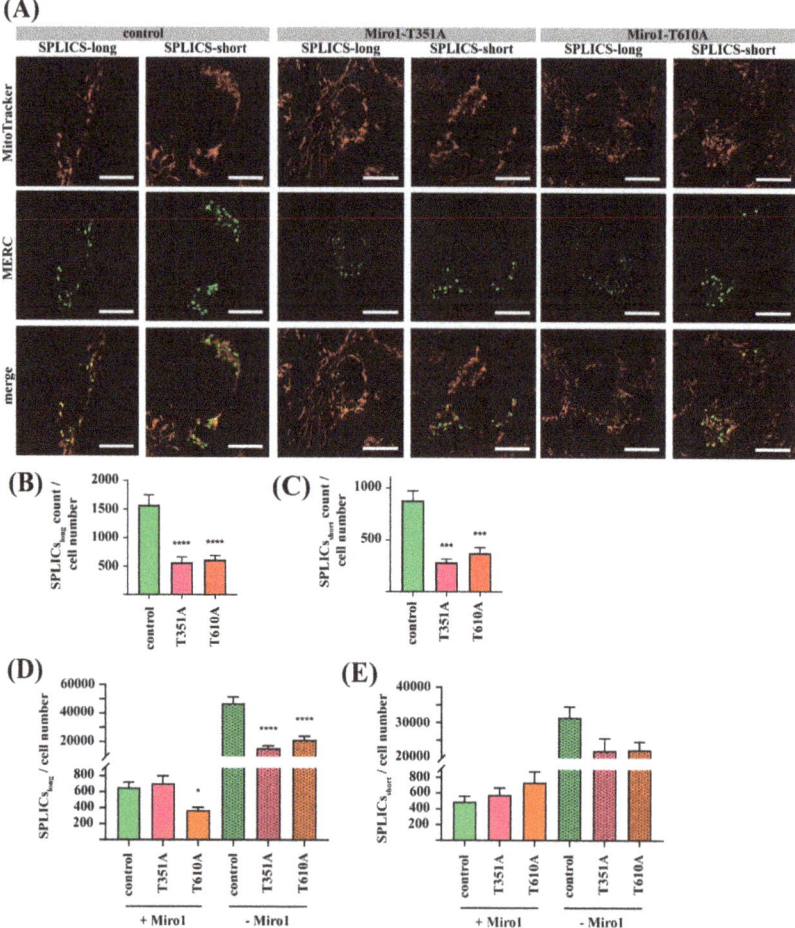

**Figure 5.** (**A**) Immortalized fibroblasts were transfected either with the SPLICS-long, or with the SPLICS-short construct. After 12 h, cells were stained with MitoTracker deep red FM for live cell imaging, using a 63x objective; scale bars indicate 20 μm. (**B**) Quantification of wide MERCs (from SPLICS-long signal) and (**C**) narrow MERCs (from SPLICS-short signal) per cell. Fibroblasts transfected with (**D**) SPLICS-long or (**E**) SPLICS-short constructs were fixed and stained with an antibody against Miro1. Afterwards, cells were imaged with a 63× objective and SPLICS signals with and without Miro1 were quantified. All data indicated as mean ± SEM. Significance was assessed using a Kruskal-Wallis test ($n = 3$; ~16 cells analyzed per fibroblast line per experiment). * $p < 0.05$; *** $p < 0.0001$; **** $p < 0.00001$.

### 3.6. LC3-Dependent Autophagy is Impaired in Miro1-T351A and Miro1-T610A Fibroblasts

MERCs play a crucial role not only in calcium homeostasis, but also in the regulation of mitophagy [8]. In our previous study describing the Miro1 mutations R272Q and R450C, we found changes in mitochondrial quality control mechanisms in patient-derived fibroblasts. Hence, we investigated autophagy pathways in the T351A and T610A fibroblasts. Fibroblasts were transfected with mito-dsRed and eGFP-LC3 for subsequent treatment with the mitochondrial uncoupler CCCP or Bafilomycin A1, an inhibitor of lysosomal degradation (Figure 6A). Co-localization of mitochondria with LC3 puncta indicated mitophagy. In control fibroblasts, CCCP treatment leads to an increased co-localization of mitochondria and LC3 puncta, indicating increased mitophagy. Inhibition of lysosomal degradation by Bafilomycin A1 also leads to an increase of co-localization events in control fibroblasts. In contrast, neither of the treatments results in changes of mitochondria-LC3 co-localization in T351A- or T610A-fibroblasts (Figure 6B).

This result points to an inhibition of the autophagy flux in these mutant lines. Therefore, we were interested in further analysis of the LC3-dependent autophagy pathway. Formation of LC3-dependent autophagosomes requires transfer of the lipids phosphatidylethanolamine (PE) and phosphatidylserine (PS) at MERCs [34]. PS is transformed into PE and together with LC3 gets integrated into the ER membrane to form autophagosomes. Therefore, the translocation of the 18:1 NBD-PS signal from mitochondria to the cytosol serves as readout for autophagosome formation [8,10,26]. We loaded fibroblasts with the fluorescent labeled lipid 18:1 NBD-PS and starved them without FBS to induce LC3/ATG5-dependent autophagy [34]. Afterwards, we quantified the 18:1 NBD-PS signal, which was not co-localized with mito-dsRed-labeled mitochondria (Figure 6C). In control fibroblasts, FBS starvation induced autophagosome formation, while both mutant cell lines showed no effect on autophagosome number under stress conditions (Figure 6D), indicating an inhibition of autophagosome formation.

In our previous study we showed that Miro1-mutant fibroblasts with the mutations R272Q or R450C displayed an increased lysosomal turnover of Rab9 [10], a marker protein for ATG5 / LC3-independent autophagy. Within this pathway, autophagosomes are not derived from the ER membrane at MERCs, but derive from the Golgi apparatus, mediated by Rab9 [35]. Hence, we quantified Rab9 protein levels under Bafilomycin A1 treatment. Interestingly, Bafilomycin A1 treatment has no effect on Rab9 levels in control fibroblasts, but increased Rab9 in both mutant lines (Figure 6E,F). Together, these results suggest that T351A and T610A mutant fibroblasts might use the Rab9-dependent autophagy pathway while the LC3-dependent pathway is impaired.

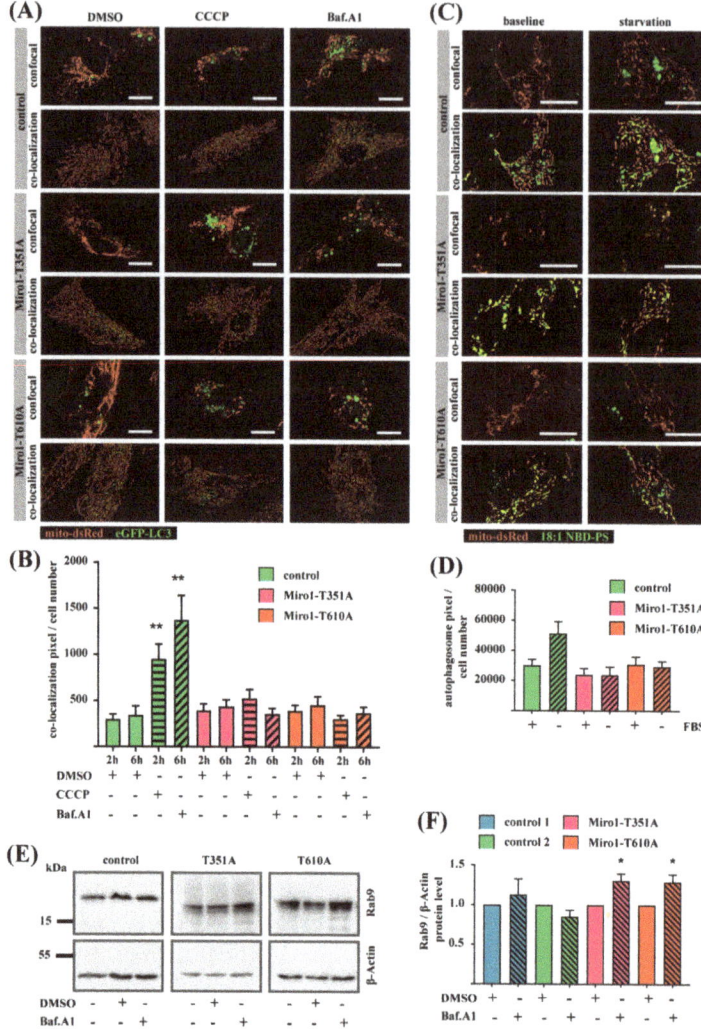

**Figure 6.** (**A**) Fibroblasts were transfected with mito-DsRed and eGFP-LC3 and treated with 25 µM CCCP for 2 h or with 10 nM BafilomycinA1 for 6 h. Microscopy images were obtained with a 40× objective. In the co-localization panel, the mitochondria are indicated in green and the LC3 puncta are indicated in red. Co-localization events of mitochondria and LC3 puncta are indicated in yellow. Scale bars indicate 20 µm. (**B**) Quantification of co-localization events of mitochondria and LC3 puncta from (A) normalized to cell number. Significance was calculated using the Mann-Whitney test ($n = 3$; ~24 cells analyzed per fibroblast line, per condition and per experiment). (**C**) Fibroblasts were transfected with mito-DsRed and after 24 h loaded with 18:1 NBD-PS. Fibroblasts were then starved without FBS for 2 h before live cell imaging, using a 63× objective. The co-localization panel shows mitochondria in red and 18:1 NBD-PS signal in green. Co-localization of mitochondria and 18:1 NBD-PS is indicated in yellow. Autophagosomes were identified as 18:1 NBD-PS signal, which did not co-localize with the mito-DsRed signal. (**D**) Quantification of autophagosomes from microscopy images shown in (C). Significance calculated with Mann-Whitney test ($n = 3$; 10 cells analyzed per line, condition and per experiment). (**E**) Western blot image of Rab9 and β-Actin in immortalized fibroblasts. (**F**) Quantification of relative Rab9 protein levels normalized to β-Actin. Significance calculated by Mann-Whitney test ($n = 4$–$6$). All data indicated as mean ± SEM. * $p < 0.05$; ** $p < 0.001$.

## 4. Discussion

Miro1 is a crucial sensor for cytosolic calcium levels and is furthermore involved in the regulation of calcium homeostasis at the contact sites between mitochondria and the ER. MERCs are an emerging topic in the field of PD research and a number of PD-associated proteins were found to be involved in the regulation of MERCs, i.e., PINK1, Parkin, and LRRK2 [5–7,36]. Already in 2011, Kornmann and colleagues showed that Miro1 plays a role at the contact sites in mammalian Cos-7 cells [37]. Moreover, in yeast cells devoid of the Miro1 orthologue Gem1, the number of MERCs was significantly decreased [37]. This confirms our previous observation of reduced MERCs in the Miro1 mutants R272Q and R450C, which also displayed a reduced amount of total Miro1 protein [10]. However, while the two mutations T351A and T610A described in the current study did not show reduced Miro1 protein levels in fibroblasts, a decrease in the number of MERCs and impaired calcium homeostasis is suggested to be a shared hallmark across all currently known PD-associated Miro1 mutations.

In addition to altered MERC numbers and calcium dyshomeostasis, we showed here that there is a shift in the proportion of wide and narrow MERCs in patient-derived fibroblasts. First, it is worth noting that in all fibroblast lines (independent of the genotype) the majority of MERCs were devoid of Miro1. This observation is in line with previous studies showing that Miro1 acts as a regulatory protein at the MERCs but is not required for the assembly of MERCs [37]. However, all four mutant fibroblast lines, R272Q, R450C (Supplementary data 1A–C), T351A, and T610A contained significantly fewer Miro1-positive MERCs compared to control fibroblasts. Furthermore, co-localization analyses revealed that also less Miro1 was recruited to mitochondria and the ER compartments compared to control cells in all four Miro1 mutants (Supplementary Data 1D). These results raise the question whether the mutations in Miro1 interfere with the localization of Miro1 to MERCs and destabilize the contact sites between mitochondria and ER.

Electron microscopy revealed that MERCs are formed with varying distances between ER and mitochondria [38]. Different mechanisms regulate the distance of the cleft between ER and mitochondria at MERCs suggesting that wide and narrow MERCs are involved in distinct cellular processes. While the smooth ER forms connections with mitochondria at a distance of 8–10 nm, the rough ER forms mitochondria connections at 50–60 nm [39]. Moreover, the distance between ER and mitochondria membranes at MERCs changes as a result of metabolic alterations. Starvation increased the distance of MERCs and over-nutrition decreased the distance in mice liver [38,40].

With the SPLICS method, Cieri and colleagues could additionally show that the distance of MERCs is regulated during processes such as ER stress, mitochondrial elongation, fragmentation, and mitophagy [33]. Earlier studies showed that MERCs, which facilitate calcium transfer between ER and mitochondria via a complex of IP3R, Grp75, and VDAC [41], have a cleft width of ~15–20 nm [42,43]. MERC clefts that are narrower than 7 nm or wider than 25 nm inhibit the formation of the protein complex required for calcium transfer [38,40,44]. Accordingly, the SPLICS-short signal, which visualizes MERCs with a cleft of ~10 nm [33], is indicative of effective calcium transfer between ER and mitochondria. From our results we therefore conclude that the impaired calcium homeostasis could result from the reduction of narrow MERCs that was consistently observed in all four Miro1-mutant fibroblast lines (Supplementary Data 2C).

The SPLICS-long construct visualizes MERCs with a width of ~50 nm [33], which have been associated with the formation of LC3/ATG5-dependent autophagosomes [34]. The Miro1 mutations R272Q and R450C do not display a reduction of these wide MERCs (Supplementary Data 2B), which is in line with our previous observation that autophagosome formation and LC3-dependent mitophagy is indeed increased in fibroblasts with those mutations [10]. In contrast, the mutations T351A and T610A show a considerable decrease of wide MERCs alongside an impaired flux of LC3-dependent autophagy. It is tempting to speculate that the differences of wide and narrow MERCs observed in the R272Q and R450C, and the T351A and T610A mutations are related to the different mitophagy phenotypes in both sets of mutations. Differential effects of mutations have previously also been observed in fibroblasts derived from patients with monogenic PD [45]. This phenomenon warrants further investigation in neuronal models with Miro1 mutations.

However, co-localization analysis of SPLICS with Miro1 revealed that especially the SPLICS-long signal without Miro1 puncta was significantly reduced in T351A and T610A mutant fibroblasts. This result raised the question how mutant Miro1 could interfere with the amount of Miro1-negative MERCS. MERCS represented by SPLICS-long signals were previously associated with mitophagy. Conditions, which facilitate mitophagy, e.g., tunicamycin treatment, knockdown of Mfn2, activation of Parkin or Drp1-induced mitochondrial fragmentation reduced the amount of SPLICS-long signal [33]. Therefore, one could assume that the observed alterations of the mitophagy pathway are not only affecting MERCS containing Miro1, but alter MERCS architecture in general.

With the identification and functional characterization of two novel mutations in Miro1, we provided further evidence for *RHOT1* as a risk gene for PD. Moreover, our observation of altered abundance and composition of MERCs further emphasizes their critical involvement in the pathogenesis of PD.

**Supplementary Materials:** The following are available online at http://www.mdpi.com/2077-0383/8/12/2226/s1, Supplementary data 1: Reduced localization of mutant Miro1-R272Q and Miro1-R450C to MERCs; Supplementary data 2: Miro1-R272Q and Miro1-R450C cause alterations of MERC types

**Author Contributions:** Conceptualization, D.G., A.G., and R.K.; methodology, C.B.-E. and D.G.; software, P.A.; formal analysis, C.B.-E. and D.G.; investigation, C.B.-E., D.G., F.M., E.G., S.I., and J.T.; resources, P.S.; writing—original draft preparation, D.G.; writing—review and editing, C.B.-E., L.F.B., E.G., J.T., A.G., and R.K.; supervision, D.G., A.G., and R.K.; project administration, D.G. and R.K.; funding acquisition, D.G., L.F.B., A.G., and R.K.

**Funding:** The current project was supported by a research grant to R.K., A.G., and E.G. within the CORE program of the Fonds National de la Recherche de Luxembourg (FNR; MiRisk-PD, C17/BM/11676395). R.K. acknowledges funding from the FNR within the PEARL ((FNR/P13/6682797/Krüger) and NCER-PD programme, the German Research Council (KR2119/8-1), the European Union's (EU) Horizon2020 research and innovation program (WIDESPREAD; CENTRE-PD; grant agreement No. 692320), and the Federal Ministry for Education and Research (BMBF; Mito-PD 031A 430 A). A.G. received funding from the FNR within the ATTRACT program (Model IPD, FNR9631103). E.G. was supported by the FNR as part of the PD-Strat project within the ERA-NET ERACoSysMed framework (INTER/11651464).

**Acknowledgments:** We thank all patients and control individuals, who made this study possible by donating their cells for research. Furthermore, we thank Christine Klein (Institute of Neurogenetics, University of Lübeck, Germany) to provide the patient-derived fibroblasts for this study. We obtained the control fibroblasts from the Neuro-Biobank of the University of Tübingen that is supported by the Hertie Institute and the DZNE (Tübingen, Germany). The SPLICS constructs were a kind gift of Tito Cali, Department of Biomedical Sciences, University of Padova, Italy.

**Conflicts of Interest:** The authors declare no conflict of interest.

## References

1. Larsen, S.B.; Hanss, Z.; Krüger, R. The genetic architecture of mitochondrial dysfunction in Parkinson's disease. *Cell Tissue Res.* **2018**, *373*, 21–37. [CrossRef] [PubMed]
2. Hsieh, C.-H.; Shaltouki, A.; Gonzalez, A.E.; Bettencourt da Cruz, A.; Burbulla, L.F.; St Lawrence, E.; Schüle, B.; Krainc, D.; Palmer, T.D.; Wang, X. Functional Impairment in Miro Degradation and Mitophagy Is a Shared Feature in Familial and Sporadic Parkinson's Disease. *Cell Stem Cell* **2016**, *19*, 709–724. [CrossRef] [PubMed]
3. Lynes, E.M.; Simmen, T. Urban planning of the endoplasmic reticulum (ER): how diverse mechanisms segregate the many functions of the ER. *Biochim. Biophys. Acta* **2011**, *1813*, 1893–1905. [CrossRef] [PubMed]
4. Rowland, A.A.; Voeltz, G.K. Endoplasmic reticulum-mitochondria contacts: Function of the junction. *Nat. Rev. Mol. Cell Biol.* **2012**, *13*, 607–625. [CrossRef] [PubMed]
5. Lee, K.-S.; Huh, S.; Lee, S.; Wu, Z.; Kim, A.-K.; Kang, H.-Y.; Lu, B. Altered ER-mitochondria contact impacts mitochondria calcium homeostasis and contributes to neurodegeneration in vivo in disease models. *Proc. Natl. Acad. Sci. USA* **2018**, *115*, E8844–E8853. [CrossRef] [PubMed]
6. Calì, T.; Ottolini, D.; Negro, A.; Brini, M. Enhanced parkin levels favor ER-mitochondria crosstalk and guarantee Ca(2+) transfer to sustain cell bioenergetics. *Biochim. Biophys. Acta* **2013**, *1832*, 495–508. [CrossRef]

7. Basso, V.; Marchesan, E.; Peggion, C.; Chakraborty, J.; von Stockum, S.; Giacomello, M.; Ottolini, D.; Debattisti, V.; Caicci, F.; Tasca, E.; et al. Regulation of ER-mitochondria contacts by Parkin via Mfn2. *Pharmacol. Res.* **2018**, *138*, 43–56. [CrossRef]
8. Nemani, N.; Carvalho, E.; Tomar, D.; Dong, Z.; Ketschek, A.; Breves, S.L.; Jaña, F.; Worth, A.M.; Heffler, J.; Palaniappan, P.; et al. MIRO-1 Determines Mitochondrial Shape Transition upon GPCR Activation and Ca2+Stress. *Cell Rep.* **2018**, 1005–1019. [CrossRef]
9. Lee, S.; Lee, K.-S.; Huh, S.; Liu, S.; Lee, D.-Y.; Hong, S.H.; Yu, K.; Lu, B. Polo Kinase Phosphorylates Miro to Control ER-Mitochondria Contact Sites and Mitochondrial Ca$^{2+}$ Homeostasis in Neural Stem Cell Development. *Dev. Cell* **2016**, *37*, 174–189. [CrossRef]
10. Grossmann, D.; Berenguer-Escuder, C.; Bellet, M.E.; Scheibner, D.; Bohler, J.; Massart, F.; Rapaport, D.; Skupin, A.; Fouquier d'Hérouël, A.; Sharma, M.; et al. Mutations in RHOT1 disrupt ER-mitochondria contact sites interfering with calcium homeostasis and mitochondrial dynamics in Parkinson's disease. *Antioxid. Redox Signal.* **2019**, *31*, 1213–1234. [CrossRef]
11. Speijer, D. Evolution of peroxisomes illustrates symbiogenesis. *BioEssays* **2017**, *39*, 1–8. [CrossRef] [PubMed]
12. Schwede, T.; Kopp, J.; Guex, N.; Peitsch, M.C. SWISS-MODEL: An automated protein homology-modeling server. *Nucleic Acids Res.* **2003**, *31*, 3381–3385. [CrossRef] [PubMed]
13. Peng, J.; Xu, J. RaptorX: exploiting structure information for protein alignment by statistical inference. *Proteins* **2011**, *79* Suppl. 1, 161–171. [CrossRef]
14. Pettersen, E.F.; Goddard, T.D.; Huang, C.C.; Couch, G.S.; Greenblatt, D.M.; Meng, E.C.; Ferrin, T.E. UCSF Chimera—A visualization system for exploratory research and analysis. *J. Comput. Chem.* **2004**, *25*, 1605–1612. [CrossRef] [PubMed]
15. UniProt Consortium. UniProt: a hub for protein information. *Nucleic Acids Res.* **2015**, *43*, D204–D212. [CrossRef]
16. Dobson, L.; Reményi, I.; Tusnády, G.E. CCTOP: a Consensus Constrained TOPology prediction web server. *Nucleic Acids Res.* **2015**, *43*, W408–W412. [CrossRef]
17. Pires, D.E.V.; Ascher, D.B.; Blundell, T.L. mCSM: Predicting the effects of mutations in proteins using graph-based signatures. *Bioinformatics* **2014**, *30*, 335–342. [CrossRef]
18. Pires, D.E.V.; Ascher, D.B.; Blundell, T.L. DUET: A server for predicting effects of mutations on protein stability using an integrated computational approach. *Nucleic Acids Res.* **2014**, *42*, W314–W319. [CrossRef]
19. Sim, N.-L.; Kumar, P.; Hu, J.; Henikoff, S.; Schneider, G.; Ng, P.C. SIFT web server: Predicting effects of amino acid substitutions on proteins. *Nucleic Acids Res.* **2012**, *40*, W452–W457. [CrossRef]
20. Adzhubei, I.; Jordan, D.M.; Sunyaev, S.R. Predicting functional effect of human missense mutations using PolyPhen-2. *Curr. Protoc. Hum. Genet.* **2013**, *76*. Chapter 7, Unit 7.20. [CrossRef]
21. McLaren, W.; Gil, L.; Hunt, S.E.; Riat, H.S.; Ritchie, G.R.S.; Thormann, A.; Flicek, P.; Cunningham, F. The Ensembl Variant Effect Predictor. *Genome Biol.* **2016**, *17*, 122. [CrossRef] [PubMed]
22. Hecht, M.; Bromberg, Y.; Rost, B. Better prediction of functional effects for sequence variants. *BMC Genomics* **2015**, *16*, S1. [CrossRef] [PubMed]
23. Calì, T.; Ottolini, D.; Vicario, M.; Catoni, C.; Vallese, F.; Cieri, D.; Barazzuol, L.; Brini, M. splitGFP Technology Reveals Dose-Dependent ER-Mitochondria Interface Modulation by α-Synuclein A53T and A30P Mutants. *Cells* **2019**, *8*, 1072. [CrossRef] [PubMed]
24. Burbulla, L.F.; Schelling, C.; Kato, H.; Rapaport, D.; Woitalla, D.; Schiesling, C.; Schulte, C.; Sharma, M.; Illig, T.; Bauer, P.; et al. Dissecting the role of the mitochondrial chaperone mortalin in Parkinson's disease: Functional impact of disease-related variants on mitochondrial homeostasis. *Hum. Mol. Genet.* **2010**, *19*, 4437–4452. [CrossRef]
25. Krebiehl, G.; Ruckerbauer, S.; Burbulla, L.F.; Kieper, N.; Maurer, B.; Waak, J.; Wolburg, H.; Gizatullina, Z.; Gellerich, F.N.; Woitalla, D.; et al. Reduced basal autophagy and impaired mitochondrial dynamics due to loss of Parkinson's disease-associated protein DJ-1. *PLoS ONE* **2010**, *5*, e9367. [CrossRef]
26. Hailey, D.W.; Rambold, A.S.; Satpute-Krishnan, P.; Mitra, K.; Sougrat, R.; Kim, P.K.; Lippincott-Schwartz, J. Mitochondria supply membranes for autophagosome biogenesis during starvation. *Cell* **2010**, *141*, 656–667. [CrossRef]
27. Schwarz, J.M.; Cooper, D.N.; Schuelke, M.; Seelow, D. MutationTaster2: Mutation prediction for the deep-sequencing age. *Nat. Methods* **2014**, *11*, 361–362. [CrossRef]

28. Chang, K.T.; Niescier, R.F.; Min, K.-T. Mitochondrial matrix Ca$^{2+}$ as an intrinsic signal regulating mitochondrial motility in axons. *Proc. Natl. Acad. Sci. USA* **2011**, *108*, 15456–15461. [CrossRef]
29. Saotome, M.; Safiulina, D.; Szabadkai, G.; Das, S.; Fransson, A.; Aspenstrom, P.; Rizzuto, R.; Hajnoczky, G. Bidirectional Ca$^{2+}$-dependent control of mitochondrial dynamics by the Miro GTPase. *Proc. Natl. Acad. Sci. USA* **2008**, *105*, 20728–20733. [CrossRef]
30. Parekh, A.B.; Putney, J.W. Store-operated calcium channels. *Physiol. Rev.* **2005**, *85*, 757–810. [CrossRef]
31. Vaccaro, V.; Devine, M.J.; Higgs, N.F.; Kittler, J.T. Miro1-dependent mitochondrial positioning drives the rescaling of presynaptic Ca 2+ signals during homeostatic plasticity. *EMBO Rep.* **2017**, *18*, 231–240. [CrossRef] [PubMed]
32. Kirichok, Y.; Krapivinsky, G.; Clapham, D.E. The mitochondrial calcium uniporter is a highly selective ion channel. *Nature* **2004**, *427*, 360–364. [CrossRef] [PubMed]
33. Cieri, D.; Vicario, M.; Giacomello, M.; Vallese, F.; Filadi, R.; Wagner, T.; Pozzan, T.; Pizzo, P.; Scorrano, L.; Brini, M.; et al. SPLICS: A split green fluorescent protein-based contact site sensor for narrow and wide heterotypic organelle juxtaposition. *Cell Death Differ.* **2018**, *25*, 1131–1145. [CrossRef] [PubMed]
34. Hamasaki, M.; Furuta, N.; Matsuda, A.; Nezu, A.; Yamamoto, A.; Fujita, N.; Oomori, H.; Noda, T.; Haraguchi, T.; Hiraoka, Y.; et al. Autophagosomes form at ER-mitochondria contact sites. *Nature* **2013**, *495*, 389–393. [CrossRef] [PubMed]
35. Nishida, Y.; Arakawa, S.; Fujitani, K.; Yamaguchi, H.; Mizuta, T.; Kanaseki, T.; Komatsu, M.; Otsu, K.; Tsujimoto, Y.; Shimizu, S. Discovery of Atg5/Atg7-independent alternative macroautophagy. *Nature* **2009**, *461*, 654–658. [CrossRef] [PubMed]
36. Valadas, J.S.; Esposito, G.; Vandekerkhove, D.; Miskiewicz, K.; Deaulmerie, L.; Raitano, S.; Seibler, P.; Klein, C.; Verstreken, P. ER Lipid Defects in Neuropeptidergic Neurons Impair Sleep Patterns in Parkinson's Disease. *Neuron* **2018**, *98*, 1155–1169.e6. [CrossRef]
37. Kornmann, B.; Osman, C.; Walter, P. The conserved GTPase Gem1 regulates endoplasmic reticulum-mitochondria connections. *Proc. Natl. Acad. Sci. USA* **2011**, *108*, 14151–14156. [CrossRef]
38. Giacomello, M.; Pellegrini, L. The coming of age of the mitochondria-ER contact: a matter of thickness. *Cell Death Differ.* **2016**, *23*, 1417–1427. [CrossRef]
39. Wang, P.T.C.; Garcin, P.O.; Fu, M.; Masoudi, M.; St-Pierre, P.; Panté, N.; Nabi, I.R. Distinct mechanisms controlling rough and smooth endoplasmic reticulum contacts with mitochondria. *J. Cell Sci.* **2015**, *128*, 2759–2765. [CrossRef]
40. Jiang, Q.-X.; Thrower, E.C.; Chester, D.W.; Ehrlich, B.E.; Sigworth, F.J. Three-dimensional structure of the type 1 inositol 1,4,5-trisphosphate receptor at 24 A resolution. *EMBO J.* **2002**, *21*, 3575–3581. [CrossRef]
41. Szabadkai, G.; Bianchi, K.; Várnai, P.; De Stefani, D.; Wieckowski, M.R.; Cavagna, D.; Nagy, A.I.; Balla, T.; Rizzuto, R. Chaperone-mediated coupling of endoplasmic reticulum and mitochondrial Ca$^{2+}$ channels. *J. Cell Biol.* **2006**, *175*, 901–911. [CrossRef] [PubMed]
42. Csordás, G.; Renken, C.; Várnai, P.; Walter, L.; Weaver, D.; Buttle, K.F.; Balla, T.; Mannella, C.A.; Hajnóczky, G. Structural and functional features and significance of the physical linkage between ER and mitochondria. *J. Cell Biol.* **2006**, *174*, 915–921. [CrossRef] [PubMed]
43. Csordás, G.; Várnai, P.; Golenár, T.; Roy, S.; Purkins, G.; Schneider, T.G.; Balla, T.; Hajnóczky, G. Imaging interorganelle contacts and local calcium dynamics at the ER-mitochondrial interface. *Mol. Cell* **2010**, *39*, 121–132. [CrossRef] [PubMed]
44. Filadi, R.; Pozzan, T. Generation and functions of second messengers microdomains. *Cell Calcium* **2015**, *58*, 405–414. [CrossRef] [PubMed]
45. Grünewald, A.; Gegg, M.E.; Taanman, J.-W.; King, R.H.; Kock, N.; Klein, C.; Schapira, A.H.V. Differential effects of PINK1 nonsense and missense mutations on mitochondrial function and morphology. *Exp. Neurol.* **2009**, *219*, 266–273. [CrossRef]

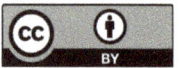 © 2019 by the authors. Licensee MDPI, Basel, Switzerland. This article is an open access article distributed under the terms and conditions of the Creative Commons Attribution (CC BY) license (http://creativecommons.org/licenses/by/4.0/).

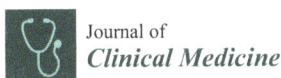 

Article

# Altered Bioenergetics of Blood Cell Sub-Populations in Acute Pancreatitis Patients

Jack C. Morton [1], Jane A. Armstrong [2], Ajay Sud [2], Alexei V. Tepikin [1], Robert Sutton [2] and David N. Criddle [1],*

[1] Department of Cellular and Molecular Physiology, Institute of Translational Medicine, University of Liverpool, Liverpool L69 3BX, UK; jack.morton87@gmail.com (J.C.M.); kiev@liverpool.ac.uk (A.V.T.)
[2] Department of Clinical Cancer Medicine, Institute of Translational Medicine, University of Liverpool, Liverpool L69 3BX, UK; janearm@liverpool.ac.uk (J.A.A.); suda@liverpool.ac.uk (A.S.); sutton@liv.ac.uk (R.S.)
* Correspondence: criddle@liv.ac.uk; Tel.: +44-151-794-5304; Fax: +44-151-794-5327

Received: 8 November 2019; Accepted: 12 December 2019; Published: 13 December 2019

**Abstract:** Acute pancreatitis (AP) is a debilitating, sometimes fatal disease, marked by local injury and systemic inflammation. Mitochondrial dysfunction is a central feature of pancreatic damage in AP, however, its involvement in circulating blood cell subtypes is unknown. This study compared mitochondrial bioenergetics in circulating leukocytes from AP patients and healthy volunteers: 15 patients with mild to severe AP were compared to 10 healthy controls. Monocytes, lymphocytes and neutrophils were isolated using magnetic activated cell sorting and mitochondrial bioenergetics profiles of the cell populations determined using a Seahorse XF24 flux analyser. Rates of oxygen consumption (OCR) and extracellular acidification (ECAR) under conditions of electron transport chain (ETC) inhibition ("stress" test) informed respiratory and glycolytic parameters, respectively. Phorbol ester stimulation was used to trigger the oxidative burst. Basal OCR in all blood cell subtypes was similar in AP patients and controls. However, maximal respiration and spare respiratory capacity of AP patient lymphocytes were decreased, indicating impairment of functional capacity. A diminished oxidative burst occurred in neutrophils from AP patients, compared to controls, whereas this was enhanced in both monocytes and lymphocytes. The data demonstrate important early alterations of bioenergetics in blood cell sub-populations from AP patients, which imply functional alterations linked to clinical disease progression.

**Keywords:** acute pancreatitis; mitochondrial dysfunction; Seahorse bioenergetics; respiration; glycolysis; inflammation; leukocytes

---

## 1. Introduction

Acute pancreatitis (AP) is a multifaceted disease, caused predominantly by gallstones and alcohol excess, which involves local injury and systemic inflammation. In severe disease, this may develop into a systemic inflammatory response syndrome, remote organ injury and death of the patient. The incidence of AP is 13–45 per 100,000 cases per year, and imposes a significant healthcare burden [1,2]. However, there is an incomplete understanding of the underlying pathophysiology, with current predictors of disease outcome inadequate and no specific therapy available. Damage to the pancreatic acinar cell is considered the initiating event of AP, manifested by premature zymogen activation, vacuolisation, mitochondrial dysfunction and necrotic cell death [3,4]. Bile acids, non-oxidative ethanol metabolites, and cholecystokinin hyperstimulation disrupt acinar cell calcium signalling and induce mitochondrial damage, via opening of the mitochondrial permeability transition pore (MPTP), causing loss of membrane potential, rundown of nicotinamide adenine dinucleotide (NADH), and fall of adenosine triphosphate (ATP) production, leading to necrosis [5–10].

However, comparatively little is known about mitochondrial dysfunction in circulating blood cells during AP. This may partly reflect the significant challenge posed by the isolation of patient blood cells in a reliable state for such bioenergetics measurements. In recent years, there has been increasing focus on the roles of immune cell subsets in the systemic inflammatory response in AP [11,12]. For example, neutrophil infiltration is evident in the pancreas within minutes of the onset of AP and exerts a significant role in disease severity [11,13]. Previously, elevated mitochondrial respiration was reported in a total population of peripheral blood mononuclear cells obtained from patients with mild AP, suggesting inefficient mitochondria, although no alteration of ATP production occurred [14]. However, whether specific bioenergetics alterations occur in blood cell subtypes during clinical AP is currently unknown. Detailed investigations of mitochondrial dysfunction can be achieved by measuring bioenergetics changes in cell populations using Seahorse flux analysis [15,16]. We have recently demonstrated that oxidative stress, which is elevated in clinical AP [17], altered the bioenergetic profiles of isolated pancreatic acinar cells determining cell death patterns [18].

In the present study, we have investigated the bioenergetics profiles of leukocyte sub-types isolated from AP patient blood samples, comparing results to those obtained from healthy volunteers. Our data show distinct alterations of mitochondrial bioenergetics in blood cell sub-types that occur during early clinical AP, pointing to a modified functional capacity of circulating blood cells during the inflammatory response.

## 2. Experimental Section

### 2.1. Blood Collection and Cell Isolation

Patients aged ≥18 years with a first attack of acute pancreatitis were recruited on the day of admission to the Royal Liverpool University Hospital for donation of blood and linked clinical data into the National Institute for Health Research Liverpool Pancreas Biomedical Research Unit Acute Pancreatitis Biobank, as approved by the regional ethics committee (REC 10/H1308/31 and 15/YH/0193). Patients with acute pancreatitis of any aetiology with two of three diagnostic features (serum amylase ≥3× upper limit of normal, typical pain, pancreatic inflammation on cross-sectional imaging) with written informed consent were eligible for inclusion, but patients who were unable to consent, had a history of recurrent acute or chronic pancreatitis or a history of pancreatic surgery or malignancy were excluded. Samples were collected prospectively within 24 h of admission from consenting patients who had presented within 72 h of onset of pain, together with clinical data that allowed severity stratification according to the 2012 Revised Atlanta Classification [19] after discharge. Blood samples were also collected from healthy volunteers (control group) aged ≥18 years; individuals with diabetes or a history of pancreatic disease were excluded. Collection, processing, storage, monitoring and usage of samples followed pre-defined standard operating procedures adhering to Good Clinical Practice.

Blood samples (one 8.5 mL/tube) were collected in a K2EDTA tube (Vacuette, Greiner Bio-One GmbH, Kremsmünster, Austria) and processed within an hour of collection using an established protocol [19]. All isolation procedures were designed and carefully executed to prevent activation of blood cells. In brief, following collection blood samples were centrifuged at 500× $g$ (acceleration 6 and no brake; Thermo Fisher Scientific, Waltham, MA, USA), the buffy layer removed and diluted with RPMI-140 (Sigma, Poole, UK) to 24 mL, then applied to a Histopaque density gradient (specific gravity 1.077/1.113, at room temperature; Alere, Waltham, MA, USA) and centrifuged at 700× $g$ (acceleration 6, no brake and at room temperature; Thermo Fisher Scientific, Waltham, MA, USA). Three distinct bands were present; the uppermost band contained peripheral blood mononuclear cells (PBMCs), the middle band polymorphonuclear cells (PMNs) and the lower band contained red blood cells (RBCs). The PBMCs and PMNs were collected separately. Red cell lysis buffer (Sigma, Poole, UK) was added to the PMNs, improving the purity of the cell population by lysing the RBCs.

The mononuclear cells were suspended in 80 µL of MACs buffer (PBS, 2 mM EDTA and 0.5% BSA; pH 7.2 and sterile filtered) and 20 µL CD61 human microbeads (Miltenyi, Bergisch Gladbach, Germany) at 4 °C for 15 min. The CD61 microbeads, which bind to CD61+ platelets, were then applied to a MS column (Miltenyi, Bergisch Gladbach, Germany) in a MiniMACS magnet (Miltenyi, Bergisch Gladbach, Germany) according to manufacturer's instructions. The column was discarded (removing any platelets from the PBMCs) and the flow through collected and re-suspended in 80 µL of MACs buffer and 20 µL CD14 human microbeads (Miltenyi, Bergisch Gladbach, Germany). CD14+ monocytes were purified from the PBMC fraction using superparamagnetic iron-dextran microbead-labelled anti-CD14 antibodies. Cells retained in the column were collected by elution with MACs buffer after removal from the magnetic field. Lymphocytes, in comparison, were present in the through flow. Isolation yielded cell populations with >90% purity and viability as determined by fluorescence-activated cell sorting and Trypan Blue exclusion, respectively (Table S1).

*2.2. Assessment of Monocyte, Lymphocyte and Neutrophil Bioenergetics*

Purified monocytes, lymphocytes and neutrophils were re-suspended in XF assay buffer (Dulbecco's Modified Eagle Medium (DMEM), 2 mM sodium pyruvate, 2 mM L-Glutamine and 10 mM D-glucose in ddH2O, pH 7.4 and sterile filtered), and then plated (250,000 cells/well) in 200 µL on CellTak (BD Biosciences, Poole, UK) coated assay plates and allowed to attach for 30 min at 37 °C in a non-$CO_2$ incubator. The cellular bioenergetics of the isolated cells were determined using the XF24 analyser (Agilent, Boston, MA, USA) [18–20]. Real-time, non-invasive measurements of OCR and ECAR were obtained which correlated to mitochondrial function and glycolysis, respectively. Using the mitochondrial respiratory function "stress" test protocol, inhibitors of the mitochondrial electron transport chain (ETC) (oligomycin, 0.5 µg/mL; carbonyl cyanide-4-trifluoromethoxy phenylhydrazone (FCCP), 0.6 µM; rotenone and antimycin, 1 µM; Sigma, Poole, UK) and an activator of the oxidative burst (phorbol 12-myristate 13-acetate (PMA), 100 ng/mL; Sigma, Poole, UK) were sequentially injected to assess the following respiratory parameters: oxygen consumption rate (OCR) basal respiration, maximal respiration, spare respiratory capacity ATP turnover capacity, proton leak, non-mitochondrial respiration, and PMA-induced oxidative burst, extracellular acidification rate (ECAR) baseline, glycolytic reserve and PMA-induced ECAR.

The mean basal respiration was determined at the 5th OCR measurement, before addition of the inhibitors or activators. ATP turnover capacity and proton leak were determined following injection of oligomycin, which blocks the ATP synthase, and then maximal respiration following FCCP, an uncoupler of the electron transport chain. The difference between the basal OCR and maximal OCR represents the Spare Respiratory Capacity OCR of the mitochondria. Antimycin A, an inhibitor of Complex III, and rotenone, an inhibitor of Complex I, were used in conjunction to completely inhibit mitochondrial electron transport: the remaining OCR is attributed to non-mitochondrial OCR. Basal OCR, proton leak OCR, and the maximal OCR were calculated after correction for the non-mitochondrial OCR for each assay. Finally, the oxidative burst OCR was determined cell following cell stimulation with PMA, a protein kinase C (PKC) activator that increases nicotinamide adenine dinucleotide phosphate (NADPH) oxidase activity. The ECAR measures were recorded in parallel to OCR measurements. Baseline ECAR was determined at the 5th ECAR reading and Glycolytic Reserve calculated by subtraction of the baseline ECAR reading from that obtained after addition of oligomycin. The optimal concentrations of the inhibitors and activator used for the assessment of mitochondrial function were as previously determined [21]. All XF assays were performed in sterile DMEM (5 mM D-glucose, 4 mM L-glutamine and 1 mM sodium pyruvate; pH 7.4).

*2.3. Statistics*

For each blood sample, 3–5 replicates were used for all bioenergetics determinations, and the data are presented as mean ± standard error of the mean (SEM). Statistical significance was determined using a Student's t-test or Mann Whitney U test, with $p \leq 0.05$ taken as indicating significant difference from control.

## 3. Results

### 3.1. Characteristics of Patients and Healthy Controls Included in the Analysis

For the study blood samples were collected from 15 AP patients. Of these, 12 were classified as mild AP, 1 was moderate and 2 patients had severe AP according to the revised Atlanta Classification [22]. The mean age of the patients was 57.2, with 11 females (mean age of 54.3 years) and 4 males (mean age of 65.3 years). The aetiology of AP in patients was: 12 biliary, 2 idiopathic, 1 alcoholic and 1 ERCP. Amylase, platelets and WBC counts (neutrophils, lymphocytes, monocytes, eosinophils and basophils) were recorded for each patient at admission by the hospital staff (Table 1). Further details of AP patient co-morbidities and Body Mass Index (BMI) are included in Table S2. For comparison, blood samples were collected from 10 healthy volunteers, of which half were male and half female. The overall mean age was 32.9 years, with female mean age of 34.4 years and male mean age of 31.4 years.

### 3.2. Bioenergetics Differences in OCR Between Healthy Volunteers and AP Patients

Application of a mitochondrial respiratory function "stress" test protocol allowed measurement of standard respiratory parameters (basal respiration, maximal respiration, spare respiratory capacity, ATP turnover capacity, proton leak and non-mitochondrial respiration) in monocytes, lymphocytes and neutrophils, providing a comparison between AP patient and healthy volunteers. The protocol illustrated in Figure 1A shows OCR changes caused by sequential injection of mitochondrial inhibitors (oligomycin, FCCP, rotenone/antimycin), followed by an activator of the oxidative burst PMA used to derive comparative bioenergetics parameters.

The blood cell sub-types exhibited distinct bioenergetics profiles (Figure 1B–D). The basal OCR values after 5 min equilibration were 51.92 ± 4.9 and 60.19 ± 6.9 in monocytes, 29.62 ± 2.6 and 22.54 ± 2.1 in lymphocytes, and −14.19 ± 6.7 and −4.6 ± 5.7 pmol/min in neutrophils in healthy volunteers and AP patients, respectively. There were no significant differences in basal respiration between AP patient and healthy volunteers for any of the blood cell types. However, when the "stress" test was applied, differences in bioenergetics were revealed. Thus, changes of OCR induced by inhibition of the electron transport chain showed that lymphocytes from AP patients exhibited a substantially decreased maximal respiration (Figure 2B; $p \leq 0.001$) and spare respiratory capacity (Figure 2C; $p \leq 0.001$) compared to lymphocytes from healthy controls.

There was a trend for reduced spare respiratory capacity in monocytes from AP patients compared to healthy volunteers, although this did not attain significance (Figure 2C). Furthermore, no significant differences in ATP turnover capacity (Figure 2D) or proton leak (Figure 2E) were detected between AP patient and healthy control blood cells. However, a significantly reduced non-mitochondrial respiratory component was found in AP patient neutrophils compared to controls (Figure 2F).

Table 1. Demographics, aetiology and blood cell details of acute pancreatitis (AP) patients obtained on admission for the study.

| Patient | Severity (1 = Mild, 2 = Moderate & 3 = Severe) | Aetiology (ERCP = Endoscopic Retrograde Cholangiopancreatography) | Sex (M = Male, F = Female) | Age | Amylase | Platelets ($\times 10 > 9$/L, N: 150–400) | White Blood Cells ($\times 10 > 9$/L, N: 3.5–11) | Neutrophils ($\times 10 > 9$/L, N: 2.0–7.5) | Lymphocytes ($\times 10 > 9$/L, N: 1.0–3.5) | Monocytes ($\times 10 > 9$/L, N: 0.2–0.8) | Eosinophils ($\times 10 > 9$/L, N: 0.0–0.4) | Basophils ($\times 10 > 9$/L, N: 0.0–0.2) |
|---|---|---|---|---|---|---|---|---|---|---|---|---|
| AP779 | 1 | Biliary | M | 59 | 2634 | 228 | 10.8 | 8.3 | 1.5 | 0.8 | 0.1 | 0.1 |
| AP784 | 3 | Idiopathic | F | 77 | 1240 | 293 | 25.6 | 22.7 | 1.4 | 1.5 | 0 | 0.1 |
| AP785 | 1 | Biliary | M | 74 | 527 | 233 | 19.4 | 17.3 | 0.6 | 1.3 | 0.1 | 0 |
| AP788 | 1 | Biliary | F | 20 | 1692 | 197 | 12.3 | 8.7 | 2.2 | 1.3 | 0 | 0 |
| AP796 | 1 | Biliary | F | 64 | 1485 | 246 | 13.1 | 10.2 | 1.6 | 1.2 | 0 | 0 |
| AP797 | 1 | Biliary | M | 63 | 2168 | 245 | 11.3 | 10.2 | 0.4 | 0.6 | 0 | 0 |
| AP799 | 1 | Biliary | F | 28 | 1968 | 278 | 8.9 | 7 | 1.4 | 0.5 | 0 | 0.1 |
| AP805 | 2 | Biliary | F | 80 | 1577 | 303 | 10.3 | 9.1 | 0.8 | 0.3 | 0 | 0 |
| AP806 | 1 | Alcohol | M | 65 | 1265 | 188 | 10.7 | 8 | 1.3 | 1.2 | 0.1 | 0.1 |
| AP812 | 1 | Idiopathic | F | 21 | 492 | 194 | 12 | 6.7 | 4.1 | 1 | 0.2 | 0 |
| AP821 | 1 | Biliary | F | 33 | 2333 | 335 | 12.9 | 9.9 | 1.9 | 0.2 | 0.1 | 0.1 |
| AP828 | 1 | Biliary | F | 77 | 1792 | 237 | 23 | 21.4 | 1.3 | 0.3 | 0.1 | 0.1 |
| AP837 | 3 | Biliary | F | 91 | 1450 | 190 | 12.4 | 11.8 | 0.4 | 0.9 | 0 | 0 |
| AP839 | 1 | Biliary | F | 49 | 2293 | 264 | 9.5 | 6 | 2.5 | 0.3 | 0.1 | 0 |
| AP842 | 1 | ERCP | F | 57 | 2184 | 229 | 10.5 | 9.6 | 0.6 | | 0 | 0 |

185

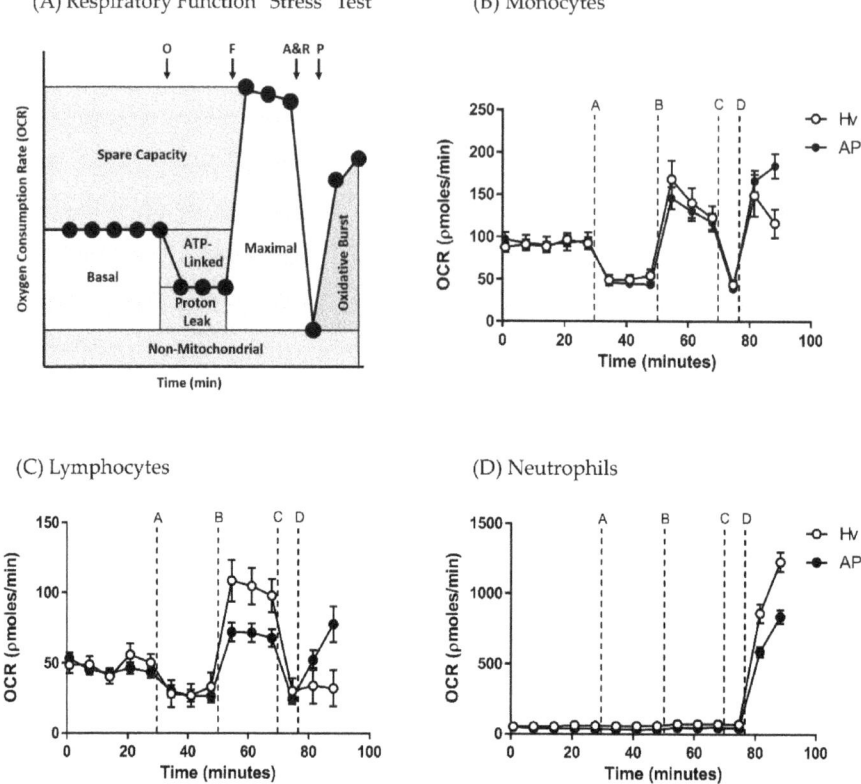

**Figure 1.** Bioenergetics changes in blood cell subtypes from acute pancreatitis (AP) patients and healthy volunteers (Hv). (**A**) Changes in oxygen consumption rates (OCR) with time in response to a mitochondrial respiratory function "stress" test using sequential applications of A = oligomycin 0.5 µg/mL, B = carbonyl cyanide-4-trifluoromethoxy phenylhydrazone (FCCP: F) 0.6 µM, C = antimycin (A) 1 µM and rotenone (R) 1 µM, and D = phorbol 12-myristate 13-acetate (P) 100 ng/mL to measure standard respiratory parameters in (**B**) monocytes, (**C**) lymphocytes and (**D**) neutrophils. Values are expressed as means ± standard error of the mean (SEM) with biological repeats of $N = 10$ (Hv) and 15 (AP).

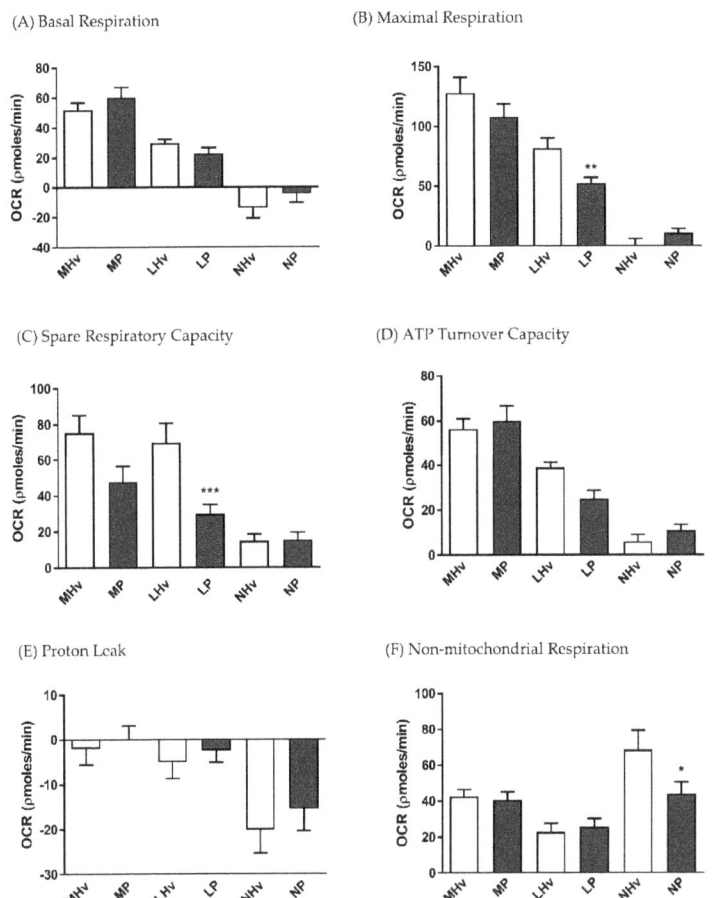

**Figure 2.** Mean changes in bioenergetics parameters determined in blood cell subtypes from acute pancreatitis (P) patients and healthy volunteers (Hv). Changes in oxygen consumption rates (OCR) obtained in monocytes (M), lymphocytes (L) and neutrophils (L) are shown in response to a mitochondrial respiratory function "stress" test to measure standard respiratory parameters (**A–F**). Values are expressed as means ± SEM with biological repeats of $N = 10$ (Hv) and 15 (AP). Significant changes in blood cells from AP patients compared to healthy controls are denoted as * $p \leq 0.05$, ** $p \leq 0.01$ and *** $p \leq 0.001$. (MHv, LHv, NHv = monocytes, lymphocytes and neutrophils from healthy volunteers, respectively; MP, LP, NP = monocytes, lymphocytes and neutrophils from patients).

### 3.3. Analysis of Mitochondrial Bioenergetics Differences in ECAR Between Healthy Volunteers and AP Patients

The basal ECAR values after 5 min equilibration were 12.27 ± 1.4 and 5.94 ± 0.8 in monocytes, 2.69 ± 0.4 and 3.11 ± 0.5 in lymphocytes, and 13.47 ± 1.1 and 8.92 ± 0.7 mpH/min in neutrophils in healthy volunteers and AP patients, respectively. Both monocyte and neutrophil basal ECARs were significantly decreased in AP patients compared to their respective healthy volunteer controls (Figure 3A; $p \leq 0.001$). However, no significant differences in glycolytic reserve, measured as the change in ECAR following application of oligomycin, were apparent in any blood cell sub-type.

(A) Basal ECAR

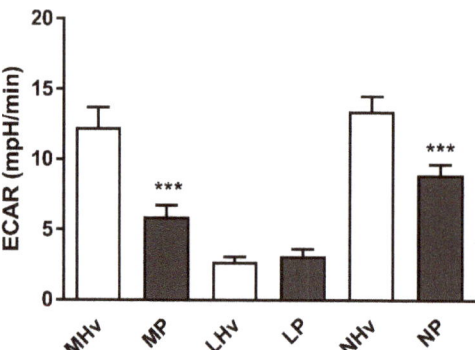

(B) Glycolytic Reserve

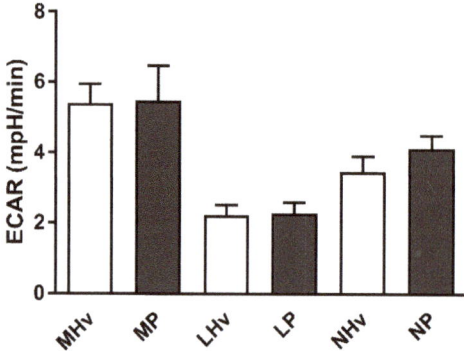

**Figure 3.** Mean changes in bioenergetics parameters determined in blood cell subtypes from acute pancreatitis patients and healthy volunteers. Changes in extracellular acidification rates (ECAR) obtained in monocytes (M), lymphocytes (L) and neutrophils (L) from patients (P) and healthy volunteers (Hv) are shown on basal glycolysis (**A**) and in response to mitochondrial inhibition to measure glycolytic reserve (**B**). Values are expressed as means ± SEM with biological repeats of $N = 10$ (Hv) and 15 (AP). Significant changes in blood cells from AP patients compared to healthy controls are denoted as *** $p \leq 0.001$.

*3.4. Analysis of the Oxidative Burst in Healthy Volunteers and AP Patients*

Both monocytes and lymphocytes from AP patients exhibited significantly increased PMA-induced oxidative respiratory bursts (Figure 4A; $p \leq 0.01$) and accompanying ECAR increases (Figure 4B; $p \leq 0.001$) compared to those from healthy volunteers. In contrast, neutrophils from AP patients had a significantly decreased PMA-induced oxidative respiratory burst compared to healthy volunteer neutrophils (Figure 4A; $p \leq 0.001$), mirrored by a reduced PMA-induced ECAR increase (Figure 4B; $p \leq 0.001$).

(A) PMA-induced OCR Response

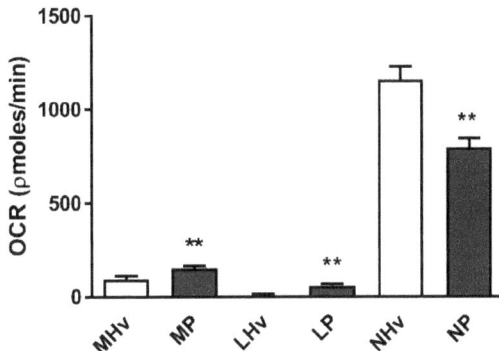

(B) PMA-induced ECAR Response

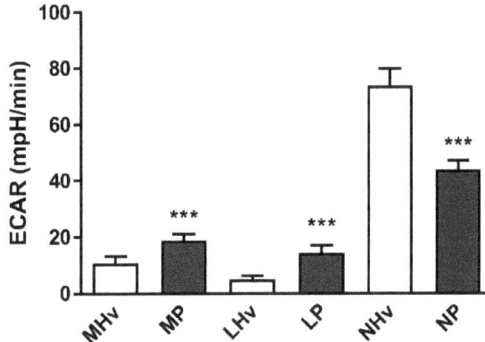

Figure 4. Mean changes in bioenergetics linked to the oxidative burst in blood cell subtypes from acute pancreatitis (P) patients and healthy volunteers (Hv). Changes in (A) oxygen consumption rates (OCR) and (B) extracellular acidification rates (ECAR) obtained in monocytes (M), lymphocytes (L) and neutrophils (L) in response to phorbol 12-myristate 13-acetate (PMA) to measure bioenergetics changes during the oxidative burst (A,B). Values are expressed as means ± SEM with biological repeats of $N = 10$ (Hv) and 15 (AP). Significant changes in blood cells from AP patients compared to healthy controls are denoted as ** $p \leq 0.01$ and *** $p \leq 0.001$.

## 4. Discussion

This study has demonstrated distinct alterations of mitochondrial bioenergetics in blood cell sub-types that occur during clinical AP, pointing to a modified functional capacity during the inflammatory response. Differences between patient and healthy volunteer blood cell respiration were only apparent, however, following manipulation of the ETC or stimulation with PMA, with no significant differences in basal OCR detected. Relatively little is known about bioenergetics changes in circulating blood cells that occur during clinical AP. Previously, a study showed that leukocytes from mild AP patients exhibited an approximate 1.5 fold elevation of endogenous respiration compared to controls with no associated change in ATP production [14]. This reflected a summation of activity in a population of peripheral blood mononuclear cells rather than changes in discrete subsets. Our study now indicates that bioenergetics profiles of monocytes, lymphocytes and neutrophils undergo complex alterations during the early course of AP, with subset-specific changes that do not simply reflect a generalized depression of mitochondrial activity. Thus, lymphocyte respiration was diminished in AP patients, with substantially reduced maximal respiration and spare respiratory capacity, whereas these parameters were unaltered in monocytes and neutrophils.

Previously, it has been suggested that prospective monitoring of lymphocyte signalling profiles might assist predicting AP outcome: a variety of alterations in severe alcoholic AP patients with organ dysfunction was detected, linked to increased infection risk and sustained inflammation [23]. Our findings in lymphocytes from predominantly mild AP patients show a markedly reduced spare respiratory capacity. This bioenergetic parameter is considered an important indication of mitochondrial capacity to meet metabolic demands under stress conditions and is decreased in pathophysiological situations, including cardiac and neurodegenerative damage [24–26]. Common features of disease progression may be present in inflammatory states, which are reflected by alterations of blood cell subtype bioenergetics profiles. For example, similarities between inflammation in AP and sepsis have been reported [27], with defects in oxidative metabolism found in leukocytes from sepsis patients, including a substantial reduction of maximum oxygen consumption [28]. A compromise of lymphocyte function in AP linked to altered bioenergetic capacity would likely increase as the disease progresses and cellular stress augments. Oxidative stress is elevated in AP patients, coupled with a decrease of antioxidant capacity [17]. Oxidative stress strongly modified pancreatic acinar cell bioenergetics, thereby determining local cell fate [18,20], while mitochondrial bioenergetic function of human peripheral blood leucocytes was susceptible to oxidative injury, an effect that was greater in aged individuals [29]. Interestingly, mitochondrial dynamics have recently been shown to modulate lymphocyte fate through metabolic programming linked to bioenergetics changes. Thus, in activated effector T cells, which mediate protective immunity against pathogens, fission-dependent cristae expansion was associated with reduced ETC efficiency and promotion of aerobic glycolysis [30]. Although our study found a decreased maximal respiration in AP patient lymphocytes, this was not associated with a fall in ATP turnover capacity, suggesting maintenance of basal function. Accordingly, there was no associated increase in basal glycolysis, implying a defect of oxidative phosphorylation that did not trigger a switch in metabolic pathway. In agreement, no significant alteration of ATP production was detected in peripheral blood mononuclear cells from mild AP patients [14], while peripheral blood mononuclear cells from septic paediatric patients, which had a significantly reduced spare respiratory capacity, exhibited no differences in basal or ATP-linked oxygen consumption [31].

Our study demonstrated a diminished oxidative burst in neutrophils from AP patients, with significantly reduced OCR and ECAR responses to PMA stimulation compared to controls. Neutrophils play an important role in the early phase of AP, participating in digestive enzyme activation and progression to severe disease [13]. They utilise an oxidative burst via the activation of NADPH oxidase, which consumes oxygen and forms superoxide radicals [32]. Accordingly, depletion of neutrophils was protective in mild and severe experimental AP induced by caerulein [33] and by taurocholate [34], respectively. Alterations of neutrophil bioenergetics have been reported in other diseases. For example, changes in neutrophil oxidative bursts have been associated with autoimmune diseases such as multiple sclerosis, arthritis and recurrent infection [19], while diminution of neutrophil activity involving a reduced oxidative burst in response to formyl peptides, impaired phagocytosis and associated ROS production may underlie an increased susceptibility to bacterial infection in elderly individuals [35]. In AP patient neutrophils, both baseline ECAR and non-mitochondrial OCR were also reduced: the sum of the bioenergetics alterations would indicate that normal activity of neutrophils is compromised in AP patients, or alternatively, that at the time of measurement these immune cells had already performed their inflammatory role. A future study including measurement of neutrophil bioenergetics changes at multiple time-points would assist clarification.

In contrast, an increased oxidative burst was detected in both monocytes and lymphocytes from AP patients compared to controls. This supports monocyte/macrophage involvement as a principal, important feature of early events in AP [11]. For example, blockade of monocyte chemoattractant protein synthesis was protective against experimental AP in mice [36], while application of antibodies against macrophage migration inhibitory factor improved AP survival in rats [37]. The increased oxidative burst capacity detected in AP patients may reflect an upregulation of NADPH oxidases in circulating monocytes, a feature which occurs in acute respiratory distress syndrome in response to ethanol [38]. Marked elevations of mitochondrial superoxide have recently been reported in peripheral blood mononuclear cells from mild AP patients [14]. Monocytes and macrophages are part of the innate immune system and exhibit a high degree of plasticity. Activated pro-inflammatory macrophages (M1) release copious amounts of cytokines, including interleukin 6 (IL6), IL12, IL1β and tumour necrosis factor alpha (TNFα), early in the inflammatory response and in AP make a significant contribution to the systemic inflammatory response syndrome linked to organ dysfunction and death [12]. Recently extra-acinar protease activation within macrophages during endocytosis of zymogen-containing vesicles has been shown to participate in the systemic inflammatory response and determine AP severity [39]. In our study, the PMA-induced ECAR response of AP patient monocytes was also greater than those of healthy volunteers, indicating an enhanced glycolytic component of ATP production during the respiratory burst with prioritisation of cellular oxygen to generate free radicals. A concurrent decrease of basal ECAR in monocytes was also found, implying a reduced glycolytic component contributing to basal energy production during AP, although the basis for this is presently unclear.

Previously separation of blood cell subtypes for evaluation of mitochondrial function has been questioned since this may increase time before performing the assays [14] and potentially disrupt cellular interactions necessary for cell activation [40]. Here, we have shown that successful isolation and separation of AP patient blood cells is achievable for detailed bioenergetics investigations: basal OCR values were not different between AP patient and control groups for all subtypes, indicating no detrimental changes due to cell isolation procedures. Alterations of mitochondrial function have been observed with aging [41] and a limitation of the present study is that the healthy volunteer group was younger than the AP group. However, the subset-specific changes detected did not appear to simply reflect a generalized depression of mitochondrial activity that might be expected as a consequence of aging, and point to more precise changes: our results demonstrated differential alterations of bioenergetics linked to the oxidative burst in leukocyte subtypes from AP patients, and further revealed an important reduction of respiratory capacity in AP patient lymphocytes. These changes occurred early in the development of clinical AP, advancing our understanding of pathophysiological events in the inflammatory response. Detection of specific bioenergetics alterations of blood cell subtypes from patient samples may provide a more detailed picture of on-going mitochondrial dysfunction during AP and potentially assist prediction of outcome.

## 5. Conclusions

Our data show distinct alterations of mitochondrial bioenergetics in blood cell sub-types that occur during early clinical AP, pointing to a modified functional capacity of circulating blood cells during the inflammatory response.

**Supplementary Materials:** The following are available online at http://www.mdpi.com/2077-0383/8/12/2201/s1, Table S1: The isolation of blood cell populations obtained >90% (A) purity and (B) viability, as determined by fluorescence-activated cell sorting and Trypan Blue exclusion, respectively; Table S2: Details of (A) co-morbidities and (B) BMI from AP patients.

**Author Contributions:** Conceptualization, A.V.T., D.N.C., R.S.; Investigation, Methodology, A.S., J.A.A., J.C.M.; Formal Analysis, J.A.A., J.C.M.; Funding Acquisition & Resources, A.V.T., D.N.C., R.S.; Supervision, A.V.T., D.N.C., R.S.; Original Draft Preparation, D.N.C.; Review & Editing, A.V.T., D.N.C., J.A.A., J.C.M., R.S.

**Funding:** This research was funded by the Wellcome Trust (102381/Z/13/Z) and Medical Research Council (MR/N011384/1).

**Conflicts of Interest:** The authors declare that they have no conflicts of interest with the contents of this article.

## References

1. Peery, A.F.; Crockett, S.D.; Murphy, C.C.; Lund, J.L.; Dellon, E.S.; Williams, J.L.; Jensen, E.T.; Shaheen, N.J.; Barritt, A.S.; Lieber, S.R.; et al. Burden and cost of gastrointestinal, liver, and pancreatic diseases in the united states: Update 2018. *Gastroenterology* **2019**, *156*, 254–272. [CrossRef] [PubMed]
2. Yadav, D.; Lowenfels, A.B. The epidemiology of pancreatitis and pancreatic cancer. *Gastroenterology* **2013**, *144*, 1252–1261. [CrossRef] [PubMed]
3. Kruger, B.; Albrecht, E.; Lerch, M.M. The role of intracellular calcium signaling in premature protease activation and the onset of pancreatitis. *Am. J. Pathol.* **2000**, *157*, 43–50. [CrossRef]
4. Raraty, M.; Ward, J.; Erdemli, G.; Vaillant, C.; Neoptolemos, J.P.; Sutton, R.; Petersen, O.H. Calcium-dependent enzyme activation and vacuole formation in the apical granular region of pancreatic acinar cells. *Proc. Natl. Acad. Sci. USA* **2000**, *97*, 13126–13131. [CrossRef] [PubMed]
5. Voronina, S.G.; Barrow, S.L.; Simpson, A.W.; Gerasimenko, O.V.; da Silva Xavier, G.; Rutter, G.A.; Petersen, O.H.; Tepikin, A.V. Dynamic changes in cytosolic and mitochondrial atp levels in pancreatic acinar cells. *Gastroenterology* **2010**, *138*, 1976–1987. [CrossRef] [PubMed]
6. Criddle, D.N.; Murphy, J.; Fistetto, G.; Barrow, S.; Tepikin, A.V.; Neoptolemos, J.P.; Sutton, R.; Petersen, O.H. Fatty acid ethyl esters cause pancreatic calcium toxicity via inositol trisphosphate receptors and loss of atp synthesis. *Gastroenterology* **2006**, *130*, 781–793. [CrossRef] [PubMed]
7. Booth, D.M.; Murphy, J.A.; Mukherjee, R.; Awais, M.; Neoptolemos, J.P.; Gerasimenko, O.V.; Tepikin, A.V.; Petersen, O.H.; Sutton, R.; Criddle, D.N. Reactive oxygen species induced by bile acid induce apoptosis and protect against necrosis in pancreatic acinar cells. *Gastroenterology* **2011**, *140*, 2116–2125. [CrossRef]
8. Mukherjee, R.; Mareninova, O.A.; Odinokova, I.V.; Huang, W.; Murphy, J.; Chvanov, M.; Javed, M.A.; Wen, L.; Booth, D.M.; Cane, M.C.; et al. Mechanism of mitochondrial permeability transition pore induction and damage in the pancreas: Inhibition prevents acute pancreatitis by protecting production of atp. *Gut* **2016**, *65*, 1333–1346. [CrossRef]
9. Wen, L.; Voronina, S.; Javed, M.A.; Awais, M.; Szatmary, P.; Latawiec, D.; Chvanov, M.; Collier, D.; Huang, W.; Barrett, J.; et al. Inhibitors of orai1 prevent cytosolic calcium-associated injury of human pancreatic acinar cells and acute pancreatitis in 3 mouse models. *Gastroenterology* **2015**, *149*, 481–492. [CrossRef]
10. Criddle, D.N. Reactive oxygen species, ca(2+) stores and acute pancreatitis; a step closer to therapy? *Cell Calcium* **2016**, *60*, 180–189. [CrossRef]
11. Xue, J.; Sharma, V.; Habtezion, A. Immune cells and immune-based therapy in pancreatitis. *Immunol. Res.* **2014**, *58*, 378–386. [CrossRef]
12. Mayerle, J.; Sendler, M.; Hegyi, E.; Beyer, G.; Lerch, M.M.; Sahin-Toth, M. Genetics, cell biology, and pathophysiology of pancreatitis. *Gastroenterology* **2019**, *156*, 1951–1968. [CrossRef]
13. Gukovskaya, A.S.; Vaquero, E.; Zaninovic, V.; Gorelick, F.S.; Lusis, A.J.; Brennan, M.L.; Holland, S.; Pandol, S.J. Neutrophils and nadph oxidase mediate intrapancreatic trypsin activation in murine experimental acute pancreatitis. *Gastroenterology* **2002**, *122*, 974–984. [CrossRef]
14. Chakraborty, M.; Hickey, A.J.; Petrov, M.S.; Macdonald, J.R.; Thompson, N.; Newby, L.; Sim, D.; Windsor, J.A.; Phillips, A.R. Mitochondrial dysfunction in peripheral blood mononuclear cells in early experimental and clinical acute pancreatitis. *Pancreatology* **2016**, *16*, 739–747. [CrossRef]
15. Brand, M.D.; Nicholls, D.G. Assessing mitochondrial dysfunction in cells. *Biochem. J.* **2011**, *435*, 297–312. [CrossRef]
16. Kramer, P.A.; Chacko, B.K.; George, D.J.; Zhi, D.; Wei, C.C.; Dell'Italia, L.J.; Melby, S.J.; George, J.F.; Darley-Usmar, V.M. Decreased bioenergetic health index in monocytes isolated from the pericardial fluid and blood of post-operative cardiac surgery patients. *Biosci. Rep.* **2015**, *35*, e00237. [CrossRef]
17. Tsai, K.; Wang, S.S.; Chen, T.S.; Kong, C.W.; Chang, F.Y.; Lee, S.D.; Lu, F.J. Oxidative stress: An important phenomenon with pathogenetic significance in the progression of acute pancreatitis. *Gut* **1998**, *42*, 850–855. [CrossRef]
18. Armstrong, J.A.; Cash, N.J.; Ouyang, Y.; Morton, J.C.; Chvanov, M.; Latawiec, D.; Awais, M.; Tepikin, A.V.; Sutton, R.; Criddle, D.N. Oxidative stress alters mitochondrial bioenergetics and modifies pancreatic cell death independently of cyclophilin d, resulting in an apoptosis-to-necrosis shift. *J. Biol. Chem.* **2018**, *293*, 8032–8047. [CrossRef]

19. Kramer, P.A.; Chacko, B.K.; Ravi, S.; Johnson, M.S.; Mitchell, T.; Darley-Usmar, V.M. Bioenergetics and the oxidative burst: Protocols for the isolation and evaluation of human leukocytes and platelets. *J. Vis. Exp.* **2014**, *85*, E51301. [CrossRef]
20. Armstrong, J.A.; Cash, N.J.; Morton, J.C.; Tepikin, A.V.; Sutton, R.; Criddle, D.N. Mitochondrial targeting of antioxidants alters pancreatic acinar cell bioenergetics and determines cell fate. *Int. J. Mol. Sci.* **2019**, *20*, 1700. [CrossRef]
21. Chacko, B.K.; Kramer, P.A.; Ravi, S.; Johnson, M.S.; Hardy, R.W.; Ballinger, S.W.; Darley-Usmar, V.M. Methods for defining distinct bioenergetic profiles in platelets, lymphocytes, monocytes, and neutrophils, and the oxidative burst from human blood. *Lab. Investig.* **2013**, *93*, 690–700. [CrossRef]
22. Banks, P.A.; Bollen, T.L.; Dervenis, C.; Gooszen, H.G.; Johnson, C.D.; Sarr, M.G.; Tsiotos, G.G.; Vege, S.S.; Acute Pancreatitis Classification Working Group. Classification of acute pancreatitis—2012: Revision of the atlanta classification and definitions by international consensus. *Gut* **2013**, *62*, 102–111. [CrossRef]
23. Oiva, J.; Mustonen, H.; Kylanpaa, M.L.; Kyhala, L.; Kuuliala, K.; Siitonen, S.; Kemppainen, E.; Puolakkainen, P.; Repo, H. Acute pancreatitis with organ dysfunction associates with abnormal blood lymphocyte signaling: Controlled laboratory study. *Crit. Care* **2010**, *14*, R207. [CrossRef]
24. Sansbury, B.E.; Jones, S.P.; Riggs, D.W.; Darley-Usmar, V.M.; Hill, B.G. Bioenergetic function in cardiovascular cells: The importance of the reserve capacity and its biological regulation. *Chem. Biol. Interact.* **2011**, *191*, 288–295. [CrossRef]
25. Yadava, N.; Nicholls, D.G. Spare respiratory capacity rather than oxidative stress regulates glutamate excitotoxicity after partial respiratory inhibition of mitochondrial complex i with rotenone. *J. Neurosci.* **2007**, *27*, 7310–7317. [CrossRef]
26. Kramer, P.A.; Darley-Usmar, V.M. The emerging theme of redox bioenergetics in health and disease. *Biomed. J.* **2015**, *38*, 294–300.
27. Kylanpaa, M.L.; Repo, H.; Puolakkainen, P.A. Inflammation and immunosuppression in severe acute pancreatitis. *World J. Gastroenterol.* **2010**, *16*, 2867–2872. [CrossRef]
28. Cheng, S.C.; Scicluna, B.P.; Arts, R.J.; Gresnigt, M.S.; Lachmandas, E.; Giamarellos-Bourboulis, E.J.; Kox, M.; Manjeri, G.R.; Wagenaars, J.A.; Cremer, O.L.; et al. Broad defects in the energy metabolism of leukocytes underlie immunoparalysis in sepsis. *Nat. Immunol.* **2016**, *17*, 406–413. [CrossRef]
29. Tsai, K.; Hsu, T.G.; Lu, F.J.; Hsu, C.F.; Liu, T.Y.; Kong, C.W. Age-related changes in the mitochondrial depolarization induced by oxidative injury in human peripheral blood leukocytes. *Free Radic. Res.* **2001**, *35*, 395–403. [CrossRef]
30. Buck, M.D.; O'Sullivan, D.; Klein Geltink, R.I.; Curtis, J.D.; Chang, C.H.; Sanin, D.E.; Qiu, J.; Kretz, O.; Braas, D.; van der Windt, G.J.; et al. Mitochondrial dynamics controls t cell fate through metabolic programming. *Cell* **2016**, *166*, 63–76. [CrossRef]
31. Weiss, S.L.; Selak, M.A.; Tuluc, F.; Perales Villarroel, J.; Nadkarni, V.M.; Deutschman, C.S.; Becker, L.B. Mitochondrial dysfunction in peripheral blood mononuclear cells in pediatric septic shock. *Pediatr. Crit. Care Med.* **2015**, *16*, e4–e12. [CrossRef]
32. Karlsson, A.; Nixon, J.B.; McPhail, L.C. Phorbol myristate acetate induces neutrophil nadph-oxidase activity by two separate signal transduction pathways: Dependent or independent of phosphatidylinositol 3-kinase. *J. Leukoc. Biol.* **2000**, *67*, 396–404. [CrossRef]
33. Sandoval, D.; Gukovskaya, A.; Reavey, P.; Gukovsky, S.; Sisk, A.; Braquet, P.; Pandol, S.J.; Poucell-Hatton, S. The role of neutrophils and platelet-activating factor in mediating experimental pancreatitis. *Gastroenterology* **1996**, *111*, 1081–1091. [CrossRef]
34. Abdulla, A.; Awla, D.; Thorlacius, H.; Regner, S. Role of neutrophils in the activation of trypsinogen in severe acute pancreatitis. *J. Leukoc. Biol.* **2011**, *90*, 975–982. [CrossRef]
35. Sauce, D.; Dong, Y.; Campillo-Gimenez, L.; Casulli, S.; Bayard, C.; Autran, B.; Boddaert, J.; Appay, V.; Elbim, C. Reduced oxidative burst by primed neutrophils in the elderly individuals is associated with increased levels of the cd16bright/cd62ldim immunosuppressive subset. *J. Gerontol. A Biol. Sci. Med. Sci.* **2017**, *72*, 163–172. [CrossRef]
36. Bhatia, M.; Ramnath, R.D.; Chevali, L.; Guglielmotti, A. Treatment with bindarit, a blocker of mcp-1 synthesis, protects mice against acute pancreatitis. *Am. J. Physiol. Gastrointest. Liver Physiol.* **2005**, *288*, G1259–G1265. [CrossRef]

37. Sakai, Y.; Masamune, A.; Satoh, A.; Nishihira, J.; Yamagiwa, T.; Shimosegawa, T. Macrophage migration inhibitory factor is a critical mediator of severe acute pancreatitis. *Gastroenterology* **2003**, *124*, 725–736. [CrossRef]
38. Yeligar, S.M.; Harris, F.L.; Hart, C.M.; Brown, L.A. Ethanol induces oxidative stress in alveolar macrophages via upregulation of nadph oxidases. *J. Immunol.* **2012**, *188*, 3648–3657. [CrossRef]
39. Sendler, M.; Weiss, F.U.; Golchert, J.; Homuth, G.; van den Brandt, C.; Mahajan, U.M.; Partecke, L.I.; Doring, P.; Gukovsky, I.; Gukovskaya, A.S.; et al. Cathepsin b-mediated activation of trypsinogen in endocytosing macrophages increases severity of pancreatitis in mice. *Gastroenterology* **2018**, *154*, 704–718. [CrossRef]
40. Schmid, D.; Burmester, G.R.; Tripmacher, R.; Kuhnke, A.; Buttgereit, F. Bioenergetics of human peripheral blood mononuclear cell metabolism in quiescent, activated, and glucocorticoid-treated states. *Biosci. Rep.* **2000**, *20*, 289–302. [CrossRef]
41. Sun, N.; Youle, R.J.; Finkel, T. The mitochondrial basis of aging. *Mol. Cell* **2016**, *61*, 654–666. [CrossRef]

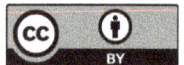

© 2019 by the authors. Licensee MDPI, Basel, Switzerland. This article is an open access article distributed under the terms and conditions of the Creative Commons Attribution (CC BY) license (http://creativecommons.org/licenses/by/4.0/).

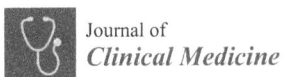 

Article

# A Humanized Bone Niche Model Reveals Bone Tissue Preservation Upon Targeting Mitochondrial Complex I in Pseudo-Orthotopic Osteosarcoma

Ivana Kurelac [1,2,*], Ander Abarrategi [3,4,5], Moira Ragazzi [6], Luisa Iommarini [7], Nikkitha Umesh Ganesh [1], Thomas Snoeks [8], Dominique Bonnet [3], Anna Maria Porcelli [7,9], Ilaria Malanchi [2,†] and Giuseppe Gasparre [1,10,†]

[1] Dipartimento di Scienze Mediche e Chirurgiche, Università di Bologna, Via Massarenti 9, 40138 Bologna, Italy; nikkitha.umesh@gmail.com (N.U.G.); giuseppe.gasparre3@unibo.it (G.G.)
[2] Tumor-Host Interaction Lab, The Francis Crick Institute, 1 Midland Rd, London NW1 1AT, UK; ilaria.malanchi@crick.ac.uk
[3] Hematopoietic Stem Cell Laboratory, The Francis Crick Institute, 1 Midland Road, London NW1 1AT, UK; aabarrategi@cicbiomagune.es (A.A.); dominique.bonnet@crick.ac.uk (D.B.)
[4] Regenerative Medicine Lab, CICbiomaGUNE, Paseo Miramón 182, 20014 Donostia, Spain
[5] Ikerbasque, Basque Foundation of Science, Maria Diaz de Haro 3, 48013 Bilbao, Spain
[6] Anatomia Patologica, Azienda Unità Sanitaria Locale–IRCCS di Reggio Emilia, Viale Risorgimento 80, 42123 Reggio Emilia, Italy; moira.ragazzi@ausl.re.it
[7] Dipartimento di Farmacia e Biotecnologie, Università di Bologna, Via Selmi 3, 40126 Bologna, Italy; iommarini.luisa@gmail.com (L.I.); annamaria.porcelli@unibo.it (A.M.P.)
[8] In Vivo Imaging Operations, The Francis Crick Institute, 1 Midland Road, London NW1 1AT, UK; thomas.snoeks@crick.ac.uk
[9] Centro Interdipartimentale di Ricerca Industriale Scienze della Vita e Tecnologie per la Salute, Università di Bologna, Via Tolara di Sopra 41/E, 40064 Ozzano dell'Emilia, Italy
[10] Centro di Ricerca Biomedica Applicata (CRBA), Università di Bologna, Via Massarenti 9, 40138 Bologna, Italy
\* Correspondence: ivana.kurelac@unibo.it
† Co-last authors.

Received: 9 November 2019; Accepted: 9 December 2019; Published: 11 December 2019

**Abstract:** A cogent issue in cancer research is how to account for the effects of tumor microenvironment (TME) on the response to therapy, warranting the need to adopt adequate in vitro and in vivo models. This is particularly relevant in the development of strategies targeting cancer metabolism, as they will inevitably have systemic effects. For example, inhibition of mitochondrial complex I (CI), despite showing promising results as an anticancer approach, triggers TME-mediated survival mechanisms in subcutaneous osteosarcoma xenografts, a response that may vary according to whether the tumors are induced via subcutaneous injection or by intrabone orthotopic transplantation. Thus, with the aim to characterize the TME of CI-deficient tumors in a model that more faithfully represents osteosarcoma development, we set up a humanized bone niche ectopic graft. A prominent involvement of TME was revealed in CI-deficient tumors, characterized by the abundance of cancer associated fibroblasts, tumor associated macrophages and preservation of osteocytes and osteoblasts in the mineralized bone matrix. The pseudo-orthotopic approach allowed investigation of osteosarcoma progression in a bone-like microenvironment setting, without being invasive as the intrabone cell transplantation. Additionally, establishing osteosarcomas in a humanized bone niche model identified a peculiar association between targeting CI and bone tissue preservation.

**Keywords:** mitochondrial complex I; osteosarcoma; orthotopic models; tumor microenvironment

## 1. Introduction

Developing treatments that target cancer metabolic reprogramming is gaining momentum, but it is often neglected that these approaches are not specific only to proliferating cancer cells. Metabolic therapies inevitably exert a systemic effect, influencing also the non-neoplastic cells, including tumor microenvironment (TME), which in turn may completely redirect the final outcome of the disease. Indeed, emerging literature warns that cancer cell metabolism may have crucial consequences on the phenotype of different non-malignant cell types within the tumor [1]. For example, tumor cells may engage in metabolic strategies such as nutrient competition to avoid immune cytotoxicity [2]. On the other hand, targeting cancer metabolic reprogramming may trigger compensatory responses leading to TME-related resistance mechanisms [3]. Thus, strategies directed against cancer metabolism need to be tested in models that allow a proper assessment of the TME effect on tumor progression.

The bone microenvironment has recently been recognized as essential in determining the fate of osteosarcoma development [4,5], even to the extent that targeting TME has been suggested as an efficient strategy to fight the disease [6,7]. In this context, it is interesting to note that studies evaluating the efficacy of antimetabolic therapies in osteosarcoma, such as those against mitochondrial complex I (CI), suggest the TME may play a role in defining the response to treatment [3,8,9]. In line with these findings, we have recently reported that targeting CI arrests progression of osteosarcomas, converting them into low-proliferative, oncocytoma-like lesions, and demonstrated that the loss of hypoxia inducible factor 1-alpha (HIF-1α) is accountable for the antitumorigenic effects of CI dysfunction [3]. However, the latter was associated with an abundance of tumor associated macrophages (TAMs), whose depletion improved the anti-cancer efficacy of metformin, a known CI inhibitor [3]. Thus, even though targeting CI is being recognized as a valid anti-cancer strategy associated with various antitumorigenic effects [10–15], at the same time CI inhibitors seem to elicit conflicting consequences on TME which alter the therapy response [16].

In murine xenografts, TME is usually taken into account by an orthotopic implant, which consents cancer cell proliferation within the native environment. For some tumor types, this approach is relatively simple, as in the case of injecting breast cancer cells in the mouse mammary fat-pad [17], or in hepatocellular carcinoma setting, where orthotopic tumor models involve a minor surgery [18]. The establishment of in situ osteosarcomas is particularly challenging, as the surgical procedures to reach the tibia or femur are invasive, and the injection is difficult due to bone stiffness, requiring drilling bone plateau and potentially resulting in the leakage of cancer cells [19,20]. Engineering approaches today may be used to create ectopic grafts resembling bone tissue environment [5], allowing not only tumor progression in the native tissue, but also generation of human TME, which is important in the setting where human cancer cells are being investigated [21]. Such approaches are becoming crucial for appropriate investigation of osteosarcoma development, since the bone tumor fate was shown to be influenced by the inoculation environment [5].

Here we take advantage of new methods to humanize and modulate ectopic osteosarcoma graft, with the aim to understand whether CI-deficiency induces changes in bone specific non-neoplastic cells during cancer progression. This pseudo-orthotopic approach established that abundance of cancer associated fibroblasts (CAFs) and TAMs is a hallmark of CI-deficient TME, and identified a peculiar association between targeting CI and osteocyte/osteoblast preservation.

## 2. Materials and Methods

### 2.1. Cell Lines

Osteosarcoma 143B Tk$^-$ cells were purchased (#CRL-8303, ATCC, LGS Standards, Milan, Italy) and cultured at low passages (<50) in in Dulbecco's modified Eagle medium (DMEM) High Glucose (#ECM0749L, Euroclone, Milan, Italy), supplemented with 10% FBS (#ECS0180L, Euroclone), L-glutamine (2 mM, #ECB3000D, Euroclone), penicillin/streptomycin (1x, #ECB3001D, Euroclone) and uridine (50 µg/mL, #U3003, Sigma-Aldrich, Milan, Italy), in an incubator with a humidified atmosphere at 5% $CO_2$ and 37 °C. The cell origin was authenticated using AMPFISTRIdentifiler kit (#4322288, Applied Biosystems, Monza, Italy) and their STR profile corresponded to their putative background. Genome editing for generation of NDUFS3 knock-out was performed using zinc finger endonucleases purchased from Sigma-Aldrich (#CKOZFND15168, Milan, Italy), according to the manufacturer's instructions.

Primary human mesenchymal stroma cells (hMSCs) were purchased (#PT-2501, Lonza, Slough, UK) and grown in alpha Minimun Essential Medium (αMEM) (#32571-028, Gibco, Paisley, UK), hMSC-specific FBS (10%) (#12662-029, Gibco, Paisley, UK), penicillin/streptomycin (1x, #ECB3001D, Euroclone), and used at low passages (<5).

### 2.2. Establishing Pseudo-Orthotopic Osteosarcomas

Most steps were performed as previously described [22–24]. All pre-surgical procedures were performed in sterile conditions. Gelfoam gelatin sponges (2 cm × 6 cm × 7 mm) (Pfizer, Kalamazoo, MI, USA) were sectioned into 24 pieces, washed with ethanol 70%, rehydrated in sterile PBS and placed in a 24-well plate. hMSC cells ($5 \times 10^5$ in 50 µl) were injected with a syringe (29G) and left to attach for 4 hours in a 37 °C incubator. Culture media was added and the cells were left to grow for 7 days. On day 8 osteosarcoma cells ($10^5$ in 30 µl) were injected into the scaffolds and left to attach before adding fresh culture media. On day 9 the scaffolds were clothed following previously described protocol [22]. Each scaffold was allocated in a 15 mL tube and 8 µL of bone morphogenic protein 2 (BMP-2) (Noricum, Tres Cantos, Spain) (reconstituted in acetic acid 50 mM at 5 µg/µL) were added. Then, 30 µL of thrombin from human plasma (Sigma, Dorset, UK) (reconstituted in 2% $CaCl_2$ at 20 U/mL) and 20 µL of fibrinogen from human plasma (Sigma) (PBS reconstituted at 4 mg/100 mL) were incorporated. Solidification was allowed during 30 min in cell culture conditions before proceeding with in vivo implantation.

Surgery was performed in aseptic conditions. Five to six-week old female $Rag1^{-/-}$ FVB/n mice available at The Francis Crick Institute Biological Research Facility (London, UK) were used. The animals were treated according to institutional guidelines and regulations and experiments performed in accordance with UK Home Office regulations under project license PPL number P83B37B3C. A bilateral implantation was performed. In detail, 2 hours before surgical procedure caprofren (Rimadyl, Zoetis, Leatherhead, UK) anti-inflammatory and pain-killer drug was administrated to each animal, both subcutaneously and in the drinking water. Anesthesia was induced with 2.5% isoflurane and O2 at 2–4%. A wide section of fur from the back was shaved. Then skin was sterilized twice with surgiscrub. For each scaffold implantation, 0.5 cm vertical incision was made 1 cm away from the spine on each side of the animal. With forceps, a pocket under the skin was made in the incision, down the side of the animal. A scaffold was inserted, making sure it was placed deep within the pocket, and then incisions were dried and glued (3M surgical glue, Vetbond, St Paul, MN, USA). Buprenorphine (Vetergesic, Alstoe, York, UK) post-operative analgesia was administered subcutaneously. Animals were placed in a pre-warmed cage and left to recover. After surgery, animals were checked frequently for their well-being. Rimadyl in the drinking water was removed 48 hours after surgery. Mice were sacrificed either at 30 or at 60 days post implantation.

### 2.3. Micro Computed Tomography Imaging

Samples were scanned using a SkyScan-1176 µCT scanner (Bruker MicroCT, Kontich, Belgium). The X-ray source was operated at 40 kV and 600 µA, no filter was used. The scans were made over a trajectory of 180° with a 0.5° step size with a 8.57µm pixel size. The images were reconstructed using nRecon (Bruker MicroCT, Kontich, Belgium) and further analysed using CTan (Bruker MicroCT).

### 2.4. Histology

Tumor tissue was processed following standard immunohistochemistry protocols. Before embedding, the samples were decalcified with 17% EDTA (Osteosoft, #101728, Merck Millipore,

Watford, UK) for 7 days. Hematoxylin/eosin coloration was performed following standard protocol and collagen fibers staining with the Masson's Trichrome Stain Kit (#25088, Polysciences, Hirschberg an der Bergstrasse, Germany). The following primary antibodies were used: mouse monoclonal anti-HIF-1$\alpha$ (1:100, #610959, BD Biosciences, Berkshire, UK); mouse monoclonal anti-KI-67 (1:100, #M7240, Dako, Agilent, Cernusco sul Naviglio, Italy); rat anti-endomucin (1:200, #SC-65495, Santa Cruz, DBA, Segrate, Italy); mouse anti-SMA (1:750, #M0851, Dako) and rat monoclonal F4/80 (1:100, #14-4801, eBiosciences, ThermoFisher, Life Technologies, Monza, Italy). For evaluation of KI-67 positive nuclei, only cancer cells were counted at 60× magnification in one hot spot area per tumor, avoiding stromal infiltrations and necrotic tissue. Macrophages (F4/80+) were counted at of 20× magnification in three fields of view (FOV) per tumor. The macrophages located close to trabecular bone were counted by considering F4/80 positive cells touching the bone matrix. The macrophages infiltrating the tumor tissue were counted by avoiding tumor front, trabecular bone and necrotic tissue. Osteocytes and osteoblasts were counted in three consecutive FOV at 60× magnification, in proximity to the trabecular bone, starting from the hot spot area.

Immunofluorescent staining included 15 min citrate antigen retrieval (10 mM sodium citrate, pH = 6) at 95 °C, 10 min blocking with goat serum (#156046, Abcam, Cambridge, UK) at RT, 1 hour incubation with primary antibodies at RT (rat anti-endomucin (1:200, #SC-65495, Santa Cruz) and mouse anti-SMA (1:750, #M0851, Dako), 40 min incubation with Alexa Fluor (ThermoFisher, Life Technologies, Monza, Italy) secondary antibodies at RT (488-goat anti-mouse diluted 1:500 and 555-goat anti-rat diluted 1:350) and mounting with Vectashield Antifade Mounting Medium containing DAPI (#H-1200, Vector Laboratories, Peterborough, UK). Vessel size was evaluated by measuring the longer diameter of 20 endomucin positive cells per tumor and avoiding areas of collective fibroblast infiltration. Immature vessels (Endo+SMA−) were counted in five FOV at 20× magnification per tumor.

### 2.5. Flow Cytometry

Xenograft samples (approximately 50 mm$^3$) were digested immediately after the sacrifice for 40 minutes at 37 °C with Liberase TL (#5401020001, Sigma), Liberase TM (#5401135001, Sigma) and DNaseI (#DN25, Sigma) in HBSS and passed through a 100 μm strainer. Hypotonic lysis with Red Blood Cell Lysis Buffer (#11814389001, Sigma) was performed and remaining cells were washed with MACS buffer (2 mM EDTA, 0.5% BSA in PBS), blocked using FcR Blocking Reagent (#130-092-575, Miltenyi, Surrey, UK) and incubated with panels of pre-labelled antibodies. In parallel, spleen, lung and a control tumor tissue were digested together and stained for Fluorescence Minus One (FMO) reading which was considered while setting the gating strategy. The following panels were used: Panel 1 (for analysis of the tumor macrophage, neutrophil and dendritic cell contribution): anti anti-CD45-APC (clone 30-F11, #17-0451-82, eBioscience), anti-CD11b-ef450 (clone M1/70, #48-0112-82, eBioscience), anti-F4/80-FITC (clone BM8, #123108, BioLegend, London, UK), anti-Ly6G-APC780 (clone RB6-8C5, #47-5931-80, eBioscience), anti-CD11c-PE (clone n418, #12-0114-81, eBioscience); Panel 3 (for analysis of M1/M2 protumorigenic macrophages): anti-CD45-APC780 (clone 30-F11, #47-0451-80, eBioscience), anti-F4/80-ef450 (clone BM8, #48-4801-82, eBioscience), anti-CD206-APC (clone C068C2, #141707, BioLegend). All antibodies were used at 1:100 dilution, apart from the anti-CD45 which was diluted 1:300. Between 300,000-500,000 cells were stained. Dead cells were stained with DAPI and gated out for analyses. Absolute cell abundance was defined as their percentage among all live cells (%Live). Relative cell abundance was defined as their percentage among populations indicated in the figure panels. The samples were run on LSRFortessa cell analyzer (BD Biosciences) and data was analyzed by BD FACSDIVA Software (BD Bioscience) and Flow Jo (Tree Star Inc., Ashland, OR, USA) software.

### 2.6. Cytokine Profiling

Xenograft-derived cell cultures were generated by a 10-day cultivation of liberase-digested tissue in basal conditions. Supernatant (0.5 mL) was taken 2 days after medium renewal from a 500,000 cells cultured and analyzed with human Proteome Profiler Array kit (ARY005B, R&D Systems, Abingdon, UK) following manufacturer's instructions. ImageJ was used for quantification of the dot blots.

## 2.7. Statistical Analyses

GraphPad Prism version 7 (GraphPad Software Inc., San Diego, CA, USA) was used to perform statistical tests and create bar plots and graphs. Unless stated otherwise, a two-tailed unpaired Student's t-tests assuming equal variance were performed to compare averages. For each experiment, p-values (* $p < 0.05$, ** $p < 0.01$, *** $p < 0.001$) are indicated in the graphs.

## 3. Results

### 3.1. A Humanized Bone Niche Scaffold Recapitulates Mature Bone Characteristics and Serves as a Pseudo-Orthotopic Osteosarcoma Xenograft Model

A humanized bone-forming ectopic xenotransplantation model was set up by using hMSCs treated with BMP-2, and applied as pseudo-orthotopic approach to grow CI-competent (143B$^{+/+}$) and CI-deficient (143B$^{-/-}$) osteosarcoma cells in vivo (Figure 1a).

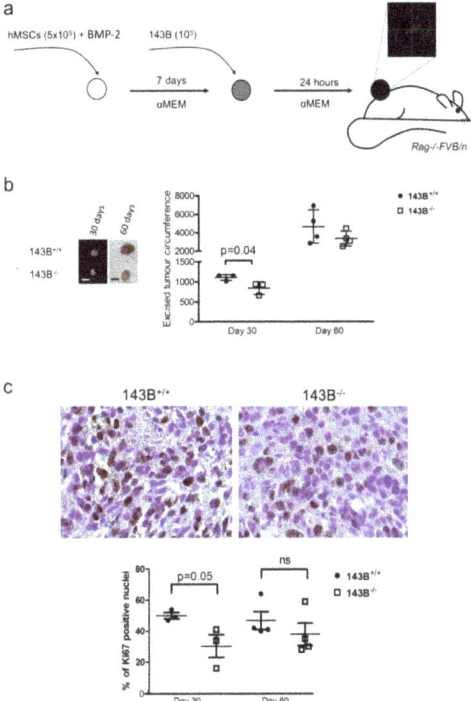

**Figure 1.** Osteosarcoma progression in the humanized bone niche model. (**a**) Experimental setting: mesenchymal stroma cells (hMSC) and osteosarcoma cells (143B) were seeded in gelfoam scaffolds (circles), treated with bone morphogenic protein (BMP-2), cultured with alpha Minimum Essential Medium (αMEM) and implanted in immunodeficient *Rag−/−/FVB/n* mice. A micro CT scan of control sample (hMSC+BMP-2) is displayed. (**b**) Xenograft size of the CI-competent (143B$^{+/+}$) and CI-deficient (143B$^{-/-}$) cells. Representative tumors are shown. Bars = 1 cm. One-tailed T-test was used to calculate statistical significance. (**c**) Quantification of Ki-67 positive nuclei. Representative images are shown for Ki-67 staining in xenografts excised at day 30. Magnification 60×. One-tailed T-test was used to calculate statistical significance.

Targeting CI reduced tumorigenic potential of 143B cells at day 30, but this antitumorigenic effect was less appreciated by day 60, when tumor size and Ki-67 proliferation index were similar between the two groups (Figure 1b,c).

Morphologically, the control sample, in which no tumor cells were injected, displayed mature spongy bone consisting of osseous trabeculae surrounded by adipose cells, blood vessels and leukocyte infiltration encompassing polymorphonuclear neutrophils (Figure 2a,b). Furthermore, lamellar bone matrix contained lacunae with typical bone-specific cell populations such as osteocytes and a thin layer of osteoblasts lined bony spicules (Figure 2b). Of note, this model allows effective humanized bone microenvironment formation [23,24].

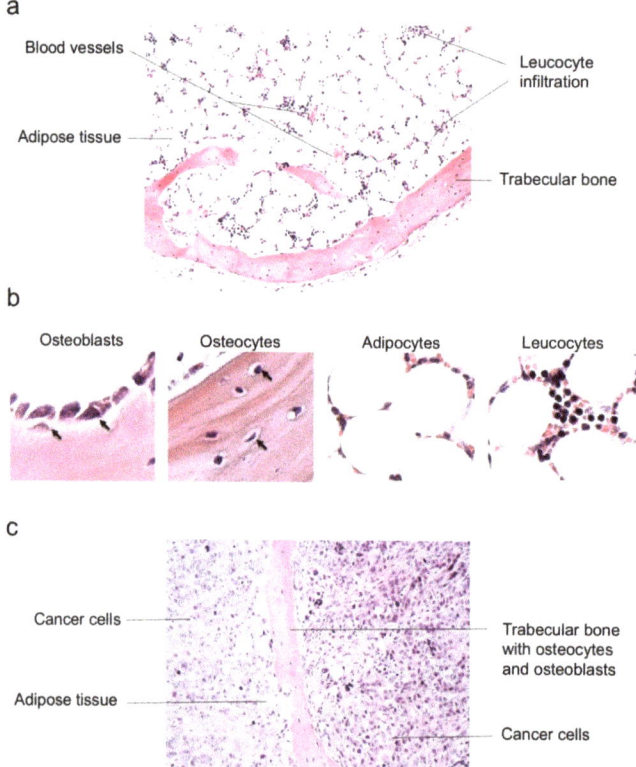

**Figure 2.** The humanized bone niche model allows investigation of bone-specific cell populations within a growing tumor. (**a**) Hematoxylin and eosin staining showing morphology within the humanized bone niche control sample. Magnification 10×. (**b**) Hematoxylin and eosin staining of the humanized bone niche control sample reveals columnar or flatter osteoblasts covering the bone surface while spindle-shaped and regular osteocytes are embedded in the mineralized bone matrix. Leukocyte infiltration encompassing some granulocytes is observed between adipocytes. Magnification 40×. (**c**) A representative image of hematoxylin and eosin stained CI-deficient osteosarcoma xenograft in which bone specific cell types may be recognized. Magnification 20×.

The masses deriving from scaffolds seeded with 143B cells displayed trabecular bone containing osteocytes and osteoblasts, as well as occasional adipose tissue areas, but were primarily occupied by neoplastic cells, indicating their high degree of aggressiveness (Figure 2c). Micro computed tomography (Micro CT) imaging identified calcified areas in the xenografts similar to native bone parenchyma, indicating the formation of a bone-like tissue (Figure S1). These observations confirmed the establishment of a mature bone tissue in which human osteosarcoma cells may progress within a bone-like microenvironment setting.

### 3.2. Tumor Associated Macrophages are the Main Hallmark of the CI-Deficient Osteosarcoma Microenvironment

With the aim to unravel the potential contribution of TME associated to CI-deficient osteosarcoma, we first carried out a detailed analysis of immune cells within the xenografts. A higher neutrophil count was detected in the control tumors, whereas TAMs were more abundant in CI-deficient masses (Figure 3a,b, Figure S2). No difference in TAM polarization from inflammatory M1 towards protumorigenic M2 population was observed, but the general contribution of M2 macrophages in the mass was higher in tumors lacking CI (Figure 3c). Interestingly, immunohistochemistry revealed TAMs were mainly located on the tumor front in the control masses, whereas in CI-deficient osteosarcomas they were also infiltrating the tumor mass and were often located in the proximity to the trabecular bone (Figure 3d).

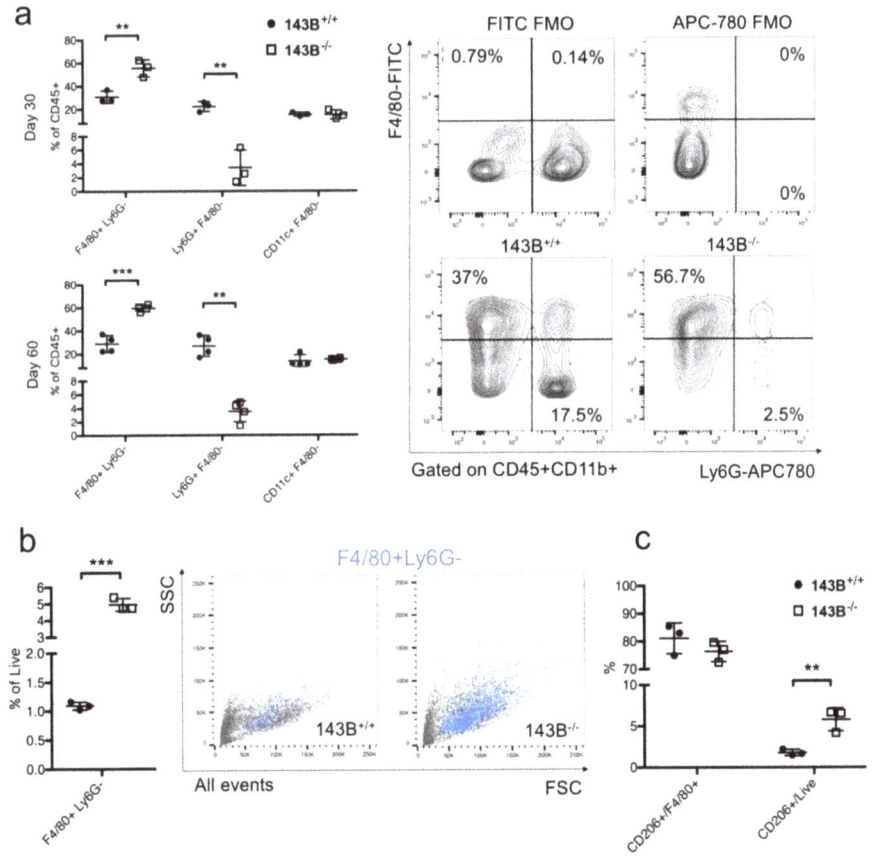

**Figure 3.** *Cont.*

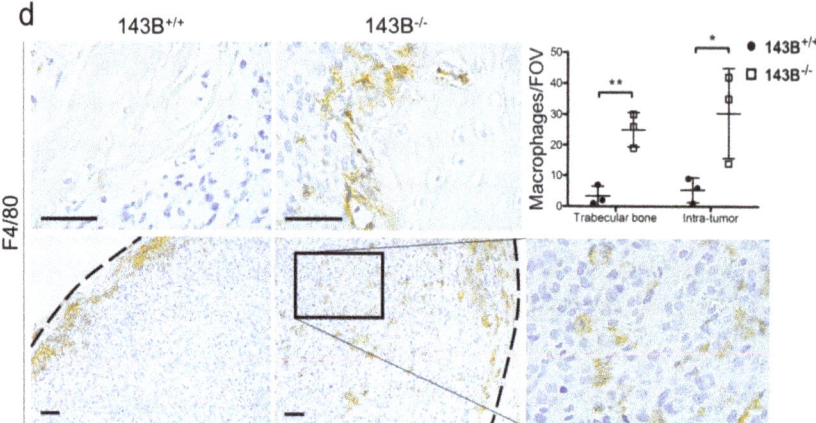

**Figure 3.** Tumor associated macrophages are a hallmark of CI-deficient osteosarcoma xenografts. (**a**) Flow cytometry analysis of innate immune system populations in 143B xenografts at day 30 ($n = 3$) and day 60 ($n = 4$) post-implantation. The contribution of macrophages (F4/80+Ly6G-), neutrophils (Lys6G+F4/80-) and dendritic cells (CD11c+F4/80-) is shown. Single values are displayed, with the error bars representing standard error of the mean. Representative contour plots with outliers are shown for evaluation of macrophage and neutrophil numbers. FMO: Fluorescence Minus One (**b**) The contribution of macrophages in 143B$^{+/+}$ (black circles) and 143B$^{-/-}$ (white squares) tumors at day 30 as evaluated by flow cytometry. Single values are displayed, with the error bars representing standard error of the mean. Representative dot-plots display contribution of macrophages (blue, F4/80+Ly6G-) among 100,000 acquired events. SSC: Side SCatter; FSC: Forward SCatter (**c**) The relative and absolute contribution of CD206+ macrophages in osteosarcoma tumors at day 30. Single values are displayed, with the error bars representing standard error of the mean. (**d**) Representative images of immunohistochemistry analysis for macrophage marker F4/80 in osteosarcoma xenografts at day 30. Scale bars: 50 µm. Dashed line indicates tumor front. The numbers of macrophages located close to trabecular bone (images in the upper panels) and infiltrating the tissue (images in the lower panels) are graphed. Single values are displayed, with the error bars representing standard error of the mean. FOV: Field of View. In each graph, statistical significance is specified with asterisks (* $p < 0.05$, ** $p < 0.01$, *** $p < 0.001$).

We next sought to understand which factors are contributing to the difference in macrophage abundance. Xenograft tissue-derived supernatants were blotted on a human cytokine array and macrophage migration inhibitory factor (MIF) was found downregulated in CI-deficient tumor-derived secretome (Figure 4a). MIF is a HIF1-responsive gene, whose downregulation has been associated with triggering a TAM-mediated alternative proangiogenic activity as a compensatory response upon anti-VEGF treatment [25].

Thus, we analyzed HIF-1α levels and localization in the xenografts, as well as their vascular architecture, since myeloid-derived proangiogenic signals have been associated with small vessels which lack pericyte marker smooth muscle actin (SMA) [26]. Whereas the control tumors expressed HIF-1α in their cancer cell nuclei, 143B$^{-/-}$ masses were characterized by a complete absence of HIF-1α staining (Figure 4b), in line with MIF downregulation. Interestingly, the lack of HIF-1α in CI-deficient tumors was associated with a higher total number of vessels, but these were significantly smaller than the ones found in controls, and were mostly lacking lumen and pericyte coating (Figure 4c), a phenotype analogue to the abnormalized vasculature typical of myeloid-derived proangiogenic signals [26].

Overall, these data identify protumorigenic macrophages as the most abundant TME component in 143B$^{-/-}$ xenografts and suggest their recruitment may be a consequence of MIF downregulation.

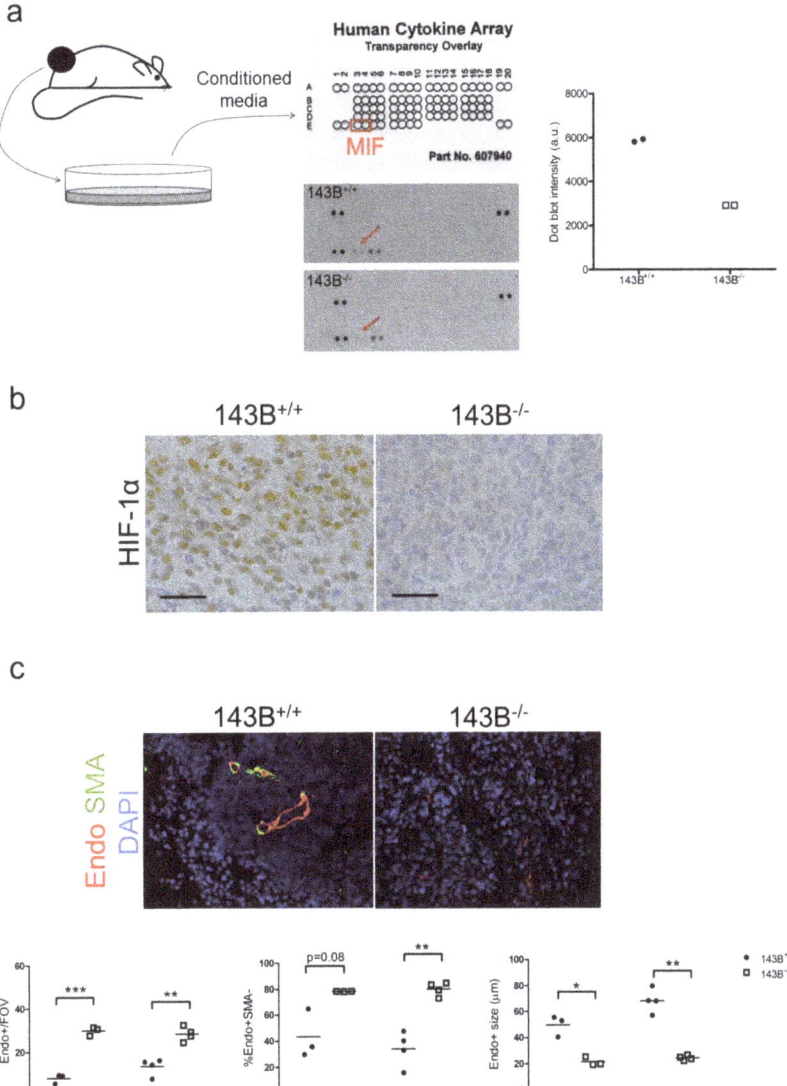

**Figure 4.** The HIF1-MIF axis is inactive in CI-deficient xenografts. (**a**) Experimental setting and results of the cytokine screening in xenograft-derived cell culture supernatants. The arrows indicate the cytokine array dot blots for MIF. Dot blot pixel intensity for MIF is graphed. (**b**) Representative images of immunohistochemistry staining for HIF-1α in osteosarcoma xenografts. Scale bars: 50 μm. (**c**) Representative images of immunofluorescent staining analyzing vessel morphology in osteosarcoma xenografts. Endo – Endomucin. Endothelial cells (Endo+), pericytes (SMA+Endo+), CAF (SMA+Endo-), nuclei (DAPI). Magnification 20×. Graphs show total number of vessels per field of view (FOV), percentage of pericyte negative vessels (%Endo+SMA−) and the average vessel size in CI-competent and CI-deficient 143B tumors. In each graph, statistical significance is specified with asterisks (* $p < 0.05$, ** $p < 0.01$, *** $p < 0.001$).

### 3.3. Osteocytes and Osteoblasts within Trabecular Bone are Preserved in the CI-Deficient Pseudo-Orthotopic Osteosarcoma Xenografts

To characterize the bone-specific TME during osteosarcoma progression, we next analyzed histology of mesenchymal cell populations in the humanized bone xenografts. A prominent involvement of the stromal cells was evident in the intra-tumoral septae specifically in CI-deficient tumors, as supported by the Masson's trichrome collagen staining and CAF marker SMA immunohistochemistry (Figure 5a,b). Despite the trabecular bone and osteoid matrix were noticeable in both groups, control xenografts were characterized by intensive necrosis which appears as tissue areas replaced by granulocytes and cellular debris with loss of nuclei. Moreover, at 60 days post implantation, osteonecrosis was evident in controls, characterized by loss of osteocytes with empty osteocytic lacunae in the mineralized bone matrix (Figure 5c). On the other hand, no necrotic tissue was observed in 143B$^{-/-}$ tumors, which displayed higher number of osteocytes and osteoblasts in the trabecular bone when compared to the controls (Figure 5c). Moreover, consistently with histology, micro CT scans of CI-deficient tumors showed higher mean intensity of the calcified volume (Figure 5d), indicating this condition is associated with lower osteolytic activity and preservation of the bone microenvironment.

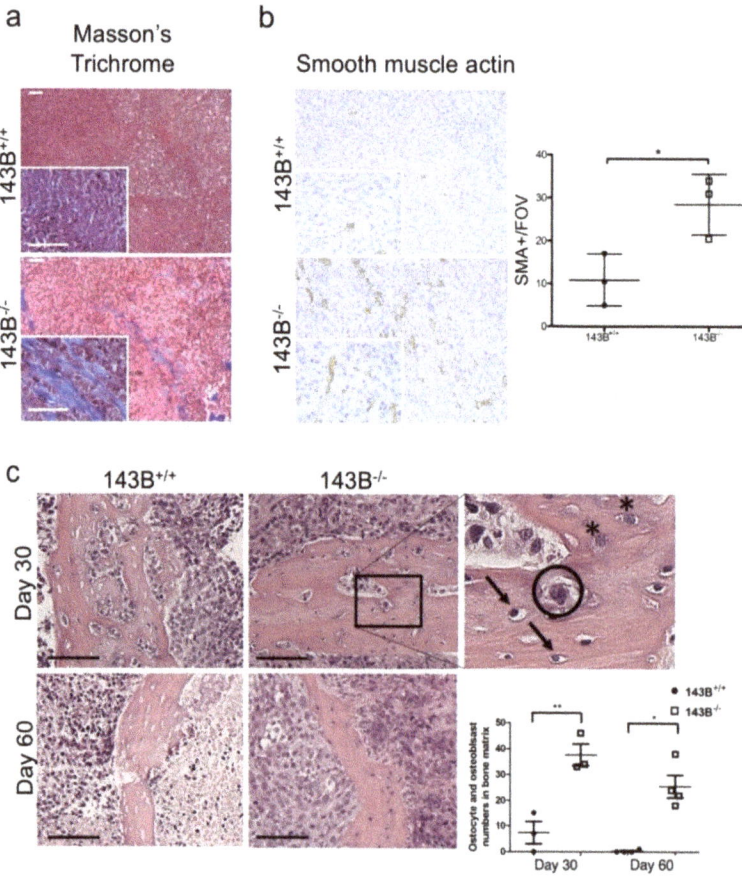

Figure 5. Cont.

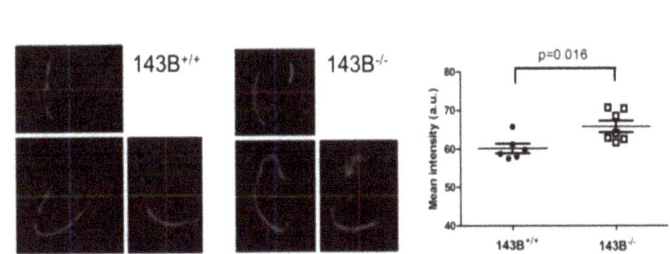

**Figure 5.** CI-deficient osteosarcomas are associated with preservation of the bone microenvironment. (**a**) Representative images of Masson's trichrome staining of the osteosarcoma xenografts. Collagen is stained in blue. Scale bars: 100 μm. (**b**) Smooth muscle actin (SMA) immunohistochemistry staining and count of SMA positive cells at 30 days post implantation in CI-competent ($143B^{+/+}$) and -deficient ($143B^{-/-}$) tumors. Magnification 20×, inserts 60×. (**c**) Representative images of hematoxylin and eosin staining of the trabecular bone in the osteosarcoma xenografts at day 30 and day 60 post implantation. The arrows indicate osteocytes, the asterisks osteoblasts, whereas the neoplastic cells are circled. Scale bars: 100 μm. The graph represents the quantification of osteocytes and osteoblasts in the osteosarcoma xenografts. (**d**) Representative micro CT scan images from CI-competent and deficient osteosarcoma tumors. Mean intensity of the calcified volume in the tumors is graphed. In each graph, statistical significance is specified with asterisks (* $p < 0.05$, ** $p < 0.01$).

## 4. Discussion

In this study, we show that by using a humanized niche model of the osteosarcoma graft, an additional level of information about the tumor histology is achieved with respect to canonical subcutaneous implant. The peculiar bone microenvironment preservation in CI-deficient tumors highlights that parenchymal cells are an important component of TME, warning they should not be neglected when investigating cancer progression. Indeed, functionally relevant cancer associated parenchyma has recently been described also in the setting of breast cancer metastases [27].

The differences regarding bone specific cell types appreciated depending on the condition tested, allow to hypothesize that osteocytes and osteoblasts may influence the response to therapies designed against CI. Targeting CI in osteosarcomas grown in the humanized bone reduced tumorigenic potential of 143B cells, albeit not as strikingly as observed in our previously described experimental settings [3,14,15]. Among other, these milder consequences may be due to the osteocyte/osteoclast-specific functions. Their preservation was particularly associated with the later stages of tumor progression, at which the antitumorigenic effect of targeting CI was less appreciated, suggesting that bone-specific non-neoplastic cells may be involved in promoting osteosarcoma survival. The possible mechanisms of growth support may be relative to essential metabolites exchange between cancer and TME cells, as previously suggested [28,29]. On the other hand, TME may sustain cancer cell proliferation by promoting angiogenesis. In this context, CI deficiency was also associated with the abundance of TAMs, that have been called into play to provide angiogenic factors when cancer cell-autonomous HIF1 signals are absent [25,26]. Indeed, the observation of TAM abundance and vasculature typical of myeloid cell proangiogenic activity in the context of the orthotopic CI-deficient xenografts corroborates our previous findings [3], suggesting that targeting CI in 143B osteosarcoma prevents HIF1-MIF activation, leading to TAM accumulation and vascular architecture remodeling.

Further investigation is required to understand the significance of these data, by using larger animal cohorts and CI inhibitors, rather than the genetic disruption of the complex, since a drug will inevitably act on TME cell populations as well [16]. Moreover, adaptive immunity should be taken into consideration by using immunocompetent models. In this context, it is important to note that a murine bone niche could be easily generated by populating the scaffold with murine MSCs. Interestingly, a study evaluating the effects of CI inhibitor metformin in immunocompetent settings reported reduced number of myeloid derived suppressor cells and TAMs in osteosarcomas [9]. The authors worked with intra-dermal grafts, therefore it would be of interest to understand what is the effect of CI inhibition on bone specific TME cells, such as osteocytes and osteoclasts. This would be particularly important since, in the bone tumor context, the fate of cancer cells in vivo depends on the type of graft that is being used as a model. For example, subcutaneous injection of transformed bone marrow mesenchymal cells is associated to development of leiomysarcoma-like tumors, while the intrabone transplantation of the same cells induced metastatic osteoblastic osteosarcoma, underlining the importance of signals elicited by the bone TME [5].

Taken together, preservation of osteocytes and osteoblasts observed upon targeting CI points to the importance of setting up appropriate tumor models, which take into consideration the origin of the cancer in question, since apart from immune cell populations, the parenchymal cells of the TME may also influence neoplastic development.

**Supplementary Materials:** The following are available online at http://www.mdpi.com/2077-0383/8/12/2184/s1, Figure S1: Micro CT scans of the mouse body sections selecting (a) soft tissue, (b) bone tissue and (c) humanized bone niche control sample, Figure S2. Gating strategies for flow cytometry analyses of (a) innate immune system cell populations and (b) CD206+ macrophages.

**Author Contributions:** Conceptualization, I.K., I.M. and G.G.; Methodology, I.K., A.A., M.R., L.I., N.U.G., T.S.; Formal Analysis, I.K., M.R., L.I., N.U.G., T.S.; Investigation, I.K., A.A., M.R., L.I., T.S.; Resources, D.B., I.M., G.G.; Data Curation, I.K., M.R., L.I., T.S.; Writing—Original Draft Preparation, I.K.; Writing—Review & Editing, A.A., A.M.P., I.M., G.G.; Visualization, I.K.; Supervision, D.B., I.M. and G.G.; Project Administration, I.K.; Funding Acquisition, I.M., A.M.P. and G.G.

**Acknowledgments:** This work was supported by EU H2020 Marie Curie project TRANSMIT GA 722605 to A.M.P. and G.G.; by Associazione Italiana Ricerca sul Cancro (AIRC) grant JANEUTICS-IG14242 and Italian Ministry of Health grant DISCO TRIP GR-2013-02356666 to G.G; and by The Francis Crick Institute which receives its core funding from Cancer Research UK (FC001112), the UK Medical Research Council (FC001112), and the Wellcome Trust (FC001112). We thank Laurie J. Gay and Flow cytometry unit from The Francis Crick Institute (UK) for technical help.

**Conflicts of Interest:** The authors declare no conflict of interest.

## References

1. Schulze, A.; Yuneva, M. The big picture: Exploring the metabolic cross-talk in cancer. *Dis. Model. Mech.* **2018**, *11*. [CrossRef] [PubMed]
2. Chang, C.-H.; Qiu, J.; O'Sullivan, D.; Buck, M.D.; Noguchi, T.; Curtis, J.D.; Chen, Q.; Gindin, M.; Gubin, M.M.; van der Windt, G.J.W.; et al. Metabolic Competition in the Tumor Microenvironment Is a Driver of Cancer Progression. *Cell* **2015**, *162*, 1229–1241. [CrossRef] [PubMed]
3. Kurelac, I.; Iommarini, L.; Vatrinet, R.; Amato, L.B.; De Luise, M.; Leone, G.; Girolimetti, G.; Umesh Ganesh, N.; Bridgeman, V.L.; Ombrato, L.; et al. Inducing cancer indolence by targeting mitochondrial Complex I is potentiated by blocking macrophage-mediated adaptive responses. *Nat. Commun.* **2019**, *10*, 903. [CrossRef] [PubMed]
4. Alfranca, A.; Martinez-Cruzado, L.; Tornin, J.; Abarrategi, A.; Amaral, T.; de Alava, E.; Menendez, P.; Garcia-Castro, J.; Rodriguez, R. Bone microenvironment signals in osteosarcoma development. *Cell. Mol. Life Sci. CMLS* **2015**, *72*, 3097–3113. [CrossRef] [PubMed]
5. Rubio, R.; Abarrategi, A.; Garcia-Castro, J.; Martinez-Cruzado, L.; Suarez, C.; Tornin, J.; Santos, L.; Astudillo, A.; Colmenero, I.; Mulero, F.; et al. Bone environment is essential for osteosarcoma development from transformed mesenchymal stem cells. *Stem Cells Dayt. Ohio* **2014**, *32*, 1136–1148. [CrossRef] [PubMed]
6. Baglio, S.R.; Lagerweij, T.; Pérez-Lanzón, M.; Ho, X.D.; Léveillé, N.; Melo, S.A.; Cleton-Jansen, A.-M.; Jordanova, E.S.; Roncuzzi, L.; Greco, M.; et al. Blocking Tumor-Educated MSC Paracrine Activity Halts Osteosarcoma Progression. *Clin. Cancer Res. Off. J. Am. Assoc. Cancer Res.* **2017**, *23*, 3721–3733. [CrossRef]
7. Verrecchia, F.; Rédini, F. Transforming Growth Factor-β Signaling Plays a Pivotal Role in the Interplay Between Osteosarcoma Cells and Their Microenvironment. *Front. Oncol.* **2018**, *8*, 133. [CrossRef]
8. Garofalo, C.; Capristo, M.; Manara, M.C.; Mancarella, C.; Landuzzi, L.; Belfiore, A.; Lollini, P.-L.; Picci, P.; Scotlandi, K. Metformin as an adjuvant drug against pediatric sarcomas: Hypoxia limits therapeutic effects of the drug. *PLoS ONE* **2013**, *8*, e83832. [CrossRef]

9. Uehara, T.; Eikawa, S.; Nishida, M.; Kunisada, Y.; Yoshida, A.; Fujiwara, T.; Kunisada, T.; Ozaki, T.; Udono, H. Metformin induces CD11b+-cell-mediated growth inhibition of an osteosarcoma: Implications for metabolic reprogramming of myeloid cells and anti-tumor effects. *Int. Immunol.* **2019**, *31*, 187–198. [CrossRef]
10. Sullivan, L.B.; Luengo, A.; Danai, L.V.; Bush, L.N.; Diehl, F.F.; Hosios, A.M.; Lau, A.N.; Elmiligy, S.; Malstrom, S.; Lewis, C.A.; et al. Aspartate is an endogenous metabolic limitation for tumour growth. *Nat. Cell Biol.* **2018**, *20*, 782–788. [CrossRef]
11. Birsoy, K.; Wang, T.; Chen, W.W.; Freinkman, E.; Abu-Remaileh, M.; Sabatini, D.M. An Essential Role of the Mitochondrial Electron Transport Chain in Cell Proliferation Is to Enable Aspartate Synthesis. *Cell* **2015**, *162*, 540–551. [CrossRef] [PubMed]
12. Griss, T.; Vincent, E.E.; Egnatchik, R.; Chen, J.; Ma, E.H.; Faubert, B.; Viollet, B.; DeBerardinis, R.J.; Jones, R.G. Metformin Antagonizes Cancer Cell Proliferation by Suppressing Mitochondrial-Dependent Biosynthesis. *PLoS Biol.* **2015**, *13*, e1002309. [CrossRef] [PubMed]
13. Zhou, X.; Chen, J.; Yi, G.; Deng, M.; Liu, H.; Liang, M.; Shi, B.; Fu, X.; Chen, Y.; Chen, L.; et al. Metformin suppresses hypoxia-induced stabilization of HIF-1α through reprogramming of oxygen metabolism in hepatocellular carcinoma. *Oncotarget* **2016**, *7*, 873–884.
14. Iommarini, L.; Kurelac, I.; Capristo, M.; Calvaruso, M.A.; Giorgio, V.; Bergamini, C.; Ghelli, A.; Nanni, P.; De Giovanni, C.; Carelli, V.; et al. Different mtDNA mutations modify tumor progression in dependence of the degree of respiratory complex I impairment. *Hum. Mol. Genet.* **2014**, *23*, 1453–1466. [CrossRef] [PubMed]
15. Gasparre, G.; Kurelac, I.; Capristo, M.; Iommarini, L.; Ghelli, A.; Ceccarelli, C.; Nicoletti, G.; Nanni, P.; De Giovanni, C.; Scotlandi, K.; et al. A mutation threshold distinguishes the antitumorigenic effects of the mitochondrial gene MTND1, an oncojanus function. *Cancer Res.* **2011**, *71*, 6220–6229. [CrossRef]
16. Kurelac, I.; Umesh Ganesh, N.; Iorio, M.; Porcelli, A.M.; Gasparre, G. The multifaceted effects of metformin on tumor microenvironment. *Semin. Cell Dev. Biol.* **2019**. [CrossRef]
17. Kocatürk, B.; Versteeg, H.H. Orthotopic injection of breast cancer cells into the mammary fat pad of mice to study tumor growth. *J. Vis. Exp. JoVE* **2015**, *96*, e51967. [CrossRef]
18. Reiberger, T.; Chen, Y.; Ramjiawan, R.R.; Hato, T.; Fan, C.; Samuel, R.; Roberge, S.; Huang, P.; Lauwers, G.Y.; Zhu, A.X.; et al. An orthotopic mouse model of hepatocellular carcinoma with underlying liver cirrhosis. *Nat. Protoc.* **2015**, *10*, 1264–1274. [CrossRef]
19. Sasaki, H.; Iyer, S.V.; Sasaki, K.; Tawfik, O.W.; Iwakuma, T. An improved intrafemoral injection with minimized leakage as an orthotopic mouse model of osteosarcoma. *Anal. Biochem.* **2015**, *486*, 70–74. [CrossRef]
20. Geller, D.S.; Singh, M.Y.; Zhang, W.; Gill, J.; Roth, M.E.; Kim, M.Y.; Xie, X.; Singh, C.K.; Dorfman, H.D.; Villanueva-Siles, E.; et al. Development of a Model System to Evaluate Local Recurrence in Osteosarcoma and Assessment of the Effects of Bone Morphogenetic Protein-2. *Clin. Cancer Res. Off. J. Am. Assoc. Cancer Res.* **2015**, *21*, 3003–3012. [CrossRef]
21. Abarrategi, A.; Mian, S.A.; Passaro, D.; Rouault-Pierre, K.; Grey, W.; Bonnet, D. Modeling the human bone marrow niche in mice: From host bone marrow engraftment to bioengineering approaches. *J. Exp. Med.* **2018**, *215*, 729–743. [CrossRef] [PubMed]
22. Abarrategi, A.; Perez-Tavarez, R.; Rodriguez-Milla, M.A.; Cubillo, I.; Mulero, F.; Alfranca, A.; Lopez-Lacomba, J.L.; García-Castro, J. In vivo ectopic implantation model to assess human mesenchymal progenitor cell potential. *Stem Cell Rev. Rep.* **2013**, *9*, 833–846. [CrossRef] [PubMed]
23. Abarrategi, A.; Foster, K.; Hamilton, A.; Mian, S.A.; Passaro, D.; Gribben, J.; Mufti, G.; Bonnet, D. Versatile humanized niche model enables study of normal and malignant human hematopoiesis. *J. Clin. Investig.* **2017**, *127*, 543–548. [CrossRef] [PubMed]
24. Passaro, D.; Abarrategi, A.; Foster, K.; Ariza-McNaughton, L.; Bonnet, D. Bioengineering of Humanized Bone Marrow Microenvironments in Mouse and Their Visualization by Live Imaging. *J. Vis. Exp. JoVE* **2017**, *126*, e55914. [CrossRef]
25. Castro, B.A.; Flanigan, P.; Jahangiri, A.; Hoffman, D.; Chen, W.; Kuang, R.; De Lay, M.; Yagnik, G.; Wagner, J.R.; Mascharak, S.; et al. Macrophage migration inhibitory factor downregulation: A novel mechanism of resistance to anti-angiogenic therapy. *Oncogene* **2017**, *36*, 3749–3759. [CrossRef]
26. De Palma, M.; Biziato, D.; Petrova, T.V. Microenvironmental regulation of tumour angiogenesis. *Nat. Rev. Cancer* **2017**, *17*, 457–474. [CrossRef]

27. Ombrato, L.; Nolan, E.; Kurelac, I.; Mavousian, A.; Bridgeman, V.L.; Heinze, I.; Chakravarty, P.; Horswell, S.; Gonzalez-Gualda, E.; Matacchione, G.; et al. Metastatic-niche labelling reveals parenchymal cells with stem features. *Nature* **2019**, *572*, 603–608. [CrossRef]
28. Pavlides, S.; Whitaker-Menezes, D.; Castello-Cros, R.; Flomenberg, N.; Witkiewicz, A.K.; Frank, P.G.; Casimiro, M.C.; Wang, C.; Fortina, P.; Addya, S.; et al. The reverse Warburg effect: Aerobic glycolysis in cancer associated fibroblasts and the tumor stroma. *Cell Cycle Georget. Tex.* **2009**, *8*, 3984–4001. [CrossRef]
29. Yang, L.; Achreja, A.; Yeung, T.-L.; Mangala, L.S.; Jiang, D.; Han, C.; Baddour, J.; Marini, J.C.; Ni, J.; Nakahara, R.; et al. Targeting Stromal Glutamine Synthetase in Tumors Disrupts Tumor Microenvironment-Regulated Cancer Cell Growth. *Cell Metab.* **2016**, *24*, 685–700. [CrossRef]

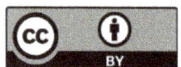 © 2019 by the authors. Licensee MDPI, Basel, Switzerland. This article is an open access article distributed under the terms and conditions of the Creative Commons Attribution (CC BY) license (http://creativecommons.org/licenses/by/4.0/).

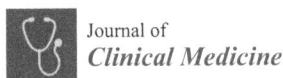 

Article

# FAD/NADH Dependent Oxidoreductases: From Different Amino Acid Sequences to Similar Protein Shapes for Playing an Ancient Function

Lucia Trisolini [†], Nicola Gambacorta [†], Ruggiero Gorgoglione [†], Michele Montaruli, Luna Laera, Francesco Colella, Mariateresa Volpicella, Anna De Grassi * and Ciro Leonardo Pierri *

Laboratory of Biochemistry, Molecular and Structural Biology, Department of Biosciences, Biotechnologies, Biopharmaceutics, University of Bari, Via E. Orabona 4, 70125 Bari, Italy; luciat202@gmail.com (L.T.); nicogamba23@hotmail.it (N.G.); rugorgo@gmail.com (R.G.); michele.montaruli@gmail.com (M.M.); laeraluna@gmail.com (L.L.); francesco.colella.92@gmail.com (F.C.); mariateresa.volpicella@uniba.it (M.V.)
* Correspondence: anna.degrassi@uniba.it (A.D.G.); ciroleopierri@gmail.com or ciro.pierri@uniba.it (C.L.P.); Tel.: +39-080-544-3614 (A.D.G. & C.L.P.); Fax: +39-080-544-2770 (A.D.G. & C.L.P.)
† These authors declared the equally contribution.

Received: 11 October 2019; Accepted: 18 November 2019; Published: 2 December 2019

**Abstract:** Flavoprotein oxidoreductases are members of a large protein family of specialized dehydrogenases, which include type II NADH dehydrogenase, pyridine nucleotide-disulphide oxidoreductases, ferredoxin-NAD+ reductases, NADH oxidases, and NADH peroxidases, playing a crucial role in the metabolism of several prokaryotes and eukaryotes. Although several studies have been performed on single members or protein subgroups of flavoprotein oxidoreductases, a comprehensive analysis on structure–function relationships among the different members and subgroups of this great dehydrogenase family is still missing. Here, we present a structural comparative analysis showing that the investigated flavoprotein oxidoreductases have a highly similar overall structure, although the investigated dehydrogenases are quite different in functional annotations and global amino acid composition. The different functional annotation is ascribed to their participation in species-specific metabolic pathways based on the same biochemical reaction, i.e., the oxidation of specific cofactors, like NADH and $FADH_2$. Notably, the performed comparative analysis sheds light on conserved sequence features that reflect very similar oxidation mechanisms, conserved among flavoprotein oxidoreductases belonging to phylogenetically distant species, as the bacterial type II NADH dehydrogenases and the mammalian apoptosis-inducing factor protein, until now retained as unique protein entities in *Bacteria/Fungi* or *Animals*, respectively. Furthermore, the presented computational analyses will allow consideration of FAD/NADH oxidoreductases as a possible target of new small molecules to be used as modulators of mitochondrial respiration for patients affected by rare diseases or cancer showing mitochondrial dysfunction, or antibiotics for treating bacterial/fungal/protista infections.

**Keywords:** flavoprotein oxidoreductases; apoptosis-inducing factor (AIF); type II NADH dehydrogenase (NDH-2); thioredoxin reductase (TrxR1); dihydrolipoamide dehydrogenase (DLD); ubiquinone; molecular modeling; protein shape; antibiotics; mitochondrial respiration

## 1. Introduction

*Flavoprotein Dehydrogenases*

Several oxidative pathways depend on the ability of cells to oxidize NADH (reduced form of nicotinamide adenine dinucleotide cofactor), $FADH_2$ (reduced form of flavin adenine dinucleotide cofactor), and ubiquinol ($UQH_2$) by using dedicated enzymes known as FAD flavoproteins or flavoprotein oxidoreductases [1–3]. Flavoprotein oxidoreductases include pyridine nucleotide-disulphide oxidoreductases (glutathione reductases, trypanothione reductases, lipoamide dehydrogenases, mercuric reductases, thioredoxin reductases, alkyl hydroperoxide reductases), ferredoxin-NAD+ reductases (rubredoxin reductases, putidaredoxin reductases, terpredoxin reductases, and components of benzene 1,2-dioxygenases, toluene 1,2-dioxygenases, chlorobenzene dioxygenases, and biphenyl dioxygenases), NADH oxidases, and NADH peroxidases ( Inter PRO_ID: IPR023753) [4–6]. A widely studied subgroup within flavoprotein oxidoreductases consists of type II NADH dehydrogenases (known as NDH-2 in *Bacteria* and NDI in *Fungi*, [5]).

The great attention dedicated to type II NADH dehydrogenases is due to the fact that these proteins are widely present in bacteria, archaea, *Protista*, *Fungi*, and *Plants*, and appear to have no counterpart in *Animals* [7–9].

Thus, type II NADH dehydrogenases are considered crucial targets for antimicrobial therapies [10]. Conversely, it was recently shown that animal apoptosis-inducing factor (AIF) proteins are rotenone-sensitive NADH/ubiquinone oxidoreductases [11,12], raising the question about the opportunity to draw antibiotics against NDH-2 without considering a putative overlapping function with AIF.

All the cited flavoproteins are involved in the oxidation of NADH, through the reduction of FAD to FADH2 and its re-oxidation to FAD through the reduction of ubiquinone (UQ) to UQH2. Accordingly, both NDH-2- and AIF-crystallized structures show in their core a FAD molecule close to a NADH molecule. Notably, NDI from *Fungi* also shows a UQ molecule very close to the FAD molecule.

In some organisms, among the above cited species, complex I is missing (in some *Fungi*, i.e., in *Saccharomy cescerevisiae* [13], and, more in general, in *Bacteria*, as in *Staphylococcusaureus* [14]) and NDH-2 is the only active NADH dehydrogenase.

Impaired NADH oxidation in cells may determine a high NADH/NAD+ ratio, with a following increase in the production of reactive oxygen species (ROS), which may trigger apoptosis [15,16]. Thus, the regulation and maintenance of the proper NADH/NAD+ as well as the $FADH_2/FAD$ and $UQH_2/UQ$ ratios may be crucial for cell viability.

The presence of a FAD and a NADH molecule in both NDH-2/NDI and AIF proteins lets us suppose that AIF has a common functional ancestor with NDH-2 [6,17,18].

It was also recently proposed that the AIF bioenergetics function may be crucial for NADH oxidation alternative pathways [11,12], as well as for the mediation of caspase-independent apoptosis [19–21]. Indeed, AIF is anchored to the inner mitochondrial membrane protruding towards the mitochondrial intermembrane space of healthy cells [22]. After critical events governing the activation of various apoptotic pathways, allowing mitochondrial outer membrane permeabilization (MOMP), a protease (calpain or cathepsin) cleaves the AIF N-terminal domain (at residue number 102 [22]) and the cut C-terminal domain is released from the inner mitochondrial membrane, crosses the outer mitochondrial membrane, and translocates to the nucleus after association with macrophage migration inhibitory factor (MIF). In the nucleus, the AIF C-terminal domain associated with MIF mediates apoptosis participating in chromatin condensation and large-scale (~50 kb) DNA degradation [19,23,24].

In this paper, we show that NDH-2/NDI from *Bacteria/Fungi* ( 5kmr.pdb from *Caldalkalibacillus thermarum* [10], 4g73.pdb from *S. cerevisiae* [25], and AIF from *Mammalia* ( 4bur.pdb from *Homo sapiens* [26]) share a very similar overall structure, able to accommodate FAD and NADH cofactors at similarly located binding regions. The shared cofactors and the corresponding binding regions indicate that the three enzymes should be able to drive the same oxidative reaction. Indeed, NDH-2 transfers an electron from NADH via FAD to UQ, without proton pumping [7,10]. At the same time, it is commonly accepted that NDI is able to transfer an electron from NADH via FAD to an UQ structurally related cofactor, behaving as a final electron acceptor [13]. Notably, along the crystallized multi-cofactor–NDI protein complex from *S. cerevisiae*, it is also possible to observe two UQ molecules in two close binding sites partially in contact with the FAD binding region [25]. Starting from the two observed poses, it was proposed that $UQ_I$ (i.e., the UQ molecule closest to FAD) may interact with FAD that behaves as an intermediate molecule for electron transfer, and that NADH may transfer electrons via the FAD–UQ$_I$ complex to UQ$_{II}$

Similarly, AIF-crystallized structure hosts a FAD and two NADH molecules (4bur.pdb, [26]) and was recently proposed to be a rotenone-sensitive NADH: ubiquinone oxidoreductase [11,12]. Nevertheless, no semiquinone intermediate could be detected in the available AIF-crystallized structures, although such a neutral radical is expected to be produced after the transfer of a single electron. Our computational approach-based multistep analyses (according to [27]) for the comparison of sequences and crystallized structures of NDH-2/NDI and AIF proteins, has allowed the proposal of a putative binding region involved in direct interactions with UQ.

Furthermore, our comparative analysis has allowed an understanding that other FAD-dependent dehydrogenases, crucial for cell viability too, beyond AIF, NDI, and NDH-2, show a similar overall structure or protein shape [28,29].

Starting from this observation, it was possible to group the sampled/investigated structures in three main groups: AIF-like protein structures, NDH-2-like/NDI-like protein structures (each with specific features), and lipoamide dehydrogenase-like structures. All the members of the three main groups show a similarly located FAD-binding region, and for all of them, it is possible to propose a region putatively involved in NADH or UQ binding.

Last, but not least, our analyses allowed an exploration of putative binding regions located on AIF/NDI/NDH-2 like proteins, possibly involved in the binding of other protein subunits (i.e., cytochrome C, CytC), cofactors (i.e., Coenzyme A, CoA), and substrates (i.e., oxygen or H$_2$S), as well as shedding light on possible species-specific FAD/NADH-dependent oxidoreductase-binding regions. Those binding regions may be targeted in the future with new high-affinity drugs, preventing side effects due to the simultaneous targeting of similarly located cofactor binding regions shared by bacterial/fungal/mammalia NDH-2/NDI/AIF-like proteins.

## 2. Materials and Methods

### 2.1. Protein SequenceSampling and Multiple Sequence Alignment (MSA)

AIF/NDH-2/NDI homologous sequences were collected from the RefSeq protein database using blastp searches (with default parameters). The sequence from *H. sapiens* AIF (NP_004199), *S. cerevisiae* NDI (NP_013586.1), and *C. thermarum* NDH-2 (WP_007502350.1) were used as queries to search for homologous sequences in selected species of animals, *Fungi*, *Plants*, and *Bacteria*. The selected taxonomic groups from *Bacteria* are *Bacillales* (TAX_ID 1385), *Enterobacteriales* (TAX_ID 91347), *Rhodospirillales* (TAX_ID 204441), *Rhodobacterales* (TAX_ID 204455), *Thermales* (gram-negative, TAX_ID 68933), and *Rhizobiales* (gram-negative, TAX_ID 356). Then, our searches were performed through other taxonomic groups, such as *Metazoa* (*Nematoda* (TAX_ID 6231), *Mammalia* (TAX_ID 40674), *Arthropoda* (TAX_ID 6656), *Anthozoa* (TAX_ID 6101)), *Fungi* (*Saccharomycetales*, TAX_ID 4892), and *Plants* (TAX_ID 3193), according to protocols described in [30]. The sampled sequences were retained whether they showed E-values lower than $10^{-25}$, query coverage higher than 70%, and the percentage of identical amino acids greater than 30%.

An MSA of the sampled sequences was built by using ClustalW implemented in the sequence editor package Jalview [31]. Redundant sequences with 100% identical amino acids were removed from the MSA.

### 2.2. Crystal Structure Sampling Via Folding Recognition

AIF/NDH-2/NDI homologus protein-crystallized structures were searched by using the folding recognition method implemented in pGenThreader [32]. The retrieved 49 crystal structures (those with "Certain" or "High" confidence level, according to [32] and [27]) were aligned, superimposed, and compared by using PyMOL [33].

Cofactor-binding regions were highlighted for comparative purposes by selecting residues within 4 Å from the cofactor crystallized in the sampled structures. When necessary, cofactors were also inserted in some crystal structures by comparative analyses and superimposition by using PyMOL according to what previously reported [27,30,34–39].

## 2.3. Phylogenetic Analysis

The analysis of the evolutionary relationships among the homologous sequences sampled by Blastp or among the sequences of the available homologous crystallized structures sampled by Folding Recognition was conducted using MEGA5 [40] starting from the MSA of the above cited 120 homologous protein sequences and from the MSA of the above cited 49 crystallized structure sequences.

In detail, the two trees were built from the ungapped MSA applying the maximum likelihood method with the JTT model for the amino acid substitutions and a gamma distribution (five discrete gamma categories) for the rates among sites. A total of 100 bootstrap samplings were applied to test the robustness of the tree (similar to what was described in [30]).

## 3. Results

### 3.1. Evolutionary Relationships among the Sampled AIF/NDH-2/NDI Homologous Sequences

Although it is commonly accepted that all NDH-2/NDI dehydrogenase sequences might share a common ancestral sequence, based on their conserved similar function and overall structure [13], it has recently been proposed that AIF has a function similar to NDH-2/NDI, i.e., that it is a rotenone-sensitive NADH:UQ oxidoreductase [11,12].

However, the spread of these oxidoreductases in distant taxonomic groups of species and their evolutionary relationships are currently unknown. Thus, we searched for proteins sharing sequence similarity with AIF or NDH-2 or NDI in representative species selected from bacteria, *Plants*, *Fungi*, and animals, and we found 120 putative homologous proteins. The evolutionary relationships among all these proteins showed two main clusters referring to AIF-homologous proteins and NDH-2/NDI-homologous proteins, whereas the latter were further divided into two main subclusters (Figure 1). AIF-homologous proteins were detected in members from all four taxonomic groups while NDH-2-homologous proteins were detected in bacterial and fungal species, and NDI-homologous proteins were detected in fungal, plant, and animal species (Figure 1).

In detail, close to the *Mammalia* AIF sequences, it is possible to observe a group of *Nitrosomonadales* and *Thermales* sequences that group into a subcluster adjacent to the AIF subcluster *Metazoan* sequences. Then, in the same tree-region, a bit more distant but related to the AIF-like sequence cluster, it is possible to observe a sequence cluster hosting *Bacillales*, *Sulfolobales*, and *Plant* sequences (i.e., XP_022741237.1_Durio_zibethinus, Figure 1).

On the other side of the tree, it is possible to observe a cluster of *Bacillales* NDH-2-like sequences clustering together with NDH-2-like sequences from *Fungi* together with two subgroups of *Bacteria* sequences (the first consisting of *Enterobacteriales*, *Rhodospirillales*, *Rhodobacterales*, and *Rhizobiales*, and the second consisting of *Thermales*, *Flavobacteriales*, and *Cytophagales* sequences) related to NDH-2-like *Bacillales* sequences. Finally, a last subgroup containing *Fungi*, *Plant*, and *Anthozoa* NDI-like sequences is detectable, in the same tree region but separated from the NDH-2-like sequence cluster (Figure 1).

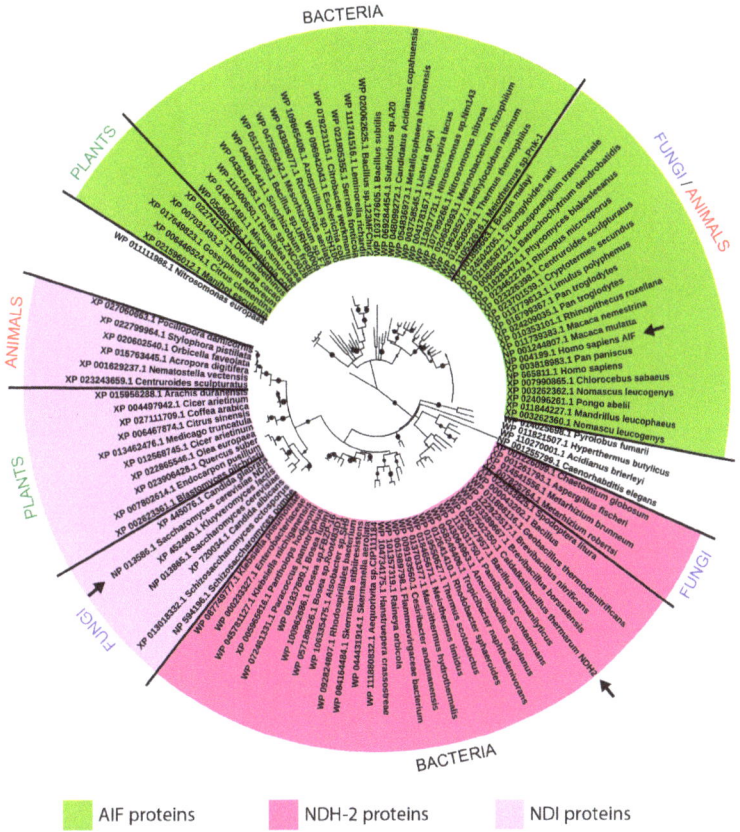

**Figure 1.** Phylogenetic tree of AIF/NDI/NDH-2-homologous sequences. Maximum likelihood phylogenetic tree of AIF/NDH2/NDI-homologous protein sequences selected from representative species of bacteria, *Fungi*, *Plants*, and animals. Each one of the tree leaves reports the corresponding organism and RefSeq protein accession number. Arrows indicate the query-protein sequences used for sampling all the other homologous sequences. Nodes supported by bootstrap values greater than 0.7 are indicated as black dots.

*3.2. Sequence Features of the Sampled AIF/NDH-2/NDI Protein Sequences*

It was expected that the proposed specialization in species-specific biochemical pathways should reflect the existence of further well-conserved sequence features observable by building a MSA, despite the global highly variable percentage of identical residues (in the 15% to 99% range) shared by the sampled full-length sequences (Supplementary Table S1).

In fact, by inspecting the MSA of AIF/NDI/NDH-2-sampled homologs, it is possible to recognize 10 amino acid conserved motifs. Some of those motifs, i.e., the two glycine-rich motifs (respectively the first and fifth sequence motif grouped in Figure 2) and the eighth motif, are conserved in all the investigated sequences, underlining a putative common involvement in the protein function/mechanism. The other sequence motifs show a high degree of amino acid conservation within specific taxonomic groups, reflecting a species-specific acquired function or substrate/cofactor specificity/affinity (Figure 2).

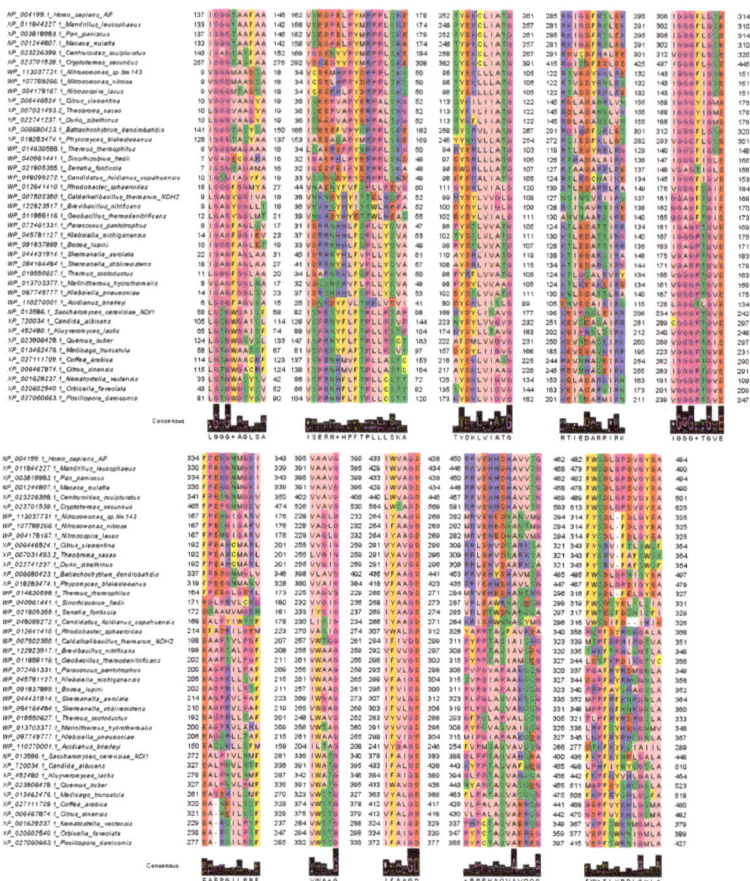

**Figure 2.** AIF/NDI/NDH-2-conserved sequence motifs. Sequence motifs detected by comparing the sampled AIF/NDI/NDH-2 homologous sequences sampled by blastp. The highlighted motifs reveal crucial protein regions involved in cofactor binding and/or the protein function mechanism. The jalviewzappo color style was used for coloring amino acids. Logo representation is also reported to highlight the most conserved residues.

In detail, the most conserved protein regions, at the first and the fifth motifs, consist of two glycine-rich regions strongly conserved in all the sampled sequences. As an example, in metazoa, the two glycine-rich motifs are at the level of residues 137-IGGGTAAFA-146 and 306-IGGGFLGSE-314 (*H. sapiens* numbering) and align with residues 9-LGAGYGGIV-17 and 161-IGGAGFTGE-169 in *Bacteria* (*C. thermarum* numbering) and 59-LGSGWGAIS-67 and 234-VGGGPYGVE-242 in *Fungi* (*S. cerevisiae* numbering) (Figure 2). It is interesting to note that the first highlighted motif hosts an aromatic residue in half of the sampled sequences, whereas the sixth motif always hosts an acidic residue and a further aromatic residue in most of the sampled sequences.

The second highlighted sequence motif, located at residues 162-VSEDPELPYMRPPLSKE-178 (*H. sapiens* numbering), close to the first glycine-rich motif, appears to be conserved in specific taxonomic groups within the sampled *Mammalia* AIF sequences. This motif appears to be conserved, with few differences in the AIF-like sequences sampled through *Arthropoda, Fish, Fungi, Plants*, and AIF-closest sampled *Bacteria* sequences (Figure 2). The motif 162-VSEDPELPYMRPPLSKE-178 (*H. sapiens* numbering) of AIF-like sequences aligns with the motif 37-NKNDYHYITTELHQPAA-53 (*C. thermarum* numbering) observed in NDH-2 from *Bacillales* and other *Bacteria* (i.e., 31-IDRRNHHLFQPLLYQVAT-48, *Paracoccus pantotrophus* numbering), such as in *Rhodobacterales, Rhizobiales, Enterobacteriales, Thermales,* and *Rhodospirillales*. These motifs align with the NDI highly conserved motif 83-SPRSYFLFTPLLPS-96 (*S. cerevisiae* numbering) observed in *Fungi* and NDI-like sequences sampled from *Plants*, i.e., 82-SPRNYFAFTPLLPS-95 (*Medicago truncatula* numbering).

Two further highly conserved motifs, i.e., the third and fourth, consist of residues 252-TYEKCLIATG-261 (*H. sapiens* numbering), with the last glycine conserved in all the sampled sequences, and 285-RKIGDFRS-292 (*H. sapiens* numbering), respectively. The third motif 252-TYEKCLIATG-261 (*H. sapiens* numbering) is conserved in all the sampled *Mammalia* AIF sequences. The same motif with few variations is observed in *Arthropoda* 258-TYEKCLIATG-267, AIF-like sequences from *Bacteria* 96-TYEKLLLATG-105 (*Nitrosomonas nitrosa* numbering), *Plants* 113-SYKILIIATG-122 (*Citrus clementina* numbering), *Fungi* 258-QYSRVLIATG-267 (*Batrachochytrium dendrobatidis* numbering), and several groups of AIF-like proteins from *Bacteria*, i.e., *Nitrosomonadales* 96-TYEKLLLATG-105 (*N. nitrosa* numbering), and NDH-2-like sequences from *Rhodospirillales* 100-SYDRLVLATG-109 (*Roseomonasaerilata* numbering), *Thermales* 94-RYERLLLATG-103 (*Thermus thermophilus* numbering), *Rhodobacterales* 111-GYDHLVIALG-120, *Rhizobiales* 97-DYDRLLLATG-106 (*Sinorhizobiumfredii* numbering), *Enterobacteriales* 98-EWDRLLLATG-107 (*Serratia fonticola* numbering), *Sulfolobales* 96-EFEKALIATG-105 (*Candidatusacidianus* numbering), and *Bacillales* 99-HYDYLVVGLG-108 (*C. thermarum* numbering).

A very similar motif is also observed in NDI-like sequences from *Fungi* 214-KYDYLVVGVG-223 (*S. cerevisiae* numbering), *Plants* 216-AYDKLVIASG-225 (*Coffeaarabica* numbering), and *Anthozoa* 125-IYDKLVIGVG-134 (*Nematostella vectensis* numbering).

The fourth motif 285-RKIGDFRS-292 (*H. sapiens* numbering) aligns with a different conserved motif in NDH-2 sequences from *Rhodobacterales* 124-KTLEDATT-131 (*P. pantotrophus* numbering), *Enterobacterales* 130-KTLEDATT-137 (*Klebsiella michiganensis* numbering), and *Rhizobiales* 126-KTLEDATT-133 (*Bosealupini* numbering), with few variations in *Rhodospirillales* 138-KTIEDARQ-145 (*Skermanella aerolata* numbering), *Thermales*, and *Bacillales* 128-RSINSVRL-135 (*Pseudochelatococcus contaminans* numbering) or 127-NSINSVRI-134 (*C. thermarum* numbering).

This motif is also observed with few variations in NDI from *Fungi* 196-KEIPNSLEI-204 (*S. cerevisiae* numbering), NDI-like sequences from *Plants* 185-KEVEDAQK-192 (*M. truncatula* numbering), and *Anthozoa* 153-KELADARK-160 (*N. vectensis* numbering).

The five last conserved motifs are detectable in all the sampled sequences.

A sixth motif conserved with specific variations in at least two great taxonomic groups consists of amino acids 334-FPEKGNMGKI-343 (AIF, *H. sapiens* numbering) highly conserved in AIF from *Mammalia* and *Arthropoda* (341-FPETGNMGKV-350, *Centruroides sculpturatus* numbering) and AIF-like proteins from some *Plants* (192-FPEAHCMARL-201, *C. clementina* numbering), *Fungi* (319-FPEEGNMANV-328, *Phycomyces blakeseeanus* numbering), and *Bacteria* (167-FPESGIGARV-176, *N. nitrosa* numbering).

The sixth motif 334-FPEKGNMGKI-343 (AIF, *H. sapiens numbering*) aligns with a highly conserved motif observed in *Fungi* NDI, i.e., 272-EALPIVLNMF-281 (*S. cerevisiae* numbering), and in NDI-like proteins from *Plants* (327-EALPNVLPMF-336, *Quercus suber* numbering) and *Anthozoa* (229-EA-RQILPSF-237, *N. vectensis* numbering).

The above cited motifs align with a highly conserved motif detectable in NDH-2 from *Bacillales* 198-EAAPTVLPGF-207 (*C. thermarum* numbering), from *Rhodobacterales* 200-EAGPRILPAF-209 (*P. pantotrophus* numbering), from *Enterobacteriales* 206-EAGPRLLSVF-215 (*K. michiganensis* numbering), from *Rhodospirillales* 214-EAGPRVLPAF-223 (*S. aerolata* numbering), from *Rhizobiales* 202-EAGPRILPSF-211 (*B. lupini* numbering), and *Thermales* 192-EAGPRLLSAF-201 (*Thermus scotoductus* numbering)

The seventh motif consists of residues 395-VAAVG-399 (*H. sapiens* numbering) aligning with, NDH-2 from *Bacteria*, i.e., 257-VWTGG-299 (*C. thermarum* numbering) or NDI from *Fungi* 336-IWATG-340 (*S. cerevisiae* numbering). Notably, the final G is conserved in all the sampled sequences.

The eighth motif consists of residues 433-IWVAGD-438 (*H. sapiens* numbering) aligning with NDH-2 from *Bacteria*, i.e., 294-IFIVGD-299 (*C. thermarum* numbering) or NDI from *Fungi* 378-IFAIGD-383 (*S. cerevisiae* numbering). Notably, the final GD dipeptide is conserved in all the sampled sequences.

The ninth motif consists of residues 450-RRVEHHDHAVAVSG-459 (*H. sapiens* numbering) that aligns with a different motif conserved with few variations in NDI-sequences from *Fungi* 388-GLPPTAQVAHQEA-400 (*S. cerevisiae* numbering) and NDH-2 sequences from *Bacteria* 311-PYPPTAQIAIQHG-323 (*C. thermarum* numbering).

The tenth motif consists of residues 482-FWSDLGPDVGYEA-494 (*H. sapiens* numbering) that aligns with a similar motif conserved with few variations in NDI-sequences from *Fungi* 436-FKPFKYNDLGALA-448 (*S. cerevisiae* numbering) and NDH-2 sequences from *Bacteria* 339-MTPFKPHIRGTVA-351 (*C. thermarum* numbering). Notably the last alanine residue is conserved in all the sampled sequences.

*3.3. Comparative Analysis of AIF, NDH-II, NDI, and the pGenTHREADER-Suggested Template Proteins for Comparative Modeling*

3.3.1. Superimposition of AIF, NDI, and NDH-2

Given the existence of the crystallized structures of the human AIF (4bur.pdb), *S. cerevisiae* NDI (4g73.pdb), and the *C. thermarum* NDH-2 (5kmr.pdb), we compared their structures by superimposition and we observed that beyond the shared motifs the investigated proteins show a highly similar overall protein structure and shape (Figure 3).

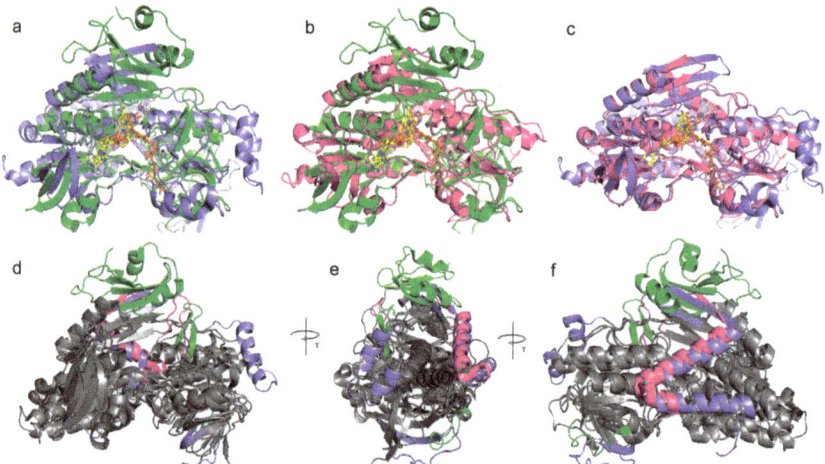

**Figure 3.** Comparative analysis of AIF/NDI/NDH-2 3D structure. Panels (**a**,**b**,**c**) Lateral view of superposition of *H. sapiens* AIF (in green cartoon, 4bur.pdb) and *S. cerevisae* NDI (in blue cartoon, 4g73.pdb) that gives a root mean square deviation(RMSD) of 2.891 Å; *H. sapiens* AIF (4bur.pdb) and *C. thermarum* NDH2 (in magenta cartoon, 5kmr.pdb) that gives an RMSD of 1.891 Å; *S. cerevisae* NDI (4g73.pdb) and *C. thermarum* NDH2 (5kmr.pdb) that gives an RMSD of 1.384 Å. Panel (**d**,**e**,**f**) Three 90-degree rotation of the alignment view of 4bur, 4g74, and 5kmr. In the grey cartoon representation, the common features highlighted by the superposition of the three structures. Specific AIF/NDI/NDH-2 structural features highlighted by the proposed superposition are reported in green, blue, and magenta cartoon representations. All the three aligned proteins are represented in complex with the FAD (orange sticks, panels **a**–**c**), NAD$^+$ (yellow sticks, panels **a**–**c**), and UQ (white sticks, panels **a** and **c**) cofactors, when the cited cofactors were present in the reported crystallized structures.

The main differences between the three crystallized structures are in the C-terminal domain and in some loops. Indeed, the AIF structure has a longer C-terminal domain containing an extra helix domain (residues 497–612, *H. sapiens* 4bur.pdb numbering) at variance with the shorter C-terminal domains of NDI (residues 458–513, *S. cerevisiae* 4g73.pdb numbering) and NDH-2 (residues 363–396, *C. thermarum* 5kmr.pdb numbering).

Furthermore, AIF, NDI, and NDH-2 show one or two specific loops. AIF-specific loops are observed at the level of residues 210–222 and 440–451 (4bur.pdb numbering, Figure 3), whereas two specific loops are observed in the NDI structure at the level of residues 138–163 and 413–435 (4g73.pdb numbering, Figure 3). A specific loop is observed at the level of residues 302–312 of NDH-2 (5kmr.pdb numbering, Figure 3).

3.3.2. Sampling of Homologous-Crystallized Structures by Folding Recognition Methods

Along the Blastp sequence sampling, it was also noticed that several dehydrogenases out of the sampled homologous protein sequences were annotated as dehydrogenases with different specific functions. i.e., among the sampled homologous AIF/NDH-2/NDI proteins, it was possible to detect a FAD-dependent pyridine-nucleotide disulfide oxidoreductase [41] from *N. nitrosa* (WP_107789266.1) and a ferredoxine reductase [42] from *Nitroso spiralacus* (WP_004178167.1), grouping in a subcluster adjacent to AIF sequences sampled from Mammalia. Another example is observed in a cluster adjacent to AIF-like sequences, where it is possible to observe a monodehydroascorbate reductase [43] from *D. zibethinus* (XP_022741237.1) proposed to be located within peroxisomes.

To verify if some structures of the above cited proteins were available in the protein data bank and showed an overall structure similar to AIF/NDH-2/NDI protein structures, we searched for AIF/NDH-2/NDI 3D-homologous structures by using the fold recognition tools implemented in pGenTHREADER.

In this way, several FAD/NAD(P)H-dependent dehydrogenase-crystallized structures, proposed to have a structure homologous to that observed for AIF, NDI, and NDH-2, were sampled. The sampled structures from different species were available in the protein data bank under different functional annotations (Table 1).

**Table 1.** List of the investigated homologous crystallized structures and specific structural features. The proteins sampled using pGenTHREADER together with the RMSD between coordinates of the sampled structure backbones superimposed to the structure of the three query sequences (AIF (4bur.pdb); NDI (4g73.pdb); and NDH-2 (5kmr.pdb)) are reported. The best hit of each reported structure sampled by Blastp in *H.sapiens*, *C. thermarum*, and *S. cerevisiae* is also reported. For each best hit E-value, %ID and query coverage are also reported. Abbreviations: AIF, apoptosis-inducing factor; DH, dehydrogenase; LD, lipoamide dehydrogenase; DLD, dihydrolipoyl dehydrogenase or dihydrolipoamide dehydrogenase; OX, oxidase; RED, reductase; GLR1, glutathione disulfide reductase; Trx, Thioredoxin; mt, mitochondrial; TRR1, Trx-disulfide reductase; RYL-552, 5n.a.fluoron.a.3n.a.methyln.a.2n.a.{4n.a.(4n.a.(trifluoromethoxy)benzyl)phenyl]quinolimn.a.4(1H)n.a.one}; SL827, N~2~-((2-amino-5-bromopyridin-3-yl)sulfonyl)-N-(4-methoxyphenyl)-N~2~-methylglycinamide; KPC, ketopropylthioethanesulphonate; CytC, Cytochrome C.

| | Functional Annotation | Res. N. | Organism | Crystallized cofactors | Crystallized Inhibitors | AIF (4bur) | NDH2 (5kmr) | NDI (4g73) | *H. sapiens* Blast Best Hits | | | | | *C. thermarum* Blast Best Hit | | | | | *S. cerevisiae* S288C Blast Best Hit | | | | |
|---|---|---|---|---|---|---|---|---|---|---|---|---|---|---|---|---|---|---|---|---|---|---|---|
| | | | | | | | RMSD (Å) | | Protein Name | Accession | Query cover | E-val | %ID | Protein Name | Accession | Query cover | E-val | %ID | Protein Name | Accession | Query cover | E-val | %ID |
| | | | | | | | | | AIF-like structures | | | | | | | | | | | | | | |
| 4bur | AIF | 511 | *H.sapiens* | FAD/NADH | n.a. | 0 | 3.12 | 2.22 | mt isoform AIF-α/β | NP_665811.1 | 100% | 0.0 | 100% | n.a. | n.a. | n.a. | n.a. | n.a. | lec1sp | NP_015308 | 25% | 0.98 | 25.55% |
| 5fs6 | AIF | 474 | *H.sapiens* | FAD | n.a. | 1.06 | 2.71 | 1.82 | mt isoform AIF | NP_004199.1 | 99% | 0.0 | 99.61% | n.a. | n.a. | n.a. | n.a. | n.a. | n.a. | n.a. | n.a. | n.a. | n.a. |
| 5vnl0 | NADH OX | 449 | *L.brevis* | FAD/NAD(H)O2 | n.a. | 2.28 | 2.03 | 2.18 | proton transport protein Sec23A | NP_006355.2 | 100% | 0.0 | 100% | CoA-disulfide reductase | WP_007505374.1 | 2% | 3×10⁻⁸⁶ | 50.00% | CTPase-activating protein SEC23 | NP_015607.1 | 98% | 0.0 | 49.80% |
| 1xhc | NADH OX /nitrile RED | 555 | *P. furiosus* | FAD | n.a. | 1.799 | 2.443 | 2.458 | AIF-3 isoform 2 | NP_001018070.1 | 77% | 9×10⁻²⁰ | 28.47% | CoA-disulfide RED | WP_007505374.1 | 98% | 9×10⁻⁹² | 35.83% | AifAp | NP_014472.1 | 54% | 9×10⁻¹¹ | 26.36% |
| 2fcz0 | NADH OX | 473 | *S. pyrogenis* | FAD | n.a. | 1.53 | 1.859 | 1.658 | AIF-3 isoform 1 | NP_653305.1 | 67% | 2×10⁻¹⁸ | 25.75% | CoA-disulfide RED | WP_007505374.1 | 92% | 2×10⁻⁷⁴ | 31.29% | GLR1 | NP_015234.1 | 40% | 8×10⁻¹⁰ | 27.09% |
| 2cdu | NADPH OX | 452 | *L. sanfranscensis* | FAD/ADP | n.a. | 2.226 | 2.2 | 2.095 | mt isoform AIF | NP_004199.1 | 56% | 2×10⁻¹¹ | 25.46% | CoA-disulfide RED | WP_007505374.1 | 96% | 3×10⁻⁷⁴ | 31.52% | GLR1 | NP_015234.1 | 39% | 3×10⁻⁸ | 27.66% |
| 1nhs | NADH PerOX | 447 | *E. fcudis* | FAD | n.a. | 1.738 | 1.932 | 2.041 | AIF-3 isoform 1 | NP_653305.1 | 55% | 7×10⁻²² | 27.17% | CoA-disulfide RED | WP_007505374.1 | 98% | 9×10⁻⁹² | 35.83% | GLR1 | NP_015234.1 | 39% | 8×10⁻⁸ | 22.40% |
| 3kd | Ferredoxin RED | 409 | *E. coli* | FAD | n.a. | 1.949 | 2.842 | 2.606 | AIF-3 isoform 1 | NP_653305.1 | 89% | 8×10⁻⁵¹ | 30.24% | CoA-disulfide RED | WP_007505374.1 | 80% | 6×10⁻²⁶ | 29.48% | GLR1 | NP_015234.1 | 35% | 2×10⁻³ | 24.03% |
| 3fg2 | Ferredoxin RED | 404 | *R. palustris* | FAD | n.a. | 1.633 | 2.087 | 2.340 | AIF-3 isoform 1 | NP_653305.1 | 91% | 6×10⁻⁴⁷ | 29.22% | CoA-disulfide RED | WP_007505374.1 | 77% | 7×10⁻²² | 24.15% | GLR1 | NP_015234.1 | 32% | 4×10⁻³ | 25.90% |
| 2pgw | Ferredoxin RED | 401 | *Pseudomonas sp. KKS102* | FAD | n.a. | 1.986 | 2.362 | 2.365 | AIF-3 isoform 1 | NP_001018070.1 | 91% | 5×10⁻²⁷ | 28.39% | CoA-disulfide RED | WP_007505374.1 | 52% | 3×10⁻¹⁴ | 29.78% | lec1sp | NP_015081 | 24% | 6×10⁻³ | 28.85% |
| 2v3a | Rubredoxin RED | 381 | *P. aeruginosa* | FAD | n.a. | 2.278 | 3.067 | 6.698 | AIF 2 | NP_001185625.1 | 61% | 3×10⁻⁵ | 24% | CoA-disulfide RED | WP_007505374.1 | 71% | 2×10⁻²³ | 27.02% | n.a. | n.a. | n.a. | n.a. | n.a. |
| 3kij | NAD+reduced oxonoicoRED | 378 | *C. acetobutylicum* | FAD | n.a. | 2.498 | 2.745 | 2.335 | AIF-3 isoform 2 | NP_001018070.1 | 95% | 5×10⁻²⁷ | 23.41% | CoA-disulfide RED | WP_007505374.1 | 89% | 1×10⁻²¹ | 23.69% | mRNA-binding ubiquitin-specific protease UBP3 | NP_011078.3 | 7% | 0.77 | 53.57% |
| 3ctb | Toluene 2,3-Dioxygenase RED | 400 | *P. putida* | FAD | n.a. | 1.914 | 1.979 | 2.146 | AIF-3 isoform 1 | NP_653305.1 | 87% | 7×10⁻⁴⁴ | 33.14% | CoA-disulfide RED | WP_007505374.1 | 43% | 9×10⁻¹⁵ | 33.33% | AifAp | NP_014472.1 | 48% | 6×10⁻⁴ | 25.35% |
| 1q1r | Putidaredoxin RED | 421 | *P. putida* | FAD | n.a. | 1.581 | 2.85 | 3.069 | AIF-3 isoform 3 | NP_001139760.1 | 87% | 5×10⁻⁴⁰ | 28.95% | CoA-disulfide RED | WP_007505374.1 | 72% | 9×10⁻²⁵ | 27.74% | GLR1 | NP_015234.1 | 38% | 2×10⁻⁴ | 21.64% |
| 3oc4 | Pyridine nucleotide-disulfide oxidoRED | 422 | *E. faecalis* | FAD | n.a. | 3.143 | 2.451 | 3.207 | AIF-3 isoform 1 | NP_653305.1 | 62% | 4×10⁻¹³ | 25.26% | CoA-disulfide RED | WP_007505374.1 | 95% | 4×10⁻⁴⁵ | 26.57% | GLR1 | NP_015234.1 | 51% | 1×10⁻⁵ | 23.36% |
| 3iwa | Pyridine Nucleotide-disulphideoxido RED | 397 | *D. vulgaris* | n.a. | n.a. | 2.243 | 3.06 | 2.664 | AIF-3 isoform 2 | NP_001018070.1 | 68% | 8×10⁻²⁴ | 28.66% | CoA-disulfide RED | WP_007505374.1 | 95% | 5×10⁻⁸² | 33.55% | GLR1 | NP_015234.1 | 99% | 3×10⁻⁹ | 22.49% |
| 3egb | Pyridyne Nucleotide Coenzyme A Disulfide RED | 444 | *B.anthracis* | FAD/CoA | n.a. | 2.17 | 2.37 | 2.341 | glycerol-3-phosphate DH, mt [Homo sapiens] | NP_000899.3 | 10% | 0.8 | 39.38% | CoA-disulfide RED | WP_007505374.1 | 91% | 5×10⁻¹³⁷ | 47.05% | lec1sp | NP_015081 | 60% | 1×10⁻⁵ | 23.51% |
| 4fc9 | CoA disulfide RED | 453 | *B. horikoshii* | FAD/CoA | n.a. | 2.148 | 2.223 | 2.488 | AIF-3 isoform 1 [Homo sapiens] | NP_653305.1 | 70% | 1×10⁻²² | 27.55% | CoA-disulfide RED | WP_007505374.1 | 96% | 3×10⁻¹⁰⁵ | 39.28% | GLR1 | NP_015234.1 | 64% | 2×10⁻¹² | 24.36% |
| 3ics | CoA disulfide RED | 555 | *B. anthracis* | ADP/FAD/CoA | n.a. | 1.845 | 1.958 | 1.98 | DLD, mt isoform 4 | NP_001276681.1 | 51% | 2×10⁻⁹ | 26.46% | CoA-disulfide RED | WP_007505374.1 | 75% | 3×10⁻⁸³ | 32.13% | thioesulfate sulfurtransferase RDL2 | NP_014929.3 | 10% | 1×10⁻³ | 29.73% |
| 3ntd | CoA-dependent persulfide RED | 565 | *S. suflica* | FAD/CoA | n.a. | 1.92 | 1.95 | 1.95 | AIF mt isoform AIF-α/β | NP_665811.1 | 47% | 6×10⁻¹⁰ | 28.01% | CoA-disulfide RED | WP_007505374.1 | 82% | 1×10⁻⁸⁵ | 31.57% | DLD | NP_116635.1 | 45% | 2×10⁻⁷ | 25.87% |
| | | | | | | | | | Type II NADH DH-like structures | | | | | | | | | | | | | | |
| 5kmr | Type II NADH DH | 405 | *C. thermarum* | FAD/NAD | n.a. | 3.12 | 0 | 1.31 | AIF 2 | NP_001185625.1 | 72% | 2×10⁻¹⁰ | 25.34% | NAD(P)FAD-dependent oxidoRED | WP_007422560.1 | 100% | 0.0 | 100.00% | NADH-ubiquinone RED (H(+)-translocating) NDI1 | NP_013865.1 | 80% | 7×10⁻²⁹ | 28.29% |
| 5n11 | FlavoCysC sulfide DH | 393 | *T. paraluteus* | CytC, CoPC, FAD | n.a. | 2.82 | 3.33 | 2.96 | n.a. | n.a. | n.a. | n.a. | n.a. | NAD(P)FAD-dependent oxidoRED | WP_007505419.1 | 74% | 5×10⁻²² | 26.33% | n.a. | n.a. | n.a. | n.a. | n.a. |
| 5na1 | NADH-dependent quinone oxidoRED | 398 | *S. aureus* | FAD | n.a. | 2.63 | 0.82 | 1.39 | n.a. | n.a. | n.a. | n.a. | n.a. | NAD(P)FAD-dependent oxidoRED | WP_007422560.1 | 97% | 3×10⁻¹³⁰ | 46.48% | nucleoside triphosphate pyrophosphohydrolase HAM1 | NP_126031 | 12% | 0.59 | 34.69% |

**Table 1.** *Cont.*

| | Functional Annotation | Res. N. | Organism | Crystallized cofactors | Crystallized Inhibitors | AIF (4bur) | NDH2 (5kmr) | NDI (4g73) | H. sapiens Blast Hits | | | | | C. thermarum Blast Best Hit | | | | | S. cerevisiae S288C Blast Best Hit | | | | |
|---|---|---|---|---|---|---|---|---|---|---|---|---|---|---|---|---|---|---|---|---|---|---|---|
| | | | | | | | | | | | | | | | | | | | | | | | |
| | | | | | | RMSD (Å) | | | Protein Name | Accession | Query cover | E-val | %ID | Protein Name | Accession | Query cover | E-val | %ID | Protein Name | Accession | Query cover | E-val | %ID |
| 5jwc | Type II NADH DH | 495 | *P. falciparum* | FAD | RYL-552 | 3.88 | 1.68 | 0.85 | AIF 2 | NP_001185625.1 | 6% | 1.7 | 44.44% | NAD(P)/FAD-dependent oxidoRED | WP_042685568.1 | 49% | $1 \times 10^{-11}$ | 22.68% | NADH-UQ RED (H(+)-translocating) NDI1 | NP_013865.1 | 94% | $8 \times 10^{-40}$ | 30.32% |
| 3byw | Sulfide-quinone oxidoRED | 429 | *arcticus* | FAD,DCQ,H2S | n.a. | 3.52 | 2.75 | 2.86 | sulfide:quinone oxidoRED, mt (Homo sapiens) | NP_001258142.1 | 68% | $3 \times 10^{-12}$ | 23.70% | NAD(P)/FAD-dependent oxidoRED | WP_075076419.1 | 75% | $4 \times 10^{-15}$ | 22.82% | NADH-UQ RED (H(+)-translocating) NDI2 | NP_010108.1 | 55% | $1 \times 10^{-9}$ | 27.27% |
| | | | | | | | | | **Ndi1 - NADH DH like structures** | | | | | | | | | | | | | | |
| 4g73 | Ndi1 - NADH DH | 502 | *S. cerevisiae* | FAD/NAD/UQ5 | n.a. | 2.22 | 1.31 | 0.0 | n.a. | n.a. | n.a. | n.a. | n.a. | NAD(P)/FAD-dependent oxidoRED | WP_075032560.1 | 86% | $1 \times 10^{-30}$ | 25.93% | NADH-UQ RED (H(+)-translocating) NDI1 | NP_013586.1 | 97% | 0.0 | 99.80% |
| 5yjw | Ndi1 - NADH DH | 454 | *S. cerevisiae* | FAD | Stigmatellin | 2.12 | 1.32 | 0.49 | n.a. | n.a. | n.a. | n.a. | n.a. | NAD(P)/FAD-dependent oxidoRED | WP_075032560.1 | 90% | $7 \times 10^{-31}$ | 25.93% | NADH-UQ RED (H(+)-translocating) NDI1 | NP_013586.1 | 100% | 0.0 | 100.00% |
| | | | | | | | | | **Other DH** | | | | | | | | | | | | | | |
| 4m5z | LD | 465 | *M. tuberculosis* | FAD | SU827 | 4.28 | 4.341 | 1.974 | DLD, mt isoform 1 | NP_000099.2 | 98% | $8 \times 10^{-67}$ | 35.82% | DLD | WP_075033768.1 | 96% | $2 \times 10^{-120}$ | 44.81% | DLD | NP_116635.1 | 96% | $3 \times 10^{-86}$ | 37.63% |
| 6aon | DLD | 473 | *B. pertussis* | n.a. | n.a. | 4.84 | 2.03 | 3.76 | DLD, mt isoform 1 | NP_000099.2 | 98% | $7 \times 10^{-141}$ | 46.74% | DLD | WP_075033768.1 | 98% | $1 \times 10^{-106}$ | 40.46% | DLD | NP_116635.1 | 97% | $3 \times 10^{-143}$ | 47.81% |
| 4jq9 | DLD | 471 | *E. coli* | FAD | n.a. | 3.61 | 2.168 | 2.238 | DLD, mt isoform 1 | NP_000099.2 | 94% | $9 \times 10^{-141}$ | 43.61% | DLD | WP_075076013.1 | 95% | $3 \times 10^{-121}$ | 43.74% | DLD | NP_116635.1 | 93% | $3 \times 10^{-100}$ | 40.79% |
| 6awa | DLD | 475 | *P. putida* | FAD/AMP | n.a. | 3.47 | 2.6 | 2.67 | DLD, mt isoform 1 | NP_000099.2 | 96% | $1 \times 10^{-135}$ | 50.43% | DLD | WP_075076013.1 | 97% | $6 \times 10^{-121}$ | 43.19% | DLD | NP_116635.1 | 93% | $1 \times 10^{-81}$ | 46.47% |
| 5j5z | DLD | 477 | *H. sapiens* | FAD | n.a. | 3.23 | 2.77 | 3.13 | DLD, mt isoform 1 | NP_000099.2 | 95% | 0.0 | 99.97% | DLD | WP_075076013.1 | 92% | $2 \times 10^{-108}$ | 42.30% | DLD | NP_116635.1 | 93% | 0.0 | 57.17% |
| 1zmd | DLD | 474 | *H. sapiens* | FAD/NAD | n.a. | 3.27 | 2.83 | 2.77 | DLD, mt isoform 1 (Homo sapiens) | NP_000099.2 | 100% | 0.0 | 99.79% | DLD | WP_075076013.1 | 96% | $2 \times 10^{-110}$ | 42.52% | DLD | NP_116635.1 | 98% | 0.0 | 57.59% |
| 5u25 | DLD | 478 | *N. gonorrhoeae* | FAD | n.a. | 3.68 | 2.44 | 2.47 | DLD, mt isoform 1 | NP_000099.2 | 75% | $7 \times 10^{-98}$ | 39.48% | DLD | WP_075076013.1 | 77% | $2 \times 10^{-112}$ | 41.76% | DLD | NP_116635.1 | 76% | $2 \times 10^{-96}$ | 40.17% |
| 3urh | DLD | 491 | *R. melitoti* | FAD | n.a. | 3.376 | 2.29 | 1.732 | DLD, mt isoform 1 | NP_000099.2 | 95% | $1 \times 10^{-129}$ | 55.08% | DLD | WP_075076013.1 | 94% | $3 \times 10^{-117}$ | 42.58% | DLD | NP_116635.1 | 94% | $2 \times 10^{-143}$ | 51.37% |
| 1lvl | LD | 458 | *P. putida* | FAD/NADH | n.a. | 3.664 | 2.976 | 4.089 | DLD, mt isoform 1 | NP_000099.2 | 98% | $5 \times 10^{-90}$ | 38.09% | DLD | WP_075076013.1 | 99% | $2 \times 10^{-132}$ | 43.94% | DLD | NP_116635.1 | 98% | $1 \times 10^{-81}$ | 36.86% |
| 1ebd | DLD | 455 | *G. stearothermophilus* | FAD/Nhyd nolipoamide acetyltransferase | n.a. | 3.22 | 2.19 | 3.69 | DLD, mt isoform 1 | NP_000099.2 | 98% | $3 \times 10^{-119}$ | 43.89% | DLD | WP_075076013.1 | 99% | 0.0 | 68.65% | DLD | NP_116635.1 | 98% | $3 \times 10^{-101}$ | 43.29% |
| 2yqu | LD | 455 | *T. thermophilus* | FAD | n.a. | 3.884 | 3.448 | 2.97 | DLD, mt isoform 1 | NP_000099.2 | 98% | $4 \times 10^{-140}$ | 46.41% | DLD | WP_075076013.1 | 99% | $1 \times 10^{-115}$ | 43.41% | DLD | NP_116635.1 | 99% | $2 \times 10^{-143}$ | 48.00% |
| 3lad | Lipoamide dehydrogenase | 476 | *A. vinelandii* | FAD | n.a. | 4.442 | 2.221 | 2.995 | DLD, mt isoform 1 | NP_000099.2 | 96% | $3 \times 10^{-130}$ | 49.36% | DLD | WP_075076013.1 | 98% | $3 \times 10^{-117}$ | 42.55% | DLD | NP_116635.1 | 98% | $3 \times 10^{-135}$ | 44.61% |
| 2rv2 | Glutathione amide RED | 463 | *C. gracile* | FAD | n.a. | 2.813 | 2.396 | 2.046 | DLD, mt isoform 1 | NP_000628.2 | 95% | $9 \times 10^{-142}$ | 48.80% | DLD | WP_075076013.1 | 98% | $2 \times 10^{-64}$ | 30.25% | GLR1 | NP_015234.1 | 96% | $1 \times 10^{-141}$ | 46.12% |
| 6n7i | Glutathione RED | 451 | *S. pyogenes* | Riboflavin/FAD | n.a. | 3.7 | 2.74 | 1.98 | DLD, mt isoform 1 | NP_000628.2 | 99% | $9 \times 10^{-160}$ | 52.48% | NAD(P)/FAD-dependent oxidoRED | WP_042684715.1 | 88% | $1 \times 10^{-53}$ | 29.70% | GLR1 | NP_015234.1 | 98% | $9 \times 10^{-149}$ | 48.70% |
| 5vdn | Glutathione RED | 449 | *Y. pestis* | FAD | n.a. | 3.73 | 2.41 | 2.66 | glutathione RED, mt isoform 1 | NP_006283.2 | 96% | $4 \times 10^{-161}$ | 53.90% | DLD | WP_075076013.1 | 95% | $5 \times 10^{-61}$ | 32.09% | GLR1 | NP_015234.1 | 96% | $9 \times 10^{-149}$ | 50.75% |
| 4j56 | Trx RED | 504 | *P. falciparum* | FAD/Trx | n.a. | 3.45 | 3.33 | 2.01 | Trx RED 2, mt isoform 1 | NP_001392229.1 | 91% | $6 \times 10^{-146}$ | 45.13% | DLD | WP_075076013.1 | 89% | $3 \times 10^{-51}$ | 26.23% | GLR1 | NP_015234.1 | 89% | $3 \times 10^{-74}$ | 33.47% |
| 1xdi | Flavoprotein Disulfide RED | 499 | *M. tuberculosis* | FAD | KPC | 4.29 | 2.975 | 3.65 | DLD, mt isoform 1 | NP_000099.2 | 91% | $2 \times 10^{-35}$ | 25.49% | DLD | WP_075033768.1 | 91% | $2 \times 10^{-47}$ | 29.12% | DLD | NP_116635.1 | 92% | $8 \times 10^{-35}$ | 26.10% |
| 1mo9 | NAD(P)H2-ketopropyl coenzyme M oxidoRED/carboxylase (2-KPCC) | 523 | *X. autotrophicus* | FAD | n.a. | 4.724 | 2.996 | 3.091 | DLD, mt isoform 1 | NP_000099.2 | 87% | $4 \times 10^{-127}$ | 22.88% | NAD(P)/FAD-dependent oxidoRED | WP_042684715.1 | 69% | $2 \times 10^{-30}$ | 28.65% | DLD | NP_116635.1 | 86% | $2 \times 10^{-22}$ | 22.13% |
| 4k7z | Mercuric RED | 467 | *P. aeruginosa* | FAD/NADP | n.a. | 3.807 | 3.341 | 3.498 | DLD, mt isoform 1 | NP_000099.2 | 97% | $2 \times 10^{-54}$ | 29.32% | DLD | WP_075076013.1 | 94% | $3 \times 10^{-71}$ | 35.68% | DLD | NP_116635.1 | 95% | $3 \times 10^{-51}$ | 29.44% |
| | | | | | | | | | **Outliers** | | | | | | | | | | | | | | |
| 4up3 | Trx RED | 312 | *E. histolytica* | FAD/NADPH | n.a. | 3.59 | 3.76 | 3.76 | (E-actin) monooxygenase MICAL2 isoform f | NP_001269997.1 | 13% | 0.2 | 30.23% | Trx-disulfide RED | WP_075032607.1 | 99% | $8 \times 10^{-68}$ | 37.50% | TRR1 | NP_010640.1 | 98% | $4 \times 10^{-138}$ | 60.83% |
| 5sh3 | Trx RED | 315 | *H. influenzae* | FAD/NADP | n.a. | 2.01 | 3.06 | 4.393 | DLD, mt isoform 1 | NP_000099.2 | 9% | 2.2 | 48.28% | Trx-disulfide RED | WP_075032607.1 | 97% | $3 \times 10^{-76}$ | 39.43% | TRR1 | NP_019174.1 | 97% | $7 \times 10^{-101}$ | 49.85% |
| 1ps9 | 2,4-dienoyl-CoA RED | 671 | *E. coli* | FMN/FAD/NADP | n.a. | 2.02 | 3.93 | 2.16 | L-amino-acid OX isoform 2 | NP_001248946.1 | 6% | 3.1 | 40.48% | NADPH DH NamA | WP_075034681.1 | 49% | $1 \times 10^{-30}$ | 30.00% | NADPH DH | NP_012049.1 | 34% | $3 \times 10^{-19}$ | 26.98% |

Despite the low percentage of identical amino acids showed by sequences sampled by pGenTHREADER with AIF (4bur), NDI (4g73), and NDH-2 (5kmr) sequences (ranging between 15% and 30%, Supplementary Table S2), the sampled crystallized structures showed an overall structure highly similar to that observed for AIF-, NDI-, and NDH-2-crystallized structures. The structural similarity among the sampled structures was quantified by visual inspection and by estimating the RMSD of AIF/NDI/NDH-2 3D coordinates and coordinates of the sampled structures (ranging between 0.8 and 4.5 Å, Table 1).

Cartoon representations of the superimposed AIF, NDI, and NDH-2, and all the pGenTHREADER-sampled structures are reported in Figure 4.

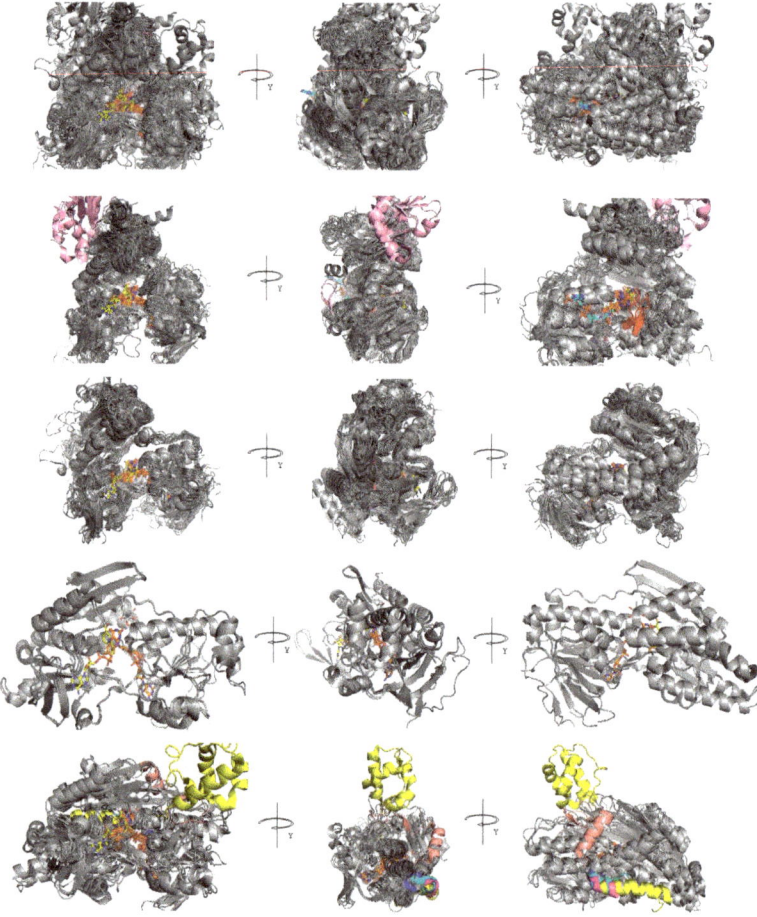

**Figure 4.** Comparative analysis of AIF/NDI/NDH-2/DLD structures. First row: Superimposition of all the sampled 49 crystallized structures (see Table 1). Second to fifth row: superimposition of all the AIF-like proteins, DLD-like proteins, NDI-like proteins, and NDH-2-like proteins, respectively. All the sampled proteins are reported as grey cartoon representations. Specific protein features are colored according to what is reported in the main text at each row. FAD, NADH, UQ, and CoA are reported as orange, yellow, white, and cyan sticks, respectively, where available at the reported crystallized structures, according to Table 1.

Although a common structural trend among all the sampled structures is observed, it is possible to recognize at least three main groups with specific structural features consisting of AIF-like proteins, NDH-2/NDI-like proteins (each with specific features), and lipoamide dehydrogenase-like proteins. The features of each cited group reflect their distribution in the phylogenetic tree (Supplementary Figure S1) built starting from the MSA of the sequences sampled by pGenTHREADER, where it is possible to observe three main groups consisting of AIF-like proteins (including ferredoxin reductases and pyridine nucleotide disulphide CoA NADPH dehydogeanses), NDI-like/NDH-2-like proteins; and other FAD-dependent dehydrogenases (including lipoamide dehydrogenases, thioredoxin reductases, and glutathione reductases).

In detail, the AIF-like protein group contains 20 of the 49 sampled structures. The functional annotation of these 20 sampled structures includes AIF, NADH-oxidase, ferredoxin reductase, rubredoxin reductase, putidaredoxin reductase, and pyridine nucleotide CoA disulfide reductase. The overall structure of those 18 structures overlaps with the human AIF, with an RMSD ranging between 1.06 and 3.1 Å (Table 1). The good superimposition allows to highlight a common cavity hosting a FAD molecule in 14 crystallized structures, a NADH molecule in 2 crystallized structures, and a CoA molecule in 2 crystallized structures, according to Table 1.

A peculiar β-sheet motif located at residues 190–200 of the human AIF (Figure 4) is observed as a specific AIF feature.

Two further structures, namely 3ics.pdb and 3ntd.pdb, annotated as CoA-disulfide reductases, may be associated to the AIF-like protein group. Both the structures host a FAD molecule and a CoA molecule similar to what was observed for 4fx9.pdb and 3cgb.pdb. Nevertheless, both 3ics.pdb and 3ntd.pdb show a 100-aa longer C-terminal domain (residues 461–554 for 3ics.pdb; 471–565 for 3ntd.pdb). Notably, 5vn0.pdb also hosts an oxygen molecule within 3.5 Å from FAD.

The NDH-2/NDI-like protein group contains 7 of the 49 sampled protein structures. Five structures are from bacterial proteins and the other two are from fungal proteins.

The functional annotation of the five sampled bacterial protein structures includes typeII NADH dehydrogenase and sulphide: UQ oxido reductases (Table 1). The related overall structures overlap with the *C. thermarum* NDH-2, with an RMSD ranging between 0.82 and 3.33 Å. The good superimposition allows to highlight a common cavity hosting a FAD molecule in all the five sampled crystallized structures and a NADH molecule in one crystallized structure, according to Table 1.

Notably, 3hyw.pdb hosts a quinone derivative (decylubiquinone, DCQ) and an $H_2S$ molecule (within 3.5 Å from FAD), whereas 5n1t.pdb (a type II NADH dehydrogenase from *Thioalkalivibrio paradoxus*) was crystallized in complex with CytC and copper chaperone [44]. The main differences between the five structures are at the level of their C-terminus portion. Notably, 5jwc.pdb [45] shows a 70-aa long extra loop (residues 363–433, 5jwc.pdb numbering (Figure 4)).

The two NDI-like proteins are both NADH dehydrogenases crystallized from *S. cerevisiae*. The overall structure of the two proteins (as expected from two crystals of the same protein, crystallized in the presence of similar ligands, i.e., UQ-like molecule and stigmatellin) is very similar, with an estimated RMSD of 0.49 Å. From their superimposition, a common cavity hosting an FAD molecule and a NADH molecule is observed. 4g73.pdb hosts a quinone derivative, whereas 5yjw.pdb [46] hosts a stigmatellin bound at the same level of the quinone-binding region. Notably, stigmatellin is known as a competitive NADH-dehydrogenase inhibitor [47] (Figure 4).

The third group of FAD-dependent dehydrogenases contains 19 dehydrogenase structures, with an overall structure more similar to the ones shown by AIF-like proteins. The functional annotation of these 19 sampled structures includes lipoamide dehydrogenases, glutathione amide reductases, thioredoxin reductases, flavoprotein disulfide reductases, mercuric reductases, and NADPH:2-ketopropyl-coenzyme M oxidoreductase/carboxylases (2-KPCC).

The overall structure of those 19 proteins overlap with the human AIF, with an RMSD ranging between 3.22 and 4.84 Å. The further good superimposition allows to highlight a similarly located common cavity hosting a FAD molecule in 16 crystallized structures and a NADH molecule in 2 crystallized structures, according to Table 1.

Notably, 4m52.pdb hosts a sulfonamide derivative [48] located 9 Å far from the FAD molecule (at a region 3 Å far from the UQ-binding region observed in proteins of the previous groups) whereas 1mo9.pdb hosts a ketopropylthioethanesulphonate [49] bound at the same level of the CoA molecule-binding region observed in the first group of protein structures (Figure 4).

Three further structures, namely 4up3.pdb, 5u63.pdb, and 1ps9.pdb annotated as thioredoxin reductases (the first two) or 2,4-dienoyl-CoA reductase (the latter), may be associated to the AIF-like protein group.

Indeed, all the structures host a FAD molecule and a NAD(P)+ molecule. Nevertheless, 4up3 and 5u63 completely lack a region corresponding to the AIF C-terminal domain, shown by all the AIF-like proteins (residues 491-C-ter, 4bur residues numbering, Supplementary Figure S3), whereas 1ps9 contains a different greater domain in correspondence of the N-terminal domain (residues 1–331, 1ps9 residues numbering). 4up3, 5u63, and 1ps9 were maintained in our comparative analyses as outliers for comparative purposes.

*3.4. FAD and NADH Binding Regions*

Beyond the highly similar overall structures shared between AIF (4bur.pdb), NDH-2 (5kmr.pdb), and NDI (4g73.pdb), highlighting a similarly located binding region for FAD and NADH, we also observed that the three superimposed crystal structures also bind those cofactors with glycine residues of the fifth sequence motif and a set of conserved aromatic/basic/acidic residues (Figures 4 and 5) located among the fifth and ninth sequence motif.

The variability observed in the composition of FAD- and NADH-binding regions does not alter the ability of those pockets in efficiently binding the two cofactors, as much as most of the sampled FAD/NADH dependent dehydrogenase structures show a FAD (32 out of the 49 compared crystal structures, see Table 1) and a NADH (8 out of the 49 compared crystal structures, see Table 1, in correspondence of $NADH_b$, according to NADH cofactor nomenclature reported in [26]) molecule at a very similar position (Figure 5D; Supplementary Table S3).

In general, all the investigated dehydrogenase 3D structures show several conserved residues, aligning with residues of the proposed 10 sequence motifs (Figure 2 and Supplementary Figure S2), interacting with FAD and NADH cofactors (Supplementary Table S3), despite the relatively low overall percentage of identical residues (15%–30% range, Supplementary Table S2, on the full length sequences) shared with AIF/NDI/NDH-2 sequences.

*3.5. UQ Binding Site Comparative Analyses between AIF and NDH-2*

Given the crystallization of an UQ-like molecule both in *S. cerevisiae* NDI (4g73.pdb) and in the sulphide: quinone oxidoreductase from *Aquifex aeolicus* (3hyw.pdb), it is also possible to propose residues putatively involved in the UQ binding in orthologous NDH-2/NDI-like proteins sampled from *Bacteria/Fungi* (Table 1).

Notably, for an investigation of the UQ-binding region from *Fungi* NDI-like proteins, it will be sufficient to superpose the crystallized dehydrogenase from *S. cerevisiae* to a comparative model of the fungal protein under investigation and highlight residues within 4 Å from the ubiquinone obtained from the *S. cerevisiae* NDI-crystallized structure (the ones in correspondence of $UQ_I$, according to UQ cofactor nomenclature reported in [25]).

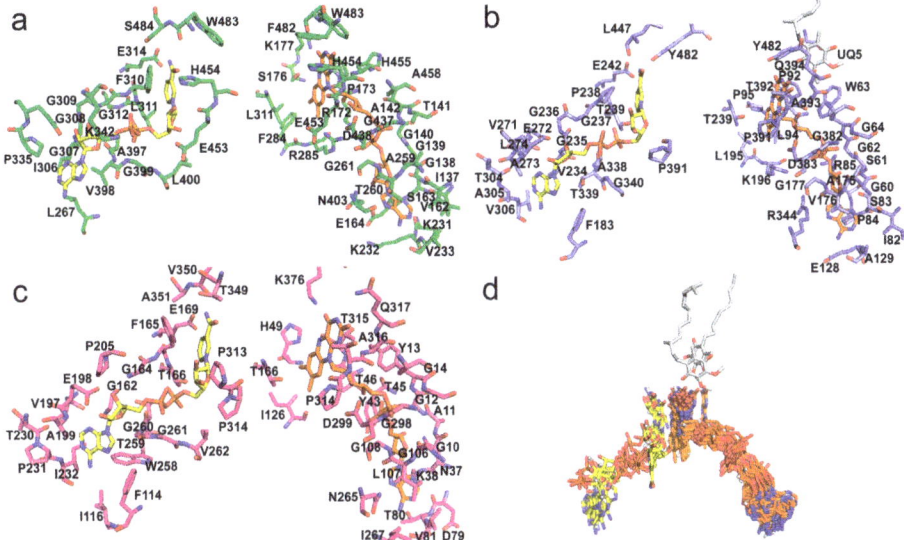

**Figure 5.** AIF/NDI/NDH-2 cofactor-binding regions. Panels (**a**–**c**) Residues within 4 Å from NADH (yellow sticks, corresponding to $NADH_a$ according to NADH cofactor nomenclature reported in [26]) or FAD (orange sticks) for AIF (green sticks from 4bur.pdb), NDI (blue sticks from 4g73.pdb), and NDH-2 (magenta sticks from 5kmr.pdb) are reported and labeled. Panel (**d**) Zoomed-in view of cofactor coordinates from all the investigated proteins obtained by superimposing the sampled crystallized structures (see Table 1). UQ (from 4g73.pdb, corresponding to $UQ_I$, according to UQ cofactor nomenclature reported in [25]) and DCQ (from 3hyw.pdb) are reported as white sticks. See Supplementary Figure S7 for visualizing the other cofactors observed along the superimposition of the investigated crystallized FAD/NADH oxidoreductases (i.e., heme C, CoA, $O_2$, and $H_2S$).

Residues forming the UQ-binding region in NDH-2-like crystallized structures were proposed by superimposing the sampled NDH-2-like structures (Table 1) on *A. aeolicus* sulphide: quinone oxidoreductase and by highlighting residues within 4 Å from DCQ crystallized in complex with the structure of sulphide: quinone oxidoreductase from *A. aeolicus* (Supplementary Table S4).

Notably, residues involved in the UQ-binding region in NDI from *Fungi* and NDH-2-like proteins from *Bacteria* are located between the 9th and 10th sequence motifs and the C-terminal portion.

Given the highly similar overall structure observed between AIF, DLD, and NDH-2/NDI-like proteins and based on recent findings about AIF proteins [11,12], it is proposed that UQ-like molecules may participate in the function of AIF-like proteins and DLD-like proteins. Residues proposed to participate in UQ-like molecule-binding regions in AIF-like proteins and DLD-like proteins were highlighted by selecting residues within 4 Å from the two UQ-like molecules entrapped within AIF-like proteins and DLD-like proteins, after superimposition of the two protein sets with 4g73 and 3hyw (Supplementary Table S4).

Notably, residues involved in the potential UQ-binding region in AIF-like proteins and DLD-like proteins from *Bacteria*, *Metazoa*, and *Plants* are located between 8th, 9th, and 10th sequence motifs and the protein C-terminal portions.

*3.6. Small Molecules and Other Cofactor-Binding Regions*

It should be noticed that most of the crystallized structures among the AIF-like proteins, NDI-like proteins, and NDH-2-like proteins host other small molecules and cofactors in dedicated binding regions or are crystallized in complex with other small proteins (Table 1).

For example, NADH oxidases (among AIF-like proteins) from *Lactobacillus brevis* (5vn0.pdb) and *Lactobacillus sanfrancensis* (2cdu.pdb) host an oxygen molecule and an ADP molecule, respectively; 4 disulphide oxidoreductases from *Bacillus anthracis* (3cgb.pdb and 3ics.pdb), *Pyrococcus horikoshii* (4fx9.pdb), and *Shewanella ioihica* (3ntd.pdb), among AIF-like proteins, host a CoA molecule at a similarly located binding region; the NDH-2-like protein from *T. paradoxus* (5n1t.pdb) was crystallized in complex with CytC and COPC, whereas NDI from *S. cerevisiae* was crystallized in complex with stigmatellin (5yjw); and finally, the NDH-2-like protein from *Plasmodium falciparum* (5jwc) was crystallized in complex with RYL-552 (5n.a.fluoron.a.3n.a.methyln.a.2n.a.{4n.a.(4n.a.(trifluoromethoxy)benzyl)phenyl} quinolinn.a.4(1H)n.a.one).

Notably, also DLD-like proteins were crystallized in complex with small molecules, cofactors, and small proteins, i.e., lipoamide DH from *Mycobacterium tubercolosis* (4m52.pdb) was crystallized in complex with sulphonamide; DLD from *Pseudomonas putida* (6awa.pdb) hosts an AMP molecule; glutathione reductase from *Streptococcus pyogenes* (6n7f.pdb) hosts a riboflavin molecule; NADPH:2-ketopropyl-coenzyme M oxidoreductase from *Xhantobacter autotrophicus* (1mo9.pdb) hosts a ketopropylthioethanesulphonate molecule; whereas DLD from *Geobacillus stearothermophilus* (1ebd.pdb) and thioredoxin reductase from *P. falciparum* (4j56) were crystallized in complex with a fragment of dihydrolipoamide acetyltransferase and thioredoxin, respectively.

While AMP, ADP, riboflavin, and stigmatellin were crystallized in binding regions generally involved in cofactor binding, or overlapping regions, it was observed that disulfide reductases, among AIF-like proteins, host a CoA molecule in a specific binding region consisting of the residues shown in Supplementary Table S5.

Conversely, it was observed that RYL-552 (a quinolinic derivative, see Table 1 and [45]) within NDH-2-like protein from *P. falciparum* (5jwc), SL827 (a sulphonamide derivative, see Table 1 and [48]) within lipoamide DH from *M. tubercolosis* (4m52.pdb), and ketopropylthioethanesulphonate within NADPH:2KPCC oxidoreductase from *Xanthobacterautotrophicus* (1mo9.pdb, [49]) are located at dedicated binding regions involving several species-specific residues not involved in the binding of NADH/FAD/UQ cofactors.

Notably, RYL-552 binds three different binding regions within 5jwc far from the NADH/FAD/UQ cofactor-binding area. While two of those regions appear to be poorly resolved, the third ones appears to be a specific binding cavity [45]. By superimposing 5jwc with the analyzed AIF, NDI, and NDH-2, it appears that NDH-2 and NDI might form several interactions with RYL-552 involving 8 and 11 residues, respectively, that appear to be further well conserved in the sampled NDH-2 and NDI-like proteins (although in the latter, the overlapping binding region appears more buried from the local secondary structure), at variance with the AIF showing a lower number of interacting residues (just four, see Supplementary Table S6 and Supplementary Figure S4). Although AIF-like proteins do not show a well-defined binding pocket in correspondence of RYL-552, at variance with DLD-like proteins showing a sterically hindered/buried region in correspondence withRYL-552, it cannot be excluded that RYL-552 analogs may also bind AIF similarly located accessible binding cavities (Supplementary Figure S4 and Supplementary Figure S5).

The SL827 (a sulphonamide derivative) binding region observed in the lipoamide DH 4m52 consists of few amino acids that appear to be conserved in DLD-like proteins and AIF-like proteins. Notably, by superimposing 4m52 with AIF, NDI, and NDH-2, it appears that NDH-2 and NDI, in correspondence with the sulphonamide derivative binding region, shows a buried region occupied by an a-helical region that most likely will not allow the sulphonamide derivative to penetrate NDI and NDH-2 cofactor-binding regions or affect NDI/NDH-2 activity (Supplementary Figure S4).

Conversely, AIF-like proteins (i.e., 4bur) and DLD-like proteins show an accessible cavity in correspondence with the sulphonamide derivative binding region observed in 4m52 (Supplementary Table S7), making us to purpose that sulphonamide derivatives may target both DLD-like and AIF-like proteins.

The ketopropylthioethanesulphonate (KPC)-binding region observed in 1mo9 (the 2KPCC) consists of few amino acids that appear to be conserved in DLD-like proteins and AIF-like proteins, similar to what observed for sulphonamide. Thus, also, in this case, NDI and NDH-2 show a buried region not accessible to KPC, whereas AIF-like proteins (i.e., 4bur) and DLD-like proteins show an accessible cavity in correspondence with the KPC-binding region observed in 1mo9 (Supplementary Table S7).

Notably, by superimposing DLD-like proteins with disulfide reductases it is possible to observe that the sulphonamide derivative and the KPC bind DLD-like proteins in correspondence of theCoA-binding region detected in disulfide reductases (Supplementary Figure S4).

*3.7. Small Protein Subunit-Binding Regions*

Some of the sampled dehydrogenases were also crystallized in complex with other related protein subunits. i.e., it was observed that flacocytochromecsulphide dehydrogenase from *T. paradoxus* (5n1t.pdb) was crystallized in complex with CytC and a dimeric copper-binding protein (COPC), whereas thioredoxin reductase from *P. falciparum* (4j56.pdb) and DLD from *G.stearothermophilus* (1ebd.pdb), among DLD-like structures, were crystallized in complex with thioredoxin and dihydrolipoamide acetyltransferase, respectively.

By superimposing flavoCytC: sulphide dehydrogenase from *T. paradoxus* with AIF and NDI, it is possible to highlight a binding region of AIF and NDI that is aligned with the flavoCytC: sulphide dehydrogenase protein region involved in interactions with CytC. We observed that the two regions consist of several amino acids located at (or very close to) the 1st, 3rd, 9th, and 10th sequence motifs and at the C-terminal region (Supplementary Table S8 and Figure 6).

From the DLD from *G.stearothermophilus* (1ebd.pdb) crystallized in complex with dihydrolipoamide acetyltransferase, it appears that the 41-aa-long dihydrolipoamide acetyl transferase binding domain may bind at the DLD monomer–monomer interface at the 1ebd C-terminal domain. Some residues close to the 9th and 10th sequence motifs are involved in acetylase binding (Supplementary Table S9)

Similarly, by superimposing one of the sampled thioredoxin reductases to the thioredoxin reductase from *P. falciparum*(4j56.pdb) crystallized in complex with thioredoxin, it is possible to predict a putative binding region for thioredoxin in all the sampled thioredoxin reductases. Notably, by superimposing 4j56 to 4bur, 4g73, and 5kmr, it appears that several residues of 4bur are in the interaction range (below 4 Å) from thioredoxin, whereas 4g73 and 5kmr do not show more than four residues below 4 Å from thioredoxin (Supplementary Table S10).

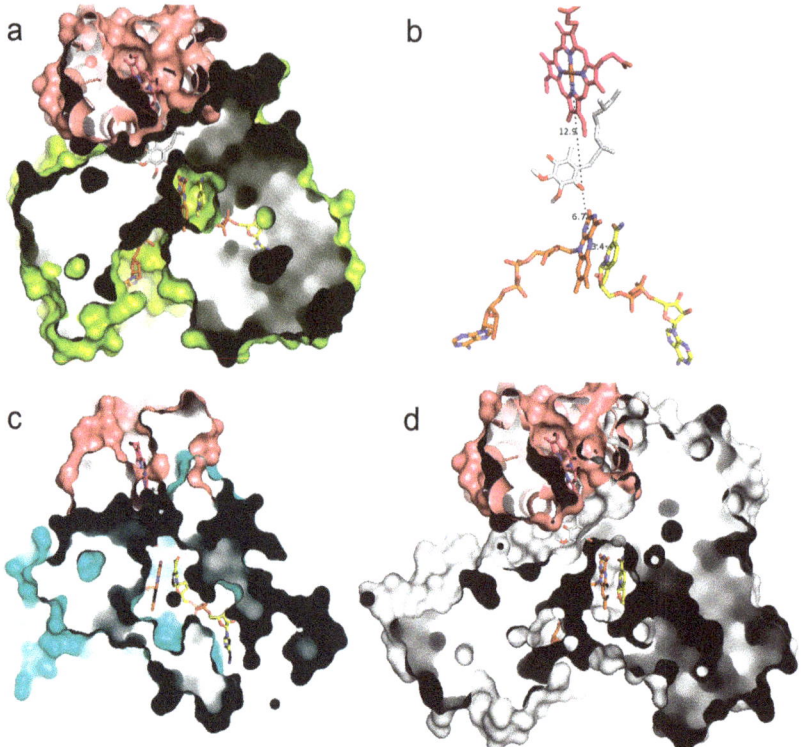

**Figure 6.** AIF/NDI/NDH-2 possible protein–protein interaction surfaces. Panel (**a**) Zoomed-in views of the crystallized heterodimeric structure of flavoprotein dehydrogenase (yellow surf representation) and CytC (pink surf representation) from *T. paradoxus* (5n1t.pdb) is reported in complex with FAD, (orange sticks), the heme C center in magenta sticks and NADH and UQ (yellow and white sticks, respectively, obtained by superimposition with 4g73 (see methods)). Panel (**b**) FAD, NADH, heme C center (from 5n1t.pdb), and UQ (superimposed from 4g73.pdb) are reported in stick representations. Intermolecular distances are reported by dashed lines and are labeled. Panel (**c,d**) 3D models of a putative heterodimeric structure of AIF (4bur.pdb) or NDI (4g73) proteins (cyan or white cartoon, respectively) in complex with CytC from *T. paradoxus* (5n1t.pdb). FAD, NADH, and UQ are reported in stick representations (see previous panels for colors).

## 4. Discussion

Among the investigated FAD-dependent dehydrogenases, it is possible to recognize AIF, NADH oxidases/nitrile reductases, ferredoxin reductases, rubredoxin reductases, toluene 2,3-dioxygenase reductases, putidaredoxin reductases, pyridine nucleotide-CoA disulfide oxidoreductases, NDH-2 and NDI, flavocytochrome c sulfide dehydrogenases, sulfide: quinone oxidoreductases, DLD, glutathione amide reductases, thioredoxin reductases, mercuric reductases, and NADPH:2-ketopropyl-CoM oxidoreductase/carboxylases.

Among the 49 sampled dehydrogenase structures, 20 show an AIF-like structure, 5 show an NDH-2-like structure, 2 show an NDI-like structure, and 19 show a DLD-like structure.

By superimposing all the investigated dehydrogenase structures, it is possible to observe that all of them have the same overall structure. Moreover, 46 out of the 49 investigated dehydrogenases host a FAD molecule in the same position, whereas 9 of the 49 host an NADH molecule in the same position.

Notably, 3 out of the 49 dehydrogenase structures host a UQ-like molecule, whereas 4 out of the 49 host a CoA molecule at two dedicated similarly located binding regions.

*4.1. A Similarly Located FAD/NADH-Binding Region for All the Investigated Flavoprotein Oxidoreductases and New Clues about a Putative UQ-Binding Region*

Our analysis has allowed to predict the exact localization of NADH and FAD-binding regions among orthologous sequences of the investigated AIF-like, NDI-like, and NDH-2-like proteins. NADH and FAD-binding regions are also similarly located within DLD-like proteins. Furthermore, based on NDI and NDH-2 available structures, MSA, and recently published functional studies about AIF dehydrogenase activity [11], it may be speculated that AIF proteins may also bind a UQ molecule to participate to oxidative pathways crucial for mitochondrial respiration. Notably, our analysis has allowed to propose the existence of a putative binding region for UQ within the different investigated FAD/NADH-dependent oxidoreductases, including AIF-like proteins, that do not show a solved UQ molecule in the available crystallized structures. Considering DLD, it was already proposed that UQ might be reduced by lipoamide DH [50], although there is no evidence of a putative DLD UQ-binding region. Based on our comparative analyses, it may be speculated that the UQ-binding region within DLD is at the same level of the UQ-binding region highlighted within AIF after superimposition with NDI/NDH-2.

*4.2. Concerns about the Opportunity to Draw New Inhibitors to be Used as Antibiotic/Antiparasitic Drugs, Directed Against the Investigated FAD/NADH Dehydrogenases*

New insights have been acquired about the investigated species-specific FAD/NADH dependent oxidoreductases that raise the question about the opportunity to draw new antibiotic/antiparasitic drugs directed against the cited FAD/NADH-dependent oxidoreductases.

Currently, some of the described FAD/NADH-dependent oxidoreductases are considered in microbiology a crucial target of antibiotics or chemotherapeutics (i.e., those structurally related to RYL-552, a quinolinic derivative or to SL827, a sulphonamide derivative [10,48,51–53]) because those enzymes play a fundamental role for the ATP synthesis and oxidative pathways in most microorganisms. The lack of NDH-2-orthologous enzymes in *Mammalia* was retained an important proof of the selective action of potential drug development [10,54–57].

Although RYL-552 and SL827 appear to target specific binding regions within NDH-2/NDI and DLD bacterial proteins, respectively, given the high structural similarity and the similarly located cofactor-binding regions highlighted in the investigated FAD/NADH-dependent oxidoreductases, it will be necessary to ascertain the absence of interactions with the human AIF/DLD-accessible cavities, before using RYL-552/SL827 structurally related ligands in new preclinical/clinical trials.

Similarly, SL827 and KPC analogs were proposed as chemicals for selective targeting of *M. tuberculosis* DLD and *X. autotrophicus* NADPH-CoM oxidoreductase. However, human DLD/AIF proteins show accessible cavities in correspondence of theSL827/KPC-binding regions observed within *M. tuberculosis* DLD and *X. autotrophicus* NADPH-CoM oxidoreductase. Thus, for SL827/KPC structurally related ligands, it will also be necessary to exclude putative interactions with human AIF/DLD proteins to guarantee the microorganism selectivity of both molecules and to avoid undesirable side effects due to interactions with the human mitochondrial FAD/NADH-dependent oxidoreductases. Notably, antibiotics that might be considered structurally related to SL827, such as sulfamethoxazole/trimethoprim and sulfisoxazole, although commercialized for several years, are known for their serious side effects [58]. It cannot be excluded that those adverse reactions may be ascribed to interactions between the cited antibiotics and AIF/DLD human proteins.

Finally, it should also be noticed that CoA disulfide reductases, structurally related to AIF/DLD-like proteins, host a CoA molecule in correspondence of the SL827/KPC-binding region. The presence of a CoA molecule in CoA disulfide redutases, at the level of the SL827/KPC-binding region observed in the homologous AIF/DLD-like proteins, raises the question about possible competitive effects between SL827/KPC structurally related ligands and disulfide reductases CoA-binding regions that may decrease the efficiency and selectivity of SL827/KPC structurally related ligands.

*4.3. New Clues in Support of AIF Participation in Mitochondrial Respiration*

Based on the performed comparative analyses, it was possible to propose that flavoprotein oxidoreductase interaction surfaces are involved in the binding of other protein subunits involved in respiratory mechanisms (i.e., a putative AIF-binding region for CytC, after comparison with flavocytochrome c sulfide DH from *T. paradoxus*).

Considering (a) the role played by NDH-2/NDI-like proteins in bacterial/fungal respiration [7,25], (b) the direct interaction between a *T. paradoxus* flavoprotein oxidoreductase and a CytC-like protein [44], and (c) the recently proposed rotenone sensitive NADH:UQ oxidoreductase activity of AIF [11,12], it could be speculated that a direct interaction between AIF and CytC and other mitochondrial copper-binding proteins of the inner membrane [59–61] might also exist in *Metazoan* mitochondria, with several implications regarding AIF participation in mitochondrial respiration. These data are coherent with previous observations about alternative respiratory protein complexes [62–65].

Concerning the above reported hypothesis, we should recall that the incomplete NADH consumption along mitochondrial respiration assays performed in the presence of high concentrations of rotenone and other respiratory protein–complex inhibitors, as well as the protective role played by AIF in the maintenance of respiratory chain complexes, are well documented [22,66–68].

Thus, it appears that other mitochondrial enzymes may contribute to the buffering of altered $NAD^+/NADH$ ratios by oxidizing alternatively cytosolic NADH or mitochondrial matrix NADH, and here, we might speculate that AIF, being anchored to the mitochondrial inner membrane, protruding into the intermembrane space, may participate in the regulation of the $NAD^+/NADH$ or $FAD/FADH2$ (maybe $UQ/UQH2$) ratio. AIF participation in the regulation of redox signaling between mitochondria and other cell compartments may be crucial above all in those tissues in which the G3P shuttle [69], nicotinamide nucleotide transhydrogenase (NNT) [70], NADH-b5 oxidoreductase [71,72], or malate/aspartate shuttle [15,73,74] do not work properly or when the cited proteins, mitochondrial oxidative phosphorylation complex subunits, or matrix proteins are mutated or downregulated [75,76]. If AIF behaves as a NADH dehydrogenase, able to oxidize cytosolic NADH, it may also participate in reprogramming metabolic pathways, providing new clues towards the full comprehension of the puzzling Warburg effect condition [77].

Notably, quinoline 3-sulfonamides were recently proposed to be a class of high-affinity (bioactive in the nM range) lactic dehydrogenase inhibitors [78] that may be employed in cancer therapies. However, quinoline 3-sulfonamides are ligands structurally related both to RYL-552 and, although at a lower extent, to quinone-related structures (i.e., stigmatellin or menaquinone) known to be able to inhibit or bind NDI/NDH-2-like proteins. Thus, it appears that it will be necessary in the near future to ascertain putative activity/affinity of quinoline 3-sulfonamides for NDI/NDH-2 and also for AIF/DLD-like proteins.

Based on the above reported observations, the redox path proposed in Figure 7, and the available crystallized structures, we propose that NDH-2, NDI, and AIF proteins may have two binding regions for NADH and two further binding regions for UQ-analogous molecules to work correctly, according to what proposed by [25,26]. The need for having two molecules for each cofactor may reflect the necessity to bind to specific binding pockets with different affinities for the entry/exit of oxidized/reduced cofactors, similar to what proposed for other quinol-dependent oxidases [30,79].

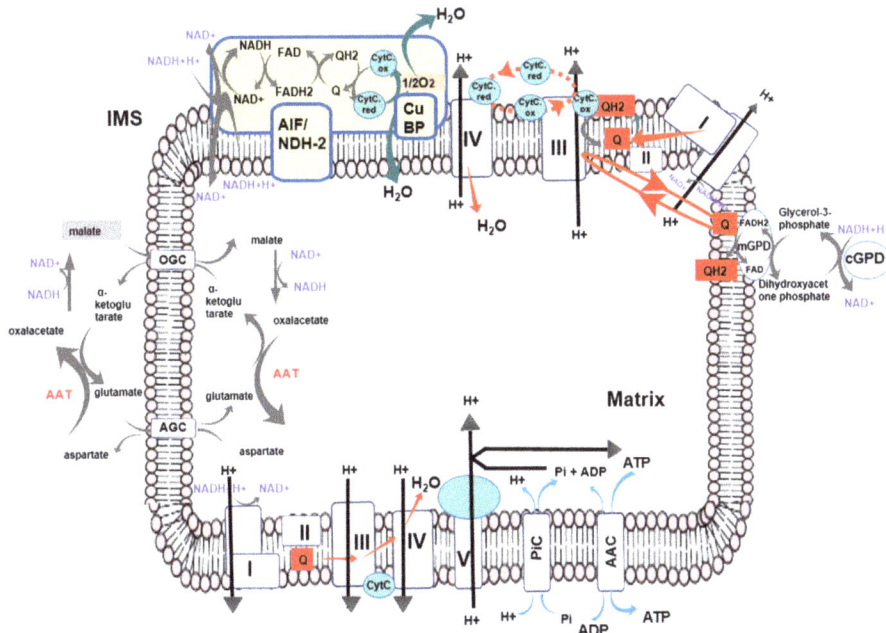

**Figure 7.** Scheme representation describing the putative participation of AIF to mitochondrial respiration. Cofactors involved in the reaction $NAD^+$ to NADH, FAD to FADH2, a quinone derivative (Q) to the corresponding quinol derivative (QH2), and CytC.ox to CytC.red are indicated by labels. Respiratory chain complexes (I, II, III, and IV) and the ATP-synthase, ADP/ATP Carrier (AAC), phosphate carrier (PiC), malate/aspartate shuttle protein members (with the two carriers OGC and AGC) and the glycerol-3-phosphate dehydrogenase (GPD) shuttle members are reported to show a putative context of action in mitochondrial redox pathways for AIF. A putative copper-binding protein (CuBP) is also indicated. IMS = Intermembrane Space.

Notably, Ferreira et al. [26] proposed that a high $NADH/NAD^+$ ratio may facilitate the formation of the AIF: NADH complex, which may trigger AIF dimerization and cell death induction, through the cleavage of the first 102 residues of AIF [22,26], the following release of $AIF_{\Delta 1-102}$ from mitochondria, and its translocation to the nucleus, where AIF (complexed with MIF [24]) mediates chromatinolysis. This hypothesis was based on AIF-crystallized structures solved by Ferreira et al. [26]. In detail, Ferreira et al. have provided a crystal structure of AIF in the presence of one FAD molecule (that they called the oxidized $hAIF_{\Delta 1-102ox}$, available as a single monomer under the PDB code 4bv6.pdb, [26]), and one further AIF structure in the presence of both FAD and NADH (that they called the reduced $hAIF_{\Delta 1-102rd}$: NAD(H), available as a dimer of homodimers under the PDB code 4bur.pdb, [26]).

Both the obtained crystallized structures 4bur and 4bv6 lack a protein region at the level of the protein segment including residues 509–560, defined by the authors as the apoptogenic segment [26]. In detail, 4bur lacks the 517–552 region (see 4bur, chain B), whereas 4bv6 lacks atomic coordinates for the 546–558 protein region (see the single chain of 4bv6). It should be noticed that the missing regions are close to the $NADH_b$-binding region (according to NADH cofactor nomenclature reported in [26])and in correspondence with the$UQ_{II}$NDH-2-binding region (according to UQ cofactor nomenclature reported in [25]).

In light of these observations and according to [26], it might also be speculated that NADH presence (i.e., a high $NADH/NAD^+$ ratio) can make more exposed/accessible AIF redox catalytic sites for UQ-like ligands that may participate in the re-oxidation of NADH mediated by FAD. Conversely, a high NAD$^+$/NADH ratio may induce conformational changes that lower the affinity of NADH and UQ-like molecules for AIF catalytic pockets.

Nevertheless, Miseviciene et al. [12] showed that AIF has quinone reductase activity (expressed as the $k_{cat}/K_m$ ratio) $10^2$- to $10^4$-fold lower than that of cytochrome P450 reductase and NAD(P)H: quinone oxidoreductase (NQO1) and $10^1$- to $10^2$-fold lower than that of *Mammalian* thioredoxin reductase but is comparable with the activity of glutathione reductase from various sources (see [12] and references therein).

However, the low quinone reductase activity exerted by the recombinant AIF investigated by Miseviciene et al. may also in part be ascribed to the fact that Miseviciene et al. used for their analyses the AIF$_{\Delta 1-77}$ protein domain [12] instead of the AIF$_{\Delta 1-52}$ protein domain, be the latter the complete protein domain responsible for redox activity [22,80]. It will be necessary to use AIF$_{\Delta 1-52}$ recombinant protein for checking/re-estimating AIF quinone reductase activity and compare it with the recently quinone reductase activity mediated by the *Mammalian* complex I [81].

Concerning the dimerization process, it should also be noticed that, beyond missing residues at the 509–560 AIF region, both 4bur and 4bv6 [12] crystallized structures lack the first 124 and thus it cannot be excluded that the missing fragments at the C-terminal domain (at the level of residues 509–560) and at the N-terminal domain may facilitate a non-physiological multimerization process.

In support of the lack of clarity about dimerization processes and cofactor access, it is observed that in correspondence of the protein region containing the missing portions in 4bur/4bv6 (residues 509–560), 4bv6 also shows the crystallized C-terminal region (Ile610, 4bv6 residues numbering) located between the two termini (Pro545 and Asp559, 4bv6 residues numbering) of the non-solved portion. Furthermore, the mercuric reductase (4k7z.pdb) from *P. aeruginosa* hosts a mercuric ion in a region partially overlapping with the AIF 546-558 (4bv6 residues numbering) protein region.

All these observations make possible to hypothesize the putative involvement of a metal ion that might locate at the level of the AIF 546-558 (4bv6 residues numbering) missing residues. The presence of a metal ion working as a further cofactor might reveal crucial for the correct protein function and/or redox mechanism.

More in general solving the structure of the missing fragments at the N-/C-terminal regions and at the level of 509-560 AIF protein region will help in elucidating conformational changes responsible both for cofactor entry in the AIF catalytic site and dimerization/multimerization processes.

On this concern it should finally be noticed that the proposed distance between FAD and UQ (obtained by superimposition as previously described) as well as the distance between UQ and CytC (obtained by superimposition as previously described) in AIF would be below 13 Å, which is in the useful distance-range for allowing electron tunneling [30], although the proposed AIF-UQ-binding region appears to be less accessible than its counterpart in NDH-2 and NDI. Also, the presence of an oxygen molecule (obtained by superimposition with 5vn0.pdb, as previously described) as well as an H$_2$S molecule (3hyw.pdb) in the investigated crystallized structures (see Supplementary Figure S7) makes us think that several investigated flavoprotein dehydrogenases may show in the future other unsuspected abilities.

*4.4. Pieces of Evidence about the Possible Targeting of AIF for the Development of New Treatments for Mitochondrial Dysfunction in Rare Diseases*

If AIF participation to mitochondrial respiration would be ascertained, AIF protein may be considered as a target for the stimulation of mitochondrial function for the development of new treatments for diseases characterized by mitochondrial dysfunction.

If an UQ structurally related ligand-binding region would be highlighted experimentally on the recombinant protein, according to what reported above, we would expect that several UQ structurally related drugs used for the treatment of mitochondrial diseases may improve patient conditions by stimulating mitochondrial function through AIF. On this concern, it could be speculated that UQ structurally related approved drugs, like EPI-743, Idebenone [82], and KH176 [83], may exert their effect also by targeting the AIF UQ-derivative-binding region.

At the moment, it is proposed that EPI-743 and Idebenone may act on complex I [47,84] whereas KH-176 would interact with the thioredoxin system [83].

Nevertheless, if complex I subunits are mutated, above all, if mutations are located close to the proposed CoQ-binding region, it would be difficult that a greater availability of the cited cofactors (or structurally related ligands) might rescue complex I defect, acting directly on the same complex I activity.

Conversely, because of the similarity between KH-176 (and its precursors, i.e., Trolox), EPI-743, Idebenone, and UQ, it may be speculated that KH-176, EPI-743, and Idebenone may target an UQ analog-binding region in a functional protein participating to mitochondrial respiration.

According to [83], the most probable binding region of KH-176 could be located within the thioredoxin reductase (TrxR1). Nevertheless, TrxR1 shows a highly similar overall structure with AIF-like proteins and appears to be even more similar to DLD-like proteins (Supplementary Figure S6). Thus, it might be speculated that KH-176 may also target AIF and DLD, beyond TrxR1, at the proposed similarly located UQ-binding region (Supplementary Table S4).

*4.5. Conclusions*

The presented computational strategy, based on the combination of sequence database screening and fold recognition methods, will allow clinicians and biomedical researchers to identify/highlight "structurally related proteins", shared from *Bacteria*, *Protista*, *Fungi*, *Metazoan*, and *Plants*, not detectable using only sequence alignment-based search tools, to choose the target of new drugs under investigation with greater confidence aiming to reduce off-target effects.

The possibility to target a species/specific enzyme becomes crucial in the battle against antibiotic resistance. Indeed, it is known that several *Bacteria* have become resistant to antibiotics directed against enzymes involved in cell wall synthesis, cell membrane function, protein and nucleic acid biosynthesis, and antimetabolites.

To overcome the problems related to antimicrobial resistance, medical scientists are starting to target the cellular energy-generating machinery [78] and, in general, enzymes regulating crucial respiration/oxidative pathways in pathogenic microorganisms [54,85–87].

Notably, new chemicals directed against FAD/NADH oxidoreductases are already approved drugs and/or are being tested in preclinical/clinical trials [53,82,83]. Given our findings, clinicians and biomedical researchers could now test drugs designed for the targeting of FAD/NADH oxidoreductases (NDH-2/TrxR1 like, from *Bacteria*, *Fungi*, or *Protista*) on human mitochondria to exclude deleterious interactions with human mitochondrial proteins (i.e., AIF, DLD, and TrxR1), ascribable to the common origin shared by mitochondria from *Metazoans* and *Protista* [88] and, in general by mitochondria and *Bacteria* [89,90].

At the same time, the proposed strategy will allow clinicians and biomedical researchers to link putative adverse effects, following the administration of new drugs directed against bacterial/fungal/protista FAD/NADH oxidoreductase (NDH-2/TrxR1-like) proteins to unpredicted interactions with human structurally related AIF/DLD/TrxR1.

Furthermore, the proposed comparative analyses might help clinicians and medical researchers to evaluate the possibility of considering FAD/NADH oxidoreductases as a possible target of new small molecules that are able to modulate mitochondrial respiration in patients affected by rare diseases or cancers characterized by a severe mitochondrial dysfunction.

## 5. Patents

The presented data are part of the Italian patent: Pierri et al., 2019; Computational methods for the identification of FAD/NADH dehydrogenases binding regions for drug design and discovery; IT Patent 102019000022545.

*J. Clin. Med.* **2019**, *8*, 2117

**Supplementary Materials:** The following are available online at http://www.mdpi.com/2077-0383/8/12/2117/s1, Figure S1: Phylogenetic tree of the crystallized AIF/NDH-2/NDI-homologous proteins, Figure S2: AIF/NDI/NDH-2 conserved sequence motifs within other homologous FAD/NADH-dependent crystallized dehydrogenases, Figure S3: 3D structure of FAD/NADH-dependent dehydrogenases used as outliers, Figure S4: Cartoon representation of the superimposition of AIF, DLD, NDH-2, NADPH-CoMoxidoreductase, CoA disulfide reductase, and NDI in the presence of cofactors NADH, FAD, UQ, and CoA and inhibitors RYL-552, SL827, and KPC, Figure S5: Surf representation of the superimposition of AIF, DLD, NDH-2, and NDI and putative interactions with the quinoline derivative RYL-552, Figure S6: Comparative analysis of AIF/DLD/TrxR1-crystallized structures, Figure S7: Zoomed-in view of FAD/NADH/UQ/HemeC/CoA/$O_2$/$H_2S$ ligand coordinates from all the investigated proteins obtained by superimposing the sampled crystallized structures (see Table 1), Table S1: Similarity/identity matrix of the listed 41 protein sequences sampled by Blastp and used for generating Figure 2 about sequence motifs, Table S2: Similarity/identity matrix of the listed 49 protein sequences sampled by pGenTHREADER, Table S3: FAD and NADH-binding residues of the crystallized structures reported in Table 1 after their superimposition, Table S4:UQ/DCQ-binding residues of the crystallized structures reported in Table 1 after their superimposition, Table S5: CoA-binding residues of the crystallized CoA disulfide reductases reported in Table 1, Table S6: RYL-552-binding residues of the crystallized NDH-2 (5jwc) from *P. falciparum*, Table S7: SL827 and KPC-binding residues within the crystallized DLD (4m52) from *M.tuberculosis* and NADPH-CoM oxidoreductase (1mo9) from *X.autotrophicus*, Table S8:CytC and CopC (copper-binding proteins)-binding residues of the crystallized NDH-2 dehydrogenase (5n1t) from *T. paradox*, Table S9: Lipoamide acetylase-binding residues of the crystallized DLD (1ebd) from *G.stearothermophilus*, Table S10: Thioredoxin reductase-binding residues of the crystallized Trx red (4j56) from *P. falciparum*.

**Author Contributions:** The author(s) have made the following declarations about their contributions: Conceptualization, A.D.G. and C.L.P.; Data curation, L.T., N.G., R.G., M.M., L.L. and F.C.; Formal analysis, L.T. and N.G.; Methodology, R.G., M.M., M.V., A.D.G. and C.L.P.; Supervision, M.V., A.D.G. and C.L.P.; Writing—original draft, M.V., A.D.G. and C.L.P.; Writing—review & editing, M.V., A.D.G. and C.L.P.

**Acknowledgments:** Authors would like to thank the Italian Association for Mitochondrial Research (www.mitoairm.it) and Mitocon (www.mitocon.it), IT resources made available by ReCaS, a project funded by the MIUR (Italian Ministry for Education, University and Re-search) in the "PON Ricerca e Competitività 2007–2013-Azione I-Interventi di rafforzamentostrutturale" PONa3_00052, Avviso 254/Ric, University of Bari ("Fondi Ateneo ex-60%" 2016"; "ProgettoCompetitivo 2018" and "FFABR 2017-2018"). Authors would also like to thank MIUR for having funded the project "Salute, alimentazione, qualità della vita": individuazione di un set di biomarker dell'apoptosi" for an innovative industrial PhD course—PON RI 2014-2020, CUP H92H18000160006. Authors would also like to thank Giovanni Lentini (Pharmaceutical Chemist); Luigi Leonardo Palese (Biochemist); Giuseppe Petrosillo (Biochemist), Domenico Marzulli (Biochemist); Fabrizio Bossis (Chemist), Francesco Busto (Biotechnologist) and Elena Marvulli (Biotechnologist) for stimulating discussions. This paper is dedicated to the memory of our Michele Montaruli, coauthor of this paper, that passed away, aged 38, too soon, after having devoted his young life to generosity, studying and teaching.

**Conflicts of Interest:** The authors declare no conflict of interest. The funders had no role in the design of the study; in the collection, analyses, or interpretation of data; in the writing of the manuscript, or in the decision to publish the results.

## Abbreviations

| | | | |
|---|---|---|---|
| AIF | Apoptosis-inducing factor | DH | dehydrogenase |
| LD | lipoamide dehydrogenase | DLD | dihydrolipoyl dehydrogenase or dihydrolipoamide dehydrogenase |
| OX | oxidase | RED | reductase |
| GLR1 | glutathione disulfide reductase | Trx | Thioredoxin |
| mt | mitochondrial | TRR1 | Trx-disulfide reductase 1 |
| MSA | multiple sequence alignment | RMSD | root-mean-square deviation |
| MIF | migration inhibitory factor | RYL-552 | 5n.a.fluoron.a.3n.a.methyln.a.2n.a.{4n.a.(4n.a.(trifluoromethoxy)benzyl)phenyl} quinolinn.a.4(1H)n.a.one) |
| SL827 | N~2~-((2-amino-5-bromopyridin-3-yl) sulfonyl)-N-(4-methoxyphenyl)- N~2~-methylglycinamide | KPC | Ketopropylthioethanesulphonate |
| CytC | cytochrome c | $NAD^+$ | nicotinamide adenine dinucleotide |
| FAD | flavin adenine dinucleotide | UQ | ubiquinone |
| CoA | Coenzyme A | | |

## References

1. Verdin, E. NAD⁺ in aging, metabolism, and neurodegeneration. *Science* **2015**, *350*, 1208–1213. [CrossRef] [PubMed]
2. Bogachev, A.V.; Baykov, A.A.; Bertsova, Y.V. Flavin transferase: The maturation factor of flavin-containing oxidoreductases. *Biochem. Soc. Trans.* **2018**, *46*, 1161–1169. [CrossRef] [PubMed]
3. Harold, L.K.; Antoney, J.; Ahmed, F.H.; Hards, K.; Carr, P.D.; Rapson, T.; Greening, C.; Jackson, C.J.; Cook, G.M. FAD-sequestering proteins protect mycobacteria against hypoxic and oxidative stress. *J. Biol. Chem.* **2019**, *294*, 2903–2912. [CrossRef] [PubMed]
4. Eggink, G.; Engel, H.; Vriend, G.; Terpstra, P.; Witholt, B. Rubredoxin reductase of Pseudomonas oleovorans. Structural relationship to other flavoprotein oxidoreductases based on one NAD and two FAD fingerprints. *J. Mol. Biol.* **1990**, *212*, 135–142. [CrossRef]
5. Ross, R.P.; Claiborne, A. Molecular cloning and analysis of the gene encoding the NADH oxidase from Streptococcus faecalis 10C1. Comparison with NADH peroxidase and the flavoprotein disulfide reductases. *J. Mol. Biol.* **1992**, *227*, 658–671. [CrossRef]
6. Kuriyan, J.; Krishna, T.S.; Wong, L.; Guenther, B.; Pahler, A.; Williams, C.H.; Model, P. Convergent evolution of similar function in two structurally divergent enzymes. *Nature* **1991**, *352*, 172–174. [CrossRef]
7. Heikal, A.; Nakatani, Y.; Dunn, E.; Weimar, M.R.; Day, C.L.; Baker, E.N.; Lott, J.S.; Sazanov, L.A.; Cook, G.M. Structure of the bacterial type II NADH dehydrogenase: A monotopic membrane protein with an essential role in energy generation. *Mol. Microbiol.* **2014**, *91*, 950–964. [CrossRef]
8. Vinogradov, A.D.; Grivennikova, V.G. Oxidation of NADH and ROS production by respiratory complex I. *Biochim. Biophys. Acta* **2016**, *1857*, 863–871. [CrossRef]
9. Titov, D.V.; Cracan, V.; Goodman, R.P.; Peng, J.; Grabarek, Z.; Mootha, V.K. Complementation of mitochondrial electron transport chain by manipulation of the NAD+/NADH ratio. *Science* **2016**, *352*, 231–235. [CrossRef]
10. Blaza, J.N.; Bridges, H.R.; Aragão, D.; Dunn, E.A.; Heikal, A.; Cook, G.M.; Nakatani, Y.; Hirst, J. The mechanism of catalysis by type-II NADH:quinone oxidoreductases. *Sci. Rep.* **2017**, *7*, 40165. [CrossRef]
11. Elguindy, M.M.; Nakamaru-Ogiso, E. Apoptosis-inducing Factor (AIF) and Its Family Member Protein, AMID, Are Rotenone-sensitive NADH:Ubiquinone Oxidoreductases (NDH-2). *J. Biol. Chem.* **2015**, *290*, 20815–20826. [CrossRef] [PubMed]
12. Misevičien, L.; Anusevičius, Ž.; Šarlauskas, J.; Sevrioukova, I.F.; Čnas, N. Redox reactions of the FAD-containing apoptosis-inducing factor (AIF) with quinoidal xenobiotics: A mechanistic study. *Arch. Biochem. Biophys.* **2011**, *512*, 183–189. [CrossRef]
13. Iwata, M.; Lee, Y.; Yamashita, T.; Yagi, T.; Iwata, S.; Cameron, A.D.; Maher, M.J. The structure of the yeast NADH dehydrogenase (Ndi1) reveals overlapping binding sites for water- and lipid-soluble substrates. *Proc. Natl. Acad. Sci. USA* **2012**, *109*, 15247–15252. [CrossRef] [PubMed]
14. Sousa, F.M.; Sena, F.V.; Batista, A.P.; Athayde, D.; Brito, J.A.; Archer, M.; Oliveira, A.S.F.; Soares, C.M.; Catarino, T.; Pereira, M.M. The key role of glutamate 172 in the mechanism of type II NADH:quinone oxidoreductase of Staphylococcus aureus. *Biochim. Biophys. Acta Bioenerg.* **2017**, *1858*, 823–832. [CrossRef] [PubMed]
15. Amoedo, N.D.; Punzi, G.; Obre, E.; Lacombe, D.; De Grassi, A.; Pierri, C.L.; Rossignol, R. AGC1/2, the mitochondrial aspartate-glutamate carriers. *Biochim. Biophys. Acta* **2016**, *1863*, 2394–2412. [CrossRef]
16. Le Bras, M.; Clément, M.V.; Pervaiz, S.; Brenner, C. Reactive oxygen species and the mitochondrial signaling pathway of cell death. *Histol. Histopathol.* **2005**, *20*, 205–219.
17. Todd, A.E.; Orengo, C.A.; Thornton, J.M. Evolution of protein function, from a structural perspective. *Curr. Opin. Chem. Biol.* **1999**, *3*, 548–556. [CrossRef]
18. Todd, A.E.; Orengo, C.A.; Thornton, J.M. Evolution of function in protein superfamilies, from a structural perspective. *J. Mol. Biol.* **2001**, *307*, 1113–1143. [CrossRef]
19. Zamzami, N.; Kroemer, G. The mitochondrion in apoptosis: How Pandora's box opens. *Nat. Rev. Mol. Cell Biol.* **2001**, *2*, 67–71. [CrossRef]
20. Modjtahedi, N.; Giordanetto, F.; Madeo, F.; Kroemer, G. Apoptosis-inducing factor: Vital and lethal. *Trends Cell Biol.* **2006**, *16*, 264–272. [CrossRef]
21. Joza, N.; Pospisilik, J.A.; Hangen, E.; Hanada, T.; Modjtahedi, N.; Penninger, J.M.; Kroemer, G. AIF: Not just an apoptosis-inducing factor. *Ann. N.Y. Acad. Sci.* **2009**, *1171*, 2–11. [CrossRef] [PubMed]

22. Bano, D.; Prehn, J.H.M. Apoptosis-Inducing Factor (AIF) in Physiology and Disease: The Tale of a Repented Natural Born Killer. *EBioMedicine* **2018**, *30*, 29–37. [CrossRef] [PubMed]
23. Ravagnan, L.; Roumier, T.; Kroemer, G. Mitochondria, the killer organelles and their weapons. *J. Cell. Physiol.* **2002**, *192*, 131–137. [CrossRef] [PubMed]
24. Wang, Y.; An, R.; Umanah, G.K.; Park, H.; Nambiar, K.; Eacker, S.M.; Kim, B.; Bao, L.; Harraz, M.M.; Chang, C.; et al. A nuclease that mediates cell death induced by DNA damage and poly(ADP-ribose) polymerase-1. *Science* **2016**, *354*, aad6872. [CrossRef] [PubMed]
25. Feng, Y.; Li, W.; Li, J.; Wang, J.; Ge, J.; Xu, D.; Liu, Y.; Wu, K.; Zeng, Q.; Wu, J.W.; et al. Structural insight into the type-II mitochondrial NADH dehydrogenases. *Nature* **2012**, *491*, 478–482. [CrossRef]
26. Ferreira, P.; Villanueva, R.; Martínez-Júlvez, M.; Herguedas, B.; Marcuello, C.; Fernandez-Silva, P.; Cabon, L.; Hermoso, J.A.; Lostao, A.; Susin, S.A.; et al. Structural insights into the coenzyme mediated monomer-dimer transition of the pro-apoptotic apoptosis inducing factor. *Biochemistry* **2014**, *53*, 4204–4215. [CrossRef]
27. Pierri, C.L.; Parisi, G.; Porcelli, V. Computational approaches for protein function prediction: A combined strategy from multiple sequence alignment to molecular docking-based virtual screening. *Biochim. Biophys. Acta* **2010**, *1804*, 1695–1712. [CrossRef]
28. Han, X.; Sit, A.; Christoffer, C.; Chen, S.; Kihara, D. A global map of the protein shape universe. *PLoS Comput. Biol.* **2019**. [CrossRef]
29. Knoverek, C.R.; Amarasinghe, G.K.; Bowman, G.R. Advanced Methods for Accessing Protein Shape-Shifting Present New Therapeutic Opportunities. *Trends Biochem. Sci.* **2019**, *44*, 351–364. [CrossRef]
30. Bossis, F.; De Grassi, A.; Palese, L.L.; Pierri, C.L. Prediction of high- and low-affinity quinol-analogue-binding sites in the aa3 and bo3 terminal oxidases from Bacillus subtilis and Escherichia coli1. *Biochem. J.* **2014**, *461*, 305–314. [CrossRef]
31. Waterhouse, A.M.; Procter, J.B.; Martin, D.M.; Clamp, M.; Barton, G.J. Jalview Version 2–a multiple sequence alignment editor and analysis workbench. *Bioinformatics* **2009**, *25*, 1189–1191. [CrossRef] [PubMed]
32. Lobley, A.; Sadowski, M.I.; Jones, D.T. pGenTHREADER and pDomTHREADER: New methods for improved protein fold recognition and superfamily discrimination. *Bioinformatics* **2009**, *25*, 1761–1767. [CrossRef] [PubMed]
33. Ordog, R. PyDeT, a PyMOL plug-in for visualizing geometric concepts around proteins. *Bioinformation* **2008**, *2*, 346–347. [CrossRef] [PubMed]
34. Tavani, C.; Bianchi, L.; De Palma, A.; Passeri, G.I.; Punzi, G.; Pierri, C.L.; Lovece, A.; Cavalluzzi, M.M.; Franchini, C.; Lentini, G.; et al. Nitro-substituted tetrahydroindolizines and homologs: Design, kinetics, and mechanism of α-glucosidase inhibition. *Bioorg. Med. Chem. Lett.* **2017**, *27*, 3980–3986. [CrossRef]
35. Pierri, C.L.; Palmieri, F.; De Grassi, A. Single-nucleotide evolution quantifies the importance of each site along the structure of mitochondrial carriers. *Cell. Mol. Life Sci.* **2014**, *71*, 349–364. [CrossRef]
36. Infantino, V.; Pierri, C.L.; Iacobazzi, V. Metabolic routes in inflammation: The citrate pathway and its potential as therapeutic target. *Curr. Med. Chem.* **2018**. [CrossRef]
37. Pierri, C.L.; Bossis, F.; Punzi, G.; De Grassi, A.; Cetrone, M.; Parisi, G.; Tricarico, D. Molecular modeling of antibodies for the treatment of TNFα-related immunological diseases. *Pharmacol. Res. Perspect.* **2016**, *4*, e00197. [CrossRef]
38. Coccaro, N.; Brunetti, C.; Tota, G.; Pierri, C.L.; Anelli, L.; Zagaria, A.; Casieri, P.; Impera, L.; Minervini, C.F.; Minervini, A.; et al. A novel t(3;9)(q21.2; p24.3) associated with SMARCA2 and ZNF148 genes rearrangement in myelodysplastic syndrome. *Leuk. Lymphoma* **2018**, *59*, 996–999. [CrossRef]
39. Itkis, Y.; Krylova, T.; Pechatnikova, N.L.; De Grassi, A.; Tabakov, V.Y.; Pierri, C.L.; Aleshin, V.; Boyko, A.; Bunik, V.I.; Zakharova, E.Y. A novel variant m.641A>T in the mitochondrial MT-TF gene is associated with epileptic encephalopathy in adolescent. *Mitochondrion* **2019**, *47*, 10–17. [CrossRef]
40. Tamura, K.; Peterson, D.; Peterson, N.; Stecher, G.; Nei, M.; Kumar, S. MEGA5: Molecular evolutionary genetics analysis using maximum likelihood, evolutionary distance, and maximum parsimony methods. *Mol. Biol. Evol.* **2011**, *28*, 2731–2739. [CrossRef]
41. Harnvoravongchai, P.; Kobori, H.; Orita, I.; Nakamura, S.; Imanaka, T.; Fukui, T. Characterization and gene deletion analysis of four homologues of group 3 pyridine nucleotide disulfide oxidoreductases from Thermococcus kodakarensis. *Extremophiles* **2014**, *18*, 603–616. [CrossRef] [PubMed]

42. Seo, D.; Okabe, S.; Yanase, M.; Kataoka, K.; Sakurai, T. Studies of interaction of homo-dimeric ferredoxin-NAD(P)+ oxidoreductases of Bacillus subtilis and Rhodopseudomonas palustris, that are closely related to thioredoxin reductases in amino acid sequence, with ferredoxins and pyridine nucleotide coenzymes. *Biochim. Biophys. Acta Proteins Proteom.* **2009**, *1794*, 594–601. [CrossRef] [PubMed]
43. Park, A.K.; Kim, I.S.; Do, H.; Jeon, B.W.; Lee, C.W.; Roh, S.J.; Shin, S.C.; Park, H.; Kim, Y.S.; Kim, Y.H.; et al. Structure and catalytic mechanism of monodehydroascorbate reductase, MDHAR, from Oryza sativa L. japonica. *Sci. Rep.* **2016**, *6*, 33903. [CrossRef] [PubMed]
44. Osipov, E.M.; Lilina, A.V.; Tsallagov, S.I.; Safonova, T.N.; Sorokin, D.Y.; Tikhonova, T.V.; Popova, V.O. Structure of the flavocytochrome C sulfide dehydrogenase associated with the copper-binding protein CopC from the haloalkaliphilic sulfuroxidizing bacterium thioalkalivibrio paradoxus ArH 1. *Acta Crystallogr. D Struct. Biol.* **2018**, *74*, 632–642. [CrossRef]
45. Yang, Y.; Yu, Y.; Li, X.; Li, J.; Wu, Y.; Yu, J.; Ge, J.; Huang, Z.; Jiang, L.; Rao, Y.; et al. Target Elucidation by Cocrystal Structures of NADH-Ubiquinone Oxidoreductase of Plasmodium falciparum (PfNDH2) with Small Molecule To Eliminate Drug-Resistant Malaria. *J. Med. Chem.* **2017**, *60*, 1994–2005. [CrossRef]
46. Yamashita, T.; Inaoka, D.K.; Shiba, T.; Oohashi, T.; Iwata, S.; Yagi, T.; Kosaka, H.; Miyoshi, H.; Harada, S.; Kita, K.; et al. Ubiquinone binding site of yeast NADH dehydrogenase revealed by structures binding novel competitive- and mixed-type inhibitors. *Sci. Rep.* **2018**, *8*, 2427. [CrossRef]
47. Degli Esposti, M. Inhibitors of NADH-ubiquinone reductase: An overview. *Biochim. Biophys. Acta Bioenerg.* **1998**, *1364*, 222–235. [CrossRef]
48. Bryk, R.; Arango, N.; Maksymiuk, C.; Balakrishnan, A.; Wu, Y.T.; Wong, C.H.; Masquelin, T.; Hipskind, P.; Lima, C.D.; Nathan, C. Lipoamide channel-binding sulfonamides selectively inhibit mycobacterial lipoamide dehydrogenase. *Biochemistry* **2013**, *52*, 9375–9384. [CrossRef]
49. Nocek, B.; Jang, S.B.; Jeong, M.S.; Clark, D.D.; Ensign, S.A.; Peters, J.W. Structural basis for CO 2 fixation by a novel member of the disulfide oxidoreductase family of enzymes, 2-ketopropyl-coenzyme M oxidoreductase/carboxylase. *Biochemistry* **2002**, *41*, 12907–12913. [CrossRef]
50. Xia, L.; Björnstedt, M.; Nordman, T.; Eriksson, L.C.; Olsson, J.M. Reduction of ubiquinone by lipoamide dehydrogenase: An antioxidant regenerating pathway. *Eur. J. Biochem.* **2001**, *268*, 1486–1490. [CrossRef]
51. Nilsen, A.; LaCrue, A.N.; White, K.L.; Forquer, I.P.; Cross, R.M.; Marfurt, J.; Mather, M.W.; Delves, M.J.; Shackleford, D.M.; Saenz, F.E.; et al. Quinolone-3-diarylethers: A new class of antimalarial drug. *Sci. Transl. Med.* **2013**, *5*. [CrossRef]
52. Doggett, J.S.; Nilsen, A.; Forquer, I.; Wegmann, K.W.; Jones-Brando, L.; Yolken, R.H.; Bordón, C.; Charman, S.A.; Katneni, K.; Schultz, T.; et al. Endochin-like quinolones are highly efficacious against acute and latent experimental toxoplasmosis. *Proc. Natl. Acad. Sci. USA* **2012**, *109*, 15936–15941. [CrossRef]
53. Stickles, A.M.; Smilkstein, M.J.; Morrisey, J.M.; Li, Y.; Forquer, I.P.; Kelly, J.X.; Pou, S.; Winter, R.W.; Nilsen, A.; Vaidya, A.B.; et al. Atovaquone and ELQ-300 combination therapy as a novel dual-site cytochrome bc1 inhibition strategy for malaria. *Antimicrob. Agents Chemother.* **2016**, *60*, 4853–4859. [CrossRef] [PubMed]
54. Heikal, A.; Nakatani, Y.; Jiao, W.; Wilson, C.; Rennison, D.; Weimar, M.R.; Parker, E.J.; Brimble, M.A.; Cook, G.M. 'Tethering' fragment-based drug discovery to identify inhibitors of the essential respiratory membrane protein type II NADH dehydrogenase. *Bioorg. Med. Chem. Lett.* **2018**, *28*, 2239–2243. [CrossRef] [PubMed]
55. Sellamuthu, S.; Singh, M.; Kumar, A.; Singh, S.K. Type-II NADH Dehydrogenase (NDH-2): A promising therapeutic target for antitubercular and antibacterial drug discovery. *Expert Opin. Ther. Targets* **2017**, *21*, 559–570. [CrossRef]
56. Harbut, M.B.; Yang, B.; Liu, R.; Yano, T.; Vilchèze, C.; Cheng, B.; Lockner, J.; Guo, H.; Yu, C.; Franzblau, S.G.; et al. Small Molecules Targeting Mycobacterium tuberculosis Type II NADH Dehydrogenase Exhibit Antimycobacterial Activity. *Angew. Chem.Int. Ed. Engl.* **2018**, *57*, 3478–3482. [CrossRef]
57. Murugesan, D.; Ray, P.C.; Bayliss, T.; Prosser, G.A.; Harrison, J.R.; Green, K.; Soares De Melo, C.; Feng, T.S.; Street, L.J.; Chibale, K.; et al. 2-Mercapto-Quinazolinones as Inhibitors of Type II NADH Dehydrogenase and Mycobacterium tuberculosis: Structure-Activity Relationships, Mechanism of Action and Absorption, Distribution, Metabolism, and Excretion Characterization. *ACS Infect. Dis.* **2018**, *4*, 954–969. [CrossRef]
58. Miller, J.O.; Taylor, J.; Goldman, J.L. Severe acute respiratory failure in healthy adolescents exposed to trimethoprim-sulfamethoxazole. *Pediatrics* **2019**, *143*, e20183242. [CrossRef]

59. Inesi, G. Molecular features of copper binding proteins involved in copper homeostasis. *IUBMB Life* **2017**, *69*, 211–217. [CrossRef]
60. Terziyska, N.; Lutz, T.; Kozany, C.; Mokranjac, D.; Mesecke, N.; Neupert, W.; Herrmann, J.M.; Hell, K. Mia40, a novel factor for protein import into the intermembrane space of mitochondria is able to bind metal ions. *FEBS Lett.* **2005**, *579*, 179–184. [CrossRef]
61. Banci, L.; Bertini, I.; Cefaro, C.; Ciofi-Baffoni, S.; Gallo, A.; Martinelli, M.; Sideris, D.P.; Katrakili, N.; Tokatlidis, K. MIA40 is an oxidoreductase that catalyzes oxidative protein folding in mitochondria. *Nat. Struct. Mol. Biol.* **2009**, *16*, 198–206. [CrossRef] [PubMed]
62. Hirst, J. Open questions: Respiratory chain supercomplexes-why are they there and what do they do? *BMC Biol.* **2018**, *16*, 111. [CrossRef] [PubMed]
63. Saari, S.; Garcia, G.S.; Bremer, K.; Chioda, M.M.; Andjelković, A.; Debes, P.V.; Nikinmaa, M.; Szibor, M.; Dufour, E.; Rustin, P.; et al. Alternative respiratory chain enzymes: Therapeutic potential and possible pitfalls. *Biochim. Biophys. Acta Mol. Basis Dis.* **2019**, *1865*, 854–866. [CrossRef] [PubMed]
64. Sousa, J.S.; Calisto, F.; Langer, J.D.; Mills, D.J.; Refojo, P.N.; Teixeira, M.; Kühlbrandt, W.; Vonck, J.; Pereira, M.M. Structural basis for energy transduction by respiratory alternative complex III. *Nat. Commun.* **2018**, *9*, 1728. [CrossRef]
65. Miramar, M.D.; Costantini, P.; Ravagnan, L.; Saraiva, L.M.; Haouzi, D.; Brothers, G.; Penninger, J.M.; Peleato, M.L.; Kroemer, G.; Susin, S.A. NADH Oxidase Activity of Mitochondrial Apoptosis-inducing Factor. *J. Biol. Chem.* **2001**, *276*, 16391–16398. [CrossRef]
66. Spinazzi, M.; Casarin, A.; Pertegato, V.; Salviati, L.; Angelini, C. Assessment of mitochondrial respiratory chain enzymatic activities on tissues and cultured cells. *Nat. Protoc.* **2012**, *7*, 1235–1246. [CrossRef]
67. Wilkinson, J.C.; Wilkinson, A.S.; Galban, S.; Csomos, R.A.; Duckett, C.S. Apoptosis-Inducing Factor Is a Target for Ubiquitination through Interaction with XIAP. *Mol. Cell. Biol.* **2008**, *28*, 237–247. [CrossRef]
68. Vahsen, N.; Candé, C.; Brière, J.J.; Bénit, P.; Joza, N.; Larochette, N.; Mastroberardino, P.G.; Pequignot, M.O.; Casares, N.; Lazar, V.; et al. AIF deficiency compromises oxidative phosphorylation. *EMBO J.* **2004**, *23*, 4679–4689. [CrossRef]
69. Zheng, Y.; Qu, H.; Xiong, X.; Wang, Y.; Liu, X.; Zhang, L.; Liao, X.; Liao, Q.; Sun, Z.; Ouyang, Q.; et al. Deficiency of Mitochondrial Glycerol 3-Phosphate Dehydrogenase Contributes to Hepatic Steatosis. *Hepatology* **2019**, *70*, 84–97. [CrossRef]
70. Fisher-Wellman, K.H.; Lin, C.T.; Ryan, T.E.; Reese, L.R.; Gilliam, L.A.A.; Cathey, B.L.; Lark, D.S.; Smith, C.D.; Muoio, D.M.; Neufer, P.D. Pyruvate dehydrogenase complex and nicotinamide nucleotide transhydrogenase constitute an energy-consuming redox circuit. *Biochem. J.* **2015**, *467*, 271–280. [CrossRef]
71. Atlante, A.; Calissano, P.; Bobba, A.; Azzariti, A.; Marra, E.; Passarella, S. Cytochrome c is released from mitochondria in a reactive oxygen species (ROS)-dependent fashion and can operate as a ROS scavenger and as a respiratory substrate in cerebellar neurons undergoing excitotoxic death. *J. Biol. Chem.* **2000**, *275*, 37159–37166. [CrossRef] [PubMed]
72. Marzulli, D.; La Piana, G.; Cafagno, L.; Fransvea, E.; Lofrumento, N.E. Proton translocation linked to the activity of the bi-trans-membrane electron transport chain. *Arch. Biochem. Biophys.* **1995**, *319*, 36–48. [CrossRef] [PubMed]
73. Punzi, G.; Porcelli, V.; Ruggiu, M.; Hossain, M.F.; Menga, A.; Scarcia, P.; Castegna, A.; Gorgoglione, R.; Pierri, C.L.; Laera, L.; et al. SLC25A10 biallelic mutations in intractable epileptic encephalopathy with complex I deficiency. *Hum. Mol. Genet.* **2018**, *27*, 499–504. [CrossRef] [PubMed]
74. Wilkins, H.M.; Brock, S.; Gray, J.J.; Linseman, D.A. Stable over-expression of the 2-oxoglutarate carrier enhances neuronal cell resistance to oxidative stress via Bcl-2-dependent mitochondrial GSH transport. *J. Neurochem.* **2014**, *130*, 75–86. [CrossRef] [PubMed]
75. Craven, L.; Alston, C.L.; Taylor, R.W.; Turnbull, D.M. Recent Advances in Mitochondrial Disease. *Annu. Rev. Genomics Hum. Genet.* **2017**, *18*, 257–275. [CrossRef]
76. Zeviani, M.; Carelli, V. Mitochondrial disorders. *Curr. Opin. Neurol.* **2007**, *20*, 564–571. [CrossRef]
77. Liberti, M.V.; Locasale, J.W. The Warburg Effect: How Does it Benefit Cancer Cells? *Trends Biochem. Sci.* **2016**, *41*, 211–218. [CrossRef]
78. Billiard, J.; Dennison, J.B.; Briand, J.; Annan, R.S.; Chai, D.; Colón, M.; Dodson, C.S.; Gilbert, S.A.; Greshock, J.; Jing, J.; et al. Quinoline 3-sulfonamides inhibit lactate dehydrogenase A and reverse aerobic glycolysis in cancer cells. *Cancer Metab.* **2013**, *1*, 19. [CrossRef]

79. Abramson, J.; Riistama, S.; Larsson, G.; Jasaitis, A.; Svensson-Ek, M.; Laakkonen, L.; Puustinen, A.; Iwata, S.; Wikström, M. The structure of the ubiquinol oxidase from Escherichia coli and its ubiquinone binding site. *Nat. Struct. Biol.* **2000**, *7*, 910–917.
80. Otera, H.; Ohsakaya, S.; Nagaura, Z.I.; Ishihara, N.; Mihara, K. Export of mitochondrial AIF in response to proapoptotic stimuli depends on processing at the intermembrane space. *EMBO J.* **2005**, *24*, 1375–1386. [CrossRef]
81. Fedor, J.G.; Jones, A.J.Y.; Di Luca, A.; Kaila, V.R.I.; Hirst, J. Correlating kinetic and structural data on ubiquinone binding and reduction by respiratory complex I. *Proc. Natl. Acad. Sci. USA* **2017**, *114*, 12737–12742. [CrossRef] [PubMed]
82. Hirano, M.; Emmanuele, V.; Quinzii, C.M. Emerging therapies for mitochondrial diseases. *Essays Biochem.* **2018**, *62*, 467–481. [PubMed]
83. Beyrath, J.; Pellegrini, M.; Renkema, H.; Houben, L.; Pecheritsyna, S.; Van Zandvoort, P.; Van Den Broek, P.; Bekel, A.; Eftekhari, P.; Smeitink, J.A.M. KH176 Safeguards Mitochondrial Diseased Cells from Redox Stress-Induced Cell Death by Interacting with the Thioredoxin System/Peroxiredoxin Enzyme Machinery. *Sci. Rep.* **2018**, *8*, 6577. [CrossRef] [PubMed]
84. Fiedorczuk, K.; Letts, J.A.; Degliesposti, G.; Kaszuba, K.; Skehel, M.; Sazanov, L.A. Atomic structure of the entire mammalian mitochondrial complex I. *Nature* **2016**, *538*, 406–410. [CrossRef]
85. Hards, K.; Cook, G.M. Targeting bacterial energetics to produce new antimicrobials. *Drug Resist. Updat.* **2018**, *36*, 1–12. [CrossRef]
86. Lu, J.; Vlamis-Gardikas, A.; Kandasamy, K.; Zhao, R.; Gustafsson, T.N.; Engstrand, L.; Hoffner, S.; Engman, L.; Holmgren, A. Inhibition of bacterial thioredoxin reductase: An antibiotic mechanism targeting bacteria lacking glutathione. *FASEB J.* **2013**, *27*, 1394–1403. [CrossRef]
87. Volpicella, M.; Costanza, A.; Palumbo, O.; Italiano, F.; Claudia, L.; Placido, A.; Picardi, E.; Carella, M.; Trotta, M.; Ceci, L.R. Rhodobacter sphaeroides adaptation to high concentrations of cobalt ions requires energetic metabolism changes. *FEMS Microbiol. Ecol.* **2014**, *88*, 345–357. [CrossRef]
88. Bullerwell, C.E.; Gray, M.W. Evolution of the mitochondrial genome: Protist connections to animals, fungi and plants. *Curr. Opin. Microbiol.* **2004**, *7*, 528–534. [CrossRef]
89. Schägger, H. Respiratory chain supercomplexes of mitochondria and bacteria. *Biochim. Biophys. Acta Bioenerg.* **2002**, *1555*, 154–159. [CrossRef]
90. Archibald, J.M. Endosymbiosis and eukaryotic cell evolution. *Curr. Biol.* **2015**, *25*, R911–R921. [CrossRef]

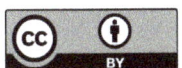

© 2019 by the authors. Licensee MDPI, Basel, Switzerland. This article is an open access article distributed under the terms and conditions of the Creative Commons Attribution (CC BY) license (http://creativecommons.org/licenses/by/4.0/).

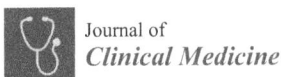 

Article

# Brain-Immune Alterations and Mitochondrial Dysfunctions in a Mouse Model of Paediatric Autoimmune Disorder Associated with Streptococcus: Exacerbation by Chronic Psychosocial Stress

Maria Antonietta Ajmone-Cat [1,†], Chiara Spinello [2,3,†], Daniela Valenti [4], Francesca Franchi [2], Simone Macrì [2], Rosa Anna Vacca [4,*] and Giovanni Laviola [2,*]

1. National Center for Drug Research and Evaluation, Istituto Superiore di Sanità, Viale Regina Elena, 299, I-00161 Rome, Italy; mariaantonietta.ajmone-cat@iss.it
2. Centre for Behavioural Sciences and Mental Health, Istituto Superiore di Sanità, Viale Regina Elena, 299, I-00161 Rome, Italy; chiara.spnll@gmail.com (C.S.); francesca.franchi@iss.it (F.F.); simone.macri@iss.it (S.M.)
3. Department of Mechanical and Aerospace Engineering, New York University Tandon School of Engineering, Brooklyn, NY 11201, USA
4. Institute of Biomembranes, Bioenergetics and Molecular Biotechnologies, National Council of Research, Via Giovanni Amendola 122/O - 70126 Bari, Italy; d.valenti@ibiom.cnr.it
* Correspondence: r.vacca@ibiom.cnr.it (R.A.V.); giovanni.laviola@iss.it (G.L.)
† These authors contributed equally to this work.

Received: 9 September 2019; Accepted: 18 September 2019; Published: 20 September 2019

**Abstract:** Adverse psychosocial experiences have been shown to modulate individual responses to immune challenges and affect mitochondrial functions. The aim of this study was to investigate inflammation and immune responses as well as mitochondrial bioenergetics in an experimental model of Paediatric Autoimmune Neuropsychiatric Disorders Associated with Streptococcus (PANDAS). Starting in adolescence (postnatal day 28), male SJL/J mice were exposed to five injections (interspaced by two weeks) with Group-A beta-haemolytic streptococcus (GAS) homogenate. Mice were exposed to chronic psychosocial stress, in the form of protracted visual exposure to an aggressive conspecific, for four weeks. Our results indicate that psychosocial stress exacerbated individual response to GAS administrations whereby mice exposed to both treatments exhibited altered cytokine and immune-related enzyme expression in the hippocampus and hypothalamus. Additionally, they showed impaired mitochondrial respiratory chain complexes IV and V, and reduced adenosine triphosphate (ATP) production by mitochondria and ATP content. These brain abnormalities, observed in GAS-Stress mice, were associated with blunted titers of plasma corticosterone. Present data support the hypothesis that challenging environmental conditions, in terms of chronic psychosocial stress, may exacerbate the long-term consequences of exposure to GAS processes through the promotion of central immunomodulatory and oxidative stress.

**Keywords:** PANDAS; adverse emotional experience; immunity; neuroinflammation; animal Models; mitochondrial bioenergetics

---

## 1. Introduction

Recent epidemiological, clinical, and preclinical studies suggest that immune responses to pathogens may play a remarkable role in the onset and course of a heterogeneous group of psychiatric disturbances. Several authors proposed that genetically predisposed individuals may develop a series of immune-mediated disturbances, ranging from Paediatric Autoimmune Disorders Associated with Streptococcus (PANDAS) to neuropsychiatric systemic lupus erythematosus and autoimmune encephalopathies [1–4]. Within this framework, pathogen-directed antibodies are hypothesized to cross-react with a variety of partly identified neuronal antigens for a phenomenon of molecular mimicry, thereby damaging specific brain circuits and ultimately result in behavioural abnormalities [5,6].

The acronym PANDAS was coined to define a series of disturbances with a paediatric onset—mostly characterized by the exhibition of choreic or repetitive movements—in which repeated exposures to bacterial infections (in particular of Group-A beta-Haemolytic Streptococcus, GAS) are causally linked to the exhibition of symptoms [7–12]. Recurrent exhibition of abnormal behaviours, and remitting-relapsing presence of obsessive-compulsive symptoms and/or tics are among the defining criteria of PANDAS [13,14]. Sydenham's chorea (SC) and Tourette's syndrome (TS) have been proposed to constitute instances of PANDAS [15,16].

Orlovska and co-authors provided additional support to the PANDAS hypothesis through a cohort study wherein they observed that individuals with streptococcal throat infection had elevated risks of obsessive-compulsive (OCD) and tic disorders [17]; non-streptococcal throat infection was also associated with increased risks, albeit to a lesser extent, suggesting an even wider association between immunity and neurological sequelae.

The possibility that autoimmune phenomena may contribute to the manifestation of neurological and behavioural disturbances has been corroborated by several independent preclinical studies [9,12,18]. Hoffman and colleagues demonstrated that mice repeatedly injected with Streptococcus homogenate showed locomotor alterations associated with IgG deposits in deep cerebellar nuclei [9]. We recently extended these observations and reported that analogous treatments in mice resulted, in the long term, in increased repetitive behaviours, impairments in sensorimotor gating, and indices of inflammatory processes occurring at the level of the rostral diencephalon [18,19].

Symptom fluctuations and recurrences in PANDAS seem to be influenced by various contextual features (see [13,20] for reviews), among which psychosocial factors and stress have called particular attention [21–23]. Environmental stressors contribute to vulnerability to Tourette's syndrome, and play a remarkable role in modulating the severity of clinical symptoms [24,25]. Similarly, acute psychosocial stressors have been associated with worsening of tics [20,26,27]. On the other hand, chronic psychosocial stress has been shown to influence individual adaptation to additional challenges [28].

In a translational rodent model of repeated GAS injections [19], we originally reported that neonatal exogenous corticosterone administration mitigated behavioural and immunohistochemical alterations induced by subsequent GAS injections. These compensatory effects co-occurred with modifications in hypothalamic pituitary adrenal axis (HPA) activity and remarkable increases in plasma inflammatory cytokines and chemokines. These results support the view that the HPA axis may contribute to the regulation of the immune responses involved in the pathological sequelae of PANDAS and ultimately modulate the severity of the PANDAS-related phenotype [19].

Stress and highly demanding social dynamics have been causally linked to both mental and somatic pathologies [29–35], albeit the underlying mechanisms remained elusive.

Compelling evidence indicate stress-mediated alterations in HPA activity may influence the immune system, favour peripheral inflammation as well as neuroinflammation [36], increase individual vulnerability towards subsequent immune challenges, and ultimately promote autoimmunity [37–40]. Different psychogenic stressors induce oxidative and nitrosative stress in the central nervous system (CNS) and few studies showed that the development of psychosis in immune activation translational models could be mediated by an imbalance between pro-oxidants and anti-oxidants [41]. Accordingly, several clinical, genetic, and biochemical studies highlighted a central role of impaired mitochondrial function and oxidative stress in the etiology of both neurological and neuropsychiatric diseases [42–44]. Just as the immune system represents a major source of oxidative stress, so also oxidative stress induces inflammation via the activation of nuclear factor κB (NF-κB), a key transcription factor for the modulation of inflammatory genes [41]. It is well known that dysfunction of the mitochondrial respiratory chain (MRC) machinery leads to a decrease in adenosine triphosphate (ATP) production through oxidative phosphorylation (OXPHOS) (for refs see [45]) and exposure to oxidative stress could exacerbate mitochondrial damage and induce death at the cellular level [46]. Beside regulating cellular energy-generating processes, mitochondria play a pivotal role in controlling immune cell activation and functions (see [47–50]), and may thus represent targets of inflammatory cytokines in immune-mediated diseases [51].

In the present study, we aimed at investigating the role of social stressors in the calibration of psychiatric disorders, and at identifying candidate mediators potentially serving as future therapeutic targets. Specifically, we aimed at: (i) clarifying the role of the immune system in the pathological sequelae linking streptococcal infections and psychiatric disturbances; (ii) providing additional evidence that psychosocial stress may exacerbate the symptoms occurring in response to streptococcal infection; (iii) demonstrating that mitochondrial oxidative phosphorylation apparatus may represent a candidate biological determinant, potentially representing a valid therapeutic target.

Based on the evidence discussed above, we evaluated the possibility that adverse environmental factors calibrate individual vulnerability in a validated translational mouse model of PANDAS [18,19]. To this aim, we tested the prediction that chronic psychosocial stress may worsen the brain immune response and induce oxidative stress and mitochondrial dysfunction. In the present study, we opted to focus on male mice due to the higher incidence of PANDAS observed in males compared to females (with a 4.7:1 ratio; see [8]). While we acknowledge that it would be important to extend our findings to females, we note that in the light of the innovative nature of this study, it was necessary to identify a proof-of-principle in the most promising study population (males) before planning a study involving female subjects.

## 2. Experimental Section

### 2.1. Animals and Rearing

Male SJL/J mice, postnatal day (PND) 25 on the day of arrival, were purchased from Charles River, Italy (Calco, Lecco, Italy). Upon arrival, mice were randomly housed in groups of two individuals in type-1 polycarbonate cages (33 × 13 × 14 cm). All cages were equipped with sawdust bedding, an enrichment bag (Mucedola, Settimo Milanese, Italy), metal top and ad libitum water and food pellets (Mucedola, Settimo Milanese, Italy). Mice were maintained on a reversed 12-h-light-dark cycle (light on at 7:00 PM) in an air-conditioned room (temperature 21 ± 1 °C and relative humidity 60 ± 10%).

All experimental procedures were performed in agreement with the Legislative Decree 26/14 and the European Directive 2010/63/UE on laboratory animal protection and experimentation. The study has been approved by the Italian Ministry of Health (Decree Nr. 217/2010-B).

### 2.2. Immunization Protocol

GAS homogenate was prepared as described in previous studies [9,18,19]. After preparation, streptococcus homogenate was stored at −70 °C. A blood agar plate was used to inoculate a sample of homogenate (2.5 µL), to verify that it contained no viable bacteria. Immunization protocol, described in [9] and adopted in our previous study [18], comprised five injections interspaced by a time interval of two weeks, starting on PND 28. During the first injection, Phosphate-buffered saline (PBS) mice were injected subcutaneously (s.c.) with 125 µL of an emulsion (1:1), containing PBS and Complete Freund's adjuvant (CFA; Sigma Aldrich, Milano, Italy), and GAS mice were injected with 125 µL of the same emulsion (PBS:CFA), containing 5 µL of GAS homogenate (0.52 mg/mL of total protein as determined by Bradford Assay, Biorad, (Hercules, CA, USA). Mice were then treated four additional times at 2-week intervals with 125 µL of vehicle – an emulsion (1:1) containing PBS and Incomplete Freud's Adjuvant (IFA; Sigma Aldrich, Milano, Italy) – for the PBS group, or 125 µL of PBS:IFA and 5 µL of GAS homogenate for the GAS group. To prepare the PBS/adjuvant emulsions we used the vortex method described by [52]. According to the adult and the PBS/GAS treatment received, experimental subjects were randomly assigned to four experimental groups: control vehicle-injected (PBS-no Stress), GAS homogenate/vehicle-injected (GAS-no Stress), vehicle-injected plus psychosocial stress (PBS-Stress), and GAS homogenate/vehicle-injected plus psychosocial stress (GAS-Stress).

## 2.3. Chronic Psychosocial Stress

Psychosocial stress consisted of a 4-week protocol in which mice were exposed to daily defeats and sensory contact housing (enabled by a wire mesh partition bisecting the cage into two symmetrical compartments, each with food and water available at libitum). The chronic psychosocial stress, starting at PND 56, was conducted as previously described [53,54]. Briefly, each SJL male mouse, representing the experimental subject, was transferred as intruder to the home cage of a CD1 resident mouse. The CD1 strain manifests high territorial aggression [55]. Resident and intruder mice were allowed to freely interact for a maximum of 10 min during the 1st social confrontation. After the interaction, resident and intruder mice were separated by a perforated partition, which allowed continuous sensory contact but no physical interaction. The partition was removed daily (between 9:30 AM and 12:30 PM or between 2:30 PM and 5:00 PM), for a theoretical maximum of 10 min. However, from the 2nd event onwards, because of the elevated level of aggressive behavior displayed by the resident mouse, the physical confrontation was generally interrupted shortly after its beginning. During the first active social interaction, offensive/defensive behaviors and the display of upright posture, flight behavior of the experimental SJL mice were video recorded for subsequent scoring [55,56]. Videos were scored by a trained observer using a specific software (The Observer, The observer XT 10, Noldus, PA Wageningen, The Netherland). Behaviors observed are part of the aggressive and defensive/subordination repertoire of male mice [57,58]. In particular, the behaviors collected were: attack (forward motion of the resident mouse toward the mouse belonging to the experimental group; the motion is combined with direct physical contact), defensive upright (the animal stands on the hind-limbs and push the aggressive opponent with the forepaws, the head pulled far back), fleeing (the animal rapidly escapes from the opponent, often screaming), immobility-attack related (the animal is motionless during an attack), immobility-contact related (the animal is motionless while the opponent is in physical contact but is not attacking) and submissive behaviors (animal standing on its hind limbs while having the head pulled far back; also, the body is rigid). Furthermore, self-grooming (the mouse licks its own fur helping itself with its forepaws) were scored.

## 2.4. Experimental Design

In the four experimental groups of mice consisting of PBS-no Stress (N = 10), GAS-no Stress (N = 9), PBS-Stress (N = 10) and GAS-Stress (N = 10), the experimental design (Figure 1) comprised the following evaluations: the immune response to the injection protocol and corticosterone determination in blood sampling; assessment of neuroinflammatory and mitochondrial parameters in brain sampling/sectioning.

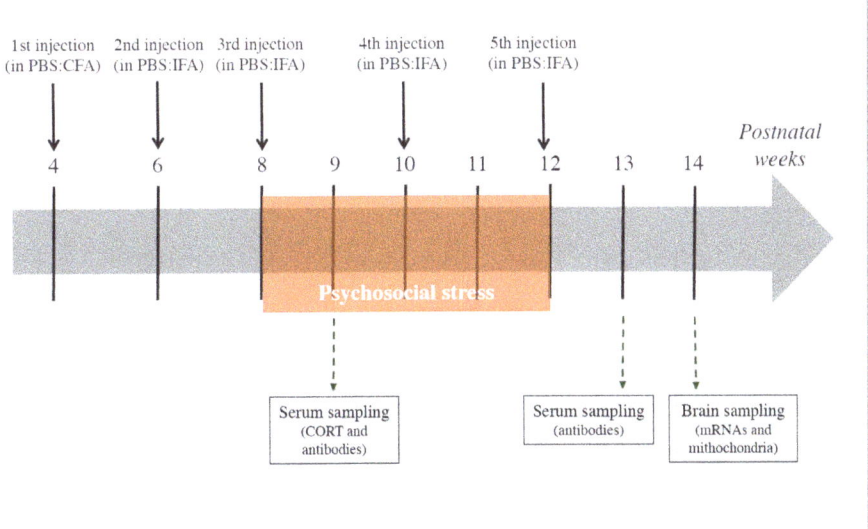

**Figure 1.** Timing of stress exposure and of the Group-A beta-haemolytic streptococcus (GAS) injections, expressed in weeks, and the experimental procedures performed. Mice (N = 9–10 per group) received 5 injections of GAS homogenate or Phosphate Buffer Saline (PBS), formulated with the indicated adjuvants (CFA = Complete Freund's adjuvant; IFA = Incomplete Freund's adjuvant). Serum samples were collected for antibody determination and corticosterone (CORT) concentration assessment; brain samples were collected for mRNA expression and mitochondrial analyses.

### 2.5. Blood Serum Sampling and Corticosterone Determination

To evaluate the effects of experimental treatments on HPA activity, we evaluated serum corticosterone concentrations at post-natal week 9, one week after the beginning of the psychosocial stress procedure. Blood samples (~20 μL) were collected through tail incision [59,60] at 9:00 PM, i.e. two hours after the beginning of the dark phase of the inverted light-dark cycle, and before the beginning of the daily stress procedure. Blood samples were allowed to clot at room temperature for 4 hours, centrifuged at 3000 rpm for 15 minutes. The serum was transferred into Eppendorf tubes and maintained at −80 °C until biochemical assays. Corticosterone concentration was assessed using a commercial radioimmunoassay (RIA) kit (ICN Biomedicals, Costa Mesa, CA, USA). Vials were counted for 2 minutes in a gamma counter (Packard Minaxi Gamma counter, Series 5000, Packard Instruments Company Inc, Meriden, CT, USA). The procedures for washing and steroid extraction followed the protocol described by Gao and colleagues [61]. One change was made to the protocol: the dry residue was resuspended using 175 μL distilled water. Afterwards, 100 μL of the medium were injected into a Shimadzu HPLC system (Shimadzu, Canby, OR, USA) coupled to an AB Sciex API 5000 Turboion-spray1triple quadrupole tandem mass spectrometer equipped with Atmospheric Pressure Chemical Ionization (APCI) Source (AB Sciex, Foster City, CA, USA). The system was controlled by AB Sciex Analyst1 software (version 1.5.1, AB Sciex, Milano, Italy). The lower limit of detection was ~0.1 pg/mg. Intra- and inter-plate coefficients of variance ranged between 3.7–8.8%. All samples were prepared and analysed within the same time period in order to prevent batch effects.

### 2.6. Analysis of Anti-Group A Streptococcal Antibodies in Serum Samples

GAS homogenates obtained as described above (see Section 2.2) were size-separated by SDS-PAGE (4–12% acrylamide) under reducing conditions and electroblotted onto nitrocellulose membranes. Immunostaining was performed by blocking the membrane overnight with 3% (*w/v*) skimmed milk in

TPBS (0.1% Tween in PBS) and incubating for 2 h with sera from mice of all experimental groups (all sera were diluted 1: 200). For this analysis, sera were collected one week after the 3rd and 5th injection of GAS homogenate or adjuvant alone following the procedure described above (see Section 2.5). After 3 washes with TPBS, the membrane was incubated with Horseradish Peroxidase (HRP)-conjugated secondary antibody (1:1000), washed again with TPBS and PBS, and developed with a chromogenic substrate. Densitometric analysis of the overall lane intensities in the blot was performed by using Image J software (Image J2, Image J developers).

### 2.7. Brain Sampling

In order to collect brain samples, mice were rapidly decapitated, two weeks after treatment endings. This time point was chosen to investigate the possible long-term effects of treatments on brain immune and mitochondrial parameters. Samples collected were immediately sectioned on ice to obtain hippocampus, and hypothalamus. For mRNA expression analyses, brain samples were collected after decapitation, kept intact in mRNAase free tubes, flash frozen and stored at −80 °C.

For mitochondrial analysis, brain hemispheres immediately after explant were added to an ice-cold cryopreservation solution consisting of 50 mM K-MES (pH 7.1), 3 mM $K_2HPO_4$, 9.5 mM $MgCl_2$, 3 mM ATP plus 20% glycerol and 10 mg/mL BSA, and stored at −80 °C until assayed. We have previously demonstrated that mitochondria isolated from cryopreserved brain tissues show mitochondrial membrane potential, outer and inner membrane integrity and mitochondrial ATP production capacity comparable to mitochondria isolated from fresh brains [62,63].

### 2.8. Real-Time Quantitative Polymerase Chain Reaction (RT-PCR)

Dissected hypothalami and hippocampi (from N = 6 mice per experimental group) were homogenized in Tri Reagent (Sigma, St. Louis, MO, USA) and mRNA extraction was performed on supernatants.

Total RNA (1 µg) from each sample was transcribed into complementary DNA using the RT-PCR Superscript III kit (Invitrogen, Eugene, OR, USA), according to the manufacturer's instructions. RT-PCR was performed on the reverse transcription products with a SensiMix SYBR Kit (Bioline, London, UK) for hypoxanthine guanine phosphoribosyl transferase (HPRT), tumor necrosis factor-α (TNF-α), interleukin-1β (IL-1β), interleukin-10 (IL-10), inducible nitric oxide synthase (iNOS), arginase-1 (Arg-1), manganese superoxide dismutase (MnSOD), and glucocorticoid receptor (GR) mRNA expression, or with TaqMan for HPRT and CD11b, using an ABI Prism 7500 Sequence Detection System (Applied Biosystems, Foster City, CA, USA).

Primer sequences for HPRT, IL-1β, TNF-α, IL-10, iNOS, Arg-1, MnSOD, and GR were from Integrated DNA Technologies (IDT, TEMA Ricerca Bologna, Italy); accession numbers are as follows:

1. HPRT (NM_013556): forward 5′-CAGGCCAGACTTTG-TTGGAT-3′; reverse 5′-TTGCGCTCATC-TTAGGCTTT-3′;
2. IL-1β (NM_008361): forward 5′-CGACAAAATACCTGTGGCCT-3′, reverse 5′-TTCTTTGGG TATTCCTTGGG-3′;
3. TNF-α (NM_013693.3): forward 5′-AGCCCCCAGTCTGTATCCTT-3′, reverse 5′-ACAGTCCAGG TCACTGTCCC-3′;
4. IL-10 (NM_010548): forward 5′-TTAAGCTGTTTCCATTGGGG-3′, reverse 5′-AAGTGTGGC CAGCCTTAGAA-3′;
5. iNOS (NM_010927): forward 5′-CAGCTGGGCTGTACAAACCTT-3′, reverse 5′-CATTGGAAGT GAAGCGTTTCG-3′;
6. Arg-1 (NM_007482): forward 5′-GGAAAGCCAATGAAGAGCTG-3′, reverse 5′-AACACTCCCC TGACAACCAG-3′;
7. MnSOD (NC_000083.6): forward 5′-GCTCTGGCCAAGGGAGATGT-3′, reverse, 5′-GGGCTCAG GTTTGTCCAGAAA-3′;

8. GR (NM_008173.3): forward 5′-CGCCAAGTGATTGCCGC-3′, reverse 5′-TGTAGAAGGGTCA TTTGGTCATCCA-3′.

TaqMan primers for HPRT (Mn.PT.39a22214828) and CD11b (Mn.PT.58.9189361), were also from IDT.

Annealing temperature was 60 °C for all the primer pairs listed. All samples were run in triplicate, and each PCR well contained 20 µL as a final volume of reaction, including 2 µL complementary DNA corresponding to approximately 60 ng total RNA, 750 nM of each primer, and 10 µL PCR master mix. Thermal cycling conditions were as follows: 1 cycle at 95 °C for 10 min, 40 cycles at 95 °C for 15 s, and 60 °C for 1 min. The relative expression level of each mRNA was calculated using the $\Delta\Delta Ct$ method normalized to HPRT and relative to the control samples. The amplification specificity was verified by melting curve analyses.

*2.9. Measurement of Mitochondrial Respiratory Chain Complex (MRC) Activities*

Measurements of mitochondrial respiratory chain (MRC) complex activities were carried out in mitochondrial membrane-enriched fractions obtained from crude mitochondria isolated by differential centrifugation of brain homogenate as previously described [62]. To obtain mitochondrial membrane-enriched fractions, mitochondrial pellets were first frozen at −80 °C, then thawed at 2–4 °C, suspended in 1 ml of 10 mM Tris-HCl (pH 7.5) plus 1mg/ml BSA and exposed to ultrasound energy for 8 s at 0 °C (11 pulse 0.7 s on, 0.7 s off) at 20 kHz, intensity 2. The ultrasound-treated mitochondria were centrifuged at 600 g for 10 min, 4 °C. The supernatant was centrifuged again at 14000 g for 10 min, 4 °C and the resulting pellet was kept at −80 °C until use. The MRC complex activities were assessed spectrophotometrically essentially as in [64], by three measurements which rely on the sequential addition of reagents to measure the activities of: (i) NADH:ubiquinone oxidoreductase (complex I) followed by ATP synthase (complex V), (ii) succinate:ubiquinone oxidoreductase (complex II) and (iii) cytochrome c oxidase (complex IV) followed by cytochrome c oxidoreductase (complex III).

*2.10. Measurement of Mitochondrial ATP Production Rate*

The rate of ATP production by OXPHOS was determined in isolated mitochondria, essentially as previously described in [65]. Briefly, mitochondria isolated from total brain (0.5 mg protein) were incubated at 37°C in 2 mL of respiratory medium consisting of 210 mM mannitol, 70 mM sucrose, 20 mM Tris/HCl, 5 mM $KH_2PO_4/K_2HPO_4$, (pH 7.4) plus 5 mg/mL BSA, 3 mM $MgCl_2$, in the presence of the ATP detecting system consisting of glucose (2.5 mM), hexokinase (HK, 2 enzymatic units, e.u.), glucose 6-phosphate dehydrogenase (G6P-DH, 1 e.u.) and $NADP^+$ (0.25 mM) in the presence of glutamate (GLU) plus malate (MAL) (5 mM each) or succinate (SUCC, 5 mM) plus rotenone (ROT, 3 µM), or ascorbate (ASC, 0.5 mM) plus $N,N,N',N'$-tetramethyl-p-phenylenediamine (TMPD, 0.25 mM), as energy sources. The reduction of $NADP^+$ in the extramitochondrial phase, which reveals ATP formation from externally added adenosine diphosphate (ADP, 0.5 mM), was monitored as an increase in absorbance at 340 nm. Care was taken to use enough HK/G6P-DH coupled enzymes to ensure a non-limiting ADP-regenerating system for the measurement of ATP production.

*2.11. Measurement of Mouse Brain ATP Levels*

The brain hemisphere was subjected to perchloric acid extraction as described in [66]. In brief, tissues were homogenized in 600 µL of pre-cooled 10% perchloric acid and then centrifuged at 14000 g for 10 min, 4 °C. The amount of tissue ATP was determined in KOH neutralized extracts by spectrofluorimetric measurements (with excitation wavelength of 334 and emission wavelength of 456 nm) following the formation of NADPH, which reveals ATP, in the presence of the ATP detecting system consisting of glucose (2.5 mM), hexokinase (HK, 2 e.u.), glucose 6-phosphate dehydrogenase (G6P-DH, 1 e.u.), and $NADP^+$ (0.25 mM) [67].

## 2.12. T-Maze

Animals were screened for perseverative behaviours in the T-maze test through the same procedure adopted in our previous study [19]. The T-maze provides an inverse index of perseverative behaviour whereby, in this test, rodents have the natural tendency to alternate their choices in a binary-test paradigm (spontaneous alternation) [68]. The apparatus was an enclosed T-shaped maze, composed of three equally sized arms (50 × 16 cm). Mice performed ten sessions, in the housing room, during five consecutive days (2 sessions per day). The experimental session consisted of two choice trials, beginning with the mouse in the start compartment, facing the wall of the apparatus. Mice were allowed to explore the apparatus for a maximum of two minutes, or until it completed the trial (entering one of the two alternative arms). Immediately after the mouse entered one arm, such instance was scored as the first choice and the door of the arm was closed. After a few seconds, the animal was gently removed from the arm, placed again in the starting compartment, and allowed to perform a second-choice trial. If the subject entered the arm opposite to the previously chosen one, an instance of alternation was scored. The percentage of alternations (the number of alternations divided by the number of completed sessions times 100) was scored for each mouse.

## 2.13. Statistical Analyses

All statistical analyses were conducted using the software Statview 5.0 (Abacus Concepts, Piscataway, NJ, USA). The experimental design entailed two between subject factors (psychosocial stress, two levels; and Treatment, two levels: PBS vs. GAS) and one within-subject factor (repeated measures with a variable number of levels, depending on the specific parameter). Thus, the general experimental model consisted of a 2 (psychosocial Stress) × 2 (PBS/GAS treatment) × k (repeated measurements) repeated measures ANOVA for split-plot designs. Tukey's post-hoc tests were used for between-group comparisons and Cohen's d factor to measure the effect size between groups. Data are expressed as mean ± SEM or SD were specified. Statistical significance was set at $p < 0.05$.

## 2.14. Data Statement

All data set produced in the present study are available upon request.

## 3. Results

### 3.1. Evaluation of Anti-GAS Antibody Responses in Sera from Mice Injected with GAS Homogenates and Exposed (or not) to Chronic Psychosocial Stress

To investigate the presence of GAS-specific antibodies in sera from treated mice, we loaded 10 microliters of GAS homogenates onto SDS-PAGE, transferred to nitrocellulose, and tested with pools of sera from animals treated with three (Figure 2A) or five (Figure 2B) injections of: GAS homogenate (GAS), GAS homogenate and psychosocial stress (GAS-Stress), adjuvant alone (Adj), or adjuvant and psychosocial stress (Adj-Stress). Western Blot analyses of GAS homogenates using sera from animals treated with three (Figure 2A) or five (Figure 2B) injections of adjuvant (Adj and Adj-Stress mice) did not reveal any or very few bands. Several bands were instead detected in the lanes incubated with sera from animals receiving three (Figure 2A) or five (Figure 2B) GAS injections (GAS and GAS-Stress mice). These results indicate that sera from GAS treated mice recognize specific GAS proteins. Interestingly, this profile appeared much more marked as a consequence of the 5 injections (Figure 2C).

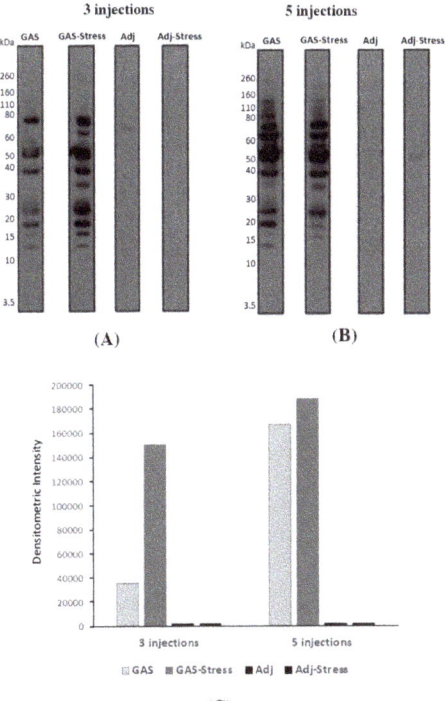

**Figure 2.** (**A**,**B**): Representative immunoblot of GAS extracts probed with pooled sera from mice either treated with 3 (**A**) or 5 doses (**B**) of GAS homogenate (GAS), GAS homogenate and psychosocial stress (GAS-Stress), adjuvant alone (Adj), or adjuvant and psychosocial stress (Adj-Stress). (**C**): Densitometric analysis of overall lane intensities from the blot shown in (**A**,**B**).

*3.2. Consequences of Psychosocial Stress on Serum Corticosterone Concentrations and Glucocorticoid Receptor mRNA Levels in Hypothalamus and Hippocampus*

To evaluate the consequences of chronic psychosocial stress on HPA function, we evaluated serum basal corticosterone concentrations one week after the beginning of the psychosocial stress procedure. We observed that corticosterone concentrations were significantly reduced in all Stress-treated subjects irrespective of exposure to GAS (Stress condition: $F(1,26) = 4.859$, $p < 0.036$; no Stress group: $41.296 \pm 4.236$ ng/mL; Stress group: $28.754 \pm 3.255$ ng/mL; Cohen's d: 3.320).

Given the key role of glucocorticoid receptors (GRs) in regulating corticosterone secretion and mediating its effects on general metabolism, we analyzed the regulation of GRs in the hypothalamus and hippocampus of experimental subjects. These two limbic regions were selected due to their relevance in the response to peripheral immune activation and social stress, as well as in the behavioural abnormalities already evidenced in the PANDAS model [19].

As shown in Figure 3A, hypothalamic mRNA GRs levels were indistinguishable across experimental groups two weeks after the end of treatments.

Conversely, hippocampal GR mRNAs levels were affected by GAS treatment and chronic stress condition (GAS by Stress interaction, $F(1,18) = 17.607$, $p = 0.001$, Figure 3B). Specifically, both chronic stress and GAS exposure independently increased GR concentrations compared to PBS no-Stress subjects. Yet, experimental subjects exposed to both treatments at the same time were indistinguishable from PBS no-Stress controls.

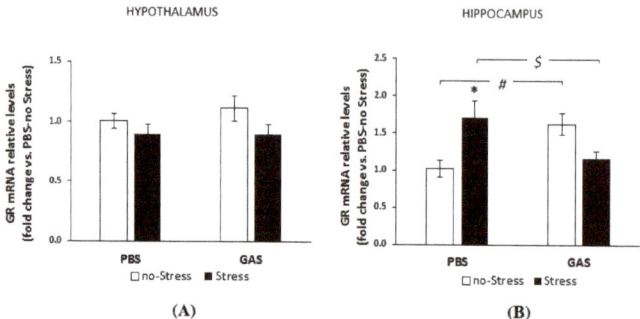

**Figure 3.** Glucocorticoid receptor (GR) mRNA expression in GAS-Stress mice and relative controls. RT-PCR were performed with mRNAs extracted from hypothalamus (**A**) and hippocampus (**B**) of control mice (PBS-no Stress), Group-A beta-haemolytic streptococcus injected mice (GAS-no Stress), psychosocial stressed mice (PBS-Stress), and mice exposed to haemolytic streptococcus and psychosocially stressed (GAS-Stress) at two weeks from treatment endings. Relative expression of GR mRNA in each area is presented as fold change over the expression measured in control mice (PBS-no Stress), taken as 1, and calculated using the 2-$\Delta\Delta$Ct method, normalized to hypoxanthine guanine phosphoribosyl transferase (HPRT), as detailed in the Materials and Methods section. Data are mean ± SEM, N= 4–6 per group. \$ $p < 0.05$: GAS-Stress vs. PBS-Stress; # $p < 0.05$: GAS-no Stress vs. PBS-no Stress; * $p < 0.05$ PBS-no Stress vs. PBS-Stress. Cohen's d measures are reported in Table S1A.

### 3.3. Behavioural Profile Exhibited during the First Active Social Confrontation

We have previously reported that the functional state of the HPA axis at the time of GAS exposure markedly affected GAS-induced neurobehavioral phenotype [19]. To deepen our investigation on the interaction between GAS exposure and environmental stress, we adopted a chronic psychosocial stress model [55]. Specifically, SJL male mice were randomly paired to resident males of the CD1 strain to attain exposure to a gradient of territorial aggression, reportedly high in CD1 [55,56,69]. Thus, half the mice exposed to repeated injections of either vehicle or GAS starting early in adolescence, were later on randomized to psychosocial stress during four weeks according to an established protocol [70]. The Stress condition started by maintaining the two pair members, which had agonistic confrontation on a daily basis, co-housed but prevented from physical interaction. According to the procedure, mice were indeed separated by a transparent and perforated partition allowing continuous sensory contact, thus mimicking a lifelong stress threat.

As reported in Table 1, data collected during the 1st active agonistic confrontation of the psychosocial stress procedure showed that GAS-Stress mice were exposed to significantly higher levels of aggressive behavior than PBS-Stress mice (Treatment by Time interaction ($F(1,37) = 4.338$, $p = 0.044$, for frequency; $F(1,37) = 3.578$, $p = 0.066$, for duration). Accordingly, GAS-Stress mice attained a Defensive upright posture more often and much earlier than controls (Treatment ($F(1,37) = 3.545$, $p = 0.0676$, for frequency; $F(1,38) = 4.907$, $p = 0.0328$, for latency). For Immobility attack-related, a Treatment ($F(1,38) = 3.777$, $p = 0.0785$, for frequency; $F(1,36) = 3.279$, $p = 0.0785$, duration, respectively), were evidenced with increased levels being characteristic of GAS-Stress subjects. A quite similar profile appeared for Immobility contact-related (Treatment: $F(1,37) = 3.982$, $p = 0.0534$ for frequency; $F(1,37) = 5.402$, $p = 0.0257$, for duration).

T-maze test showed, in accordance with our predictions, that repeated GAS immunizations resulted in impaired spontaneous alternation (Treatment: $F(1,35) = 28.326$, $p < 0.001$). Specifically, regardless of exposure to stress, GAS treated mice exhibited reduced spontaneous alternations compared to controls. Furthermore, although exposure to stress apparently influenced the effects of GAS (Stress condition × Treatment: $F(1,35) = 5.025$, $p = 0.0314$), post-hoc tests failed to reveal significant differences between stressed and control individuals within the respective treatment group (PBS-no Stress: 78.020 ± 2.902;

PBS-Stress: 60.937 ± 5.642; GAS-no Stress: 36.607 ± 7.359; GAS-Stress: 44.885 ± 4.377; values are means ± SD; N = 9–10 per group. Cohen's d for PBS-no Stress, GAS-no Stress: 7.404; PBS-no Stress, GAS-Stress: 8.923; PBS-Stress, GAS-Stress: 3.179; GAS-no Stress, GAS-Stress: 1.367).

**Table 1.** Analysis of the behavioural profile during the 1st active agonist confrontation in the psychosocial stress procedure. Submissive behaviours = crouched posture + submissive posture. Duration = time spent (s) performing the behaviour, expressed as a mean of two 5-min intervals. Values are means ± SD; N = 9–10 per group. * $p < 0.05$, ^ trend, df = degrees of freedom.

| Behaviour | Parameter | GAS-Stress | PBS-Stress | F (df) | p | Cohen's d |
|---|---|---|---|---|---|---|
| Attack received | Duration | 6.559 ± 1.135 | 4.996 ± 0.957 | 3.578 (1,37) | 0.07 Treat × Time ^ | 1.489 |
| | Frequency | 9.974 ± 1.866 | 7.175 ± 1.422 | 4.338 (1,37) | 0.04 Treat × Time * | 1.687 |
| Defensive upright posture | Duration | 23.724 ± 3.616 | 16.925 ± 3.482 | 1.707 (1,38) | 0.20 | 1.915 |
| | Frequency | 10.575 ± 1.729 | 6.079 ± 1.076 | 3.545 (1,37) | 0.07 Treat ^ | 3.122 |
| | Latency | 212.518 ± 36.059 | 337.022 ± 43.116 | 4.907 (1,38) | 0.03 Treat * | 3.132 |
| Self-grooming | Duration | 13.048 ± 2.366 | 12.784 ± 2.318 | 0.007 (1,38) | 0.93 | 0.113 |
| | Frequency | 3.350 ± 0.452 | 2.900 ± 0.477 | 0.707 (1,38) | 0.41 | 0.968 |
| Immobility attack-related | Duration | 8.967 ± 2.156 | 2.923 ±.1.181 | 3.279 (1,36) | 0.08 Treat ^ | 3.477 |
| | Frequency | 3.475 ± 0.791 | 2.350 ± 0.648 | 3.777 (1,38) | 0.06 Treat ^ | 1.556 |
| Immobility contact-related | Duration | 13.3 ± 3.650 | 3.988 ± 1.022 | 5.402 (1,37) | 0.03 Treat * | 3.474 |
| | Frequency | 2.950 ± 0.636 | 1.447 ± 0.375 | 3.982 (1,37) | 0.05 Treat ^ | 2.879 |
| Submissive behaviours | Duration | 55.198 ± 6.601 | 45.790 ± 7.840 | 0.843 (1,38) | 0.36 | 1.298 |
| | Frequency | 24.550 ± 3.890 | 17.700 ± 3.069 | 1.911 (1,38) | 0.17 | 1.955 |
| Fleeing | Duration | 7.909 ± 1.452 | 6.480 ± 1.233 | 0.381 (1,37) | 0.54 | 1.061 |
| | Frequency | 9.650 ± 1.743 | 6.350 ± 1.212 | 1.607 (1,38) | 0.21 | 2.198 |
| | Latency | 285.654 ± 39.534 | 349.358 ± 46.590 | 1.087 (1,38) | 0.30 | 1.474 |

### 3.4. Chronic Psychosocial Stress Increased Inflammatory Genes Expression in the Brain of GAS Mice

By using RT-PCR technique, we then investigated the relative levels of typical markers known to be regulated under stress and inflammatory conditions, and playing a central role in mechanisms of neuronal and synaptic plasticity, whose modulation could affect brain function and behaviour. Specifically, we addressed the regulation of the pro-inflammatory cytokines IL-1β and TNF-α, the immunomodulatory cytokine IL-10, the inflammatory/oxidative stress-related enzymes iNOS, Arg-1, MnSOD, and the macrophage/microglial marker CD11b, in the hypothalamus and hippocampus of the experimental subjects. As mentioned above, these two limbic regions were selected for their relevance in the response to peripheral immune activation and social stress, as well as in behavioural abnormalities already evidenced in the PANDAS model [19].

All data (mean ± SEM) on transcript levels obtained two weeks after the end of treatment, alongside with the statistical analyses, are reported in Figure 4 (hypothalamus) and Figure 5 (hippocampus).

In the hypothalamus (Figure 4), ANOVA yielded a significant effect for GAS and Stress single treatments on IL-1β mRNA levels (panel A), with both treatments inducing increased IL-1β expression (GAS: $F(1,15) = 5.863$, $p = 0.029$; Stress: $F(1,15) = 4.401$, $p = 0.053$). The combination of GAS and Stress treatments did not add any change to the profile ($F(1,15) = 0.723$, $p = 0.409$).

As shown in Figure 4B, no changes in TNF-α mRNA levels due to GAS exposure ($F(1,14) = 2.909$, $p = 0.110$) were found. In contrast, PBS-Stress mice had higher transcript levels than PBS-no Stress mice ($F(1,14) = 4.572$, $p = 0.05$). Interestingly, the combination of GAS and Stress completely abated the up-regulatory effect of Stress alone (GAS by Stress interaction: $F(1,14) = 7.597$, $p = 0.015$).

A similar profile was found for IL-10 (Figure 4C): while GAS exposure per se did not modify IL-10 mRNA levels, Stress treatment upregulated the cytokine transcripts ($F(1,14) = 2.558$, $p = 0.132$) compared to no-Stress controls. Also in this case, the combination of GAS and Stress completely abated the upregulation induced by Stress alone (GAS by Stress interaction: $F(1,14) = 6.248$, $p = 0.025$). iNOS mRNA levels (Figure 4D) were neither modified by the two treatments *per se* nor by their interaction.

As shown in Figure 4E, no changes in Arg-1 mRNA levels due to GAS exposure were observed. In contrast, values for PBS-Stress mice were markedly increased ($F(1,14) = 14.07$, $p = 0.002$). In this case, we failed to observe any interaction between GAS and Stress ($F(1,14) = 2.650$, $p = 0.125$).

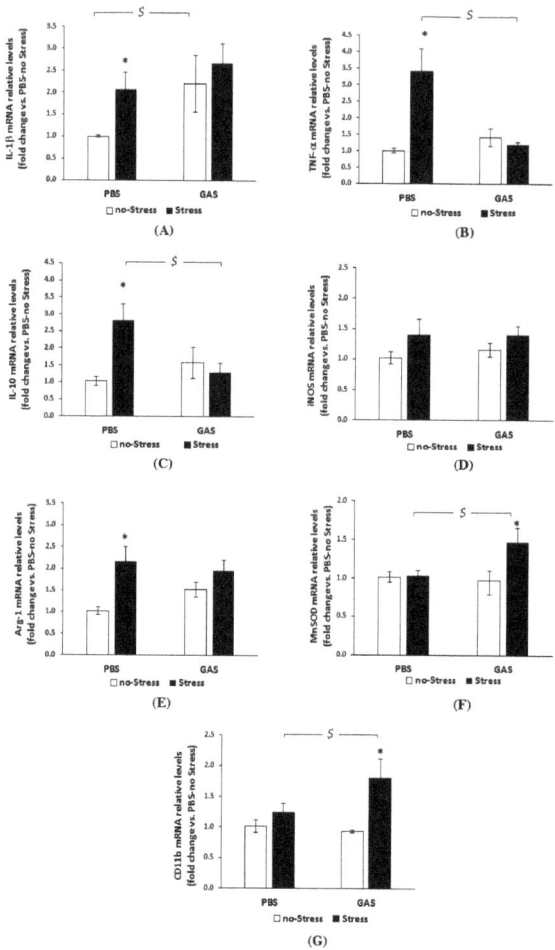

**Figure 4.** mRNA relative levels of inflammatory and oxidative stress-related markers in hypothalamus of GAS-Stress mice and relative controls. RT-PCR analysis was performed with mRNAs extracted from hypothalamus of control mice (PBS-no Stress), Group-A beta-haemolytic streptococcus injected mice (GAS-no Stress), psychosocially stressed mice (PBS-Stress) and mice exposed to haemolytic streptococcus and psychosocially stressed (GAS-Stress), at two weeks from treatment endings. Expression of each gene is presented as fold change over the expression measured in the hypothalamus of control mice (PBS-no Stress), taken as 1. The relative expression level of each mRNA was calculated using the 2-ΔΔCt method, normalized to hypoxanthine guanine phosphoribosyl transferase (HPRT), as detailed in the Materials and Methods section. Data are mean ± SEM, N = 4–6 per group. (**A**) IL-1β mRNA levels: $ $p < 0.05$ for GAS-no Stress vs. PBS-no Stress; * $p < 0.05$ for PBS-Stress vs. PBS-no Stress. (**B**) TNF-α mRNA levels: $ $p < 0.05$ for GAS-Stress vs. PBS-Stress; * $p < 0.05$ for PBS-Stress vs. PBS-no Stress. (**C**) IL-10 mRNA levels: $ $p < 0.05$ for GAS-Stress vs. PBS-Stress; * $p < 0.05$ for PBS-Stress vs. PBS-no Stress. (**D**) iNOS mRNA levels. (**E**) Arg-1 mRNA levels: * $p < 0.01$ for PBS-Stress vs. PBS-no Stress. (**F**) MnSOD mRNA level: $ $p < 0.05$ for GAS-Stress vs. PBS-Stress; * $p < 0.05$ for GAS-Stress vs. GAS-no Stress. (**G**) CD11b mRNA levels: $ $p < 0.05$ for GAS-Stress vs. PBS-Stress; * $p < 0.05$ for GAS-Stress vs. GAS-no Stress. Cohen's d measures are reported in Table S1A.

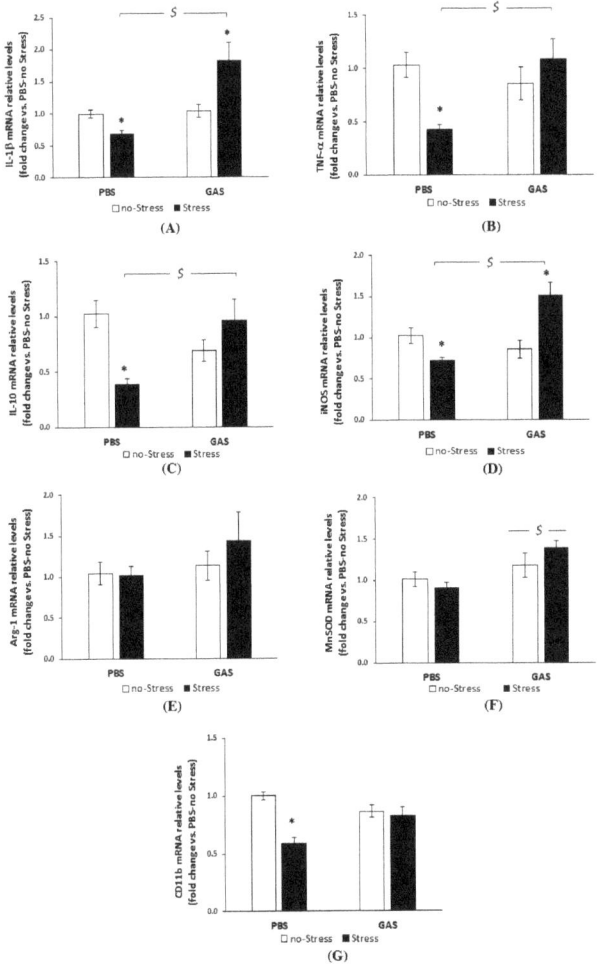

**Figure 5.** mRNA relative levels of inflammatory and oxidative stress-related markers in the hippocampus of GAS-Stress mice and relative controls. RT-PCR analysis was performed with mRNAs extracted from hippocampus of control mice (PBS-no Stress), Group-A beta-haemolytic streptococcus exposed mice (GAS-no Stress), psychosocially stressed mice (PBS-Stress) and mice exposed to haemolytic streptococcus and psychosocially stressed (GAS-Stress), at two weeks from treatment endings. Expression of each gene is presented as fold change over the expression measured in the hippocampus of control mice (PBS-no Stress), taken as 1. The relative expression level of each mRNA was calculated using the 2-ΔΔCt method, normalized to hypoxanthine guanine phosphoribosyl transferase (HPRT), as detailed in the Materials and Methods section. Data are mean ± SEM, $n$ = 4–6 per group. (**A**) IL-1β mRNA levels: \$ $p < 0.01$ for GAS- Stress vs. PBS-Stress; * $p < 0.05$ for GAS-Stress vs. GAS-no Stress and for PBS-Stress vs. PBS-no Stress. (**B**) TNF-α mRNA levels: \$ $p < 0.05$ for GAS-Stress vs. PBS-Stress; * $p < 0.05$ for PBS-Stress vs. PBS-no Stress. (**C**) IL-10 mRNA levels: \$ $p < 0.05$ for GAS-Stress vs. PBS-Stress; * $p < 0.05$ for PBS-Stress vs. PBS-no Stress. (**D**) iNOS mRNA level: \$ $p < 0.01$ for GAS-Stress vs. PBS-Stress; * $p < 0.01$ for GAS-Stress vs. GAS-no Stress and $p < 0.05$ for PBS-Stress vs. PBS-no Stress. (**E**) Arg-1 mRNA levels. (**F**) MnSOD mRNA level: \$ $p < 0.05$ for PBS vs. GAS. (**G**) CD11b mRNA levels: * $p < 0.01$ for PBS-Stress vs. PBS-no Stress and vs. GAS-Stress. Cohen's d measures are reported in Table S1A.

In the absence of a main effect of GAS on MnSOD mRNA levels (Figure 4F) ANOVA indicated that the Stress group as a whole was higher than control ($F(1,13) = 5.692$, $p = 0.0329$). Further, a significant GAS by Stress interaction ($F(1,13) = 5.411$, $p = 0.0368$) revealed that the upregulation of mRNA transcripts was specific to the GAS-Stress group.

No main effect of GAS on CD11b (Figure 4G) mRNA levels was found. ANOVA yielded an effect of Stress as a whole ($F(1,17) = 7.770$, $p = 0.0126$), and a GAS by Stress interaction ($F(1,17) = 2.727$, $p = 0.117$); Tukey post hoc indicated that the upregulation of mRNA transcripts due to Stress was again specific to GAS-Stress mice.

To summarize, two weeks after the last GAS injection, among the transcripts analysed in the hypothalamus, only IL-1β transcripts were reliably modified by GAS inoculation per se. Chronic psychosocial Stress per se upregulated both typical pro-inflammatory (IL-1β and TNF-α) and anti-inflammatory genes (IL-10 and Arg-1) while leaving unaltered the expression of the pro- and anti-oxidant enzymes iNOS and MnSOD and the phagocytic marker CD11b. When mice, previously inoculated with GAS, were faced with stress adverse experience, also MnSOD and CD11b resulted up-regulated. In contrast, TNF-α and IL-10 were down-regulated compared to Stress alone, suggesting the activation of the oxidative defense system in the combined condition, and a more pronounced or longer lasting inflammatory macrophage/microglial activation.

Noteworthy, in the hippocampus (Figure 5), GAS and Stress elicited a differential regulation of these inflammatory genes compared to the hypothalamus. Indeed, repeated GAS inoculation alone did not significantly or reliably alter the expression levels of the genes analysed (panels A–G). This suggests that, at this time point, the inflammatory reaction to the GAS stimulus was already subsided in this region, at least in term of the mRNA regulation of the panel of genes assayed.

Unlike GAS per se, Stress alone significantly reduced IL-1β, TNF-α, IL-10, iNOS, and CD11b mRNA levels (Figure 5, panels A–D, and G respectively), as revealed by post hoc analyses (see the Figure legend).

Interestingly, in the absence of significant GAS-related changes per se, the combination of GAS and Stress reverted the Stress-induced down-regulatory effect, indicating a relevant interaction of the two treatments. Indeed, GAS-Stress mice showed comparable TNF-α, IL-10, and CD11b levels than PBS-no Stress subjects, and higher IL-1β and iNOS levels (GAS by Stress interaction for TNF-α: $F(1,19) = 9.695$, $p = 0.0057$; for IL-10: $F(1,16) = 14.502$, $p = 0.0015$; for IL-1β: $F(1,20) = 16.754$, $p = 0.0006$; for iNOS: $F(1,20) = 24.628$, $p < 0.0001$; for CD11b: $F(1,19) = 16.789$, $p = 0.0006$).

Unlike the other genes analyzed, Arg-1 mRNA levels (Figure 5E) were unaffected, irrespective of both treatments and their combination.

Considering MnSOD expression (Figure 5F), ANOVA yielded a significant effect for GAS exposure ($F(1,15) = 9.999$, $p = 0.006$), with GAS group as a whole being higher than controls (for post hoc, see figure legend). Stress *per se* or its combination with previous GAS inoculation, did not affect the profile.

As a whole, these data suggest that Psychosocial Stress mostly induced a down-regulated basal immune profile at the hippocampal level, while the combination with GAS exposure was associated with an increased, longer-lasting, pro-inflammatory oxidative condition in the hippocampus.

### 3.5. Psychosocial Stress Affects Mitochondrial OXPHOS Machinery and Reduces Energy Status in the Brain of GAS Immunized Mice

We first examined whether GAS and Stress treatments, separately or in interaction, could affect the MRC complex activity in mice brain mitochondria (Figure 6). Measurements of MRC complex I-IV as well as ATP synthase (complex V) activities showed no significant changes in all MRC activities in both PBS-Stress and GAS-no Stress treated mice, respect to control (PBS-no Stress) group. Interestingly, GAS treatment in mice exposed to psychosocial stress (GAS-Stress group) resulted in a significant reduction in the activity of complex IV and V compared to control mice ($F(1,12) = 16.12$, $p = 0.002$; $F(1,12) = 95.28$, $p = 0.001$, respectively). Importantly, chronic stress plus GAS treatments did not alter the mitochondrial content in the brain tissue being 4.70 ± 0.6 and 4.66 ± 0.3 mg the amount of mitochondrial proteins obtained respectively from untreated and GAS-Stress groups ($p > 0.5$), from brain hemisphere tissues with comparable wet weights ($0.24 \pm 0.1$ g).

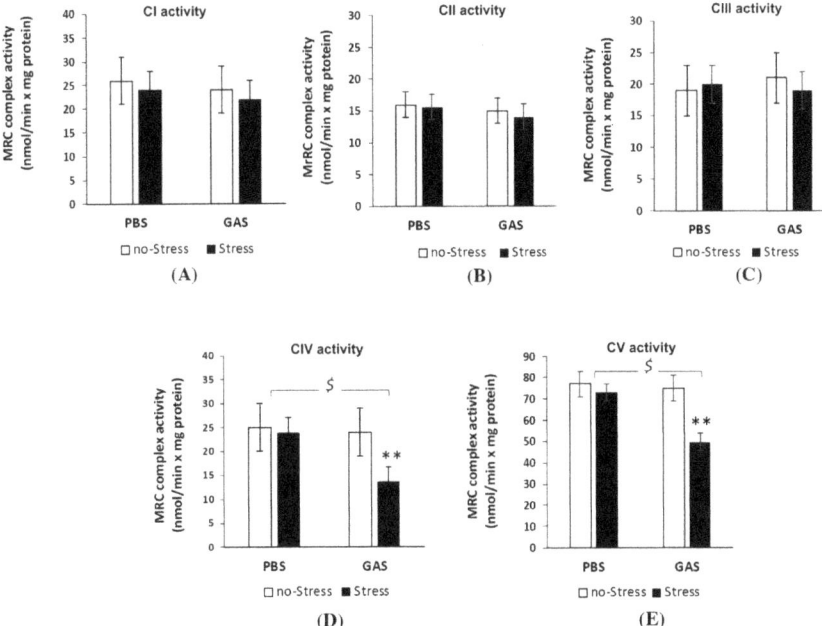

**Figure 6.** Mitochondrial respiratory chain (MRC) complex activities in brain of GAS-Stress mice and relative controls. The activities of the MRC (**A**) complex I, (**B**) complex II, (**C**) complex III, (**D**) complex IV and (**E**) complex V (ATP synthase) were measured spectrophotometrically in mitochondrial membrane enriched fractions from cryopreserved brain hemispheres of wt littermates control mice (PBS-no Stress), Group-A beta-haemolytic streptococcus exposed mice (GAS-no Stress), psychosocially stressed mice (PBS-Stress) and psychosocially stressed mice exposed to haemolytic streptococcus (GAS-Stress), at two weeks from treatment endings. Complex activities are expressed as nmol/min × mg protein. Data are mean rates ± SD obtained from three independent experiments. For MRC complex IV and V activities $ p < 0.05$ for PBS-Stress vs. GAS-Stress; ** $p < 0.01$ for GAS no-Stress vs. GAS-Stress. Cohen's d measures are reported in Table S1B.

In order to investigate whether the MRC defective complex activities found in GAS-Stress mice group was accompanied by an impairment of bioenergetic efficiency, the mitochondrial ATP synthesis was measured following the relative contribution of the individual MRC complexes of the OXPHOS apparatus in the mitochondrial ATP production i.e. by adding the respiratory substrates of either complex I (GLU/MAL), complex II (SUCC) or complex IV (ASC/TMPD), as energy sources (Figure 7). Consistently with the data obtained from MRC activity measurements, GAS-Stress mice showed a significant reduction in mitochondrial ATP synthesis only when using as energy source the respiratory substrates of complex IV (Figure 7C); after post hoc comparison on GAS-Stress vs. PBS-no Stress mice: $F(1,12) = 4.60, p = 0.04$. No significant differences among all mice groups were found in the complex I- and II-dependent rate of mitochondrial ATP production from brain mitochondria. These results suggest that specific components of the respiratory apparatus resulted selectively affected by GAS in psychosocial stressed mice and contributed to the shortage in mitochondrial ATP production.

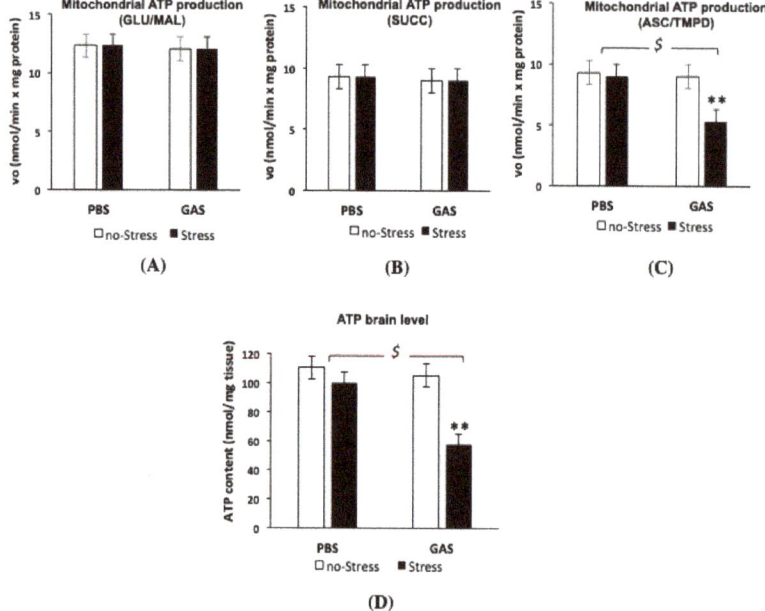

**Figure 7.** Mitochondrial ATP production and ATP level in the brain of GAS-Stress mice and relative controls. The rate of mitochondrial ATP production was measured in mitochondria isolated from cryopreserved brain hemispheres in the presence of the respiratory substrates of (**A**) complex I glutamate plus malate (GLU/MAL), (**B**) complex II succinate (SUCC) plus rotenone or (**C**) complex IV ascorbate plus TMPD (ASC/TMPD). Values are mean rates ± SD obtained from three independent experiments and expressed as nmol/min × mg protein. Values are mean rates ± SD obtained from three independent experiments and expressed as nmol/min × mg protein. (**D**) The ATP level was measured as described in Material and Methods. Values are mean rates ± SD obtained from three independent experiments and expressed as nmol/mg protein. For the panels C and D $ $p < 0.05$ for PBS-Stress vs. GAS-Stress. ** $p < 0.01$ for GAS no-Stress vs. GAS-Stress. Cohen's d measures are reported in Table S1C.

Interestingly, the levels of ATP assayed in the brain of all four groups were strongly lowered in GAS-Stress group as compared to the other groups (Figure 7D, $F(1,16) = 18.36$, $p = 0.001$), thus suggesting that alterations in mitochondrial ATP production by GAS in psychosocial stress conditions affected the whole brain energy status.

## 4. Discussion

The validated translational mouse model of PANDAS, adopted in the present study, has been extensively characterized from a behavioural and biochemical point of view in our previous studies [18,19]. Consistently with the hypothesis of the infectious and autoimmune pathogenesis of PANDAS (see [71]), we reported that repeated exposures to GAS induce an antibody-mediated response (also confirmed in the present study) and behavioural alterations homologous to clinical symptoms observed in PANDAS (impaired sensorimotor gating, and abnormal repetitive and perseverative behaviours). The behavioural phenotypes exhibited by GAS mice represent the preclinical analogue of core clinical symptoms observed in PANDAS and obsessive-compulsive syndrome [11,72,73], and are useful for studying their neurobiological basis. For example, increased behavioural rigidity, reflected in impairments in spontaneous alternations, could be due to alterations in forebrain structures (prefrontal cortex and dorsal striatum) [74] and imbalances in dopaminergic [75] and serotonergic [76] neurochemical systems.

We previously reported that the behavioural changes observed in GAS mice were associated with immune-mediated brain alterations, as indicated by the presence of inflammatory infiltrates and activated microglia at the level of the rostral diencephalon (see [19,71] for a detailed discussion). In the same rodent model, we observed that neonatal corticosterone administration contrasted both behavioural and immunohistochemical alterations induced by later GAS exposure. These compensatory effects co-occurred with persistent modifications in HPA activity and remarkable plasma increases of several cytokines and chemokines, supporting the view that the HPA axis may contribute to the regulation of the immune responses involved in the pathological sequelae of PANDAS and ultimately modulate the severity of the PANDAS-related phenotype.

On this basis, herein, we further characterized the sequelae of repeated exposures to a GAS homogenate during development (between late infancy and young adulthood) on behaviour, neuroinflammatory and brain oxidative stress responses, and mitochondrial functional aspects later at adulthood, and addressed the modulatory effects of chronic psychosocial stress on the same parameters.

With the aim of a translational approach, and to model a chronic psychosocial stress condition [55,56,69], GAS mice and their controls were exposed to a gradient of territorial aggression by resident male mice. Specifically, compared to PBS-injected control mice, during the first active social confrontation, GAS mice were the recipients of consistently higher levels of aggressive behavior (in terms of Attacks received). GAS mice also showed a characteristic behavioural repertoire, consisting of a shortened latency to and an increased frequency of defensive upright postures, and time spent in immobility. The observed behavioral profile of chronic stress condition is consistent with recent literature on this translational model of adverse emotional experience [70], and on the reported interaction of chronic stress with central immune dysregulation [77]. We believe that this profile of increased aggression received by GAS mice during the first confrontation may relate to the fact that the homogenate injection resulted in an overt inflammatory profile. The latter may have signalled a state of vulnerability to the resident mouse which, in turn, may have increased its degree of aggression. Whilst this aspect is worth additional investigation, we note that the differential attacks received by Stress and GAS mice during the first day have unlikely extended to the following days of stress exposure. This tenet stems from the fact that, after the first day, during the following days, direct attacks were physically prevented by the experimenter, which interrupted the session upon the first occurrence of aggressive interaction. Ultimately, although future studies are needed to clarify this aspect, we suggest that the increased aggression received by GAS mice on day one may be due to a short-term effect of GAS homogenate on individual phenotype, but that – in the light of the experimental paradigm adopted—such differential profile is unlikely to explain the observed findings.

Consistently with our previous histochemical observations, suggestive of GAS-induced central immune activation, here we found increased hypothalamic mRNA levels of the pro-inflammatory cytokine IL-1β in GAS mice, analysed two weeks after the last GAS inoculation, revealing a long-lasting central inflammatory effect of peripheral immunization. However, the other inflammatory- or oxidative stress-related genes analysed (i.e. TNF-α, IL-10, iNOS, Arg-1, MnSOD, CD11b) were not altered compared to PBS-injected control subjects.

Interestingly, at the hippocampal level, the expression of IL-1β was not reliably modified by GAS treatment per se, as well as that of TNF-α, iNOS, and MnSOD, while the immunomodulatory cytokine IL-10 and the macrophage/microglial phagocytic marker CD11b showed a tendency to decrease compared to PBS-injected control mice.

It is worth noting that, as the above mRNA expression analyses were conducted two weeks after the last GAS inoculation, our data depict the long-lasting alteration of neuroinflammatory state consequent to repeated GAS challenges rather than the acute alteration of the genes analysed. It is well known that brain immune cells (mainly microglia and astrocytes) undergo a profound rearrangement of their functions following chronic stimulation, and acute and chronic preconditioning regimens differentially affect their responsiveness to a later inflammatory challenge, for the onset of distinct mechanisms of molecular memory ([78,79] and refs therein). Therefore, the mRNA data of inflammatory markers reflect brain immune cell adaptation to a chronic stimulation. Similar considerations apply to the analyses of inflammation-related transcripts in subjects exposed to Psychosocial Stress, two weeks after treatment termination.

Also in this case, and in line with previous experimental studies on Psychosocial Stress effects [77], we observed a region-specific modulation of central cytokine expression. The direction of mRNA regulation by Psychosocial Stress was however different from what found for GAS exposure, as it was characterized by a prominent inflammatory response in the hypothalamus, and an opposite profile in the hippocampus. Specifically, compared to PBS-injected control mice, while Stress upregulated the mRNA levels of the inflammatory genes IL-1β, TNF-α, IL-10, Arg-1, and marginally modulated iNOS and CD11b mRNAs in the hypothalamus, it downregulated the same genes (with the exception of Arg-1) in the hippocampus.

Besides their role in neuroinflammatory processes, cytokines typically participate in brain development and plasticity, by translating environmental inputs into molecular signals [80]. An imbalance between pro-inflammatory and anti-inflammatory cytokines can lead to long-lasting changes in brain anatomy and function, and therefore long-term impairments in mood, cognition, and behavior [81]. We did not analyze possible changes in brain anatomy in the GAS mouse model, but the neuroimmune and behavioural alterations found in our study further support the link between inflammatory gene regulation and behaviour.

Obvious limitations of mRNA analysis on bulk hippocampus and hypothalamus include the possible dilution of signals confined to specific sub-regions important for immune and stress responses, as well as the exclusion of additional levels of gene expression regulation; nonetheless, our data clearly indicate that GAS peripheral infection and Stress have long-term and region-specific consequences on brain immune homeostasis.

Region-specific patterns of up-regulation of distinct cytokines and differences in the extent and time-course of activation in response to peripheral and central stressors have been reported in different experimental models, albeit mechanisms conferring specificity of action remain to be fully elucidated. Among the different factors accounting for these differences, neutrophil infiltration rate, microglia/astrocyte density, blood brain barrier permeability, and relative densities of mineralocorticoid and glucocorticoid receptors may represent valid targets [82–84].

Although the identification of possible mechanisms is far beyond the scope of the present experimental investigation, the finding that GAS and chronic psychosocial Stress independently upregulated GR expression at the hippocampal but not hypothalamic level suggests that these changes might be involved in the different sensitivity of the two brain regions to HPA-related regulatory mechanisms of inflammation. This is consistent with other reports from different chronic stress models [85,86].

Furthermore, while both repeated GAS exposure and Psychosocial Stress exerted independent effects, the main translational finding of the present study resides in the fact that the latter exacerbated the effects of the former. In accordance with experimental data indicating that variations in circulating corticosteroids may influence autoimmune phenomena [87,88], we observed that chronic psychosocial stress, which exerted persistent effects on HPA axis activity (revealed by changes in hippocampal GR expression and reduced peripheral corticosterone concentrations), exacerbated the behavioural, immune and mitochondrial effects of GAS administration. The observation that the combination of GAS and Stress halted the upregulation of GR in the hippocampus, together with the reduced corticosterone concentrations found in this experimental group, suggest a persistent blunted HPA activity in these mice at the time point of our analyses.

Classical studies conducted by Levine and his group showed that psychological and physiological stress suppresses [87] and adrenalectomy potentiates [89] vulnerability to experimental autoimmune encephalomyelitis. Ultimately, it is tenable that, depending on the directionality of the long-term consequences exerted by experimental manipulations on HPA activity (increase or decrease in circulating concentrations of corticosteroids and regulation of their receptors), autoimmune responses may be either potentiated or contrasted. Complex feedforward and feedback control mechanisms of gene expression between glucocorticoids, activating GRs, and cytokines (such as IL-1β and TNF-α) have been described in different experimental models [90,91] providing an explanation for the not univocal role of glucocorticoids on inflammatory gene expression regulation. Further investigations will be needed to address these issues in our GAS-Stress model and to dissect the interactions that can take place in the two separate or combined GAS and Stress conditions.

Interestingly, the combination of GAS exposures with chronic stress-induced a significant upregulation of the hippocampal levels of IL-1β, TNF-α, and the inducible enzyme iNOS compared to PBS-injected control subjects, which was not achieved by the single treatments. GAS-Stress treatment also elicited a further upregulation of CD11b mRNA compared to Stress (in the hippocampus and hypothalamus) or GAS alone (in the hypothalamus), suggesting an increased macrophage/microglia activation in these areas.

Overall, these findings are in line with growing evidence indicating that cross-sensitization can occur between immune-induced and stress-induced pro-inflammatory cytokines, resulting in the potentiation of CNS cytokine responses [37–40]. The phenomenon of cross-sensitization suggests that a shared neural substrate, mainly identified by others in the primary immune effector cell in the nervous system i.e. microglia, may be primed by either stress or immune activation [37,38,40,92]. Whatever the underlying mechanisms may be, cross-sensitization provides a mechanism explaining how stress can exacerbate inflammatory disease processes and vice versa.

In consideration of the increasingly recognized modulatory action of cytokines and nitric oxide on mechanisms of neuronal and synaptic plasticity, our data support the view that peripheral inflammation and stress converge on pathways culminating in disruption of brain homeostatic functions and neuroinflammation. In addition, by the generation of nitrogen reactive species, iNOS can contribute to oxidative stress as shown in different tissues and experimental models [93,94], including psychogenic stress treatments [95,96].

Consistently, we observed that GAS-Stress treatment promoted the expression of MnSOD—the primary antioxidant enzyme in mitochondria—at hippocampal and hypothalamic levels; these data indicate the induction of the antioxidant defense system. MnSOD, a key component of the enzymatic antioxidant system, is upregulated by various mediators of oxidative stress, including reactive oxygen and nitrogen species and inflammatory cytokines, such as IL-1β and TNF-α [49], and its abnormalities have been documented in several clinical cases and experimental neurodegenerative processes [97].

Superoxide dismutase function is activated in the mitochondria to detoxify free radical superoxide anion with formation of less reactive peroxide anion ($H_2O_2$) [49]. However, conditions of chronic increase of MnSOD activity could result in $H_2O_2$ accumulation, thereby causing mitochondrial alterations. In particular, the MRC complex IV-cytochrome c oxidase is a target of hydrogen peroxide showing various sites of oxidative modifications, which leads to a decline in its catalytic activity [98].

Consistently with a condition of oxidative stress in the GAS-Stress mouse model, our data demonstrate that the combined exposure to GAS and stress caused a reduction of the complex IV activity and decreased complex IV-dependent ATP production. These deficits, together with a reduced ATP synthase activity, impair mitochondrial bioenergetics resulting in a deficit of brain ATP content. The defective whole brain energy status and activation of MnSOD were not elicited by the single treatments, suggesting for the first time a direct link between inflammation, mitochondrial bioenergetic deficiency and ROS production in the combined infection/stress condition.

This is, to the best of our knowledge, the first report suggesting a clear link between inflammation status and mitochondrial dysfunction in infectious GAS condition exacerbated by psychosocial stress.

Mitochondrial dysfunction is emerging as a pathological mechanism underlying various inflammatory and autoimmune diseases, which become worse when accompanied by systemic inflammation and oxidative stress [99]. Accumulating clinical and preclinical evidence indicate that mitochondria are key players in neuroinflammatory and neurodegenerative diseases, as well as a critical intersection point connecting early-life stress, brain programming and mental health [100–102]. There is growing evidence for the involvement of both mitochondrial ROS and mitochondrial metabolism in inflammatory microglia/macrophage activation [47,103,104]. Moreover, it has been recently shown that alterations of mitochondrial activity in microglia hamper the process of alternative activation, suggesting that in severe clinical neurological conditions characterized by mitochondrial dysfunctions, microglia may not be able to induce a full anti-inflammatory response, exacerbating neuroinflammation [48].

Our results in the preclinical model of PANDAS substantiate the translational hypothesis that Streptococcus infection could induce an inflammatory status in PANDS patients, exacerbated by stress conditions, with the secretion of inflammatory cytokines, which likely induce increase of ROS production and mitochondrial dysfunction, resulting in brain energy deficit, which in turn intensify the clinical symptoms severity. Previous clinical studies have demonstrated that inflammatory cytokines such as interleukin-17 disable the main function of mitochondria, the energy production by respiration, and activate autophagy in an autoimmune disease such as rheumatoid arthritis [51]. Indeed, the critical role of pro-inflammatory cytokines on mitochondrial stress signalling and proteostasis is well known [105,106]. Of note, a direct link between stress-derived corticosteroids and mitochondrial function has been demonstrated in recent studies, revealing that activated GRs, besides their genomic action, can translocate to the mitochondrial compartment and regulate mitochondrial mRNA expression, including complex 1 subunits and ATP-synthase 6 expression [107,108]. The possible regulatory function of GRs on mitochondrial activities in the GAS-Stress model will deserve further investigations.

## 5. Conclusions

Our results demonstrate that chronic psychosocial stress, which per se altered the expression of neuroinflammatory markers in the hippocampal and hypothalamic regions, exacerbated the neuroinflammatory alterations induced by experimental GAS exposures in the same areas. In addition, the combined GAS/Stress treatment elicited mitochondrial dysfunctions, brain energy deficit and upregulation of manganese superoxide dismutase (MnSOD), a mitochondrial enzyme playing a major role in modulation of mitochondrial oxidative stress.

Our findings demonstrate the negative impact of social stress on PANDAS symptomatology and provide a functional explanation to epidemiological and clinical data as well as a biological platform to investigate the impact of psychosocial stress on immune-related clinical neurological diseases.

In this study, we offered a proof of principle and a translational hypothesis that experimentally-induced alterations of HPA functionality may calibrate the individual response and vulnerability to autoimmune phenomena. Furthermore, we identified a potential translational link between environmental stress experience and the underlying mechanisms (promotion of immunomodulatory processes) capable of promoting/exacerbating the progression of the pathological phenotype. We propose that these data may inform future clinical strategies in the treatment of PANDAS.

**Supplementary Materials:** The following are available online at http://www.mdpi.com/2077-0383/8/10/1514/s1, Table S1: Effect Size measures (Cohen's d) for the comparisons shown in Figure 3, Figure 4, Figure 5 (**A**), Figure 6 (**B**) and Figure 7 (**C**). * Cohen's *d* corresponding to significant comparisons.

**Author Contributions:** G.L. and S.M. designed the studies, interpreted the results, and wrote the manuscript. G.L. supervised the study. C.S. designed the studies, performed the experiments, interpreted the results, performed statistical analyses, and revised the manuscript. F.F. carried out the behavioural characterization and performed statistical analyses. M.A.A.-C. carried out Real time PCR analyses, interpreted the results, and wrote the manuscript. R.A.V. and D.V. carried out mitochondrial analyses, interpreted the results, performed statistical analyses, and wrote the manuscript. R.A.V. provided useful suggestions and revised the manuscript.

**Funding:** This research was funded the European Community's Seventh Framework Program (FP7) under grant agreement n° 278367, the EMTICS Consortium and n° 603016, the MATRICS Consortium to G.L.

**Acknowledgments:** We thank Erika Bartolini and Immaculada Margarit for providing help with the measure of GAS-related antibodies.

**Conflicts of Interest:** The authors declare no conflict of interest.

## References

1. Benros, M.E.; Waltoft, B.L.; Nordentoft, M.; Østergaard, S.D.; Eaton, W.W.; Krogh, J.; Mortensen, P.B. Autoimmune Diseases and Severe Infections as Risk Factors for Mood Disorders. *JAMA Psychiatry* **2013**, *70*, 812. [CrossRef] [PubMed]
2. Köhler-Forsberg, O.; Petersen, L.; Gasse, C.; Mortensen, P.B.; Dalsgaard, S.; Yolken, R.H.; Mors, O.; Benros, M.E. A Nationwide Study in Denmark of the Association between Treated Infections and the Subsequent Risk of Treated Mental Disorders in Children and Adolescents. *JAMA Psychiatry* **2018**. [CrossRef] [PubMed]
3. Sperner-Unterweger, B. Immunological aetiology of major psychiatric disorders: Evidence and therapeutic implications. *Drugs* **2005**, *65*, 1493–1520. [CrossRef] [PubMed]
4. Tylee, D.S.; Sun, J.; Hess, J.L.; Tahir, M.A.; Sharma, E.; Malik, R.; Worrall, B.B.; Levine, A.J.; Martinson, J.J.; Nejentsev, S.; et al. Genetic correlations among psychiatric and immune-related phenotypes based on genome-wide association data. *Am. J. Med. Genet. B. Neuropsychiatr. Genet.* **2018**, *177*, 641–657. [CrossRef] [PubMed]
5. Khandaker, G.M.; Dantzer, R.; Jones, P.B. Immunopsychiatry: Important facts. *Psychol. Med.* **2017**, *47*, 2229–2237. [CrossRef] [PubMed]
6. Levin, M.C.; Lee, S.M.; Kalume, F.; Morcos, Y.; Dohan, F.C.; Hasty, K.A.; Callaway, J.C.; Zunt, J.; Desiderio, D.M.; Stuart, J.M. Autoimmunity due to molecular mimicry as a cause of neurological disease. *Nat. Med.* **2002**, *8*, 509–513. [CrossRef] [PubMed]
7. Brimberg, L.; Benhar, I.; Mascaro-Blanco, A.; Alvarez, K.; Lotan, D.; Winter, C.; Klein, J.; Moses, A.E.; Somnier, F.E.; Leckman, J.F.; et al. Behavioral, pharmacological, and immunological abnormalities after streptococcal exposure: A novel rat model of Sydenham chorea and related neuropsychiatric disorders. *Neuropsychopharmacology* **2012**, *37*, 2076–2087. [CrossRef] [PubMed]
8. Garvey, M.A.; Giedd, J.; Swedo, S.E. PANDAS: The search for environmental triggers of pediatric neuropsychiatric disorders. Lessons from rheumatic fever. *J. Child Neurol.* **1998**, *13*, 413–423. [CrossRef]
9. Hoffman, K.L.; Hornig, M.; Yaddanapudi, K.; Jabado, O.; Lipkin, W.I. A murine model for neuropsychiatric disorders associated with group A beta-hemolytic streptococcal infection. *J. Neurosci.* **2004**, *24*, 1780–1791. [CrossRef]
10. Snider, L.A.; Swedo, S.E. PANDAS: Current status and directions for research. *Mol. Psychiatry* **2004**, *9*, 900–907. [CrossRef]
11. Swedo, S.E.; Leonard, H.L.; Rapoport, J.L. The pediatric autoimmune neuropsychiatric disorders associated with streptococcal infection (PANDAS) subgroup: Separating fact from fiction. *Pediatrics* **2004**, *113*, 907–911. [CrossRef] [PubMed]
12. Yaddanapudi, K.; Hornig, M.; Serge, R.; De Miranda, J.; Baghban, A.; Villar, G.; Lipkin, W.I. Passive transfer of streptococcus-induced antibodies reproduces behavioral disturbances in a mouse model of pediatric autoimmune neuropsychiatric disorders associated with streptococcal infection. *Mol. Psychiatry* **2010**, *15*, 712–726. [CrossRef] [PubMed]
13. Hoekstra, P.J.; Dietrich, A.; Edwards, M.J.; Elamin, I.; Martino, D. Environmental factors in Tourette syndrome. *Neurosci. Biobehav. Rev.* **2013**, *37*, 1040–1049. [CrossRef] [PubMed]
14. Leonard, H.L.; Swedo, S.E. Paediatric autoimmune neuropsychiatric disorders associated with streptococcal infection (PANDAS). *Int. J. Neuropsychopharmacol.* **2001**, *4*, 191–198. [CrossRef] [PubMed]
15. Cardona, F.; Orefici, G. Group A streptococcal infections and tic disorders in an Italian pediatric population. *J. Pediatr.* **2001**, *138*, 71–75. [CrossRef] [PubMed]
16. Rizzo, R.; Gulisano, M.; Pavone, P.; Fogliani, F.; Robertson, M.M. Increased antistreptococcal antibody titers and anti-basal ganglia antibodies in patients with Tourette syndrome: Controlled cross-sectional study. *J. Child Neurol.* **2006**, *21*, 747–753. [CrossRef] [PubMed]
17. Orlovska, S.; Vestergaard, C.H.; Bech, B.H.; Nordentoft, M.; Vestergaard, M.; Benros, M.E. Association of Streptococcal Throat Infection with Mental Disorders: Testing Key Aspects of the PANDAS Hypothesis in a Nationwide Study. *JAMA Psychiatry* **2017**, *74*, 740–746. [CrossRef] [PubMed]
18. Macrì, S.; Ceci, C.; Onori, M.P.; Invernizzi, R.W.; Bartolini, E.; Altabella, L.; Canese, R.; Imperi, M.; Orefici, G.; Creti, R.; et al. Mice repeatedly exposed to Group-A β-Haemolytic Streptococcus show perseverative behaviors, impaired sensorimotor gating, and immune activation in rostral diencephalon. *Sci. Rep.* **2015**, *5*, 13257. [CrossRef] [PubMed]

19. Macrì, S.; Spinello, C.; Widomska, J.; Magliozzi, R.; Poelmans, G.; Invernizzi, R.W.; Creti, R.; Roessner, V.; Bartolini, E.; Margarit, I.; et al. Neonatal corticosterone mitigates autoimmune neuropsychiatric disorders associated with streptococcus in mice. *Sci. Rep.* **2018**, *8*, 10188. [CrossRef] [PubMed]
20. Conelea, C.A.; Woods, D.W. The influence of contextual factors on tic expression in Tourette's syndrome: A review. *J. Psychosom. Res.* **2008**, *65*, 487–496. [CrossRef]
21. Buse, J.; Kirschbaum, C.; Leckman, J.F.; Münchau, A.; Roessner, V. The Modulating Role of Stress in the Onset and Course of Tourette's Syndrome: A Review. *Behav. Modif.* **2014**, *38*, 184–216. [CrossRef] [PubMed]
22. Godar, S.C.; Bortolato, M. What makes you tic? Translational approaches to study the role of stress and contextual triggers in Tourette syndrome. *Neurosci. Biobehav. Rev.* **2017**, *76*, 123–133. [CrossRef] [PubMed]
23. Leckman, J.F. Tourette's syndrome. *Lancet* **2002**, *360*, 1577–1586. [CrossRef]
24. Motlagh, M.G.; Katsovich, L.; Thompson, N.; Lin, H.; Kim, Y.-S.; Scahill, L.; Lombroso, P.J.; King, R.A.; Peterson, B.S.; Leckman, J.F. Severe psychosocial stress and heavy cigarette smoking during pregnancy: An examination of the pre- and perinatal risk factors associated with ADHD and Tourette syndrome. *Eur. Child. Adolesc. Psychiatry* **2010**, *19*, 755–764. [CrossRef] [PubMed]
25. Saccomani, L.; Fabiana, V.; Manuela, B.; Giambattista, R. Tourette syndrome and chronic tics in a sample of children and adolescents. *Brain Dev.* **2005**, *27*, 349–352. [CrossRef] [PubMed]
26. Conelea, C.A.; Woods, D.W.; Brandt, B.C. The impact of a stress induction task on tic frequencies in youth with Tourette Syndrome. *Behav. Res. Ther.* **2011**, *49*, 492–497. [CrossRef] [PubMed]
27. Lin, H.; Katsovich, L.; Ghebremichael, M.; Findley, D.B.; Grantz, H.; Lombroso, P.J.; King, R.A.; Zhang, H.; Leckman, J.F. Psychosocial stress predicts future symptom severities in children and adolescents with Tourette syndrome and/or obsessive-compulsive disorder. *J. Child Psychol. Psychiatry* **2007**, *48*, 157–166. [CrossRef] [PubMed]
28. Bateson, P.; Barker, D.; Clutton-Brock, T.; Deb, D.; D'Udine, B.; Foley, R.A.; Gluckman, P.; Godfrey, K.; Kirkwood, T.; Lahr, M.M.; et al. Developmental plasticity and human health. *Nature* **2004**, *430*, 419–421. [CrossRef]
29. Bale, T.L.; Epperson, C.N. Sex differences and stress across the lifespan. *Nat. Neurosci.* **2015**, *18*, 1413–1420. [CrossRef]
30. Bartolomucci, A. Social stress, immune functions and disease in rodents. *Front. Neuroendocrinol.* **2007**, *28*, 28–49. [CrossRef]
31. Krishnan, V.; Han, M.-H.; Graham, D.L.; Berton, O.; Renthal, W.; Russo, S.J.; LaPlant, Q.; Graham, A.; Lutter, M.; Lagace, D.C.; et al. Molecular Adaptations Underlying Susceptibility and Resistance to Social Defeat in Brain Reward Regions. *Cell* **2007**, *131*, 391–404. [CrossRef] [PubMed]
32. Lassance-Soares, R.M.; Sood, S.; Chakraborty, N.; Jhamnani, S.; Aghili, N.; Nashin, H.; Hammamieh, R.; Jett, M.; Epstein, S.E.; Burnett, M.S. Chronic stress impairs collateral blood flow recovery in aged mice. *J. Cardiovasc. Transl. Res.* **2014**, *7*, 749–755. [CrossRef] [PubMed]
33. McEwen, B.S. Physiology and neurobiology of stress and adaptation: Central role of the brain. *Physiol. Rev.* **2007**, *87*, 873–904. [CrossRef] [PubMed]
34. Pryce, C.R.; Fuchs, E. Chronic psychosocial stressors in adulthood: Studies in mice, rats and tree shrews. *Neurobiol. Stress* **2017**, *6*, 94–103. [CrossRef] [PubMed]
35. Scharf, S.H.; Sterlemann, V.; Liebl, C.; Müller, M.B.; Schmidt, M.V. Chronic social stress during adolescence: Interplay of paroxetine treatment and ageing. *Neuropharmacology* **2013**, *72*, 38–46. [CrossRef] [PubMed]
36. Goshen, I.; Yirmiya, R. Interleukin-1 (IL-1): A central regulator of stress responses. *Front. Neuroendocrinol.* **2009**, *30*, 30–45. [CrossRef] [PubMed]
37. Cunningham, C.; Wilcockson, D.C.; Campion, S.; Lunnon, K.; Perry, V.H. Central and systemic endotoxin challenges exacerbate the local inflammatory response and increase neuronal death during chronic neurodegeneration. *J. Neurosci.* **2005**, *25*, 9275–9284. [CrossRef] [PubMed]
38. Frank, M.G.; Weber, M.D.; Watkins, L.R.; Maier, S.F. Stress-induced neuroinflammatory priming: A liability factor in the etiology of psychiatric disorders. *Neurobiol. Stress* **2016**, *4*, 62–70. [CrossRef]
39. Johnson, J.; O'Connor, K.; Watkins, L.; Maier, S. The role of IL-1β in stress-induced sensitization of proinflammatory cytokine and corticosterone responses. *Neuroscience* **2004**, *127*, 569–577. [CrossRef] [PubMed]
40. Perry, V.H.; Newman, T.A.; Cunningham, C. The impact of systemic infection on the progression of neurodegenerative disease. *Nat. Rev. Neurosci.* **2003**, *4*, 103–112. [CrossRef] [PubMed]

41. Barron, H.; Hafizi, S.; Andreazza, A.; Mizrahi, R. Neuroinflammation and Oxidative Stress in Psychosis and Psychosis Risk. *Int. J. Mol. Sci.* **2017**, *18*, 651. [CrossRef] [PubMed]
42. Pei, L.; Wallace, D.C. Mitochondrial Etiology of Neuropsychiatric Disorders. *Biol. Psychiatry* **2018**, *83*, 722–730. [CrossRef] [PubMed]
43. Valenti, D.; de Bari, L.; De Filippis, B.; Henrion-Caude, A.; Vacca, R.A. Mitochondrial dysfunction as a central actor in intellectual disability-related diseases: An overview of Down syndrome, autism, Fragile X and Rett syndrome. *Neurosci. Biobehav. Rev.* **2014**, *46 Pt 2*, 202–217. [CrossRef]
44. Vacca, R.A.; Bawari, S.; Valenti, D.; Tewari, D.; Nabavi, S.F.; Shirooie, S.; Sah, A.N.; Volpicella, M.; Braidy, N.; Nabavi, S.M. Down syndrome: Neurobiological alterations and therapeutic targets. *Neurosci. Biobehav. Rev.* **2019**, *98*, 234–255. [CrossRef] [PubMed]
45. Valenti, D.; Braidy, N.; De Rasmo, D.; Signorile, A.; Rossi, L.; Atanasov, A.G.; Volpicella, M.; Henrion-Caude, A.; Nabavi, S.M.; Vacca, R.A. Mitochondria as pharmacological targets in Down syndrome. *Free Radic. Biol. Med.* **2018**, *114*, 69–83. [CrossRef] [PubMed]
46. Morris, G.; Stubbs, B.; Köhler, C.A.; Walder, K.; Slyepchenko, A.; Berk, M.; Carvalho, A.F. The putative role of oxidative stress and inflammation in the pathophysiology of sleep dysfunction across neuropsychiatric disorders: Focus on chronic fatigue syndrome, bipolar disorder and multiple sclerosis. *Sleep Med. Rev.* **2018**, *41*, 255–265. [CrossRef] [PubMed]
47. De Simone, R.; Ajmone-Cat, M.A.; Pandolfi, M.; Bernardo, A.; De Nuccio, C.; Minghetti, L.; Visentin, S. The mitochondrial uncoupling protein-2 is a master regulator of both M1 and M2 microglial responses. *J. Neurochem.* **2015**, *135*, 147–156. [CrossRef] [PubMed]
48. Ferger, A.I.; Campanelli, L.; Reimer, V.; Muth, K.N.; Merdian, I.; Ludolph, A.C.; Witting, A. Effects of mitochondrial dysfunction on the immunological properties of microglia. *J. Neuroinflamm.* **2010**, *7*, 45. [CrossRef] [PubMed]
49. Li, C.; Zhou, H.-M. The Role of Manganese Superoxide Dismutase in Inflammation Defense. *Enzym. Res.* **2011**, *2011*, 387176. [CrossRef]
50. Piantadosi, C.A.; Suliman, H.B. Transcriptional control of mitochondrial biogenesis and its interface with inflammatory processes. *Biochim. Biophys. Acta Gen. Subj.* **2012**, *1820*, 532–541. [CrossRef]
51. Kim, E.K.; Kwon, J.-E.; Lee, S.-Y.; Lee, E.-J.; Kim, D.S.; Moon, S.-J.; Lee, J.; Kwok, S.-K.; Park, S.-H.; Cho, M.-L. IL-17-mediated mitochondrial dysfunction impairs apoptosis in rheumatoid arthritis synovial fibroblasts through activation of autophagy. *Cell Death Dis.* **2017**, *8*, e2565. [CrossRef] [PubMed]
52. Flies, D.B.; Chen, L. A simple and rapid vortex method for preparing antigen/adjuvant emulsions for immunization. *J. Immunol. Methods* **2003**, *276*, 239–242. [CrossRef]
53. Bartolomucci, A.; Cabassi, A.; Govoni, P.; Ceresini, G.; Cero, C.; Berra, D.; Dadomo, H.; Franceschini, P.; Dell'Omo, G.; Parmigiani, S.; et al. Metabolic consequences and vulnerability to diet-induced obesity in male mice under chronic social stress. *PLoS ONE* **2009**, *4*, e4331. [CrossRef] [PubMed]
54. Sanghez, V.; Razzoli, M.; Carobbio, S.; Campbell, M.; McCallum, J.; Cero, C.; Ceresini, G.; Cabassi, A.; Govoni, P.; Franceschini, P.; et al. Psychosocial stress induces hyperphagia and exacerbates diet-induced insulin resistance and the manifestations of the Metabolic Syndrome. *Psychoneuroendocrinology* **2013**, *38*, 2933–2942. [CrossRef] [PubMed]
55. Bartolomucci, A.; Carola, V.; Pascucci, T.; Puglisi-Allegra, S.; Cabib, S.; Lesch, K.-P.; Parmigiani, S.; Palanza, P.; Gross, C. Increased vulnerability to psychosocial stress in heterozygous serotonin transporter knockout mice. *Dis. Model. Mech.* **2010**, *3*, 459–470. [CrossRef] [PubMed]
56. Dadomo, H.; Sanghez, V.; Di Cristo, L.; Lori, A.; Ceresini, G.; Malinge, I.; Parmigiani, S.; Palanza, P.; Sheardown, M.; Bartolomucci, A. Vulnerability to chronic subordination stress-induced depression-like disorders in adult 129SvEv male mice. *Prog. Neuropsychopharmacol. Biol. Psychiatry* **2011**, *35*, 1461–1471. [CrossRef] [PubMed]
57. Zoratto, F.; Sbriccoli, M.; Martinelli, A.; Glennon, J.C.; Macrì, S.; Laviola, G. Intranasal oxytocin administration promotes emotional contagion and reduces aggression in a mouse model of callousness. *Neuropharmacology* **2018**, *143*, 250–267. [CrossRef] [PubMed]
58. Bartolomucci, A.; Pederzani, T.; Sacerdote, P.; Panerai, A.E.; Parmigiani, S.; Palanza, P. Behavioral and physiological characterization of male mice under chronic psychosocial stress. *Psychoneuroendocrinology* **2004**, *29*, 899–910. [CrossRef]

59. Macrì, S.; Pasquali, P.; Bonsignore, L.T.; Pieretti, S.; Cirulli, F.; Chiarotti, F.; Laviola, G. Moderate neonatal stress decreases within-group variation in behavioral, immune and HPA responses in adult mice. *PLoS ONE* **2007**, *2*, e1015. [CrossRef]
60. Macrì, S.; Granstrem, O.; Shumilina, M.; Antunes Gomes dos Santos, F.J.; Berry, A.; Saso, L.; Laviola, G. Resilience and vulnerability are dose-dependently related to neonatal stressors in mice. *Horm. Behav.* **2009**, *56*, 391–398. [CrossRef]
61. Gao, W.; Stalder, T.; Foley, P.; Rauh, M.; Deng, H.; Kirschbaum, C. Quantitative analysis of steroid hormones in human hair using a column-switching LC-APCI-MS/MS assay. *J. Chromatogr. B Anal. Technol. Biomed. Life Sci.* **2013**, *928*, 1–8. [CrossRef] [PubMed]
62. Valenti, D.; de Bari, L.; De Filippis, B.; Ricceri, L.; Vacca, R.A. Preservation of mitochondrial functional integrity in mitochondria isolated from small cryopreserved mouse brain areas. *Anal. Biochem.* **2014**, *444*, 25–31. [CrossRef] [PubMed]
63. De Filippis, B.; Valenti, D.; Chiodi, V.; Ferrante, A.; de Bari, L.; Fiorentini, C.; Domenici, M.R.; Ricceri, L.; Vacca, R.A.; Fabbri, A.; et al. Modulation of Rho GTPases rescues brain mitochondrial dysfunction, cognitive deficits and aberrant synaptic plasticity in female mice modeling Rett syndrome. *Eur. Neuropsychopharmacol.* **2015**, *25*, 889–901. [CrossRef] [PubMed]
64. Manente, A.G.; Valenti, D.; Pinton, G.; Jithesh, P.V.; Daga, A.; Rossi, L.; Gray, S.G.; O'Byrne, K.J.; Fennell, D.A.; Vacca, R.A.; et al. Estrogen receptor β activation impairs mitochondrial oxidative metabolism and affects malignant mesothelioma cell growth in vitro and in vivo. *Oncogenesis* **2013**, *2*, e72. [CrossRef] [PubMed]
65. De Filippis, B.; Valenti, D.; de Bari, L.; De Rasmo, D.; Musto, M.; Fabbri, A.; Ricceri, L.; Fiorentini, C.; Laviola, G.; Vacca, R.A. Mitochondrial free radical overproduction due to respiratory chain impairment in the brain of a mouse model of Rett syndrome: Protective effect of CNF1. *Free Radic. Biol. Med.* **2015**, *83*, 167–177. [CrossRef] [PubMed]
66. Khan, H.A. Bioluminometric assay of ATP in mouse brain: Determinant factors for enhanced test sensitivity. *J. Biosci.* **2003**, *28*, 379–382. [CrossRef] [PubMed]
67. Vigli, D.; Rusconi, L.; Valenti, D.; La Montanara, P.; Cosentino, L.; Lacivita, E.; Leopoldo, M.; Amendola, E.; Gross, C.; Landsberger, N.; et al. Rescue of prepulse inhibition deficit and brain mitochondrial dysfunction by pharmacological stimulation of the central serotonin receptor 7 in a mouse model of CDKL5 Deficiency Disorder. *Neuropharmacology* **2019**, *144*, 104–114. [CrossRef] [PubMed]
68. Deacon, R.M.J.; Rawlins, J.N.P. T-maze alternation in the rodent. *Nat. Protoc.* **2006**, *1*, 7–12. [CrossRef] [PubMed]
69. Zou, J.; Storm, D.R.; Xia, Z. Conditional deletion of ERK5 MAP kinase in the nervous system impairs pheromone information processing and pheromone-evoked behaviors. *PLoS ONE* **2013**, *8*, e76901. [CrossRef] [PubMed]
70. Razzoli, M.; Nyuyki-Dufe, K.; Gurney, A.; Erickson, C.; McCallum, J.; Spielman, N.; Marzullo, M.; Patricelli, J.; Kurata, M.; Pope, E.A.; et al. Social stress shortens lifespan in mice. *Aging Cell* **2018**, *17*, e12778. [CrossRef]
71. Spinello, C.; Laviola, G.; Macrì, S. Pediatric Autoimmune Disorders Associated with Streptococcal Infections and Tourette's Syndrome in Preclinical Studies. *Front. Neurosci.* **2016**, *10*, 310. [CrossRef] [PubMed]
72. Swedo, S.E.; Grant, P.J. Annotation: PANDAS: A model for human autoimmune disease. *J. Child Psychol. Psychiatry* **2005**, *46*, 227–234. [CrossRef] [PubMed]
73. Trifiletti, R.R.; Packard, A.M. Immune mechanisms in pediatric neuropsychiatric disorders. Tourette's syndrome, OCD, and PANDAS. *Child. Adolesc. Psychiatr. Clin. N. Am.* **1999**, *8*, 767–775. [CrossRef]
74. Lalonde, R. The neurobiological basis of spontaneous alternation. *Neurosci. Biobehav. Rev.* **2002**, *26*, 91–104. [CrossRef]
75. Irwin, J.; Tombaugh, T.N.; Zacharko, R.M.; Anisman, H. Alteration of exploration and the response to food associated cues after treatment with pimozide. *Pharmacol. Biochem. Behav.* **1983**, *18*, 235–246. [CrossRef]
76. Jaffard, R.; Mocaer, E.; Poignant, J.-C.; Micheau, J.; Marighetto, A.; Meunier, M.; Béracochéa, D. Effects of tianeptine on spontaneous alternation, simple and concurrent spatial discrimination learning and on alcohol-induced alternation deficits in mice. *Behav. Pharmacol.* **1991**, *2*, 37–46. [CrossRef] [PubMed]
77. Bartolomucci, A.; Palanza, P.; Parmigiani, S.; Pederzani, T.; Merlot, E.; Neveu, P.J.; Dantzer, R. Chronic psychosocial stress down-regulates central cytokines mRNA. *Brain Res. Bull.* **2003**, *62*, 173–178. [CrossRef] [PubMed]

78. Ajmone-Cat, M.A.; D'Urso, M.C.; di Blasio, G.; Brignone, M.S.; De Simone, R.; Minghetti, L. Glycogen synthase kinase 3 is part of the molecular machinery regulating the adaptive response to LPS stimulation in microglial cells. *Brain Behav. Immun.* **2016**, *55*, 225–235. [CrossRef] [PubMed]
79. Ajmone-Cat, M.A.; Mancini, M.; De Simone, R.; Cilli, P.; Minghetti, L. Microglial polarization and plasticity: Evidence from organotypic hippocampal slice cultures. *Glia* **2013**, *61*, 1698–1711. [CrossRef] [PubMed]
80. Alboni, S.; Maggi, L. Editorial: Cytokines as Players of Neuronal Plasticity and Sensitivity to Environment in Healthy and Pathological Brain. *Front. Cell. Neurosci.* **2016**, *9*, 508. [CrossRef] [PubMed]
81. Dantzer, R.; O'Connor, J.C.; Freund, G.G.; Johnson, R.W.; Kelley, K.W. From inflammation to sickness and depression: When the immune system subjugates the brain. *Nat. Rev. Neurosci.* **2008**, *9*, 46–56. [CrossRef] [PubMed]
82. Espinosa-Oliva, A.M.; de Pablos, R.M.; Villarán, R.F.; Argüelles, S.; Venero, J.L.; Machado, A.; Cano, J. Stress is critical for LPS-induced activation of microglia and damage in the rat hippocampus. *Neurobiol. Aging* **2011**, *32*, 85–102. [CrossRef] [PubMed]
83. Ji, K.-A.; Eu, M.Y.; Kang, S.-H.; Gwag, B.J.; Jou, I.; Joe, E.-H. Differential neutrophil infiltration contributes to regional differences in brain inflammation in the substantia nigra pars compacta and cortex. *Glia* **2008**, *56*, 1039–1047. [CrossRef] [PubMed]
84. Kipp, M.; Norkute, A.; Johann, S.; Lorenz, L.; Braun, A.; Hieble, A.; Gingele, S.; Pott, F.; Richter, J.; Beyer, C. Brain-region-specific astroglial responses in vitro after LPS exposure. *J. Mol. Neurosci.* **2008**, *35*, 235–243. [CrossRef]
85. Gądek-Michalska, A.; Spyrka, J.; Rachwalska, P.; Tadeusz, J.; Bugajski, J. Influence of chronic stress on brain corticosteroid receptors and HPA axis activity. *Pharmacol. Rep.* **2013**, *65*, 1163–1175. [CrossRef]
86. Mizoguchi, K.; Ishige, A.; Aburada, M.; Tabira, T. Chronic stress attenuates glucocorticoid negative feedback: Involvement of the prefrontal cortex and hippocampus. *Neuroscience* **2003**, *119*, 887–897. [CrossRef]
87. Levine, S.; Strebel, R.; Wenk, E.J.; Harman, P.J. Suppression of experimental allergic encephalomyelitis by stress. *Proc. Soc. Exp. Biol. Med.* **1962**, *109*, 294–298. [CrossRef]
88. Levine, S.; Saltzman, A. Nonspecific stress prevents relapses of experimental allergic encephalomyelitis in rats. *Brain Behav. Immun.* **1987**, *1*, 336–341. [CrossRef]
89. Levine, S.; Wenk, E.J.; Muldoon, T.N.; Cohen, S.G. Enhancement of experimental allergic encephalomyelitis by adrenalectomy. *Proc. Soc. Exp. Biol. Med.* **1962**, *111*, 383–385. [CrossRef]
90. Newton, R.; Shah, S.; Altonsy, M.O.; Gerber, A.N. Glucocorticoid and cytokine crosstalk: Feedback, feedforward, and co-regulatory interactions determine repression or resistance. *J. Biol. Chem.* **2017**, *292*, 7163–7172. [CrossRef]
91. Webster, J.C.; Oakley, R.H.; Jewell, C.M.; Cidlowski, J.A. Proinflammatory cytokines regulate human glucocorticoid receptor gene expression and lead to the accumulation of the dominant negative isoform: A mechanism for the generation of glucocorticoid resistance. *Proc. Natl. Acad. Sci. USA* **2001**, *98*, 6865–6870. [CrossRef] [PubMed]
92. Nair, A.; Bonneau, R.H. Stress-induced elevation of glucocorticoids increases microglia proliferation through NMDA receptor activation. *J. Neuroimmunol.* **2006**, *171*, 72–85. [CrossRef] [PubMed]
93. Choi, Y.J.; Kim, H.S.; Lee, J.; Chung, J.; Lee, J.S.; Choi, J.S.; Yoon, T.R.; Kim, H.K.; Chung, H.Y. Down-regulation of oxidative stress and COX-2 and iNOS expressions by dimethyl lithospermate in aged rat kidney. *Arch. Pharm. Res.* **2014**, *37*, 1032–1038. [CrossRef] [PubMed]
94. Hsieh, H.-L.; Yang, C.-M. Role of Redox Signaling in Neuroinflammation and Neurodegenerative Diseases. *Biomed. Res. Int.* **2013**, *2013*, 484613. [CrossRef] [PubMed]
95. Madrigal, J.L.; Moro, M.A.; Lizasoain, I.; Lorenzo, P.; Castrillo, A.; Boscá, L.; Leza, J.C. Inducible nitric oxide synthase expression in brain cortex after acute restraint stress is regulated by nuclear factor kappaB-mediated mechanisms. *J. Neurochem.* **2001**, *76*, 532–538. [CrossRef] [PubMed]
96. Novaes, L.S.; Dos Santos, N.B.; Dragunas, G.; Perfetto, J.G.; Leza, J.C.; Scavone, C.; Munhoz, C.D. Repeated Restraint Stress Decreases Na,K-ATPase Activity via Oxidative and Nitrosative Damage in the Frontal Cortex of Rats. *Neuroscience* **2018**, *393*, 273–283. [CrossRef] [PubMed]
97. Wong, G.H.; Goeddel, D.V. Induction of manganous superoxide dismutase by tumor necrosis factor: Possible protective mechanism. *Science* **1988**, *242*, 941–944. [CrossRef]
98. Musatov, A.; Robinson, N.C. Susceptibility of mitochondrial electron-transport complexes to oxidative damage. Focus on cytochrome c oxidase. *Free Radic. Res.* **2012**, *46*, 1313–1326. [CrossRef]

99. Hernández-Aguilera, A.; Rull, A.; Rodríguez-Gallego, E.; Riera-Borrull, M.; Luciano-Mateo, F.; Camps, J.; Menéndez, J.A.; Joven, J. Mitochondrial dysfunction: A basic mechanism in inflammation-related non-communicable diseases and therapeutic opportunities. *Mediat. Inflamm.* **2013**, *2013*, 135698. [CrossRef]
100. Hoffmann, A.; Spengler, D. The Mitochondrion as Potential Interface in Early-Life Stress Brain Programming. *Front. Behav. Neurosci.* **2018**, *12*, 306. [CrossRef]
101. Di Filippo, M.; Chiasserini, D.; Tozzi, A.; Picconi, B.; Calabresi, P. Mitochondria and the Link Between Neuroinflammation and Neurodegeneration. *J. Alzheimer Dis.* **2010**, *20*, S369–S379. [CrossRef]
102. Witte, M.E.; Mahad, D.J.; Lassmann, H.; van Horssen, J. Mitochondrial dysfunction contributes to neurodegeneration in multiple sclerosis. *Trends Mol. Med.* **2014**, *20*, 179–187. [CrossRef]
103. Naik, E.; Dixit, V.M. Mitochondrial reactive oxygen species drive proinflammatory cytokine production. *J. Exp. Med.* **2011**, *208*, 417–420. [CrossRef]
104. Park, J.; Choi, H.; Min, J.-S.; Park, S.-J.; Kim, J.-H.; Park, H.-J.; Kim, B.; Chae, J.-I.; Yim, M.; Lee, D.-S. Mitochondrial dynamics modulate the expression of pro-inflammatory mediators in microglial cells. *J. Neurochem.* **2013**, *127*, 221–232. [CrossRef]
105. Cao, Y.; Zhang, X.; Shang, W.; Xu, J.; Wang, X.; Hu, X.; Ao, Y.; Cheng, H. Proinflammatory Cytokines Stimulate Mitochondrial Superoxide Flashes in Articular Chondrocytes In Vitro and In Situ. *PLoS ONE* **2013**, *8*, e66444. [CrossRef]
106. Hahn, W.S.; Kuzmicic, J.; Burrill, J.S.; Donoghue, M.A.; Foncea, R.; Jensen, M.D.; Lavandero, S.; Arriaga, E.A.; Bernlohr, D.A. Proinflammatory cytokines differentially regulate adipocyte mitochondrial metabolism, oxidative stress, and dynamics. *Am. J. Physiol. Endocrinol. Metab.* **2014**, *306*, E1033–E1045. [CrossRef]
107. Du, J.; McEwen, B.; Manji, H.K. Glucocorticoid receptors modulate mitochondrial function. *Commun. Integr. Biol.* **2009**, *2*, 350–352. [CrossRef]
108. Hunter, R.G.; Seligsohn, M.; Rubin, T.G.; Griffiths, B.B.; Ozdemir, Y.; Pfaff, D.W.; Datson, N.A.; McEwen, B.S. Stress and corticosteroids regulate rat hippocampal mitochondrial DNA gene expression via the glucocorticoid receptor. *Proc. Natl. Acad. Sci. USA* **2016**, *113*, 9099–9104. [CrossRef]

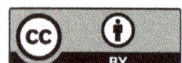

© 2019 by the authors. Licensee MDPI, Basel, Switzerland. This article is an open access article distributed under the terms and conditions of the Creative Commons Attribution (CC BY) license (http://creativecommons.org/licenses/by/4.0/).

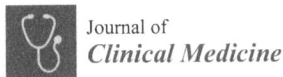 

Article

# Genes and Variants Underlying Human Congenital Lactic Acidosis—From Genetics to Personalized Treatment

Irene Bravo-Alonso [1], Rosa Navarrete [1], Ana Isabel Vega [1], Pedro Ruíz-Sala [1], María Teresa García Silva [2], Elena Martín-Hernández [2], Pilar Quijada-Fraile [2], Amaya Belanger-Quintana [3], Sinziana Stanescu [3], María Bueno [4], Isidro Vitoria [5], Laura Toledo [6], María Luz Couce [7], Inmaculada García-Jiménez [8], Ricardo Ramos-Ruiz [9], Miguel Ángel Martín [10], Lourdes R. Desviat [1], Magdalena Ugarte [1], Celia Pérez-Cerdá [1], Begoña Merinero [1], Belén Pérez [1,*] and Pilar Rodríguez-Pombo [1,*]

[1] Centro de Diagnóstico de Enfermedades Moleculares, Centro de Biología Molecular Severo Ochoa, UAM-CSIC, CIBERER, IDIPAZ, 28049 Madrid, Spain; ibravo@cbm.csic.es (I.B.-A.); rnavarrete@cbm.csic.es (R.N.); anaisabel.vega@scsalud.es (A.I.V.); prsala@cbm.csic.es (P.R.-S.); lruiz@cbm.csic.es (L.R.D.); mugarte@cbm.csic.es (M.U.); cpcerda@cbm.csic.es (C.P.-C.); bmerinero@cbmcsic.es (B.M.)
[2] Unidad de Enfermedades Mitocondriales y Enfermedades Metabólicas Hereditarias, Hospital Universitario 12 de Octubre, CIBERER, 28041 Madrid, Spain; mgarciasilva@salud.madrid.org (M.T.G.S.); emartinhernandez@salud.madrid.org (E.M.-H.); pilar.quijadaf@salud.madrid.org (P.Q.-F.)
[3] Unidad de Enfermedades Metabólicas Congénitas, Hospital Universitario Ramón y Cajal, 28034 Madrid, Spain; amaya.belanger@salud.madrid.org (A.B.-Q.); sinziana.stanescu@salud.madrid.org (S.S.)
[4] Dpto. de Pediatría, Hospital Universitario Virgen del Rocío, 28034 Sevilla, Spain; mbuenod@yahoo.es
[5] Unidad de Nutrición y Metabolopatías, Hospital Universitario La Fe, 46026 Valencia, Spain; vitoria_isi@gva.es
[6] Servicio de Neurología Infantil, Complejo Hospitalario Materno Insular, 35016 Las Palmas de Gran Canaria, Spain; mtolbra@gmail.com
[7] Unidad de Enfermedades Metabólicas, Hospital Clínico Universitario de Santiago, IDIS; CIBERER, 15706 Santiago de Compostela, Spain; Maria.Luz.Couce.Pico@sergas.es
[8] Unidad de Enfermedades Metabólicas, Hospital Universitario Miguel Servet, 50009 Zaragoza, Spain; igarciaji@salud.aragon.es
[9] Unidad de Genómica, Parque Científico de Madrid, 28049 Madrid, Spain; ricardo.ramos@fpcm.es
[10] Laboratorio de Enfermedades Mitocondriales y Neuromusculares, Instituto de Investigación del Hospital, de Octubre, CIBERER, 28041 Madrid, Spain; mamcasanueva.imas12@h12o.es
* Correspondence: bperez@cbm.csic.es (B.P.); mprodriguez@cbm.csic.es or pr.pombo@uam.es (P.R.-P.); Tel.: +34-911-964-566 (B.P.); +34-911-964-628 (P.R.-P.)

Received: 8 October 2019; Accepted: 24 October 2019; Published: 1 November 2019

**Abstract:** Congenital lactic acidosis (CLA) is a rare condition in most instances due to a range of inborn errors of metabolism that result in defective mitochondrial function. Even though the implementation of next generation sequencing has been rapid, the diagnosis rate for this highly heterogeneous allelic condition remains low. The present work reports our group's experience of using a clinical/biochemical analysis system in conjunction with genetic findings that facilitates the taking of timely clinical decisions with minimum need for invasive procedures. The system's workflow combines different metabolomics datasets and phenotypic information with the results of clinical exome sequencing and/or RNA analysis. The system's use detected genetic variants in 64% of a cohort of 39 CLA-patients; these variants, 14 of which were novel, were found in 19 different nuclear and two mitochondrial genes. For patients with variants of unknown significance, the genetic analysis was combined with functional genetic and/or bioenergetics analyses in an attempt to detect pathogenicity. Our results warranted subsequent testing of antisense therapy to rescue the abnormal splicing in cultures of fibroblasts from a patient with a defective *GFM1* gene. The discussed system facilitates the diagnosis of CLA by avoiding the need to use invasive techniques and increase our knowledge of the causes of this condition.

**Keywords:** congenital lactic acidosis; mitochondrial dysfunction; metabolomics datasets; clinical-exome sequencing; RNA analysis; antisense therapy for mitochondrial disorders; healthcare; mitochondrial morphology

## 1. Introduction

Congenital lactic acidosis (CLA) is a rare condition that is mainly due to a range of inborn errors of metabolism that result in defective mitochondrial function. Lactic acidosis results from the accumulation of lactate and protons in body fluids. A single elevated blood lactate event can have adverse consequences; naturally, sustained hyperlactatemia has an even worse prognosis [1]. CLA is associated with defects in the genes coding for enzymes involved in pyruvate oxidation, the Krebs cycle and gluconeogenesis and is a hallmark of primary mitochondrial disorders (which can involve any of ~1500 mitochondrial or nuclear genes). Since any organ or tissue can be affected by impaired energy production, the associated symptoms and signs of CLA can be very varied and the diagnostic workup is usually complex [2–4]. Certainly, the systematic screening of all target organs (heart, muscle, brain, eyes, ear, liver, endocrine system, etc.) must be performed [5], which usually involves biopsies being taken. In addition, the interpretation of the biochemical evidence provided by biomarkers is not always straightforward. Elevated blood and cerebrospinal fluid (CSF) lactate are certainly diagnostic clues that point towards CLA. Alterations in other biomarkers of mitochondrial disorders, such as pyruvate, alanine or acyl-carnitines or cofactors such as free-thiamine or CoQ10 [6–8], contribute to address the diagnosis of primary mitochondrial disorders, although are not fully specific and can be detected associated to other secondary mitochondrial dysfunctions. That is the case of CoQ10 levels [8]. The use of a scoring system based on the Consensus of Mitochondrial Disease Criteria (MDC) [9] can help, as can the use of novel computational diagnostic resources such as the Leigh Map [10] but a final diagnosis always requires a genetic analysis be performed.

Next generation sequencing (NGS) has positively influenced diagnosis rates for all heterogeneous genetic disorders. The use of extended gene panels, whole exome sequencing (WES), whole genome sequencing (WGS) and RNA sequencing, has increased diagnostic yield of mitochondrial disorders from 10%–20% in the pre-NGS era to close 50% in the NGS-era [11–14]. There is now a growing rational for performing sequencing first [15] and treating biochemical analyses as a means of understanding the clinical significance of genetic findings. Indeed, the present work confirms the diagnostic value of combining biochemical profiling and targeted DNA and/or RNA testing to deliver information that minimizes the need for invasive and/or more specialized biochemical tests that delay a diagnosis being reached.

## 2. Experimental Section

### 2.1. Patients

The study subjects were 39 patients (18 males and 21 females, all neonates or infants) who together provided a representative sample of the broad spectrum of clinical signs and symptoms of the patients with suspected CLA referred to our laboratory between 1996 and 2017 (Table S1). All were clinically suspected of having CLA but with different levels of supporting evidence (imaging, biochemical or cellular functional assay results). Most of the patients' plasma and urine samples were profiled by ion-exchange chromatography, gas-chromatography mass-spectrometry or high-performance liquid chromatography/tandem mass spectrometry, checking for amino acids, urine organic acids and plasma acyl-carnitines and other metabolic studies [16,17]. The results were compared to those for healthy controls but without specific matching for gender or nutritional status. Pyruvate carboxylase and/or pyruvate dehydrogenase activity had already been measured in 23 of the 39 patients (Table S2) but note these results were not used in the present analysis. Histochemical analyses of biopsy materials and enzymatic analyses of mitochondrial respiratory chain complexes activity had not been performed for most patients.

Written informed consent to include the patients in the study was provided by their parents. The study protocol adhered to the Declaration of Helsinki and was approved by the Ethics Committee of Universidad Autónoma de Madrid.

*2.2. Genetic Analysis*

2.2.1. Clinical Exome Sequencing

Genomic DNA was extracted from peripheral blood or fibroblast extracts using the MagnaPure system (Roche Applied Science, Indianapolis, IN, USA) and subjected to massive parallel sequencing using the Illumina® Clinical-Exome Sequencing TruSight™ One Gene Panel (Illumina, San Diego, CA, USA) as previously described [18]. A minimum coverage of 30× was achieved for 95% of the target bases (mean depth of coverage 115×).

2.2.2. Mitochondrial DNA Sequencing

DNA extracted from patient blood samples or skin fibroblasts was checked for large-scale mtDNA rearrangements and mutations according to the Illumina Human mtDNA Genome Kit. VCF files were generated and analysed using Human mtDNA Variant Processor and mtDNA Variant Analyzer software (Illumina, San Diego, CA, USA) (https://blog.basespace.illumina.com/2016/02/25/human-mtdna-analysis-in-basespace/). Sequence variants were annotated according to the MITOMAP database [19]. The mtDNA-server platform (https://mtdna-server.uibk.ac.at/index.html#!pages/home) was used to detect heteroplasmy and to assign mtDNA haplogroups [20]. To detect deletions, the mean coverage for the analysed intervals was calculated and normalized with respect to the mean coverage for all the target intervals. Deleted intervals were then detected by comparing the normalized mean coverage of the test sample with the mean coverage of the control samples.

2.2.3. Variant Prioritization and Pathogenicity Prediction of Nuclear DNA Variants

Candidate variants were filtered to be rare and disruptive to protein function. Variants were considered rare when they appeared with a minor allele frequency (MAF) of <0.5% within the GnomAD database. Variations shared by multiple patients were removed (since CLA is a rare condition it is unlikely that the same variation would be shared by many people). The filtered results only contemplated variants that affected a protein by their coding for a structural variation or their provoking an ablation, deletion, frame-shift, start loss, splice site or stop gain. Filtering also included the presence of gene variants previously associated with each patient's phenotype and which were annotated in the Human Gene Mutation Database (HGMD, professional version 2019.2) https://portal.biobase-international.com/hgmd/pro/start.php. Although variants inconsistent with a recessive mode of inheritance were initially filtered out, these samples were recovered if the changes were located in genes known to cause congenital lactic acidosis. For missense changes, potential pathogenicity was evaluated using the web platform VarSome (https://varsome.com/) [21]. This brings together data from the dbSNP, ClinVar, gnomAD, RefSeq, Ensembl, dbNSFP, Gerp, Kaviar, CIViC databases and runs the DANN, dbNSFP, FATHMM, MetaLR, MetaSVM, Mutation Assessor, PROVEAN, GERP, LRT and MutationTaster-prediction programs. To complete the analysis of the impact of missense changes on protein structure, function and conservation, the MutPred (http://mutpred1.mutdb.org/) [22] and Panther (http://pantherdb.org/tools/csnpScore.do) [23] prediction programs were also used.

Potential 3' and 5' splice sites were analysed as previously described [24] using the default settings of Alamut® Visual Interactive Bio v2.7.1 software. Those variants prioritized to be causal of CLA were confirmed by conventional Sanger sequencing using the BigDye Terminator Cycle Sequencing Kit (Applied Biosystems, Foster City, CA, USA), using both patient genomic DNA and that of the progenitors if available.

The mutation nomenclature employed followed the Human Genome Variations Society Database (HGVS v15.11. format) (http://www.HGVS.org/varnomen/). The DNA variant numbering system was based on the corresponding cDNA sequence, taking nucleotide +1 as the A of the ATG translation initiation codon in the reference sequence.

2.2.4. High-Density Genotyping

A genome-wide scan of 610,000 SNPs was conducted as previously described [25] at the Spanish National Genotyping Centre (CEGEN, www.cegen.org) using the Illumina 610-Quad Beadchip Kit (Illumina, San Diego, CA, USA) according to the manufacturer's recommendations.

2.2.5. mRNA Studies

500 ng of total RNA were extracted from dermal fibroblasts using the RNeasy Micro kit (Qiagen, Hilden, Germany) and used as a template for reverse transcription PCR (RT-PCR), making use of the NZY First-Strand cDNA synthesis kit (NZYTech, Lisbon, Portugal). PCR amplification was performed using the PCR Supreme NZY Taq II kit (NZYTech, Lisbon, Portugal) with primers designed to amplify the full-length cDNAs according to the cDNA GenBank sequences listed below.

The abundance of full length or aberrant *GFM1* transcripts was evaluated by massive parallel sequencing of cDNA amplicons. Specific amplicons were generated employing primers that included an extended tail (listed in Table S3) and used for library preparation. Libraries were completed by 2-step PCR using the Access Array Barcode Primers for Illumina Sequencers (Fluidigm Corporation, San Francisco, CA), pooled and sequenced in MiSeq (Illumina) in paired-end format of $2 \times 300$, reaching a depth of >50,000 reads.

2.3. Cellular Studies

2.3.1. Cell Culture

Control and patient dermal fibroblasts were grown under standard conditions in minimal essential medium (MEM) containing 1 g/L of glucose supplemented with 2 mmol/L glutamine, 10% foetal bovine serum (FBS) and antibiotics. The cell lines CC2509 (Lonza, Basle, Switzerland), NDHF (PromoCell, Heidelberg, Germany) and GM8680 (Coriell Institute for Medical Research, Camden, NJ, USA) were used as controls. Most experiments were performed when fibroblasts were at 80% confluence.

2.3.2. CoQ10 Measurement

Total CoQ10 was measured by liquid chromatography/tandem mass spectrometry (LC/MS/MS), using CoQ9 as an internal standard, in extracts obtained from two 100 mm plates (P100) of fibroblasts grown under standard conditions. Pelleted cells were resuspended in 125 µL of PBS and lysed by three cycles of freezing/thawing in liquid $N_2$/37 °C. Lowry's protein measurement was then performed. For the determination of CoQ10, 50 µL of CoQ9 (0.2 mg/L, internal standard) and 50 µL of 2 mg/mL p-benzoquinone were added to 100 µL of a fibroblast suspension. After 15 min incubation at room temperature, 850 µL of 1-propanol was added to the fibroblast suspension and centrifuged (12,000 rpm for 15 min at 4 °C). Supernatants were transferred to a glass tube and evaporated to dryness under an $N_2$ stream. Dried extracts were then resuspended in a water—1-propanol (2:8) solution. A calibration curve was prepared with 0.2 mg/L CoQ9 internal standard solution and concentrations of CoQ10 ranging from 0.002 to 1 µg/mL. Samples were injected into an Agilent 1290/AB Sciex 4500 LC/MS/MS device. CoQ9 and CoQ10 were separated using a Symmetry C18 HPLC column (Waters, Milford,

MA, USA) with a 2-propanol/methanol/formic acid (50:50:0.1) mobile phase and acquired by multiple reaction monitoring in positive mode (CoQ9: 796/197, CoQ10: 864/197).

2.3.3. Cellular Oxygen Consumption

The cellular oxygen consumption rate (OCR) was measured using an XF24 Extracellular Flux Analyzer (Seahorse Bioscience, Izasa Scientific) as previously described [26], except that 60,000 fibroblasts per well were seeded in XF 24-well cell culture microplates and 1 h before the assay the growth medium was replaced with 700 µL of un-buffered fresh MEM medium with 0.5% FBS. After taking an OCR baseline measurement, 50 µL of oligomycin, carbonyl cyanide-4-(trifluoromethoxy) phenylhydrazone (FCCP), rotenone and antimycin A solutions were sequentially added to each well to reach final working concentrations 6 µM, 20 µM, 1 µM and 1 µM respectively. Basal respiration was measured without substrates. Oxygen consumption coupled to ATP production (ATP-linked) was calculated as the difference between basal respiration and the proton leak state determined after the addition of oligomycin. Maximum respiration was measured by stepwise 20 µM titrations of FCCP and inhibition by rotenone and antimycin. Spare capacity was calculated as the difference between maximum and basal respiration.

2.3.4. Mitochondrial Mass and Membrane Potential

Mitochondrial mass and mitochondrial membrane potential were determined by flow cytometry using a BD FACSCanto II flow cytometer (BD Biosciences, San Jose, CA, USA). Cells were loaded with 50 nM MitoTracker green (MitoGreen, 37 °C, 30 min) (Invitrogen, Carlsbad, CA, USA) or 200 nM TMRM (tetramethylrhodamine methyl ester, 37 °C, 30 min) (Thermo Fisher Scientific, Waltham, MS, USA). Data were acquired using FACSDiva software (BD Biosciences, Franklin Lakes, NJ, USA). In each analysis, 10,000 events were recorded.

2.3.5. Mitochondrial Isolation and Western Blotting

Mitochondria were isolated using the hypotonic swelling procedure as previously described [27]. Human dermal fibroblasts were harvested, resuspended in ice-cold isolation buffer (75 mM mannitol, 225 mM sucrose, 10 mM MOPS, 1 mM EGTA and 2 mM PMSF, pH 7.2) and subjected to centrifugation at 1000× $g$ for 5 min at 4°C. The cell pellet was then resuspended in cold hypotonic buffer (100 mM sucrose, 10 mM MOPS, 1 mM EGTA and 2 mM PMSF, pH 7.2; 5 mL of buffer/g of cells), homogenized in a Dounce glass homogenizer and incubated on ice for 7 min. Cold hypertonic buffer (1.25 M sucrose and 10 mM MOPS) at 1.1 mL/g of cells and twice the cell-mix volume of isolation buffer plus 2 mg/mL of bovine serum albumin (BSA), were then added to the cell suspension. Cell debris was removed by centrifugation at 1000× $g$ for 10 min. Mitochondria were then collected by further centrifugation at 10,000× $g$ for 10 min at 4 °C. The pellet was resuspended in isolation buffer without BSA and quantified by Bradford analysis. Mitochondria were denatured in Laemmli buffer for 5 min at 50 °C. The samples were separated by SDS-PAGE and analysed by Western blotting as previously described [28]. The primary polyclonal antibodies used were—anti-total OxPhos (CI-NDUFB8, CII-SDHB, CIII-UQCRC2, CIV-MTCOI and CV-ATP5A) (ab110413; Abcam, Cambridge, UK) at a dilution of 1:250, anti-SDHA (1:5000, ab14715), anti-GFM1 (1:1000, ab173529, Abcam) and anti-MTCO1 (1:1000, ab14705). Anti-GAPDH (ab8245, Abcam) and anti-citrate synthase (C5498, Sigma) at 1:5000 were used as loading controls. Quantitative changes in band intensity were evaluated by densitometry scanning using a calibrated GS-800 densitometer (Bio-Rad, Hercules, CA, USA).

2.3.6. Transmission Electron Microscopy

Electron microscopy imaging of cells was performed as previously described [29] using a Jeol JEM-1010 (JEOL Ltd, Tokyo, Japan) electron microscope operating at 80 kV. Images were recorded with a 4k CMOS F416 camera (TVIPS, Gauting, Germany). For the morphometric analysis of mitochondria, the major and minor axes were measured of at least 50 mitochondria randomly selected from cells as previously described [29]. The aspect ratio was defined as the major axis/minor axis [30]. The minimum aspect ratio of 1 corresponded to a perfect circle.

2.3.7. Minigene Analysis and Morpholino Assay

For the in vitro evaluation of splicing alterations, a fragment of human *GFM1* was cloned into a pSPL3 minigene (Gibco BRL, Carlsbad, CA, USA). For this, gene fragments corresponding to 813 bp of intron 5 of human *GFM1* from patient or control fibroblasts were cloned into the pGEMT easy vector (Promega, Madison, WI, USA). The inserts were then excised with the restriction enzyme EcoRI and cloned into pSPL3. Automated DNA sequencing identified clones containing normal and mutant inserts in the correct orientation. Two micrograms of the wild-type or mutant minigene were transfected into COS7 using the JetPEI reagent (Polyplus Transfection, Illkirch, France). At 24 h post-transfection, the cells were harvested by trypsinization and the RNA purified with trizol. Splicing minigene-derived transcripts were amplified and sequenced using the pSPL3-specific primers SD6 and SA2.

For the morpholino assay, a 25-mer morpholino (5′-GATCACAATGCCATTCGCTCACCTG-3′) targeting NM_024996.5 *GFM1* c.689+908G>A was designed, synthesized and purified by Gene Tools (Oregon, USA). NM_000531.5, a 25-mer morpholino against *OTC* (ornithine carbamoyltransferase), was used as a negative control. The Endo-Porter® delivery reagent (Gene Tools,) was used aid in the transfection following the manufacturer's recommendations. Some 250,000 fibroblasts from patient Pt16 and from controls were seeded in a P100 and transfected with 0, 10, 20 or 30 µM of morpholino. At 24 h, the cells were harvested for the extraction of total RNA and protein.

2.3.8. Statistical Analysis

Values are expressed as means ± SEM of 'n' independently performed experiments in cultured cells. Differences between means were examined using the Student t test. Significance was set at $p < 0.05$. All calculations were performed using GraphPad Prism 6 (GraphPad Software, La Jolla, CA, USA)

## 3. Results

### 3.1. Biochemical Profile

The 39 individuals included in the study represent a heterogeneous patient population with a clinical suspicion of congenital lactic acidosis (neonatal or early childhood onset). Table S1 shows the main clinical features for each patient, annotated using Human Phenotype Ontology (HPO) terms.

For metabolic profiling, amino acid, organic acid and acyl-carnitine metabolomics were examined. Blood lactic acid concentrations at diagnosis ranged from 3.7 to 30 mM and an ≥2X increase in alanine was detected in 10 samples. Urinary organic acids were very consistently raised, with increases in α-hydroxybutyrate detected in 25 urine samples, para-hydroxy-phenyl-derivatives (4-OHphenyl-lactic, 4-OHphenyl-pyruvate or 4-OHphenyl-acetic acids) detected in 19 samples and TCA cycle intermediates detected in 14. Other metabolites such as 3-OH propionic, 3-OH isovaleric or methyl-citrate, 2- or 3-OHglutaric, 3-methylglutaric (3MGA) and 3-methylglutaconic (3-MGC) acids and dicarboxylic acids such as adipic 2-OH and 2-keto adipic acid, also appeared increased although less so. Finally, plasma acyl-carnitines of different chain-lengths showed increases over normal in 10 out of the 26 samples analysed. Since most of these metabolites could reflect immediate or downstream disturbances related to a redox-unbalance compatible with mitochondrial dysfunction, patients were considered to be likely suffering a mitochondrial disorder. To arrive at this result, patients' biochemical and clinical data were used to score the likelihood of mitochondrial disease being present according to the modified [9] Nijmegen system (mitochondrial disease criteria (MDC)) [2]. Scores of ≥8 indicate a definite disorder, 5–7 a probable disorder, 2–4 a possible disorder and below 2 no disorder (Table S2). The MDC distribution was as follows—36% (14/39) had a definite disorder, 46% returned a score indicating a probable disorder (18/39) and 15% (6/39) a score indicating a possible disorder. One patient remained unclassified (missing data). Neither increases in the metabolites thought linked to disturbances of mitochondrial fatty acid β-oxidation (such as acyl-carnitines), nor 3-OH isovaleric or 3-OH propionic related to branched-chain amino acid catabolism, nor muscle histology, nor OxPhos proteins were contemplated in the above MDC scoring.

*3.2. Genetic Analysis*

The genetic analysis followed three steps—(1) massive parallel sequencing of the clinical exome to identify pathogenic mutations in nuclear genes, (2) mitochondrial DNA analysis, (3) RNA analysis.

3.2.1. DNA Sequencing of Nuclear Genes

In 24 of the 39 patients analysed, massive-parallel sequencing of the clinical exome identified 33 nucleotide sequence variations in 19 different nuclear genes. Seventeen corresponded to genes known to cause CLA—*PDHA1* and *PDHX*, related to pyruvate metabolism; *PHKA2* related to glycogen storage diseases; *ACAD9, BCS1L, DGUOK, COQ2, FOXRED1, FARS2, GFM1, MRPS22, PDSS1, TMEM70, TRMU* and *TSFM*, all responsible for primary mitochondrial diseases; and *DLD* and *SLC19A3* related to multiple mitochondrial enzyme complex deficiencies. The remaining two were in the non-CLA-related genes *NPHS2*, responsible for nephrotic syndrome type 2 and *SLC16A1*, which encodes a monocarboxylate transporter (MCT1), that mediates the movement of lactate and pyruvate across cell membranes. In total, seven patients had homozygous variants and 11 more were potentially compound heterozygous. A further three patients carried hemizygous (two boys) or heterozygous (one girl) mutations in the X-linked genes *PHKA2* or *PDHA1* (Table 1). This first massive parallel sequencing analysis also returned three patients (Pt16, Pt19 and Pt21) with a single nucleotide change in three other genes—*GFM1, DLD* and *PDHX*—Likely to be involved with CLA. Sanger sequencing validated all the nucleotide changes identified by NGS and confirmed the segregation pattern in family members when samples were available.

Of the 33-nucleotide sequence variations identified, 19 appeared in the Human Gene Mutation Database (HGMD, professional version 2019.2) (https://portal.biobase-international.com/hgmd/pro/all.php); the other 14 were novel. Table 2 lists the variants identified after NGS analysis along with the criteria for their classification according to the joint consensus recommendation of the American College of Medical Genetics and Genomics (ACMG) and the Association for Molecular Pathology [31]. For all novel changes, the in-silico predictions were inconclusive (Table 2 and Table S4).

Table 1. Genes and variants.

| Patient | MDC | Inheritance | Gene | Phenotype MIM Number | RefSeq/Variant 1 | RefSeq/Variant 2 |
|---|---|---|---|---|---|---|
| Pt1.1 *<br>Pt1.2 | Definite | AR | ACAD9 | #611126<br>Mitochondrial Complex I Deficiency Due To ACAD9 Deficiency | NM_014049.4:<br>c.359delT<br>(p.Phe120Serfs*9) | NM_014049.4:<br>c.473C>T (p.Thr158Ile) |
| Pt2 * | Definite | AR | FOXRED1 | #256000<br>Leigh Syndrome Due To Mitochondrial Complex I Deficiency | NM_017547.3:<br>c.628T>G (p.Tyr210Asp) | NM_017547.3:<br>c.1273C>T (p.His425Tyr) |
| Pt3 | Definite | Mit | MT-ATP6 | #516060<br>Mitochondrial Complex V(ATP Synthase) Deficiency | NC_012920.1:<br>m.G8719A (p.Gly65 *) | |
| Pt4 * | Definite | AR | TMEM70 | #614052<br>Mitochondrial Complex V (ATPSynthase) Deficiency, Nuclear Type 2 | NM_017866.5:<br>c.317-2A>G | NM_017866.5:<br>c.317-2A>G |
| Pt5 | Definite | AR | DGUOK | #251880<br>Mitochondrial DNA Depletion Syndrome 3 (Hepato-cerebral Type) | NM_080916.2:<br>c.763_766dupGATT (p.Phe256*) | NM_080916.2:<br>c.763_766dupGATT (p.Phe256*) |
| Pt6 | Definite | AR | MRPS22 | #611719<br>Combined Oxidative Phosphorylation Deficiency 5 | NM_020191.2:<br>c.509G>A (p.Arg170His) | NM_020191.2:<br>c.1032_1035dupAACA (p.Leu346Asnfs*21) |
| Pt7 * | Definite | AR | TRMU | #613070<br>Liver Failure, Infantile, Transient | NM_018006.4:<br>c.680G>C (p.Arg227Thr) | NM_018006.4:<br>c.1041_1044dupTCAA (p.Asp349Serfs*58) |
| Pt8 | Definite | AR | TSFM | #610505<br>Combined Oxidative Phosphorylation Deficiency 3 | NM_001172696.1:<br>c.782G>C (p.Cys261Ser) | NM_001172696.1:<br>c.848G>A (p.Gly283Asp) |
| Pt9 * | Definite | AR | COQ2 | #607426<br>Coenzyme Q10 Deficiency, Primary, 1 | NM_015697.7:<br>c.163C>T (p.Arg55 *) | NM_015697.7:<br>c.1197delT<br>(p.Asn401Ilefs*15) |
| Pt10 * | Definite | AR | PDSS1 | #614651<br>Coenzyme Q10 Deficiency, Primary, 2 | NM_014317.3:<br>c.716T>G (p.Val239Gly) | NM_014317.3:<br>c.1183C>T (p.Arg395*) |
| Pt11 * | Definite | AR | NPHS2 | #600995<br>Nephrotic Syndrome, Type 2 | NM_014625.3:<br>c.413G>A (p.Arg138Gln) | NM_014625.3:<br>c.413G>A (p.Arg138Gln) |
| Pt12 | Definite | XL | PDHA1 | #312170<br>Pyruvate Dehydrogenase E1-Alpha Deficiency | NM_000284.3:<br>c.787C>G (p.Arg263Gly) | |
| Pt15 | Probable | AR | FARS2 | #614946<br>Combined Oxidative Phosphorylation Deficiency 14 | NM_006567.3:<br>c.737C>T (p.Thr246Met) | NM_006567.3:<br>c.1082C>T (p.Pro361Leu) |
| Pt16 * | Probable | AR | GFM1 | #609060<br>Combined Oxidative Phosphorylation Deficiency 1 | NM_024996.5:<br>c.2011C>T (p.Arg671Cys) | a.NM_024996.5:<br>c.689+908G>A<br>r.(689_690ins57)<br>(p.Gly230_231Glnins19) |

Table 1. Cont.

| Patient | MDC | Inheritance | Gene | Phenotype MIM Number | RefSeq/Variant 1 | RefSeq/Variant 2 |
|---|---|---|---|---|---|---|
| Pt17 * | Probable | AR | GFM1 | #609060 Combined Oxidative Phosphorylation Deficiency 1 | NM_024996.5: c.2011C>T (p.Arg671Cys) | NM_024996.5: c.1404delA (p.Gly469Valfs*84) |
| Pt18 | Probable | AR | DLD | #246900 Dihydrolipoamide Dehydrogenase Deficiency | NM_000108.4: c.259C>T (p.Pro87Ser) | NM_000108.4: c.946C>T (p.Arg316*) |
| Pt19 | Probable | AR | DLD | #246900 Dihydrolipoamide Dehydrogenase Deficiency | NM_000108.4: c.788G>A (p.Arg263His) | not found |
| Pt20 ** | Probable | XL | PDHA1 | #312170 Pyruvate Dehydrogenase E1-Alpha Deficiency | NM_000284.3: c.506C>T (p.Ala169Val) | = |
| Pt21 | Probable | AR | PDHX | #245349 Pyruvate Dehydrogenase E3-Binding Protein Deficiency | NM_003477.2: c.965-1G>A (p.Asp322Alafs*6) | b.NG_013368.1: g.34984192_34988219del r.642_816del (p.Asp215Alafs*19) |
| Pt22 * | Probable | AR | SLC16A1 | #616095 Monocarboxylate Transporter 1 Deficiency | NM_003051.3: c.747_750delTAAT (p.Asn250Serfs*5) | NM_003051.3: c.747_750delTAAT (p.Asn250Serfs*5) |
| Pt23 | Probable | XLR | PHKA2 | #306000 Glycogen Storage Disease IXA1 | NM_000292.2: c.1246G>A (p.Gly416Arg) | |
| Pt33 | Possible | AR | BCS1L | #124000 Mitochondrial Complex III Deficiency, Nuclear Type 1 | NM_004328.4 c.166C>T (p.Arg56*) | NM_004328.4 c.-147A>G (p.?) |
| Pt34 | Possible | Mit | MT-ND5 | #540000 Mitochondrial Myopathy, Encephalopathy, Lactic Acidosis and Stroke-Like Episodes | NC_012920.1: m.13513G>A (p.Asp393Asn) | |
| Pt35 * | Possible | AR | DLD | #246900 Dihydrolipoamide Dehydrogenase Deficiency | NM_000108.4 c.647T>C (p.Met216Thr) | NM_000108.4 c.647T>C (p.Met216Thr) |
| Pt36 * | Possible | AR | SLC19A3 | #607483 Thiamine Metabolism Dysfunction Syndrome 2 (Biotin- Or Thiamine-Responsive Type) | NM_025243.3: c.20C>A (p.Ser7*) | NM_025243.3: c.20C>A (p.Ser7*) |
| Pt39 * | Possible | AR | SLC19A3 | #607483 Thiamine Metabolism Dysfunction Syndrome 2 (Biotin- Or Thiamine-Responsive Type) | NM_025243.3: c.20C>A (p.Ser7*) | NM_025243.3: c.20C>A (p.Ser7*) |

Abbreviations: * Mendelian segregation confirmed; ** Not found in mother; Mitochondrial disease criteria (MDC); Autosomal recessive (AR); X-Linked (XL); X-Linked recessive (XLR); Mitochondrial DNA (Mit). In bold, nucleotide variations identified after complementary test; [a] RNA analysis, [b] SNP array and RNA analysis. The mutation nomenclature follows that used by Mutalyzer 2.0.29 (https://mutalyzer.nl). RefSeq number for each gene is included.

**Table 2.** Analysis of variants identified by massive-parallel sequencing and pathogenicity status.

| Gene | Variant/ Consequence | ACMG Tags | Classification | HGMD Accession | gnomaD |
|---|---|---|---|---|---|
| ACAD9 | c.359delT (p.Phe120Serfs*9) | PVS1, PM2, PP1, PP5 | Pathogenic | CD153914 | 0.0001042 |
| ACAD9 | c.473C>T (p.Thr158Ile) | PM2, PM3, PP1, PP3 | Likely pathogenic | - | 0 |
| BCS1L | c.166C>T (p.Arg56Ter) | PS3, PM4, PP3, PP5 | Likely pathogenic | CM022763 | 0.0001626 |
| BCS1L | c.-147A>G (p.?) | PM2 PM3, PP5 | VUS | CS098028 | 0 |
| COQ2 | c.1197delT (p.Asn401Ilefs*15) | PM2, PM3, PM4, PP5 | Likely pathogenic | CD071308 | 1.217e-5 |
| COQ2 | c.163C>T (p.Arg55Ter) | PM2, PM3, PM4, PP1 PS3 | Likely pathogenic | - | 0 |
| DGUOK | c.763_766dupGATT (p.Phe256Ter) | PM4, PM2, PM5, PS3, PP5 | Likely pathogenic | CI034484 | 2.031e-5 |
| DLD | c. 259C>T (p.Pro87Ser) | PM2, PM3, PP2, PP3, PP4 | VUS | - | 0 |
| DLD | c.647T>C (p.Met216Thr) | PM2, PP2, PP3 | VUS | - | 0 |
| DLD | C.788G>A (p.Arg263Hys) | PM3, PP3 | VUS | - | 0.000817 |
| DLD | c.946C>T (p.Arg316Ter) | PM2, PM4, PP3, PP4 | Likely pathogenic | - | 1.63e-05 |
| FARS2 | c.737C>T (p.Thr246Met) | BS2, BP6 | Likely benign | - | 0.004064 |
| FARS2 | c.1082C>T (p.Pro361Leu) | PP3 | VUS | CM1718796 | 0.0001339 |
| FOXRED1 | c.628T>G (p.Tyr210Asp) | PM2, PP3 | VUS | - | 0 |
| FOXRED1 | c.1273C>T (p.His425Tyr) | PM2, PP3 | VUS | - | 0 |
| GFM1 | c.1404delA (p.Gly469Valfs*84) | PVS1, PM2, PP5 | Pathogenic | CD154422 | 1.635e-5 |
| GFM1 | c.2011C>T (p.Arg671Cys) | PM2, PM3, PP2, PP3, PP5 | Likely pathogenic | CM11881 | 7.216e-5 |
| MRPS22 | c.1032_1035dupAACA (p.Leu346Asnfs*21) | PVS1, PM3, PP5 | Pathogenic | CI152171 | 9.028e-5 |
| MRPS22 | c.509G>A (p.Arg170His) | PM2, PM3, PP3, PP5 | Likely pathogenic | CM076316 | 7.221e-5 |
| NPHS2 | c.413G>A (p.Arg138Gln) | PP2, PP3, PP5 | VUS | CM000581 | 0.0005739 |
| PDHA1 | c.506C>T (p.Ala169Val) | PM2, PP2, PP3, PP5 | VUS | CM091028 | 0 |
| PDHA1 | c.787C>G (p.Arg263Gly) | PM2, PM5, PS3, PS4, PP2, PP3, PP5 | Pathogenic | CM920573 | 0 |
| PDHX | c.965-1G>A (p.Asp322Alafs*6) | PVS1, PM2, PM3, PP3, PP5 | Pathogenic | CS024024 | 4.11e-6 |

Table 2. Cont.

| Gene | Variant/ Consequence | ACMG Tags | Classification | HGMD Accession | gnomaD |
|---|---|---|---|---|---|
| PDSS1 | c.716T>G (p.Val239Gly) | PM2, PP3 (PS3 - Likely path) | VUS | - | 0 |
| PDSS1 | c.1183C>T (p.Arg395Ter) | PM2, PM4, PP3 | Pathogenic | - | 4.064e-6 |
| PHKA2 | c.1246G>A (p. Gly416Arg) | PP3, BP6 | VUS | - | 0.00432 |
| SLC16A1 | c.747_750delTAAT (p.Asn250Serfs*5) | PVS1, PM2, PP5 | Pathogenic | CD1411339 | 8.123e-6 |
| SLC19A3 | c.20C>A (p.Ser7Ter) | PM2, PM3, PM4, PP4, PP5 | Likely pathogenic | CM131528 | 0 |
| TMEM70 | c.317-2A>G (p.?) | PVS1, PM2, PP1, PP5 | Pathogenic | CS084884 | 7.605e-5 |
| TRMU | c.1041_1044dupTCAA (p.Asp349Serfs*58) | PVS1, PM2, PP5 | Pathogenic | CD155923 | 1.219e-5 |
| TRMU | c.680G>C (p.Arg227Thr) | PM2, PM3, PP3 | VUS | - | 1.624e-5 |
| TSFM | c.782G>C (p. Cys261Ser) | PS3, PM2 | Likely pathogenic | CM170018 | 4.188e-6 |
| TSFM | c.848G>A (p. Gly283Asp) | PM2, PP3 | VUS | - | 5.889e-5 |

The DNA variant numbering system was based on the cDNA sequence. Nucleotide numbering uses +1 as the A of the ATG translation initiation codon in the reference sequence, with the initiation codon as codon 1. Tags for classifying missense changes are those according the American College of Medical Genetics and Genomics (ACMG). Classification was accomplished using the VarSome web platform. Accession number from HGMD® Professional 2019.2 (https://portal.biobase-international.com/hgmd/pro/start.php?) and allele frequency from https://gnomad.broadinstitute.org/ are also included.

For the three patients with single heterozygous changes, an extended genomic analysis of large heterozygous deletions was performed using Integrative Genomics Viewer (IGV) software v2.3.98 to analyse the reads of candidate genes visually, along with high-density genotyping. For Pt21, high-density SNP array analysis identified, in heterozygous fashion, a large deletion in chromosome 11 region q14.1 (g.34984192-34988219, Gh37) encompassing part of intron 5–6 and exon 6 of *PDHX*. This was also detected in mRNA analysis (r.642_816del). No large deletions were identified in either Pt16 or Pt19.

3.2.2. Whole Mitochondrial DNA Analysis

Whole mtDNA sequencing was performed for all patients with no putative genetic diagnosis. The deep coverage inherent to this next-generation sequencing system enabled the detection of low-level heteroplasmy. In two of the analysed patients, we identified two previously reported changes—the m.8719G>A (p.Gly65Ter) in *MT-ATP6* that was found in homoplasmy and the m.13513G>A (p.Asp393Asn) in *MT-ND5* gene that results in a 28% of heteroplasmy (Table 1).

In summary, the nuclear (by clinical exome) and mitochondrial DNA analyses returned 24 patients with likely causative changes in either nuclear (22) or mitochondrial genes (2). Two other patients showed a single variation in a strong candidate gene. For the remaining 13 patients, no genetic cause could be identified.

### 3.2.3. RNA Analysis Helped Diagnose Patients and Can Be Used as Proof of Concept of Personalized Therapies

To complement the exome-based molecular analysis and to improve the interpretation of certain genetic variants, two patients' RNAs (Pt15 and Pt16) were scanned for possible aberrant transcripts. Pt15 had two single nucleotide variants in *FARS2* gene, the c.737C>T (p.Thr246Met) (predicted as benign) and the previously described c.1082C>T (p.Pro361Leu) but DNA analysis could not confirm the presence on different alleles; Pt16 bore the heterozygous c.2011C>T change in exon 16 of *GFM1*; the second variant was unknown. The lack of fibroblasts for Pt19 hampered any viable *DLD* RNA analysis.

For Pt15 (Figure 1A), cDNA analysis detected a full-length transcript containing both point changes in homozygous fashion (transcript 1) and another smaller transcript (r.49_904del) that skipped the region encompassing part of exon 2 to exon 5 (transcript 2) (Figure 1B). Thus, the genotype at the mRNA level was r.(737c>u;1082c>u); (49_904del).

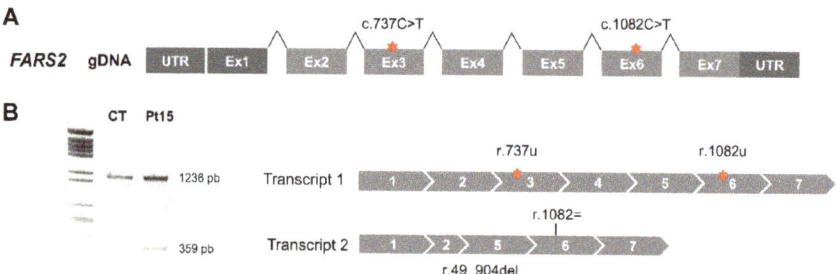

**Figure 1.** Aberrant splicing of *FARS2* in Pt15. (**A**) Diagram of the human *FARS2* gene. Red stars depict the location of nucleotide variants identified. (**B**) Agarose gel showing the results of reverse transcription polymerase chain reaction (RT-PCR) amplifications in control (CT) and patient (Pt) fibroblasts.

For Pt16, Sanger sequencing of the RT-PCR products generated using primer combinations to amplify the complete coding sequence in two overlapping fragments (F1 and F2) (Figure 2A) detected a complex profile compatible with the presence of different transcripts. Subsequent sequence analysis of the cloned RT-PCR products confirmed the presence of different transcripts (Figure 2B). Transcript 1 (from the F1 fragment) contained 57 bp of the intronic sequence between exons 5 and 6 of *GFM1*. Transcript 2.1 (from the F2 fragment) was full-length and contained the variant r.2011t (F2.1). Transcript 2.2 (from F2 fragment) skipped exon 16.

Computational tools used to analyse the impact of the change c.2011C>T on splicing events predicted a loss of an enhancer site and the activation of a silencer that would affect the binding of splicing regulatory factors SF2/ASF at position c.2007 resulting in the splicing of exon 16. The massive sequencing of cDNA and the quantization of total reads corresponding to transcripts with junction 15-17 (skipped transcript T2.2) and to full-length transcripts from controls and Pt16 fibroblasts, showed a doubling of the presence of the aberrant T2.2 in the latter patient's cells. Low levels of the skipped isoform were detected in control fibroblasts (Figure 2C). If the product of this mutant transcript, r.(1910_2070del) were translated it would lead to a frameshift creating a premature stop codon, p.(Ala637Glyfs*5), with a likely impact on EFG1 protein synthesis or stability.

The origin of the aberrant transcript containing 57 bp of the intronic sequence of intron 5 of *GFM1* was also determined and the change c.689+908G>A identified at DNA level. This change was previously proposed as responsible for the activation of a cryptic splice site and the creation of a new exon already present in the *GFM1* isoform ENST00000264263.9 (Figure S1A) [32]. Segregation pattern analysis of the progenitors' DNA corroborated the presence of c.689+908G>A and c.2011C>T in different alleles (Figure S1B). The final confirmation of the direct involvement of change c.689+908G>A in the inclusion of the 57 bp intronic sequence was obtained by minigene analysis using a recombinant pSPL3 construct containing 813 bp of the intronic 5-6 sequence. Transcriptional profile analysis of the recombinant mutant plasmid showed the 57 bp transcript seen in patient Pt16 fibroblasts (Figure S1C). No pseudo-exon inclusion was detected in control cells. Western blot analysis of the EGF1 protein encoded by *GFM1* in patient Pt16's cells showed a drastically reduced amount of protein (Figure S1D).

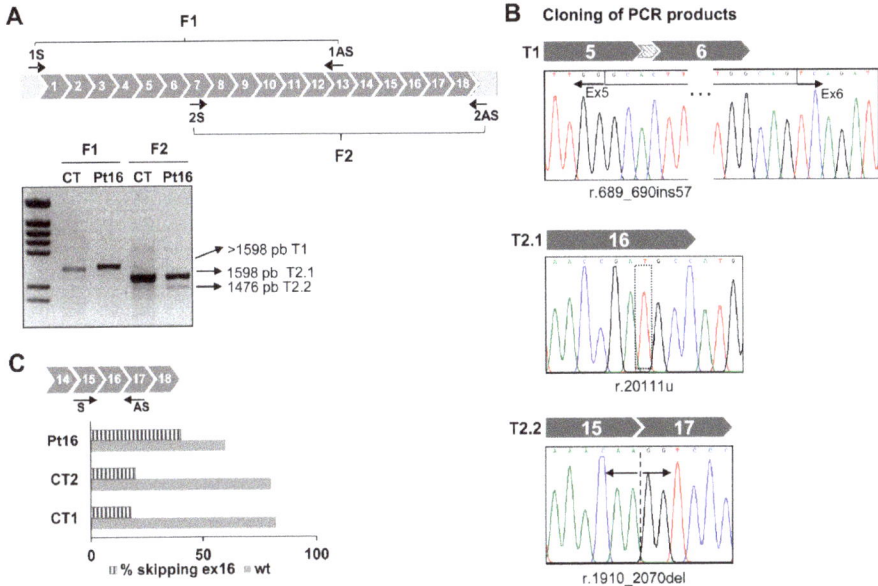

**Figure 2.** Aberrant splicing of *GFM1* in Pt16. (**A**) Diagram of *GFM1* cDNA with primers (arrows) used to amplify the complete coding region in two overlapping (F1 and F2) fragments. Agarose gel showing the results of RT-PCR amplifications in control (CT) and patient (Pt) fibroblasts. (**B**) Cloning of F1 and F2 PCR products and Sanger sequencing of regions around the nucleotide variations detected. (**C**) Distribution of reads. Data represent the percentage of *GFM1* transcript reads with exon 16 skipped (stripped bars) and full length (filled bars). Read numbers were 41,758 for Pt16, 13,581 for CT1 and 16,718 for CT2.

3.2.4. Antisense Oligonucleotide Treatment Rescues the Aberrant Splicing Event Caused by the Intronic Variant GFM1 c.689+908G>A

In an attempt to block mutant pre-mRNA access to the splicing machinery and to try to circumvent the formation of the aberrantly spliced transcript associated with change c.689+908G>A, tests were made of the ability of an antisense morpholino oligonucleotide (AON) to overlap the c.689+908G>A variation (Figure 3A). Transfection with 10 µM of the AON restored the correct splicing of *GFM1* in Pt16 fibroblasts carrying the deep-intronic variant in heterozygous fashion (Figure 3B). The AON did not alter the normal splicing of *GFM1*. Upon AON delivery, the level of EGF1 was partially restored as should correspond to the heterozygous condition of the intronic change (Figure 3C).

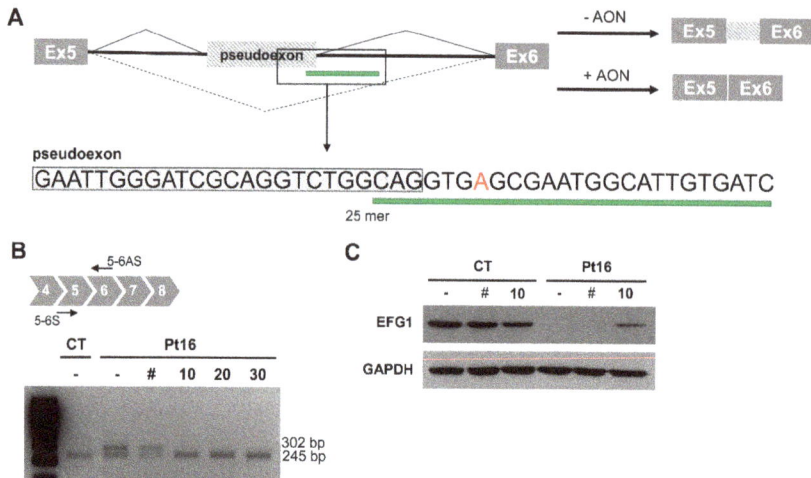

**Figure 3.** Antisense morpholino oligonucleotide-based pseudoexon skipping efficacy. (**A**) Diagram of the pseudoexon insertion caused by c.689+908G>A and the predicted effect of the antisense morpholino oligonucleotide (AON). Inset showing location and sequence of the 25mer AON. (**B**) Representative image of the RT-PCR product from mutant (Pt16) and wild type (CT) cells, non-transfected (-) and transfected with 10 µM of non-target control (#); or in the presence of different concentrations (0 to 30 µM) of GFM1-specific AON. (**C**) EFG1 rescue upon treatment with 10 µM of non-target control (#) or GFM1-specific AON.

### 3.3. Functional Studies in Patients with Novel Genotypes

#### 3.3.1. Biochemical Confirmation of Genetic Data

The pathogenicity of the changes in *DLD* carried by patients Pt18 and Pt35 was assessed by the direct measurement of dihydrolipoamide dehydrogenase activity in fibroblasts (see Table S2). The activity in the patients' cells was respectively 3% and 10% that of control cells.

CoQ10 levels were measured in the fibroblasts of patients Pt9 and Pt10, who carried changes in *COQ2* and *PDSS1* (both of which code for enzymes in the CoQ10 synthesis pathway). Reductions of 76% (11.9 ± 1.3 pmol/mg prot) were recorded for Pt9 and of 91.5% (4.2 ± 1.5 pmol/mg prot) for Pt10, both compatible with the available genotype data. Control values were 49.6 ± 10.8 pmol/mg protein.

#### 3.3.2. Mitochondrial Respiration and OxPhos Protein Analysis Confirmed Mitochondrial Dysfunction

For patients Pt15, Pt8, Pt2 and Pt10 carrying novel alleles in *FARS2*, *TSFM*, *FOXRED1* and *PDSS1* that could potentially provoke alterations in oxidative phosphorylation, assessments of possible mitochondrial dysfunction were made in terms of alterations in the OCR, mitochondrial membrane potential, OxPhos proteins and mitochondrial ultrastructure. Figure 4A shows a significant reduction detected in the ATP-linked oxygen consumption ratio, maximal OCR and reserve capacity for all patient fibroblasts. The ratio of red (TMRM) to green (MitoTracker®green) staining in fibroblasts corroborated a significant reduction in mitochondrial membrane potential in the cells of Pt8 and Pt10 (Figure 4B). In agreement with the oxygen consumption data, SDS-PAGE showed reduction in several OxPhos proteins (Figure 4C). The mitochondrial-encoded MTCO1 protein appeared reduced in mitochondrial extracts from the fibroblasts of patients Pt15 (*FARS2*) and Pt8 (*TSFM*) and the nuclear-encoded subunit of complex I, NDUFB8, was reduced in Pt15 (*FARS2*) and Pt2 (*FOXRED1*). Finally, and contrary to that previously reported [32,33], the mitochondrial extracts of Pt8 (*TSFM*) showed reduced amounts of all representative OxPhos proteins, except for complex V.

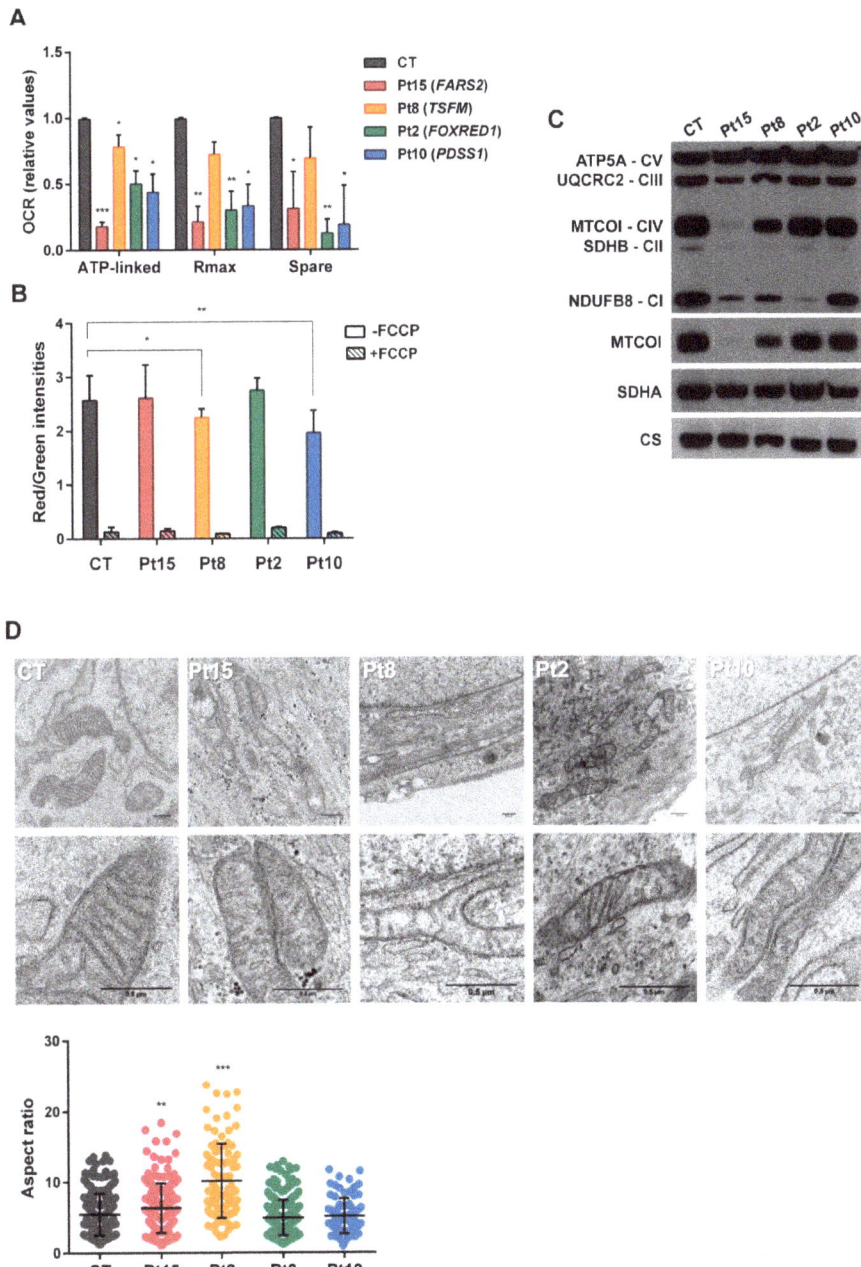

**Figure 4.** Bioenergetics of congenital lactic acidosis (CLA)-patients' fibroblasts. (**A**) Oxygen consumption rates. The data shown are for ATP-production-dependent maximal respiration (Rmax) and spare capacity (spare). Results are expressed as fold over the control concentrations and are the mean ± SD of 3–5 wells from $n = 2$–3 independent experiments. Control values are the means of two different control cell lines. (**B**) Flow cytometry analysis of mitochondrial mass (Mitotracker green) and membrane potential (TMRM staining) in the absence/presence of carbonyl cyanide-4-(trifluoromethoxy)

phenylhydrazone (FCCP). Results are the means of three independent experiments. (C) Western blots for representatives of all five respiratory complexes. Anti-MTOC1, anti-SDHA and anti-citrate synthase were also included. (D) Electron microscopy images showing defects of mitochondrial ultrastructure and cristae organization in patient fibroblasts. Mitochondrial length was analysed in control (CT) and patient (Pt) fibroblasts. Mitochondrial enlargement is expressed as the aspect ratio (major/minor mitochondrial axis ratio). Student $t$ test (* $p < 0.05$; ** $p < 0.01$; *** $p < 0.001$).

Transmission electron microscopy of the fibroblasts of patients Pt15, Pt8, Pt2 and Pt10 (Figure 4D) revealed the predominant presence of loose cristae, a condition compatible with changes in respiration capacity. Patients Pt8 and Pt15 also had a significant number of elongated mitochondria.

## 4. Discussion

This study reports how the combination of targeted-exome DNA sequencing, mtDNA analysis and functional genetics analysis identified genetic variants likely causal of CLA in 25 out of 39 patients (64%). All had a biochemical hallmark of persistent lactic acidosis and metabolites mostly related to downstream effects of an altered NADH/NAD+ redox status [6], the concentrations of which correlated with the blood lactate concentration. Based on their clinical and biochemical data, all patients received MDC scores and their nuclear and mitochondrial DNA was examined to identify genes and nucleotide variations likely responsible for pathological phenotypes. In this way, potentially biallelic changes were identified in 19 nuclear genes, 17 in genes related to congenital lactic acidosis and two in unexpected genes. Another two patients carried changes in their mitochondrial DNA compatible with their disease phenotype [34,35].

Before reporting the results of the diagnostic genetic testing to the corresponding clinicians, several lines of diagnostic evidence were taken into account. One was whether there was a confirmed causal link between a defective gene and patient phenotype. For patients Pt33, Pt5, Pt17, Pt6, Pt4, Pt3 and Pt34 carrying changes in *BCS1L*, *DGUOK*, *GFM1*, *MRPS22*, *TMEM70*, *MT-ATP6*, *MT-ND5*, the changes identified had been previously described associated with mitochondrial disorders and most of them shared phenotypic features with other patients previously reported [36–39]. The same occurred with patients Pt36, Pt39 who carried changes in *SLC19A3* and patients Pt12, Pt20 and Pt21 who had mutations in genes coding for subunits of the pyruvate dehydrogenase complex. Protein-specific functional analysis provided another line of evidence, as did the direct assay of enzymatic function in dermal fibroblasts. The latter corroborated the disease-causing nature of the nucleotide variations identified in patients Pt18 and Pt35 who carried biallelic changes in *DLD*. Further evidence was supplied by the re-phenotyping of patients to identify specific characteristics associated with defined biochemical phenotypes or by establishing a mitochondrial bioenergetics dysfunction related to the genes and changes identified. Thus, the reduced COQ10 measured in the fibroblasts of patients Pt9 and Pt10 carrying biallelic changes in *COQ2* and *PDSS1* respectively, helped confirm the deficient synthesis of coenzyme COQ10 in their fibroblasts. Because CoQ10 synthesis or thiamine transport defects are treatable conditions in which early diagnosis is essential to improve the clinical outcome [7,40,41], patients with them were immediately treated.

Access to a disease-relevant tissue is a problem in mitochondrial dysfunction analyses but epidermal fibroblasts have been reported to show potential in functional evaluations of many mitochondrial diseases [14,33,42]. In line with its role in electron transport, functional data from the fibroblasts of Pt15, Pt8, Pt2 and Pt10 confirmed the presence of impaired mitochondrial respiration and reduced amounts of representative OxPhos proteins. Thus, the diminished MTCO1 seen in patients carrying nucleotide changes in *FARS2* and *TSFM* reflect the reduced function of the transcription/translation mitochondrial machinery. The reduction in NDUFB8 protein, observed in mitochondrial extracts from patients with changes in *FOXRED1*, *FARS2* or *TSFM* might reflect the instability of this protein when not incorporated into OxPhos complex I [43]. Similar patterns have been reported in other patients with mutations in *FARS2* and *FOXRED1* [42,44]. Finally, the ultrastructure and morphology of the mitochondria and their cristae agreed with a possible alteration in mitochondrial bioenergetics function.

The present exome analysis also returned some unexpected results. For example, in patients Pt11 and Pt22, who met the criteria for mitochondrial disease with relatively high MDC scores, DNA analysis identified biallelic changes in *NPHS2* and *SLC16A1*, which might be a phenocopy of mitochondrial disease. In Pt22, respirometer tests (Figure S2) detected a notable decline in fibroblast respiratory variables compatible with mitochondrial dysfunction. However, not even whole exome sequencing returned positive results in terms of putative mutations related to mitochondrial disorders (data not shown).

The present work detected one patient, Pt16, with a single variation in a strong candidate gene and another patient, Pt15 with a possible deficiency in *FARS2* but with a nucleotide variant predicted to be benign and that did not correlate with the severity of the existing protein defect. In both patients, transcript analysis identified aberrant splicing events, probably due to disruptions of the consensus splice-site signals or to an effect on the splicing elements within the pre-mRNA. This analysis also returned important results concerning the relationship between genotype and phenotype. Thus, for patient Pt15, the new genotype deciphered by transcriptomic analysis better matched the drastic mitochondrial dysfunction observed in this patient's fibroblasts. For Pt16, in addition to characterizing the second mutation in the *GFM1* gene, an aberrant and probably unstable mRNA that skipped exon 16 was identified associated to the c.2011C>T (p.Arg671Cys) change. If translated it would produce a truncated p.(Ala637Glyfs*5) protein. Until this finding was made, the most plausible cause of the total absence of EFG1 in the fibroblasts of patients carrying the p.Arg671Cys change [33,39] was the disruption of the inter-subunit interface of the protein; this would locally destabilize the mutant protein resulting in its absence [45]. The present results, which increase the number of variants within exons causing disruptions in normal mRNA processes [46], shed new light on the effect of the nucleotide change on EFG1 expression and stability and highlight the importance of evaluating the effect of genomic variants on splicing as an integral part of the diagnostic work-up.

Overall, a genetic diagnosis was reached for 25 of the present 39 patients, obviating the need for muscle or hepatic biopsies and so forth. The highest percentage of positive results were obtained in patients with a definite mitochondrial disease, highlighting the importance of combining metabolomic, genetic and phenomic data in arriving at a diagnosis (Table 1). Although in this study, patients were initially selected based on their clinical and biochemical data, the present results support a "genome first approach" [15] be followed. In other words, genetic analyses should come first and the results of biochemical analyses and so forth, should be used in the interpretation of the genetic results.

The present work also reports the efficacy of antisense oligonucleotide therapy for rescuing normal splicing of the cryptic splice site generated by *GFM1* c.689+908G>A in patient fibroblasts. Easy to design and highly specific, antisense oligonucleotides have been used as RNA-modulators in cellular models of several genetic disorders [47] including ISCU myopathy [48]. The challenge is always to achieve the safe and efficient delivery of the therapeutic oligonucleotide to the required tissues.

## 5. Conclusions

The discussed system facilitates the diagnosis of CLA while greatly restricting the need to use invasive techniques and increases our knowledge of the causes of this condition. Identification of the genetic cause can also facilitate genetic counselling and guide the design of personalized therapeutic strategies.

**Supplementary Materials:** The following are available online at http://www.mdpi.com/2077-0383/8/11/1811/s1, Figure S1: Genomic characterization of variant c.689+908G>A and effect of the change on minigene-splicing profile, Figure S2: Oxygen consumption rates of fibroblasts from Pt22, Table S1: Clinical phenotypes. Table S2: Biochemical data, Table S3: Primers used for massive parallel sequencing of *GFM1* cDNA amplicons, Table S4: Prediction of pathogenicity by different tools.

**Author Contributions:** Conceptualization, C.P.-C., B.M., B.P. and P.R.-P. Data curation, I.B.-A., R.N., A.I.V., P.R.-S., M.T.G.S., E.M.-H., P.Q.F., A.B.-Q., S.S. and R.R.-R. Formal analysis, I.B.-A., R.N., A.I.V., P.R.-P and R.R.-R. Funding acquisition, B.P. and P.R.-P. Investigation, I.B.-A., C.P.-C., B.M., B.P and P.R.-P. Methodology, I.B.-A., R.N., A.I.V.,

P.R.-S. and R.R.-R. Project administration, B.P. and P.R.-P. Resources, M.T.G.S., E.M.H., P.Q.-F., A.B.-Q., S.S., M.B., I.V., M.L.C., L.T. and I.G.-J. Software, R.R.-R. Supervision, P.R.-P., M.A.M, L.R.D., M.U., B.M., B.P. and P.R.-P. Validation, B.P. and P.R.-P. Visualization, I.B.-A. Writing—original draft, P.R.-P. All authors contributed to manuscript revision, reading and approving the submitted version.

**Funding:** This research was funded in part by Fundación Isabel Gemio, Fundación La Caixa (LCF/PR/PR16/11110018); Spanish Ministerio de Economía y Competitividad and Fondo Europeo de Desarrollo Regional (FEDER) PI16/00573 and Regional Government of Madrid (CAM, B2017/BMD3721).

**Acknowledgments:** To Natalia Castejón for the bioinformatics analysis and Patricia Alcaide, Ascension Sanchez, Fatima Leal and Vanesa Ortega for the technical assistance. The institutional grant from the Fundación Ramón Areces to the Centro de Biología Molecular Severo Ochoa is also acknowledged.

**Conflicts of Interest:** The authors declare no conflict of interest. The funders had no role in the design of the study; in the collection, analyses or interpretation of data; in the writing of the manuscript or in the decision to publish the results.

## References

1. Kraut, J.A.; Madias, N.E. Lactic acidosis. *N. Engl. J. Med.* **2014**, *371*, 2309–2319. [CrossRef] [PubMed]
2. Morava, E.; van den Heuvel, L.; Hol, F.; de Vries, M.C.; Hogeveen, M.; Rodenburg, R.J.; Smeitink, J.A. Mitochondrial disease criteria: Diagnostic applications in children. *Neurology* **2006**, *67*, 1823–1826. [CrossRef] [PubMed]
3. Legati, A.; Reyes, A.; Nasca, A.; Invernizzi, F.; Lamantea, E.; Tiranti, V.; Garavaglia, B.; Lamperti, C.; Ardissone, A.; Moroni, I.; et al. New genes and pathomechanisms in mitochondrial disorders unraveled by NGS technologies. *Biochim. Biophys. Acta* **2016**, *1857*, 1326–1335. [CrossRef] [PubMed]
4. Gorman, G.S.; Chinnery, P.F.; DiMauro, S.; Hirano, M.; Koga, Y.; McFarland, R.; Suomalainen, A.; Thorburn, D.R.; Zeviani, M.; Turnbull, D.M. Mitochondrial diseases. *Nat. Rev. Dis. Prim.* **2016**, *2*, 16080. [CrossRef]
5. Parikh, S.; Goldstein, A.; Karaa, A.; Koenig, M.K.; Anselm, I.; Brunel-Guitton, C.; Christodoulou, J.; Cohen, B.H.; Dimmock, D.; Enns, G.M.; et al. Patient care standards for primary mitochondrial disease: A consensus statement from the Mitochondrial Medicine Society. *Genet. Med.* **2017**, *19*, 1380. [CrossRef]
6. Thompson Legault, J.; Strittmatter, L.; Tardif, J.; Sharma, R.; Tremblay-Vaillancourt, V.; Aubut, C.; Boucher, G.; Clish, C.B.; Cyr, D.; Daneault, C.; et al. A Metabolic Signature of Mitochondrial Dysfunction Revealed through a Monogenic Form of Leigh Syndrome. *Cell Rep.* **2015**, *13*, 981–989. [CrossRef]
7. Ortigoza-Escobar, J.D.; Molero-Luis, M.; Arias, A.; Oyarzabal, A.; Darin, N.; Serrano, M.; Garcia-Cazorla, A.; Tondo, M.; Hernandez, M.; Garcia-Villoria, J.; et al. Free-thiamine is a potential biomarker of thiamine transporter-2 deficiency: A treatable cause of Leigh syndrome. *Brain* **2016**, *139*, 31–38. [CrossRef]
8. Desbats, M.A.; Lunardi, G.; Doimo, M.; Trevisson, E.; Salviati, L. Genetic bases and clinical manifestations of coenzyme Q10 (CoQ 10) deficiency. *J. Inherit. Metab. Dis.* **2015**, *38*, 145–156. [CrossRef]
9. Witters, P.; Saada, A.; Honzik, T.; Tesarova, M.; Kleinle, S.; Horvath, R.; Goldstein, A.; Morava, E. Revisiting mitochondrial diagnostic criteria in the new era of genomics. *Genet. Med.* **2018**, *20*, 444–451. [CrossRef]
10. Rahman, J.; Noronha, A.; Thiele, I.; Rahman, S. Leigh map: A novel computational diagnostic resource for mitochondrial disease. *Ann. Neurol.* **2017**, *81*, 9–16. [CrossRef]
11. Wortmann, S.B.; Koolen, D.A.; Smeitink, J.A.; van den Heuvel, L.; Rodenburg, R.J. Whole exome sequencing of suspected mitochondrial patients in clinical practice. *J. Inherit. Metab. Dis.* **2015**, *38*, 437–443. [CrossRef] [PubMed]
12. Kohda, M.; Tokuzawa, Y.; Kishita, Y.; Nyuzuki, H.; Moriyama, Y.; Mizuno, Y.; Hirata, T.; Yatsuka, Y.; Yamashita-Sugahara, Y.; Nakachi, Y.; et al. A Comprehensive Genomic Analysis Reveals the Genetic Landscape of Mitochondrial Respiratory Chain Complex Deficiencies. *PLoS Genet.* **2016**, *12*, e1005679. [CrossRef] [PubMed]
13. Puusepp, S.; Reinson, K.; Pajusalu, S.; Murumets, U.; Oiglane-Shlik, E.; Rein, R.; Talvik, I.; Rodenburg, R.J.; Ounap, K. Effectiveness of whole exome sequencing in unsolved patients with a clinical suspicion of a mitochondrial disorder in Estonia. *Mol. Genet. Metab. Rep.* **2018**, *15*, 80–89. [CrossRef] [PubMed]
14. Kremer, L.S.; Bader, D.M.; Mertes, C.; Kopajtich, R.; Pichler, G.; Iuso, A.; Haack, T.B.; Graf, E.; Schwarzmayr, T.; Terrile, C.; et al. Genetic diagnosis of Mendelian disorders via RNA sequencing. *Nat. Commun.* **2017**, *8*, 15824. [CrossRef]

15. Raymond, F.L.; Horvath, R.; Chinnery, P.F. First-line genomic diagnosis of mitochondrial disorders. *Nat. Rev. Genet.* **2018**, *19*, 399–400. [CrossRef]
16. Chalmers, R.A.; Lawson, A.M. Gas Chomatography-Mass spectometry. In *Organic Acids in Man. Analytical Chemistry, Biochemistry and Diagnosis of the Organic Acidurias*; Chalmers, R.A., Lawson, A.M., Eds.; Chapman and Hall: London, UK; New York, NY, USA, 1982; pp. 81–127.
17. Ferrer, I.; Ruiz-Sala, P.; Vicente, Y.; Merinero, B.; Perez-Cerda, C.; Ugarte, M. Separation and identification of plasma short-chain acylcarnitine isomers by HPLC/MS/MS for the differential diagnosis of fatty acid oxidation defects and organic acidemias. *J. Chromatogr. B Analyt. Technol. Biomed. Life Sci.* **2007**, *860*, 121–126. [CrossRef]
18. Vega, A.I.; Medrano, C.; Navarrete, R.; Desviat, L.R.; Merinero, B.; Rodriguez-Pombo, P.; Vitoria, I.; Ugarte, M.; Perez-Cerda, C.; Perez, B. Molecular diagnosis of glycogen storage disease and disorders with overlapping clinical symptoms by massive parallel sequencing. *Genet. Med.* **2016**, *18*, 1037–1043. [CrossRef]
19. Ruiz-Pesini, E.; Lott, M.T.; Procaccio, V.; Poole, J.C.; Brandon, M.C.; Mishmar, D.; Yi, C.; Kreuziger, J.; Baldi, P.; Wallace, D.C. An enhanced MITOMAP with a global mtDNA mutational phylogeny. *Nucleic Acids Res.* **2007**, *35*, D823–D828. [CrossRef]
20. Weissensteiner, H.; Forer, L.; Fuchsberger, C.; Schopf, B.; Kloss-Brandstatter, A.; Specht, G.; Kronenberg, F.; Schonherr, S. mtDNA-Server: Next-generation sequencing data analysis of human mitochondrial DNA in the cloud. *Nucleic Acids Res.* **2016**, *44*, W64–W69. [CrossRef]
21. Kopanos, C.; Tsiolkas, V.; Kouris, A.; Chapple, C.E.; Albarca Aguilera, M.; Meyer, R.; Massouras, A. VarSome: The human genomic variant search engine. *Bioinformatics* **2018**, *35*, 1978–1980. [CrossRef]
22. Li, B.; Krishnan, V.G.; Mort, M.E.; Xin, F.; Kamati, K.K.; Cooper, D.N.; Mooney, S.D.; Radivojac, P. Automated inference of molecular mechanisms of disease from amino acid substitutions. *Bioinformatics* **2009**, *25*, 2744–2750. [CrossRef] [PubMed]
23. Tang, H.; Thomas, P.D. PANTHER-PSEP: Predicting disease-causing genetic variants using position-specific evolutionary preservation. *Bioinformatics* **2016**, *32*, 2230–2232. [CrossRef] [PubMed]
24. Bravo-Alonso, I.; Navarrete, R.; Arribas-Carreira, L.; Perona, A.; Abia, D.; Couce, M.L.; Garcia-Cazorla, A.; Morais, A.; Domingo, R.; Ramos, M.A.; et al. Nonketotic hyperglycinemia: Functional assessment of missense variants in GLDC to understand phenotypes of the disease. *Hum. Mutat.* **2017**, *38*, 678–691. [CrossRef] [PubMed]
25. Oyarzabal, A.; Martinez-Pardo, M.; Merinero, B.; Navarrete, R.; Desviat, L.R.; Ugarte, M.; Rodriguez-Pombo, P. A novel regulatory defect in the branched-chain alpha-keto acid dehydrogenase complex due to a mutation in the PPM1K gene causes a mild variant phenotype of maple syrup urine disease. *Hum. Mutat.* **2013**, *34*, 355–362. [CrossRef] [PubMed]
26. Bravo-Alonso, I.; Oyarzabal, A.; Sanchez-Arago, M.; Rejas, M.T.; Merinero, B.; Garcia-Cazorla, A.; Artuch, R.; Ugarte, M.; Rodriguez-Pombo, P. Dataset reporting BCKDK interference in a BCAA-catabolism restricted environment. *Data Br.* **2016**, *7*, 755–759. [CrossRef]
27. Mohanraj, K.; Wasilewski, M.; Beninca, C.; Cysewski, D.; Poznanski, J.; Sakowska, P.; Bugajska, Z.; Deckers, M.; Dennerlein, S.; Fernandez-Vizarra, E.; et al. Inhibition of proteasome rescues a pathogenic variant of respiratory chain assembly factor COA7. *EMBO Mol. Med.* **2019**, *11*, e9561. [CrossRef]
28. Garcia-Cazorla, A.; Oyarzabal, A.; Fort, J.; Robles, C.; Castejon, E.; Ruiz-Sala, P.; Bodoy, S.; Merinero, B.; Lopez-Sala, A.; Dopazo, J.; et al. Two novel mutations in the BCKDK (branched-chain keto-acid dehydrogenase kinase) gene are responsible for a neurobehavioral deficit in two pediatric unrelated patients. *Hum. Mutat.* **2014**, *35*, 470–477. [CrossRef]
29. Oyarzabal, A.; Bravo-Alonso, I.; Sanchez-Arago, M.; Rejas, M.T.; Merinero, B.; Garcia-Cazorla, A.; Artuch, R.; Ugarte, M.; Rodriguez-Pombo, P. Mitochondrial response to the BCKDK-deficiency: Some clues to understand the positive dietary response in this form of autism. *Biochim. Biophys. Acta* **2016**, *1862*, 592–600. [CrossRef]
30. De Vos, K.J.; Allan, V.J.; Grierson, A.J.; Sheetz, M.P. Mitochondrial function and actin regulate dynamin-related protein 1-dependent mitochondrial fission. *Curr. Biol.* **2005**, *15*, 678–683. [CrossRef]
31. Richards, S.; Aziz, N.; Bale, S.; Bick, D.; Das, S.; Gastier-Foster, J.; Grody, W.W.; Hegde, M.; Lyon, E.; Spector, E.; et al. Standards and guidelines for the interpretation of sequence variants: A joint consensus recommendation of the American College of Medical Genetics and Genomics and the Association for Molecular Pathology. *Genet. Med.* **2015**, *17*, 405–424. [CrossRef]

32. Simon, M.T.; Ng, B.G.; Friederich, M.W.; Wang, R.Y.; Boyer, M.; Kircher, M.; Collard, R.; Buckingham, K.J.; Chang, R.; Shendure, J.; et al. Activation of a cryptic splice site in the mitochondrial elongation factor GFM1 causes combined OXPHOS deficiency. *Mitochondrion* **2017**, *34*, 84–90. [CrossRef] [PubMed]
33. Emperador, S.; Bayona-Bafaluy, M.P.; Fernandez-Marmiesse, A.; Pineda, M.; Felgueroso, B.; Lopez-Gallardo, E.; Artuch, R.; Roca, I.; Ruiz-Pesini, E.; Couce, M.L.; et al. Molecular-genetic characterization and rescue of a TSFM mutation causing childhood-onset ataxia and nonobstructive cardiomyopathy. *Eur. J. Hum. Genet.* **2017**, *25*, 153–156. [CrossRef] [PubMed]
34. Tang, S.; Wang, J.; Zhang, V.W.; Li, F.Y.; Landsverk, M.; Cui, H.; Truong, C.K.; Wang, G.; Chen, L.C.; Graham, B.; et al. Transition to next generation analysis of the whole mitochondrial genome: A summary of molecular defects. *Hum. Mutat.* **2013**, *34*, 882–893. [CrossRef] [PubMed]
35. Swalwell, H.; Kirby, D.M.; Blakely, E.L.; Mitchell, A.; Salemi, R.; Sugiana, C.; Compton, A.G.; Tucker, E.J.; Ke, B.X.; Lamont, P.J.; et al. Respiratory chain complex I deficiency caused by mitochondrial DNA mutations. *Eur. J. Hum. Genet.* **2011**, *19*, 769–775. [CrossRef] [PubMed]
36. Boczonadi, V.; Ricci, G.; Horvath, R. Mitochondrial DNA transcription and translation: Clinical syndromes. *Essays Biochem.* **2018**, *62*, 321–340. [PubMed]
37. Ghezzi, D.; Zeviani, M. Human diseases associated with defects in assembly of OXPHOS complexes. *Essays Biochem.* **2018**, *62*, 271–286. [CrossRef] [PubMed]
38. Catteruccia, M.; Verrigni, D.; Martinelli, D.; Torraco, A.; Agovino, T.; Bonafe, L.; D'Amico, A.; Donati, M.A.; Adorisio, R.; Santorelli, F.M.; et al. Persistent pulmonary arterial hypertension in the newborn (PPHN): A frequent manifestation of TMEM70 defective patients. *Mol. Genet. Metab.* **2014**, *111*, 353–359. [CrossRef]
39. Brito, S.; Thompson, K.; Campistol, J.; Colomer, J.; Hardy, S.A.; He, L.; Fernandez-Marmiesse, A.; Palacios, L.; Jou, C.; Jimenez-Mallebrera, C.; et al. Long-term survival in a child with severe encephalopathy, multiple respiratory chain deficiency and GFM1 mutations. *Front. Genet.* **2015**, *6*, 102.
40. Salviati, L.; Sacconi, S.; Murer, L.; Zacchello, G.; Franceschini, L.; Laverda, A.M.; Basso, G.; Quinzii, C.; Angelini, C.; Hirano, M.; et al. Infantile encephalomyopathy and nephropathy with CoQ10 deficiency: A CoQ10-responsive condition. *Neurology* **2005**, *65*, 606–608. [CrossRef]
41. Montini, G.; Malaventura, C.; Salviati, L. Early coenzyme Q10 supplementation in primary coenzyme Q10 deficiency. *N. Engl. J. Med.* **2008**, *358*, 2849–2850. [CrossRef]
42. Vantroys, E.; Larson, A.; Friederich, M.; Knight, K.; Swanson, M.A.; Powell, C.A.; Smet, J.; Vergult, S.; De Paepe, B.; Seneca, S.; et al. New insights into the phenotype of FARS2 deficiency. *Mol. Genet. Metab.* **2017**, *122*, 172–181. [CrossRef] [PubMed]
43. Friederich, M.W.; Timal, S.; Powell, C.A.; Dallabona, C.; Kurolap, A.; Palacios-Zambrano, S.; Bratkovic, D.; Derks, T.G.J.; Bick, D.; Bouman, K.; et al. Pathogenic variants in glutamyl-tRNA(Gln) amidotransferase subunits cause a lethal mitochondrial cardiomyopathy disorder. *Nat. Commun.* **2018**, *9*, 4065. [CrossRef] [PubMed]
44. Formosa, L.E.; Mimaki, M.; Frazier, A.E.; McKenzie, M.; Stait, T.L.; Thorburn, D.R.; Stroud, D.A.; Ryan, M.T. Characterization of mitochondrial FOXRED1 in the assembly of respiratory chain complex I. *Hum. Mol. Genet.* **2015**, *24*, 2952–2965. [CrossRef] [PubMed]
45. Galmiche, L.; Serre, V.; Beinat, M.; Zossou, R.; Assouline, Z.; Lebre, A.S.; Chretien, F.; Shenhav, R.; Zeharia, A.; Saada, A.; et al. Toward genotype phenotype correlations in GFM1 mutations. *Mitochondrion* **2012**, *12*, 242–247. [CrossRef]
46. Pagani, F.; Baralle, F.E. Genomic variants in exons and introns: Identifying the splicing spoilers. *Nat. Rev. Genet.* **2004**, *5*, 389–396. [CrossRef]
47. Perez, B.; Vilageliu, L.; Grinberg, D.; Desviat, L.R. Antisense mediated splicing modulation for inherited metabolic diseases: Challenges for delivery. *Nucleic Acid Ther.* **2014**, *24*, 48–56. [CrossRef]
48. Holmes-Hampton, G.P.; Crooks, D.R.; Haller, R.G.; Guo, S.; Freier, S.M.; Monia, B.P.; Rouault, T.A. Use of antisense oligonucleotides to correct the splicing error in ISCU myopathy patient cell lines. *Hum. Mol. Genet.* **2016**, *25*, 5178–5187. [CrossRef]

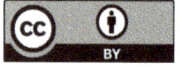

© 2019 by the authors. Licensee MDPI, Basel, Switzerland. This article is an open access article distributed under the terms and conditions of the Creative Commons Attribution (CC BY) license (http://creativecommons.org/licenses/by/4.0/).

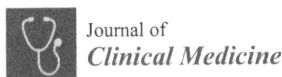

Article

# Clinical Spectrum and Functional Consequences Associated with Bi-Allelic Pathogenic *PNPT1* Variants

Rocio Rius [1,2], Nicole J. Van Bergen [1,2], Alison G. Compton [1,2], Lisa G. Riley [3,4], Maina P. Kava [5,6], Shanti Balasubramaniam [6,7,8], David J. Amor [1,2,9], Miriam Fanjul-Fernandez [2,9], Mark J. Cowley [10,11,12], Michael C. Fahey [13], Mary K. Koenig [14], Gregory M. Enns [15], Simon Sadedin [1,9], Meredith J. Wilson [16,17], Tiong Y. Tan [1,2,9], David R. Thorburn [1,2,9] and John Christodoulou [1,2,4,9,*]

1. Murdoch Children's Research Institute, Melbourne, VIC 3052, Australia; rocio.rius@mcri.edu.au (R.R.); nicole.vanbergen@mcri.edu.au (N.J.V.B.); alison.compton@mcri.edu.au (A.G.C.); david.amor@mcri.edu.au (D.J.A.); simon.sadedin@vcgs.org.au (S.S.); tiong.tan@vcgs.org.au (T.Y.T.); david.thorburn@mcri.edu.au (D.R.T.)
2. Department of Paediatrics, University of Melbourne, Melbourne, VIC 3052, Australia; miriam.fanjul@vcgs.org.au
3. Kids Research, The Children's Hospital at Westmead, Sydney, NSW 2145, Australia; lisa.riley@health.nsw.gov.au
4. Discipline of Child & Adolescent Health, Sydney Medical School, University of Sydney, Sydney, NSW 2050, Australia
5. Department of Neurology, Perth Children's Hospital, Perth, WA 6009, Australia; maina.kava@health.wa.gov.au
6. Department of Metabolic Medicine and Rheumatology, Perth Children's Hospital, Perth, WA 6009, Australia; shanti.balasubramaniam@health.nsw.gov.au
7. Genetic Metabolic Disorders Service, Western Sydney Genetics Program, The Children's Hospital at Westmead, Sydney, NSW 2145, Australia
8. Discipline of Genetic Medicine, Sydney Medical School, University of Sydney, Sydney, NSW 2145, Australia
9. Victorian Clinical Genetic Services, Melbourne, VIC 3052, Australia
10. Precision Medicine Theme, Children's Cancer Institute, Kensington, NSW 2750, Australia; MCowley@ccia.org.au
11. Kinghorn Centre for Clinical Genomics, Garvan Institute, University of New South Wales, Randwick, NSW 2010, Australia
12. School of Women's and Children's Health, University of New South Wales, Randwick, NSW 2031, Australia
13. Department of Paediatrics, Monash University, Melbourne, VIC 3168, Australia; michael.fahey@monash.edu
14. The University of Texas McGovern Medical School, Houston, TX 77030, USA; Mary.K.Koenig@uth.tmc.edu
15. Department of Pediatrics, Division of Medical Genetics, Stanford University, Stanford, CA 94305, USA; genns@stanford.edu
16. Department of Clinical Genetics, The Children's Hospital at Westmead, Sydney, NSW 2145, Australia; meredith.wilson@health.nsw.gov.au
17. Discipline of Genomic Medicine, Faculty of Medicine and Health, University of Sydney, Sydney, NSW 2006, Australia
* Correspondence: john.christodoulou@mcri.edu.au; Tel.: +613-9936-6353

Received: 9 October 2019; Accepted: 14 November 2019; Published: 19 November 2019

**Abstract:** *PNPT1* (PNPase—polynucleotide phosphorylase) is involved in multiple RNA processing functions in the mitochondria. Bi-allelic pathogenic *PNPT1* variants cause heterogeneous clinical phenotypes affecting multiple organs without any established genotype–phenotype correlations. Defects in PNPase can cause variable combined respiratory chain complex defects. Recently, it has been suggested that PNPase can lead to activation of an innate immune response. To better understand the clinical and molecular spectrum of patients with bi-allelic *PNPT1* variants, we captured detailed clinical and molecular phenotypes of all 17 patients reported in the literature, plus seven new patients, including a 78-year-old male with the longest reported survival. A functional follow-up of genomic sequencing by cDNA studies confirmed a splicing defect in a novel, apparently synonymous, variant. Patient fibroblasts showed an accumulation of mitochondrial unprocessed *PNPT1* transcripts, while blood showed an increased interferon response. Our findings suggest that functional analyses of the RNA processing function of PNPase are more sensitive than testing downstream defects in oxidative phosphorylation (OXPHPOS) enzyme activities. This research extends our knowledge of the clinical and functional consequences of bi-allelic pathogenic *PNPT1* variants that may guide management and further efforts into understanding the pathophysiological mechanisms for therapeutic development.

**Keywords:** mitochondrial; *PNPT1*; PNPase; interferon; OXPHOS; respiratory chain; mutation; splice defect

## 1. Introduction

*PNPT1* encodes for polynucleotide phosphorylase (PNPase), a conserved homotrimeric 3'-to-5' exoribonuclease predominantly localized in the mitochondrial matrix and intermembrane space [1]. It is primarily involved in mitochondrial RNA (mtRNA) processing and degradation [2].

PNPase has been suggested to play a role in RNA import into mitochondria [3,4]; however, experimental data have been contradictory and, to date, there is no general agreement about an RNA import mechanism [5]. Recent reports suggest that disrupted PNPase RNA processing could lead to the accumulation of double-stranded mtRNAs, with the possibility of triggering an altered immune response [6,7].

Patients with bi-allelic *PNPT1* pathogenic variants have shown wide clinical heterogeneity ranging from non-syndromic hearing loss to multisystemic Leigh syndrome [8,9]. To date, no clear phenotype–genotype correlations have been drawn.

In a bid to better understand the clinical phenotype and functional consequences of patients with *PNPT1*-related diseases, we reported seven new patients with bi-allelic *PNPT1* variants and expanded upon the mutational spectrum. We also conducted functional studies and performed a thorough clinical review of previously published patients with *PNPT1* variants [6,8–13].

## 2. Experimental Section

### 2.1. Patients

We report seven new patients (P1, 2, 3, 3.2, 4, 7, 8) with bi-allelic variants in *PNPT1*, and provided updates for three previously published cases (P5, 6, 9). We also conducted a PubMed search using the terms PNPase (All Fields) OR (PNPT1 (All Fields) AND ("persons" (MeSH Terms) OR "persons" (All Fields) OR "individual" (All Fields))) up to September 2019 for publications limited to human subjects to describe the clinical features of all the patients with bi-allelic *PNPT1* pathogenic variants reported in the literature to date [6,8–13].

Functional studies were conducted in samples collected from four patients (P1, 2, 3, 4) in which the *PNPT1* variants were identified by whole genome sequencing (WGS; Garvan Institute, Sydney) or whole exome sequencing (WES; Victorian Clinical Genetics Services (VCGS), Melbourne; Broad Institute, Cambridge, MA, USA; and Baylor College of Medicine, Houston, TX, USA).

This study was performed in accordance with the Helsinki Declaration and ethical standards of the responsible ethics committees. The project was approved by the Human Research Ethics Committees of the Sydney Children's Hospitals Network (ID number HREC/10/CHW/114), Melbourne Health (ID number HREC/16/MH/251), and the Royal Children's Hospital (ID number HREC/16/RCHM/150).

## 2.2. Next Generation Sequencing (NGS) and in Silico Tools

The variants in P1 were identified through whole exome sequencing (WES) performed by the Genomics Platform at the Broad Institute of Harvard and MIT (Broad Institute, Cambridge, MA, USA). The variants in P2 were identified through trio whole genome sequencing (WGS) performed at the Kinghorn Centre for Clinical Genomics (Garvan Institute, Sydney) as previously described [14]. The variants in P3 and P4 were identified through WES performed at Victorian Clinical Genetics Services (VCGS), Melbourne. P7 and P8 variants were identified through WES performed at Baylor College of Medicine, Medical Genetics Laboratories, Whole Genome Laboratory (Houston, TX, USA).

In silico prediction analyses were performed using PolyPhen-2 [15], SIFT [16], Combined Annotation Dependent Depletion CADD [17], MutationTaster [18], and Human Splicing Finder v3.1 [19]. Visualization of variants in the Pfam [20] protein domains was conducted with MutationMapper [21]. Allele frequencies were determined using the Genome Aggregation Database [22].

## 2.3. Western Blotting

Fibroblast protein extraction and Western blotting were performed using total Abcam OXPHOS human WB antibody cocktail (ab11041) and PNPase (ab96176) as previously published [10].

## 2.4. Mitochondrial Oxidative Phosphorylation (OXPHOS) Enzyme Activities

Spectrophotometric analysis of OXPHOS enzyme activities in muscle and fibroblasts was performed as previously described [23]. The mitochondrial respiratory chain complex I (CI) and complex IV (CIV) dipstick activity assays (Abcam, Melbourne, VIC, Australia) were performed using 15 µg of whole-cell lysates fibroblasts as previously published [10].

## 2.5. Fibroblast Culture, RNA Extraction, and Complementary DNA (cDNA) Studies

Cycloheximide treatment of cultured fibroblasts from P2 and controls was performed as published [24]. Cultured fibroblasts from patients P1, P2, P3, and P4, and three control lines were incubated in the presence or absence of 100 U/mL interferon α-2a Roferon-A (Roche, Sydney, Australia) in HyClone Dulbecco's Modified Eagle Medium (GE Healthcare, Rydalmere, NSW, Australia) at 37 °C and 5% $CO_2$ for 24 h.

RNA was isolated from fibroblasts using the RNeasy Plus kit (Qiagen, Hilden, Germany) following the manufacturer's instructions. Reverse transcription was performed using SuperScript III First-Strand synthesis kit (Thermo Fisher Scientific, Carlsbad, CA, USA) following the manufacturer's instructions.

## 2.6. RNA Extraction from Blood

PAXgene blood RNA tubes (PreAnalytix by Qiagen, Hombrechtikon, Switzerland) were used to collect peripheral blood samples. After collection, the tubes were left at room temperature between 2 h and 72 h before extracting RNA using the PAXgene blood RNA kit (PreAnalytix by Qiagen) following the manufacturer's instructions.

## 2.7. PCR Quantification of Unprocessed Mitochondrial Transcripts

qPCR for the quantification of unprocessed transcripts was performed with AccuPower 2X Greenstar qPCR Master Mix (Bioneer, Daejeon, Korea) using primers previously published by Matilainen and collaborators [9]. The relative accumulation of unprocessed mitochondrial transcripts was calculated using the $2^{(-\Delta\Delta Ct)}$ method [25].

## 2.8. Interferon Signature Analysis

The relative expression of six interferon-stimulated genes was analyzed by qPCR using cDNA from 40 ng RNA, TaqMan Fast Advanced Master Mix (Thermo Fisher Scientific), and Taq Man probes for *IFI27* (Hs01086370_m1), *IFI44L* (Hs00199115_m1), *IFIT1* (Hs00356631_g1), *ISG15* (Hs00192713_m1),

*RSAD2* (Hs01057264_m1), and *SIGLEC1* (Hs00988063_m1). The relative abundance was normalized to *HPRT1* (Hs03929096_g1) and *18S* (Hs999999001_s1). Median expression was used to calculate an interferon score as described by Dhir, Rice, and collaborators [6,26].

## 3. Results

A total of 24 patients with bi-allelic variants in *PNPT1* were identified in 15 families, including seven new patients (P1, 2, 3, 3.1, 4, 7, 8), three previously published individuals with additional clinical information since the previous publication (P5, 6, 9), and fourteen other patients reported in the literature (Tables S1 and S2). A total of 22 different pathogenic variants were found, of which only three were reported in more than one family. The p.(Ala507Ser) variant was reported in 27% of the families (4/15), followed by the p.(Thr531Arg) variant at 13% (2/15), and p.(Arg136His) at 13% (2/15) (Figure 1).

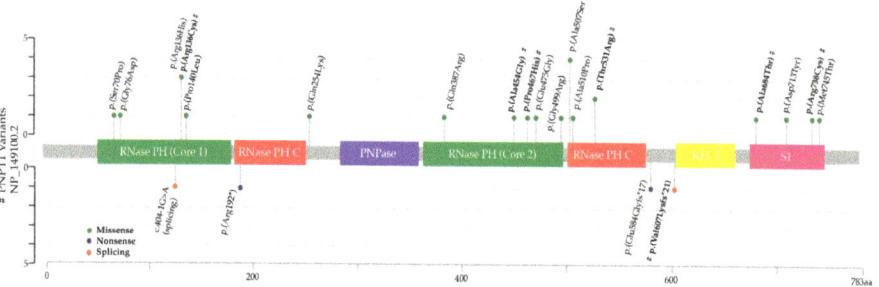

**Figure 1.** Lollipop plot depicting the polynucleotide phosphorylase (PNPase) protein and location of pathogenic variants reported in 30 alleles (15 families). Missense variants are shown above the protein. Nonsense and splicing variants are shown below. Novel variants reported in this article are marked with #.

Most of the patients (75% n = 18) presented within the first year of life. The most common initial manifestations were tone abnormalities (42% n = 10), feeding difficulties (17% n = 4), and mild to severe sensorineural hearing loss (38% n = 9). Other reported initial features were regression, choreoathetosis, visual loss, and cataracts (Table S1).

The median age at the last follow up was 8.9 years (range 1–78). Three of the patients died due to acute encephalopathy (P15 at 4 years), infection (P16 at 2.4 years), and unstated reasons (P21 at 2 years) (Table S1).

The clinical symptoms of all the reported patients to date are summarized in Figure 2 and Table S1.

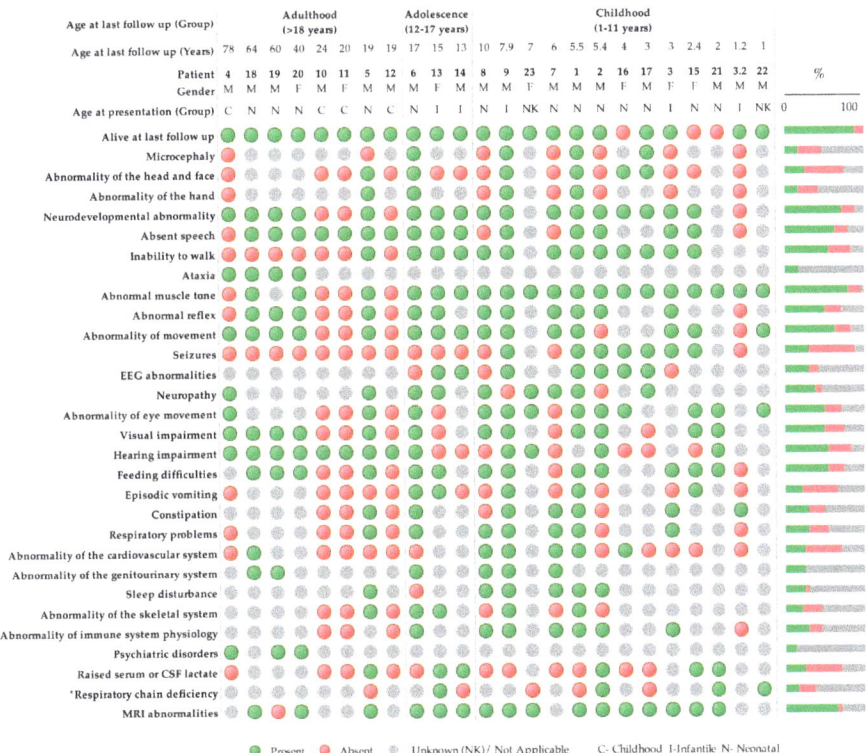

**Figure 2.** Clinical symptoms using Human Phenotype Ontology (HPO) terminology of patients with bi-allelic *PNPT1* variants ($n = 24$). Green indicates a present phenotype, red indicates an absent phenotype, and gray is unknown or not applicable. * Respiratory chain deficiencies refer to reported reductions in oxidative phosphorylation (OXPHOS) enzyme activity measured by spectrophotometric analysis in any tissue. Neonatal (0–28 days), infant (28 days–1 year), and childhood (>1 year).

### 3.1. cDNA Studies Identify a Splicing Defect in P2

The NM_033109.4:c.1818T>G heterozygous variant identified in P2 was originally believed to be synonymous p.(Val606=), however it was located 5 bp from the donor splice site and in silico studies suggested the possibility of a splicing defect (Table S2). cDNA studies performed from cultured fibroblasts grown with and without cycloheximide treatment to inhibit nonsense-mediated decay (NMD) confirmed a splicing defect resulting in a frameshift deletion and premature termination codon p.(Val607Lysfs*21), leading the transcript to be subject to degradation by NMD (Figure 3).

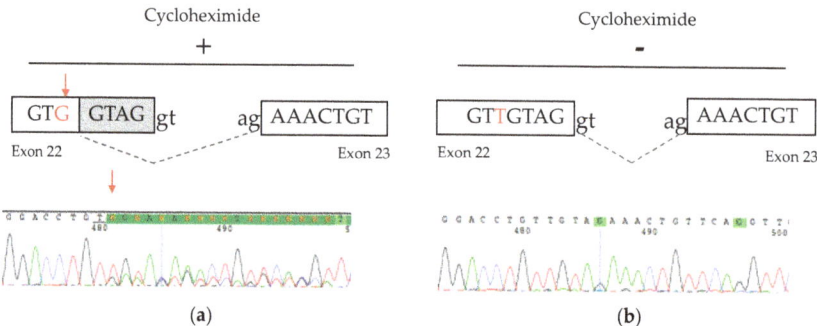

**Figure 3.** cDNA studies from P2 fibroblast cells. (**a**) Schematic representation and partial electropherogram showing the creation of a new splice site generated by the NM_033109.4:c.1818T>G variant in cells treated with cycloheximide. (**b**) Without cycloheximide treatment, the heterozygous NM_033109.4:c.1818T>G variant was not detectable, suggesting that the mutant RNA is subject to nonsense-mediated decay.

### 3.2. Mitochondrial OXPHOS Protein Expression and Activity

In the fibroblasts, there was a reduction of the mitochondrial complex IV COX II subunit and the complex I NDUFB8 subunit in patients P1–4, although the levels of other OXPHOS subunits were normal (Figure 4a). The activities of complex I and complex IV were determined using a dipstick assay. Compared to the control means, there was a relatively mild reduction in complex I by 20% (P1), 45% (P2), 50% (P4), and a modest reduction in complex IV by 40% (P1), 57% (P2), 20% (P3), and 80% (P4) (Figure 4b). P5 was a previously reported patient with *PNPT1* variants [10] and was used as a positive control.

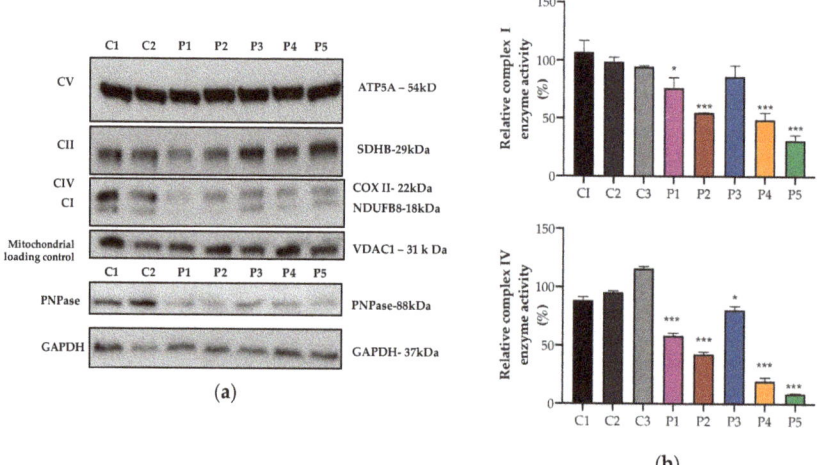

**Figure 4.** Protein expression and OXPHOS activity in fibroblasts. (**a**) Representative images of Western blot analysis performed in fibroblast proteins from controls (C) and patients (P). In the patients, there was a reduction in protein expression of PNPase (lower panel) and complex I and complex IV OXPHOS mitochondrial subunits (upper panel). (**b**) Complex I (upper panel) and complex IV (lower panel) enzyme activity was analyzed using dipstick activity assays. In the patients, there was a mild/moderate reduction in complex I and complex IV enzyme activities. The mean and variation (SEM) between three independent experiments are shown. (*** $p < 0.001$, * $p < 0.033$).

However, spectrophotometric analysis of OXPHOS enzymes was normal in fibroblasts from P1, and was only borderline low for complex IV activity relative to protein and citrate synthase in muscle from P2 (Table 1).

**Table 1.** Spectrophotometric analysis of oxidative phosphorylation (OXPHOS) enzyme activities in fibroblasts from P1 and muscle from P2.

| Enzyme | P1 (Fibroblasts) | | | P2 (Muscle) | | |
| --- | --- | --- | --- | --- | --- | --- |
| | Residual Activity (%) | CS Ratio (%) | CII Ratio (%) | Residual Activity (%) | CS Ratio (%) | CII Ratio (%) |
| I | 150 | 107 | 75 | 75 | 73 | 126 |
| II | 194 | 140 | - | 59 | 58 | - |
| III | 266 | 187 | 133 | 69 | 65 | 113 |
| IV | 91 | 67 | 47 | 34 | 34 | 59 |
| CS | 137 | | | 102 | | |

Activities of OXPHOS enzyme complexes I, II, III, IV, and citrate synthase (CS) are expressed as % relative to protein (residual activity), citrate synthase (CS ratio), and CII (CII ratio) of control samples.

### 3.3. Accumulation of Mitochondrial Unprocessed Transcripts

To assess the PNPase mitochondrial RNA processing activity, we measured the accumulation of unprocessed polycistronic mitochondrial transcripts in fibroblasts.

Compared to controls, fibroblasts from patients P1–4 showed an accumulation of aberrantly processed mitochondrial RNA transcripts (Figure 5) in line with the PNPase function in mtRNA processing. The accumulation of unprocessed transcripts in myoblasts from a patient with bi-allelic pathogenic variants in *PNPT1* was previously described [9]. Notably, our patients presented different patterns of accumulation, which were not restricted to transcripts around *MT-ND6*. Further studies may help us to understand if the differences in the accumulation of unprocessed mitochondrial transcripts are related to specific *PNPT1* variants.

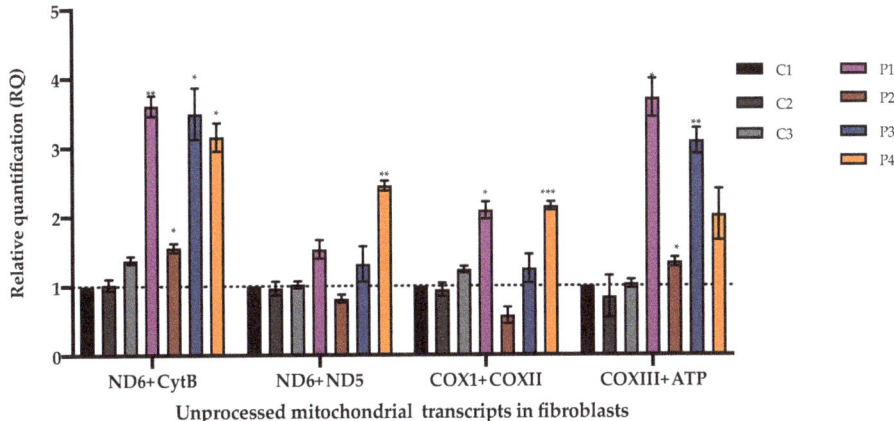

**Figure 5.** Unprocessed polycistronic mitochondrial transcripts in fibroblasts measured by qPCR. Mean and variation (SEM) between three independent experiments are shown (*** $p < 0.001$, ** $p < 0.002$, * $p < 0.033$).

### 3.4. Interferon Signature in Patients with PNPT1 Variants

Increased expression of interferon-stimulated genes has been previously described in blood from P14, P22, and P23 with bi-allelic *PNPT1* variants [6]. To assess if the PNPase defects could elicit an increased interferon response in different tissues, we calculated the interferon score in fibroblasts (P1–4) and in blood (only available from P2 and P4). In fibroblasts from P1–4 stimulated with IFN-α2a (100 U/mL), the interferon response was not different to controls (interferon score below the 1.3 threshold in fibroblasts). On the other hand, in blood from P1 and P4, a positive interferon score was identified with a median of 2.53 and 4.65, respectively (above the 1.8 threshold in blood) (Figure 6).

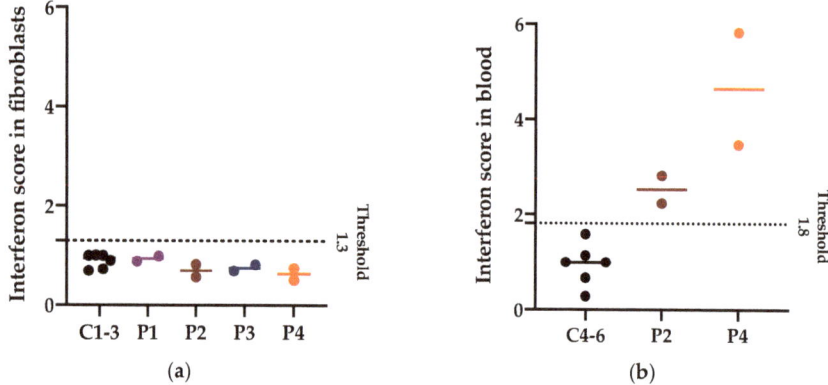

**Figure 6.** Interferon (IFN) score in fibroblasts and in blood. (**a**) Median and individual values of the IFN score in fibroblasts of three controls and patients with *PNPT1* variants (P1–4) from two independent experiments. The IFN score threshold of 1.3 corresponds to the mean IFN score of controls + 2SD. Higher values are considered positive. (**b**) Median and individual values of the IFN score in blood of three controls and patients with *PNPT1* variants (P2 and P4) from two independent experiments. The IFN score threshold of 1.8 corresponds to the mean IFN score of controls + 2SD. Higher values are considered positive.

## 4. Discussion

This cohort illustrated the marked phenotypic heterogeneity associated with bi-allelic *PNPT1* variants. Severe developmental delay and regression were the most common neurodevelopmental abnormalities. Sensorineural hearing loss, optic atrophy, tone, and movement abnormalities—including choreoathetosis, dystonia, myoclonus, and ataxia—were also amongst the most prevalent clinical features. Most patients had a history of hypotonia ($n = 19$) and four patients presented a pattern of central hypotonia with peripheral hypertonia. Brain imaging was available in 17 patients, of which 16 patients had MRI abnormalities. The most common were white matter abnormalities ($n = 8$), followed by thin corpus callosum ($n = 5$), and basal ganglia abnormalities ($n = 4$) (Figure S1).

Interestingly, most of the patients in the cohort had normal to mildly deficient OXPHOS when measured by spectrophotometric enzyme assays. This finding has several implications. First, a normal OXPHOS enzyme analysis does not rule out the diagnosis of *PNPT1*-related disease. Second, reduced OXPHOS protein expression or activity measured by dipstick assays does not always correlate with spectrophotometric assays, as shown in P1 and P2. This discrepancy could be attributed to sample preparation and differences in the methodology, which has been discussed previously [10]. Finally, in order to confirm pathogenicity, functional analyses focusing on the primary role of *PNPT1* (mtRNA processing) and interferon signaling in blood rather than fibroblasts appear to be more sensitive, and potentially more specific than evaluating the downstream effects on the OXPHOS enzyme activities.

Most of the patients with *PNPT1*-related disease have been identified through NGS approaches. The identification of an apparently synonymous variant in P2 that was later demonstrated to result in abnormal mRNA splicing highlights the importance of careful interpretation of apparently "silent" variants in NGS data, the utility of in silico tools, and the need for cDNA studies when following up potential splicing variants.

The identification of an interferon signature in blood from patients with *PNPT1* variants raises the possibility that an immune response could contribute to disease pathogenesis [6]. Further longitudinal studies could elucidate if there is a correlation between the interferon signature and disease severity, or the possibility of being a useful clinical biomarker and/or therapeutic target.

So far, little is known about possible genotype–phenotype correlations, and it is not clear what factors could be contributing to the clinical spectrum of *PNPT1*-related diseases. Studies suggest that the rate of disease progression could be, in part, related to having two deleterious variants affecting the first core domain [9]. In line with this, three patients with rapidly progressive disease and early death (median age 2.4 years) were described (Table S1), in which the variants were located in the first core domain. P21 had the p.(Arg136His) variant in a homozygous state. P15 also had the p.(Arg136His) variant but in compound heterozygosity with the p.(Pro140Leu) variant, which was also located in the first core domain. P16, who had a p.(Gly76Asp) located in the first core domain and a p.(Arg192*), was predicted to result in nonsense-mediated decay [6,9,12]. The novel variant p.(Arg136Cys) identified in P3 was an alternate amino acid change located in the same active site as described in P21 and P15, but her second pathogenic variant p.(Pro467His) was located in the second core domain. Interestingly, she is currently three years old and has a relatively slower progression. Her brother (P3.2) also seemed to be more mildly affected. Intrafamilial variability was also described in other families with *PNPT1* variants (P5, 6, 7, 8; Table S1), but bona fide genetic modifiers of disease severity have yet to be identified.

P4 had the longest survival reported to date (78 years), with a slowly progressive clinical course. He presented at 11 years old with hearing and visual loss. Subsequently, he developed blepharospasm and ptosis. Over the decades, he developed progressive ataxia, poor night vision, and external ophthalmoplegia. His hearing worsened during his 60s and, therefore, he received a cochlear implant. Eaton and collaborators [13] also described one family that presented with a slowly progressive pattern. Both affected individuals had congenital sensorineural hearing loss and developed neurological symptoms in adulthood. It is interesting to note that the pathogenic *PNPT1* variants in both these patients were distal variants located within the S1 domain. Further work and more patients are required to formally establish genotype–phenotype correlations.

Careful phenotypic analysis in rare monogenic diseases is valuable for identifying common clinical features [27,28]. In our cohort, this approach led us to describe the most common phenotypic findings associated with *PNPT1*-related disease that should increase the diagnostic suspicion of this genetic etiology, and could guide screening and management in patients with a molecular diagnosis. On the other hand, no single finding was present in 100% of the patients and, thus, the lack of any of these features does not rule out the diagnosis. Some of the clinical features have only been described in adult patients, such as obsessive–compulsive disorder (P19), depression (P4, P19), and paranoia (P20), or in single cases, such as renal artery stenosis in P9. The causal relationship of some of these findings is unknown and it remains to be seen whether some of these features are coincidental rather than linked to the pathophysiology of *PNPT1* dysfunction.

The diverse clinical heterogeneity of patients with bi-allelic *PNPT1* variants presents a diagnostic and management challenge to the clinician. As more patients are diagnosed, it is important to share detailed clinical information to understand the natural history, elucidate new insights into the mechanisms underlying the pathology, and aid with the identification of potential treatment strategies.

**Supplementary Materials:** The following are available online at http://www.mdpi.com/2077-0383/8/11/2020/s1, Table S1: Clinical phenotype of patients with bi-allelic PNPT1 variants; Table S2: In silico studies and population frequency of PNPT1 variants identified in new families; Figure S1: Brain MRI findings in patients with bi-allelic *PNPT1* variants.

**Author Contributions:** Conceptualization, J.C.; data curation, R.R., M.F.-F., M.K.K., and S.S.; formal analysis, R.R. and L.G.R.; funding acquisition, D.R.T. and J.C.; clinical evaluation and investigation, M.P.K., S.B., D.J.A., G.M.E., M.C.F., M.K.K., M.J.W., and T.Y.T.; methodology, R.R. and N.J.V.B.; software, M.J.C.; supervision, N.J.V.B., A.G.C., D.R.T., and J.C.; writing—Original draft, R.R.; writing—Review and editing, N.J.V.B., A.G.C., L.G.R., M.P.K., S.B., D.J.A., M.F.-F., M.J.C., M.C.F., M.K.K., G.M.E., S.S., M.J.W., T.Y.T., D.R.T., and J.C.

**Funding:** This research was supported by: A New South Wales Office of Health and Medical Research (OHMR) Council Sydney Genomics Collaborative grant (JC); the Australian Genomics Health Alliance (Australian Genomics) project, funded by an NHMRC Targeted Call for Research grant (GNT1113531; JC, DRT); NHMRC research fellowship 1155244 (DRT); OHMR Fellowship (MJC); and a CONACYT Postgraduate Research Scholarship (RR). Sequencing and analysis were provided by the Broad Institute of MIT and Harvard Center for Mendelian Genomics (Broad CMG) and were funded by the National Human Genome Research Institute, the National Eye Institute, the National Heart, Lung and Blood Institute grant UM1 HG008900, and, in part, by a National Human Genome Research Institute grant R01 HG009141.

**Acknowledgments:** We are grateful to the Crane and Perkins families for their generous financial support. The research conducted at the Murdoch Children's Research Institute was supported by the Victorian Government's Operational Infrastructure Support Program.

**Conflicts of Interest:** The authors declare no conflicts of interest.

## References

1. Chen, H.W.; Rainey, R.N.; Balatoni, C.E.; Dawson, D.W.; Troke, J.J.; Wasiak, S.; Hong, J.S.; McBride, H.M.; Koehler, C.M.; Teitell, M.A.; et al. Mammalian polynucleotide phosphorylase is an intermembrane space RNase that maintains mitochondrial homeostasis. *Mol. Cell. Biol.* **2006**, *26*, 8475–8487. [CrossRef]
2. Borowski, L.S.; Dziembowski, A.; Hejnowicz, M.S.; Stepien, P.P.; Szczesny, R.J. Human mitochondrial RNA decay mediated by PNPase-hSuv3 complex takes place in distinct foci. *Nucleic Acids Res.* **2013**, *41*, 1223–1240. [CrossRef] [PubMed]
3. Wang, G.; Chen, H.W.; Oktay, Y.; Zhang, J.; Allen, E.L.; Smith, G.M.; Fan, K.C.; Hong, J.S.; French, S.W.; McCaffery, J.M.; et al. PNPASE regulates RNA import into mitochondria. *Cell* **2010**, *142*, 456–467. [CrossRef] [PubMed]
4. Golzarroshan, B.; Lin, C.L.; Li, C.L.; Yang, W.Z.; Chu, L.Y.; Agrawal, S.; Yuan, H.S. Crystal structure of dimeric human PNPase reveals why disease-linked mutants suffer from low RNA import and degradation activities. *Nucleic Acids Res.* **2018**, *46*, 8630–8640. [CrossRef] [PubMed]
5. Gammage, P.A.; Moraes, C.T.; Minczuk, M. Mitochondrial Genome Engineering: The Revolution May Not Be CRISPR-Ized. *Trends Genet.* **2018**, *34*, 101–110. [CrossRef]
6. Dhir, A.; Dhir, S.; Borowski, L.S.; Jimenez, L.; Teitell, M.; Rotig, A.; Crow, Y.J.; Rice, G.I.; Duffy, D.; Tamby, C.; et al. Mitochondrial double-stranded RNA triggers antiviral signalling in humans. *Nature* **2018**, *560*, 238–242. [CrossRef]
7. Pajak, A.; Laine, I.; Clemente, P.; El-Fissi, N.; Schober, F.A.; Maffezzini, C.; Calvo-Garrido, J.; Wibom, R.; Filograna, R.; Dhir, A.; et al. Defects of mitochondrial RNA turnover lead to the accumulation of double-stranded RNA in vivo. *PLoS Genet.* **2019**, *15*, e1008240. [CrossRef]
8. Von Ameln, S.; Wang, G.; Boulouiz, R.; Rutherford, M.A.; Smith, G.M.; Li, Y.; Pogoda, H.M.; Nürnberg, G.; Stiller, B.; Volk, A.E.; et al. A mutation in PNPT1, encoding mitochondrial-RNA-import protein PNPase, causes hereditary hearing loss. *Am. J. Hum. Genet.* **2012**, *91*, 919–927. [CrossRef]
9. Matilainen, S.; Carroll, C.J.; Richter, U.; Euro, L.; Pohjanpelto, M.; Paetau, A.; Isohanni, P.; Suomalainen, A. Defective mitochondrial RNA processing due to PNPT1 variants causes Leigh syndrome. *Hum. Mol. Genet.* **2017**, *26*, 3352–3361. [CrossRef]
10. Alodaib, A.; Sobreira, N.; Gold, W.A.; Riley, L.G.; Van Bergen, N.J.; Wilson, M.J.; Bennetts, B.; Thorburn, D.R.; Boehm, C.; Christodoulou, J. Whole-exome sequencing identifies novel variants in PNPT1 causing oxidative phosphorylation defects and severe multisystem disease. *Eur. J. Hum. Genet.* **2016**, *25*, 79. [CrossRef]
11. Vedrenne, V.; Gowher, A.; De Lonlay, P.; Nitschke, P.; Serre, V.; Boddaert, N.; Altuzarra, C.; Mager-Heckel, A.M.; Chretien, F.; Entelis, N.; et al. Mutation in PNPT1, which encodes a polyribonucleotide nucleotidyltransferase, impairs RNA import into mitochondria and causes respiratory-chain deficiency. *Am. J. Hum. Genet.* **2012**, *91*, 912–918. [CrossRef] [PubMed]
12. Sato, R.; Arai-Ichinoi, N.; Kikuchi, A.; Matsuhashi, T.; Numata-Uematsu, Y.; Uemura, M.; Fujii, Y.; Murayama, K.; Ohtake, A.; Abe, T.; et al. Novel biallelic mutations in the PNPT1 gene encoding a mitochondrial-RNA-import protein PNPase cause delayed myelination. *Clin. Genet.* **2018**, *93*, 242–247. [CrossRef] [PubMed]
13. Eaton, A.; Bernier, F.P.; Goedhart, C.; Caluseriu, O.; Lamont, R.E.; Boycott, K.M.; Parboosingh, J.S.; Innes, A.M. Care4Rare Canada Consortium. Is PNPT1-related hearing loss ever non-syndromic? Whole exome sequencing of adult siblings expands the natural history of PNPT1-related disorders. *Am. J. Med. Genet. A* **2018**, *176*, 2487–2493. [CrossRef] [PubMed]

14. Riley, L.G.; Cowley, M.J.; Gayevskiy, V.; Roscioli, T.; Thorburn, D.R.; Prelog, K.; Bahlo, M.; Sue, C.M.; Balasubramaniam, S.; Christodoulou, J. A SLC39A8 variant causes manganese deficiency, and glycosylation and mitochondrial disorders. *J. Inherit. Metab. Dis.* **2017**, *40*, 261–269. [CrossRef]
15. Adzhubei, I.A.; Schmidt, S.; Peshkin, L.; Ramensky, V.E.; Gerasimova, A.; Bork, P.; Kondrashov, A.S.; Sunyaev, S.R. A method and server for predicting damaging missense mutations. *Nat. Methods* **2010**, *7*, 248–249. [CrossRef]
16. Choi, Y.; Sims, G.E.; Murphy, S.; Miller, J.R.; Chan, A.P. Predicting the functional effect of amino acid substitutions and indels. *PLoS ONE* **2012**, *7*, e46688. [CrossRef]
17. Kircher, M.; Witten, D.M.; Jain, P.; O'Roak, B.J.; Cooper, G.M.; Shendure, J. A general framework for estimating the relative pathogenicity of human genetic variants. *Nat. Genet.* **2014**, *46*, 310–315. [CrossRef]
18. Schwarz, J.M.; Rodelsperger, C.; Schuelke, M.; Seelow, D. MutationTaster evaluates disease-causing potential of sequence alterations. *Nat. Methods* **2010**, *7*, 575–576. [CrossRef]
19. Desmet, F.O.; Hamroun, D.; Lalande, M.; Collod-Beroud, G.; Claustres, M.; Beroud, C. Human Splicing Finder: An online bioinformatics tool to predict splicing signals. *Nucleic Acids Res.* **2009**, *37*, e67. [CrossRef]
20. Punta, M.; Coggill, P.C.; Eberhardt, R.Y.; Mistry, J.; Tate, J.; Boursnell, C.; Pang, N.; Forslund, K.; Ceric, G.; Clements, J.; et al. The Pfam protein families database. *Nucleic Acids Res.* **2012**, *40*, D290–D301. [CrossRef]
21. Cerami, E.; Gao, J.; Dogrusoz, U.; Gross, B.E.; Sumer, S.O.; Aksoy, B.A.; Jacobsen, A.; Byrne, C.J.; Heuer, M.L.; Larsson, E.; et al. The cBio cancer genomics portal: An open platform for exploring multidimensional cancer genomics data. *Cancer Discov.* **2012**, *2*, 401–404. [CrossRef] [PubMed]
22. Lek, M.; Karczewski, K.J.; Minikel, E.V.; Samocha, K.E.; Banks, E.; Fennell, T.; O'Donnell-Luria, A.H.; Ware, J.S.; Hill, A.J.; Cummings, B.B.; et al. Analysis of protein-coding genetic variation in 60,706 humans. *Nature* **2016**, *536*, 285–291. [CrossRef] [PubMed]
23. Frazier, A.E.; Thorburn, D.R. Biochemical analyses of the electron transport chain complexes by spectrophotometry. *Methods Mol. Biol.* **2012**, *837*, 49–62. [PubMed]
24. Calvo, S.E.; Tucker, E.J.; Compton, A.G.; Kirby, D.M.; Crawford, G.; Burtt, N.P.; Rivas, M.; Guiducci, C.; Bruno, D.L.; Goldberger, O.A.; et al. High-throughput, pooled sequencing identifies mutations in NUBPL and FOXRED1 in human complex I deficiency. *Nat. Genet.* **2010**, *42*, 851–858. [CrossRef]
25. Schmittgen, T.D.; Livak, K.J. Analyzing real-time PCR data by the comparative CT method. *Nat. Protoc.* **2008**, *3*, 1101–1108. [CrossRef]
26. Rice, G.I.; Forte, G.M.A.; Szynkiewicz, M.; Chase, D.S.; Aeby, A.; Abdel-Hamid, M.S.; Ackroyd, S.; Allcock, R.; Bailey, K.M.; Balottin, U.; et al. Assessment of interferon-related biomarkers in Aicardi-Goutières syndrome associated with mutations in TREX1, RNASEH2A, RNASEH2B, RNASEH2C, SAMHD1, and ADAR: A case-control study. *Lancet Neurol.* **2013**, *12*, 1159–1169. [CrossRef]
27. Fuchs, S.A.; Schene, I.F.; Kok, G.; Jansen, J.M.; Nikkels, P.G.J.; van Gassen, K.L.I.; Terheggen-Lagro, S.W.J.; van der Crabben, S.N.; Hoeks, S.E.; Niers, L.E.M.; et al. Aminoacyl-tRNA synthetase deficiencies in search of common themes. *Genet. Med.* **2019**, *21*, 319–330. [CrossRef]
28. Robinson, P.N. Deep phenotyping for precision medicine. *Hum. Mutat.* **2012**, *33*, 777–780. [CrossRef]

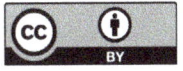 © 2019 by the authors. Licensee MDPI, Basel, Switzerland. This article is an open access article distributed under the terms and conditions of the Creative Commons Attribution (CC BY) license (http://creativecommons.org/licenses/by/4.0/).

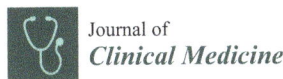 

*Review*

# Mitochondrial Dysfunction in Aging and Cancer

**Loredana Moro**

Institute of Biomembranes, Bioenergetics and Molecular Biotechnologies, National Research Council, 70126 Bari, Italy; l.moro@ibiom.cnr.it; Tel.: +39-080-544-9807

Received: 10 October 2019; Accepted: 13 November 2019; Published: 15 November 2019

**Abstract:** Aging is a major risk factor for developing cancer, suggesting that these two events may represent two sides of the same coin. It is becoming clear that some mechanisms involved in the aging process are shared with tumorigenesis, through convergent or divergent pathways. Increasing evidence supports a role for mitochondrial dysfunction in promoting aging and in supporting tumorigenesis and cancer progression to a metastatic phenotype. Here, a summary of the current knowledge of three aspects of mitochondrial biology that link mitochondria to aging and cancer is presented. In particular, the focus is on mutations and changes in content of the mitochondrial genome, activation of mitochondria-to-nucleus signaling and the newly discovered mitochondria-telomere communication.

**Keywords:** mitochondrial DNA; mitochondria-to-nucleus signaling; aging; cancer

## 1. Introduction

Mitochondria are cellular organelles that play a pivotal role in maintaining cellular homeostasis by regulating energy metabolism, cell survival and proliferation. Production of adenosine triphosphate (ATP) and the generation of intermediate metabolites are the traditional functions ascribed to mitochondria. Within the mitochondria, the tricarboxylic acid cycle (TCA cycle) generates mitochondrial metabolites and reducing equivalents, in the form of reduced nicotinamide adenine dinucleotide (NADH) and flavin adenine dinucleotide (FADH2), which enter into the mitochondrial electron respiratory chain (ETC). ETC includes four membrane-bound protein complexes and catalyzes the oxidation of reducing equivalents using oxygen as the terminal electron acceptor. The electron transfer is coupled to the transfer of protons across the inner mitochondrial membrane to generate an electrochemical gradient (mitochondrial membrane potential) required both for ATP synthesis through the ATP synthase complex, and for efficient shuttling of proteins across the inner mitochondrial membrane. Electron leakage can arise along the ETC, leading to the formation of reactive oxygen species (ROS), important second messengers in aging, cancer and other physiopathological conditions. The intermediate metabolites generated in the TCA cycle are the precursors of lipids, carbohydrates, proteins and other macromolecules [1]. Mitochondria are able to migrate within the cell, fuse and divide through rapid fusion and fission processes and undergo turnover through mitophagy, a specialized form of autophagy. Mitochondrial dynamics is regulated by the large dynamin family of GTPases, enables mitochondrial recruitment to subcellular compartments that require more energy and is important for mitochondrial quality control and for communication with the cytosol and the nucleus (reviewed in [2]). Mitochondrial fusion begins with the joining of the mitochondrial outer membrane mediated by the mitofusin proteins Mfn1 and Mfn2, followed by fusion of the mitochondrial inner membrane catalyzed by OPA1. Fusion occurs similarly for the inner and outer membrane and involves a formation of interlocking coiled coils mediated by fusion proteins on the two membranes, followed by their fusion catalyzed by GTP hydrolysis [3].

The inner membrane fusion is dependent upon the mitochondrial membrane potential [4]. The mitochondrial fission is instead mediated by the GTPase DRP1, a protein that is recruited to the outer membrane where it oligomerizes and forms a spiral around the outer and inner membrane that causes fragmentation of the mitochondrion [5,6]. Disruption of the normal fusion/fission balance results in mitochondrial dysfunction [6].

Recent evidences point to the mitochondrial content and functionality in the regulation of nuclear gene expression by affecting transcription and translation, as well as alternative splicing mechanisms [7]. Hence, mitochondrial dysfunction leading to changes in nuclear gene expression may affect the risk of degenerative diseases, cancer and aging [7–10].

Aging is the most important risk factor for cancer. According to the National Cancer Institute (NCI), the median age of a cancer diagnosis is 66 years (https://www.cancer.gov/about-cancer/causes-prevention/risk/age). At first glance, aging and cancer may seem to be two opposite processes, the first implying a slow decline of cellular and organismal functions, the second providing fitness to the cells. In reality, these two processes are strictly interconnected and share common origins. Aging is associated with the progressive accumulation of genetic and cellular damage [11,12]. However, DNA damage may confer survival and growth advantages to certain cells, which can eventually thrive and evolve into a tumorigenic phenotype. Genetic damage affecting the functionality of mitochondria has been associated with both aging and cancer.

Mitochondria have been the focus of the aging research for decades, when Harman proposed the free radical theory of aging [13,14], then revisited by Alexeyev as the mitochondrial theory of aging [15]. Both theories hypothesize that ROS are the main determinants of the loss of cellular performance observed with increasing age, with the mitochondrial theory implying mitochondria as the main producers of ROS, and consequently, mitochondria as key drivers of aging. In the last decade, knowledge of these organelles has expanded, providing more connections between mitochondrial biology and the aging process [16]. Similarly to aging, changes in mitochondrial functionality have been strictly linked to cancer [17]. Indeed, several studies have shown that mutations in mitochondrial proteins encoded by either the mitochondrial or the nuclear genome may favor cancer development and progression [8,9,18,19]. This review provides an overview of the convergent and divergent roles that mitochondrial dysfunction may play in cellular processes linked to aging and cancer, with a specific focus on mitochondrial DNA, mitochondria-to-nucleus signaling and telomere shortening.

## 2. The Mitochondrial Genome

Mitochondria are equipped with their own genome, the mitochondrial genome (mtDNA), a circular, double-stranded DNA molecule of ~16.5 kb in humans, present in one to several thousand copies per cell, depending on the tissue and cell type. The two mtDNA strands have different resolution on a cesium chloride gradient and can be separated in a heavy strand (H-strand) rich in G and a light strand (L-strand) rich in C [20]. In addition, the mtDNA has a unique regulatory region, the displacement loop (D-loop), a triple-stranded region that includes a short single-strand DNA molecule, the 7S DNA [21]. The mitochondrial genome encodes for 13 proteins belonging to the respiratory complexes I, III, IV and V, and for two rRNAs and 22 tRNAs required for mitochondrial protein synthesis. Most of the mtDNA information is encoded by the H-strand (12 proteins, 2 rRNAs, 14 tRNAs). The mtDNA is maternally inherited and depends upon nuclear-encoded proteins for its replication and transcription. Replication of mtDNA is performed by DNA polymerase γ (POLγ), twinkle helicase and mitochondrial single-stranded binding protein (mtSSB), and proceeds throughout the entire life of an organism in both dividing and terminally differentiating cells. The exact molecular mechanism involved in the regulation of mtDNA replication in response to extracellular stimuli/stress remains a poorly investigated area [22]. The mitochondrial proteome is dynamic; i.e., the protein composition and the levels of a given protein may vary depending on the tissue and cell type. Even within the same cell type the mitochondrial proteome may vary over time depending on specific external stimuli or stress conditions [23].

Though the majority of the mammalian mitochondrial proteome (about 1200 proteins) is encoded by the nuclear genome and then imported into mitochondria, the 13 proteins encoded by the mtDNA (1% of the mitochondrial proteome) play an essential role for the mitochondrial function. Mutations or depletion of the mtDNA can indeed impair the energy metabolism and alter the intracellular signaling, resulting in mitochondrial dysfunction that may affect the cell performance at various degrees, leading to "mitochondrial diseases" in extreme cases [8,9,24,25]. MtDNA accumulates mutations at a considerably higher rate than nuclear DNA [26]. Traditionally, the increased mutational load was ascribed to a lack of efficient repair systems, lack of protective histones and to the close proximity of mtDNA to the respiratory chain complexes, the main site of production of ROS. Though mtDNA lacks traditional histones, the mitochondrial transcriptional factor A (TFAM) is tightly associated to the mtDNA molecules and plays an histone-like protective role [27]. However, mitochondria lack nucleotide excision repair (NER), efficient homologous recombination, microhomology-mediated end joining (MMEJ) and non-homologous end joining (NHEJ). The short and long patch base excision repair (BER) and single strand break repair pathways are instead preserved [28]. Hundreds of mtDNA mutations have been reported leading to a variety of human disorders (www.mitomap.org). In most cases, wild-type and mutated mtDNA coexist within the same cell, a condition known as heteroplasmy, as opposed to the term homoplasmy, when all the copies of the mtDNA are identical. The severity of the mtDNA-associated disorders is dependent on the level of heteroplasmy. For example, the mitochondrial dysfunction observed in the MELAS (mitochondrial myopathy, encephalopathy, lactic acidosis and stroke-like episodes) syndrome, usually caused by a mutation within the mtDNA-encoded tRNA Leu (UUR), can be rescued by levels of wild-type mtDNA above 6% [29]. In general, a pathogenic mtDNA mutation would need to reach a threshold level of more than 60% in a given tissue or cell type to produce a measurable bioenergetic defect [30].

## 2.1. MtDNA and Aging

MtDNA point mutations and deletions are known to accumulate with age in human tissues, including brain, heart and skeletal muscles [31–34]. A debate is still ongoing to define whether accumulation of mtDNA mutations is causal or just a correlation with aging. So far, the strongest evidence favoring the hypothesis of a causal role of mtDNA changes in aging comes from the generation of homozygous knock-in mice for the catalytic subunit of POLγ that lacks proofreading activity. These mice exhibit a mtDNA mutator phenotype, with accumulation of extremely high levels of mtDNA mutations, a shortened lifespan and early onset of age-associated phenotypes, including hair graying, weight loss, reduced subcutaneous fat, osteoporosis, alopecia and kyphosis [35,36]. Of note, while an increased load of mtDNA point mutations has not been linked to the aging phenotype [37], the presence of large mtDNA deletions has been reported as a driver of premature aging in mitochondrial mutator mice [38]. These mice apparently did not exhibit a net increase in ROS levels [35], and in general, in oxidative stress markers [36]. However, Kolesar et al. [39] have recently shown that the mitochondrial protein content in the muscle tissues of Polγ-knock-out mice is significantly reduced compared with wild-type mice, which results in a net increase in ROS levels per mitochondrial proteins, and a burst in mtDNA and mitochondrial protein oxidative stress. Increased oxidative stress in the muscle of Polγ-knock-out mice has been confirmed by a subsequent study [40]. These findings support previous experimental evidences showing an anti-aging role of mitochondria-targeted catalase, an anti-oxidant enzyme [41–43]. Further experiments in mice have shown that maternally inherited mtDNA mutations may cause premature aging signs, such as alopecia, kyphosis and premature death [44,45]. In humans, HIV patients treated with nucleoside analog reverse transcriptase inhibitor antiretroviral drugs have shown signs of premature aging, including increased cardiovascular disease and bone fractures [46]. Subsequent studies have shown that these antiretroviral drugs have mitochondria as off-target sites, and in particular, they inhibit POLγ, causing mtDNA mutations and depletion that result in mitochondrial dysfunction [47]. Another example linking mtDNA to the aging phenotype comes from human subjects carrying mutations in POLγ. More than 300 pathogenic mutations in human POLγ have been identified so far (https://tools.niehs.nih.gov/polg/), and they have been linked to several disorders, including age-related pathologies such as Parkinson's disease [10,48,49].

Loss of mitochondrial fusion in the skeletal muscle of *Mfn1*- and *Mfn2*-knockout mice has been linked to increased mtDNA mutations and deletions, as well as mtDNA depletion. These molecular events precede the phenotypic changes observed in these mice, such as impaired mitochondrial functionality, abnormal mitochondria proliferation and muscle loss [50]. Overall, increased mitochondrial fusion may support longevity, as highlighted by a recent study in *C. elegans* [51]. In addition, a decline in mtDNA content has been observed in peripheral mononuclear blood cells (PMBC) during aging, and it has been linked to reduced immune response in the elderly [52,53]. Recently, a novel and very precise technique has allowed researchers to ascertain that healthy centenarians retain more mtDNA copies and less mtDNA deletions during immune cell stimulation than old people and frail centenarians [54], implying that the retention of a high amount of mtDNA is a hallmark of healthy aging.

## 2.2. MtDNA and Cancer

MtDNA mutations and changes in mtDNA content have been associated with cancer progression in a variety of cancer types (reviewed in [8,9]). A large-scale analysis performed on several cancer types of the TCGA dataset has recently confirmed that many, but not all cancers, display a significant depletion of the mtDNA content, which is directly associated with reduction in the expression of genes of the mitochondrial respiratory chain, and inversely correlated with the expression of genes of the immune response and cell cycle [55]. Some somatic mtDNA mutations were reported to favor tumorigenesis [56] and others to promote cancer metastasis [57] through an increase in ROS production [56,57]. However, a definitive link between mtDNA depletion/somatic mutations and tumorigenesis or cancer progression is still missing. Experiments in cell culture have shown that induced mtDNA depletion may restrain tumorigenesis [58,59] but support cancer cell invasion and metastasis [9,60–64]. Partial mtDNA depletion results in decreased mitochondrial membrane potential, increased DRP1 mitochondrial localization and decreased OPA1 levels, accompanied by increased mitochondrial fission, as demonstrated by enrichment in fragmented mitochondria [65]. In turn, increased mitochondrial fission alters the cytoskeleton and promotes the formation of pseudopodia-like structures, typical of invasive cells [65]. Consistently, increased mitochondrial fission has been frequently detected in carcinoma samples (reviewed in [66]). Analysis of the TCGA dataset reported a direct correlation between mtDNA depletion and reduced patients' survival [55]. An independent study performed on 8161 normal and cancer samples in the TCGA dataset showed that decreased oxidative phosphorylation is associated with poor survival across multiple cancer types and with an epithelia-to-mesenchymal (EMT) gene expression profile [67], typical of cells with acquired invasive abilities [9]. Furthermore, analysis of the Skin Cutaneous Melanoma dataset containing 367 metastatic lesions and 103 primary cancer samples demonstrated that: (i) Reduced oxidative phosphorylation was the most significant metabolic signature in the metastatic lesions compared with the primary cancers; and (ii) EMT was strongly upregulated in the metastatic cancer samples [67], supporting a role of mitochondrial dysfunction in the metastatic process. A previous study performed on 49 patients with advanced metastatic melanoma has shown that stage IV melanomas may be dependent either on glycolysis or a combination of glycolysis and oxidative phosphorylation, which may suggest a metabolic symbiosis within the same tumor [68]. In agreement with this study, Najjar et al. [69] reported that metabolic adaptation can vary in melanoma samples, with some cells exhibiting only deregulated glycolysis and others only deregulated oxidative phosphorylation. Patient-derived melanoma cell lines with a prevalent oxidative metabolism showed resistance to immunotherapy as well [69]. Recent evidences have pointed out to the horizontal transfer of whole mitochondria from host cells present in the tumor microenvironment to respiratory-deficient tumor cells, depleted of mtDNA [70]. This transfer would recover mitochondrial respiratory activity and promote tumor growth [70]. Based on these observations, it is tempting to speculate that mtDNA depletion/deletions and pathogenic mtDNA mutations may confer a selective advantage to certain cancer cells for invading and thriving in hostile microenvironments, such as the circulating system, while abating cell proliferation. Partial reconstitution of the wild-type mtDNA pool by horizontal transfer from stromal cells would allow cancer cells to recover their proliferative capacity, and thus, their full tumorigenic potential.

## 3. Retrograde Signaling in Aging and Cancer

Besides being considered as the cell's "energy hubs", mitochondria have emerged as critical "signaling hubs" in regulating cell homeostasis [71]. Communication from mitochondria to the nucleus is known as "retrograde signaling", opposed to the traditional anterograde signaling, i.e., the communication pathways from the nucleus to the mitochondria. It has been first described by Butow in yeast. That is, in yeast cells depleted of mtDNA, Butow described changes in the transcription of nuclear-encoded genes, and an increase in the transcription of genes associated with a metabolic shift from aerobic to anaerobic respiration (reviewed in [72]). Screenings performed in C. elegans have revealed that impairing the mitochondrial respiratory chain unexpectedly extends the lifespan [73]. This observation seems a paradox given that aging tissues are characterized by loss of mitochondrial fitness. Similarly, in C. elegans a transient increase of mitochondrial ROS triggers changes in gene expression that promote longevity instead of aging, sharply in contrast with the mitochondrial theory of aging [74]. These findings have been corroborated in mammals using mouse models. For example, mice heterozygous for Mclk1, a mitochondrial protein necessary for the biosynthesis of ubiquinone, show increased lifespan correlated with early impairment of the mitochondrial functionality, significant reduction of mitochondrial electron transport, ATP and NAD+ levels [75]. The reason why mitochondrial stress may counteract the aging process is still not completely understood. Some experimental evidences suggest that the retrograde signaling activated by the mitochondrial stress may play a critical role. In the context of aging, activation of the mitochondrial unfolded protein response (UPRmt) seems to be important in signaling a mitochondrial stress to the nucleus. This retrograde response is elicited by mtDNA depletion or by protein misfolding occurring in these mitochondria [76]. It was described for the first time in mammalian cells depleted of mtDNA through ethidium bromide treatment, which exhibited induction of mRNAs for mitochondrial proteases and chaperons [77]. A similar transcriptional profile was observed upon overexpression in the mitochondrial matrix of a dominant negative ornithine transcarbamylase, an enzyme essential for protein processing and folding, suggesting a link between mitochondrial dysfunction, alteration of proteostasis mechanisms and the activation of UPRmt [78]. Work in C. elegans and other organisms has identified several components of this retrograde response (for a comprehensive review, see [79]). In C. elegans, mitochondrial dysfunction reduces the mitochondrial import efficiency of the transcription factor ATFS-1, allowing it to accumulate in the nucleus where it induces the transcription of hundreds of genes, including antioxidant proteins, proteases and enzymes involved in cellular metabolism that would promote survival and recovery of the mitochondrial functionality, thus supporting longevity and lifespan [78]. However, prolonged UPRmt activation occurring in the context of a heteroplasmic mtDNA pool seems to exacerbate mitochondrial dysfunction because it would result in an accumulation of damaged mtDNA (for a detailed review see [76]).

Evidence is accumulating on the important role that mitochondrial metabolites may play as second messengers eliciting epigenetic changes in the nucleus (for comprehensive reviews see [80,81]). In this context, acetyl-CoA is one of the most studied signaling molecules. This metabolite is present in mitochondria, cytosol and the nucleus. In mitochondria, it can be produced through different metabolic pathways, including conversion of pyruvate to acetyl-CoA by the pyruvate dehydrogenase complex (PDH), fatty acid β-oxidation, amino acid metabolism, direct synthesis by a reaction of ligation of acetate with CoA catalyzed by mitochondrial acyl-CoA synthetase short-chain family member 1 (ACSS1). Mitochondrial acetyl-CoA enters into the TCA cycle together with oxaloacetate to produce citrate, which is oxidized, allowing production of ATP through the oxidative phosphorylation.

Once inside mitochondria, acetyl-CoA is unable to cross the inner mitochondrial membrane. To replenish its cytosolic and nuclear pool, citrate exported from mitochondria via the tricarboxylate carrier is converted to acetyl-CoA and oxaloacetate by the ATP-citrate lyase (ACLY) [82]. Cytosolic acetyl-CoA can participate to biosynthetic pathways, such as to fatty acids synthesis, and provides acetyls for lysine acetylation of proteins, thereby regulating their activity and localization [83]. In the nucleus, protein lysine acetylation modulates histone acetylation. It has been recently reported that the PDH complex can translocate from mitochondria to the nucleus during active cell proliferation, generating a nuclear pool of acetyl-CoA for fine-tuning histone acetylation [84]. Acetyl-CoA may thus function as a "sentinel metabolite", where under stress conditions, acetyl-CoA would be diverted to mitochondria to provide energy and mitochondria-generated products, such as ketone bodies. Instead, elevated nucleo-cytosolic levels of acetyl-CoA would signal permissive conditions for growth, biosynthesis of lipids and histone acetylation. Indeed, a recent work has reported that high cytosolic/nuclear levels of acetyl-CoA due to overexpression of ACLY promote pancreatic cancer development [85]. In aging cells, elevated nucleo-cytosolic acetyl-CoA levels function as the metabolic repressor of autophagy [86]. Consistently, brain-specific knock-down of acetyl-CoA synthetase increases lifespan in *Drosophila* [86], suggesting that mitochondrial metabolites may play opposite roles in aging and cancer.

Chronic inflammation has been linked to aging and age-related pathologies, as well as to cancer (for detailed reviews see [87,88]). The inflammation process represents an essential immunological defense system that promotes survival. It has been extensively reported that mitochondrial dysfunction can promote the release of factors, known as damage-associated molecular patterns (DAMPs), into the cytosol, which can trigger an inflammatory response by engaging pattern recognition receptors. Mitochondrial DAMPs (mtDAMPs) include several molecules/effectors, such as mtDNA and mitochondria-produced ROS, which can activate the inflammasomes, multi-protein cytosolic complexes consisting of the adaptor apoptosis-associated speck-like protein (ASC), the inflammatory cysteine protease caspase-1, NOD-, LRR- and pyrin domain-containing protein 1 (NLRP1), NLRP3, NOD-, LRR- and CARD-containing protein 4 (NLRC4), and absent in melanoma 2 (AIM2). Among different inflammasomes, mitochondrial stress has been implicated in the regulation of NLRP3 activity, with mtDNA released into the cytosol as a triggering DAMP of NLRP3 inflammasome. In macrophages, cytosolic accumulation of mtDNA upon stress activates caspase-1 and promotes the secretion of IL-1β and IL-18 through activation of the NLRP3 inflammasome [89]. This retrograde response requires mitochondria-generated ROS that would cause a release of mtDNA into the cytosol [89]. Degraded mtDNA has been shown to induce the release of pro-inflammatory cytokines in brain cells and represents a possible trigger of neurodegenerative processes [90]. Recent reports further support the role of mitochondrial ROS and mtDNA in the activation of NLRP3 in age-dependent diseases, including atherosclerosis [91–96], as well as in cancer, though the activation of inflammasomes during tumor development and progression still remains controversial and with conflicting outcomes (for a detailed review see [97]). Recent evidences point to a role of DAMPs released by dying cancer cells upon chemotherapy and inflammasome's activation in bursting an immune response that could help the removal of the remaining live cancer cells. In this context, it has been proposed that a particular class of mitocans (mitochondrial-targeted anti-cancer drugs), like vitamin E analogs, that selectively induce cell death by triggering ROS production in cancer cell mitochondria, may be promising candidates for anti-cancer therapy (reviewed in [98]).

Work from Avadhani's group has shown that mammalian cells can activate another mitochondria-to-nucleus signaling pathway upon mitochondrial respiratory stress [72,99]. This signaling pathway considers $Ca^{2+}$ as the main second messenger involved in the transmission of stress signals from mitochondria to nucleus and has been related to the response to a mitochondrial stress in the context of cancer cells. Mitochondria store large amounts of $Ca^{2+}$. Upon mitochondrial stress/dysfunction leading to reduced mitochondrial membrane potential, $Ca^{2+}$ is released into the cytosol where it can activate $Ca^{2+}$-dependent signaling. An early event of this signaling is activation of the phosphatase Calcineurin. This $Ca^{2+}$/calcineurin-mediated pathway can be ROS-dependent or -independent, in relation to the cell type. For example, it is ROS-independent in skeletal myocytes, but ROS-dependent in macrophages [60,100,101]. In turn, the $Ca^{2+}$/calcineurin signaling would activate the insulin-like growth factor receptor I (IGF1R) in a growth factor-independent manner that, by promoting the PI3-kinase/AKT pathway, would culminate in the induction of the transcription of nuclear genes (reviewed in [65,99]). Ca$^{2+}$ may also activate other pathways independently on calcineurin. From a "phenotypic" point of view, Ca$^{2+}$-mediated signaling upon mitochondrial stress results in survival, resistance to pro-apoptotic drugs, increased glycolysis and invasion of otherwise not invasive cells [8,9,61,63,99,102,103]. Taken together, these experimental evidences are consistent with a role of mild mitochondrial dysfunction in supporting health and fitness of the cells, both in aging and in cancer, through the activation of a protective retrograde signaling.

## 4. Telomeres in Aging and Cancer

Telomeres are DNA-protein structures present at both ends of each chromosome that protect the genome from interchromosomal fusion and rapid nucleolytic degradation. These specialized structures function as biological clocks: most normal cells have a limited lifespan and at each cell division, telomeres lose a portion of DNA. After a certain number of cell divisions, telomeres reach a critical minimal length and cells undergo apoptosis [104]. Telomere length decreases with the aging process and the rate of telomere shortening may indicate the pace of aging [104]. Stem cells and cancer cells express high levels of telomerase, an enzyme known as hTERT in humans (human TElomerase Reverse Transcriptase), which is able to prevent telomeres' shortening by elongating the telomeres' DNA. Most somatic cells instead do not express telomerase. In addition to its established role in regulating telomere length in the nucleus, TERT exerts a protective role within mitochondria by shuttling from the nucleus to the mitochondria upon exogenous stress [105–109]. Within mitochondria, TERT binds mtDNA and protects it from damage, thus preserving the mitochondrial function and promoting resistance to apoptosis in cancer cells [108–110]. Consistently, expression of a mutant telomerase lacking a nuclear export signal inhibits cancer cell proliferation, prevents immortalization, promotes mitochondrial dysfunction and sensitivity to ionizing radiation and hydrogen peroxide exposure, two genotoxic stresses [111–113].

Inherited mutations in genes encoding for protein components of the telomeres cause accelerated aging symptoms (cardiovascular disease, hair graying, diabetes, poor immune response) [114]. Interestingly, in a yeast model system, lack of telomerase accelerated aging independently on de-protected telomeres [115]. Overexpression of telomerase can delay aging but would increase the risk of tumor formation [116]. Consistently, 80%–90% of malignant tumors show overexpression of hTERT, which may occur via multiple mechanisms, including epigenetic modifications (h*TERT* gene promoter methylation), h*TERT* amplification or structural variants (reviewed in [117]). Overall, up-regulation of hTERT confers unlimited replicative potential to cancer cells, and is one of the distinctive hallmarks of cancer [118].

Despite overexpression of hTERT in cancer cells, increasing evidence demonstrates that telomere shortening correlates with cancer aggressiveness (reviewed in [119]), suggesting a threshold of telomere shortening in cancer. In this context, hTERT may guarantee an optimal telomere length that would prevent replicative senescence. In addition, expression of hTERT splice variants in cancer cells has been shown to confer a growth advantage and resistance to chemotherapeutic drugs independently upon telomere protection [120], supporting the notion that hTERT plays multiple roles in different pathophysiological conditions.

A recent work has shown a direct connection between mitochondrial dysfunction and telomere attrition [121]. Qian et al. have used a chemoptogenetic approach to produce short-lived singlet oxygen (a highly reactive ROS) in the mitochondrial matrix, whose destiny in the whole cells may be easily monitored. One pulse of singlet oxygen produced secondary ROS (superoxide radical anion and hydrogen peroxide) that promoted mtDNA damage, decrease in mitochondrial respiration and cell cycle arrest. Intriguingly, these secondary ROS were detected in the nucleus where they induced telomere fragility and loss, without causing general nuclear DNA strand breaks. DNA double-strand breaks were exclusively present in telomeres. In turn, telomere dysfunction promoted Ataxia-Telangiectasia Mutated (ATM)-dependent repair of DNA damage, preventing cells from undergoing apoptosis [121].

These findings highlight a novel mitochondria-telomere axis activated by mitochondrial ROS and associated with mitochondrial dysfunction that may be important both in aging and in cancer. Future studies are needed to assess whether this new retrograde signaling pathway may also activate hTERT, thus supporting cell survival in the long term, and tumorigenesis. Alternatively, since in progeroid syndrome this telomere dysfunction has been shown to impair the mitochondrial function [122], it is possible that an initial, transient mitochondrial dysfunction may cause progressive loss of cell fitness and apoptosis via induction of telomere shortening in a vicious cycle.

## 5. Conclusions

Mitochondrial function is critical for cell homeostasis, and alteration of mitochondrial performance is linked both to aging and cancer (Figure 1), two opposite processes, being aging associated with "loss of function" and cancer with "gain of fitness".

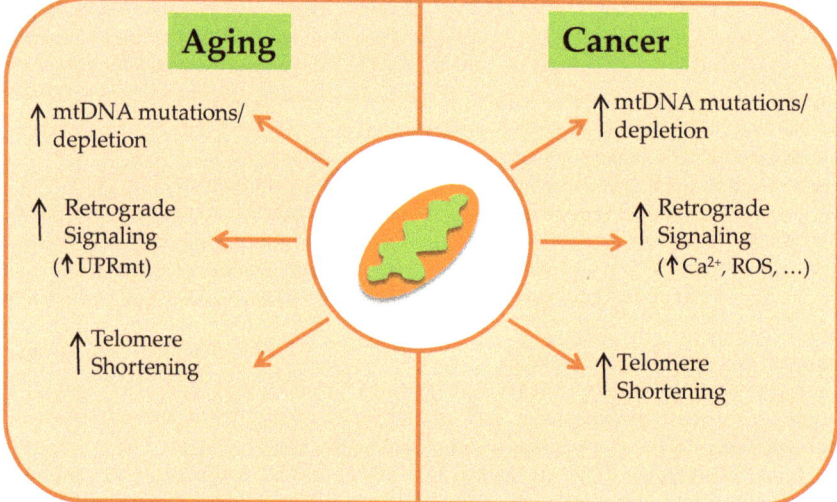

**Figure 1.** Mitochondrial dysfunction in aging and cancer. Aging and cancer share common mechanisms that include an alteration of the mitochondrial genome (mtDNA), activation of mitochondria-to-nucleus signaling pathways (retrograde signaling; see text for details) and telomere shortening. The latter is the biological clock of the cells, and beyond a limit, would cause cell cycle arrest and apoptosis, preventing the unlimited replication of normal cells. In cancer cells, expression of the telomerase hTERT would prevent excessive shortening of telomeres. Recent evidence points to mitochondrial dysfunction as a regulator of telomere shortening.

MtDNA mutations and/or decreased mtDNA content have been described in aging tissues and cancer cells. In aging, they have been associated with reduced respiration and available energy, thus decreasing the rate of anabolic reactions for biosynthesis of the cell's bricks (lipids, proteins, carbohydrates) and leading to physiological decline. Genetic studies in mouse models have provided evidence for a causal link between mtDNA depletion and the aging symptoms [35,44,45]. In cancer, some mtDNA point mutations seem to favor tumorigenesis, and other mutations would promote cancer metastasis, while mtDNA depletion correlates with poor patients' survival in certain cancers. Though there are several evidences in support of the causal role of mtDNA changes in cancer, a definitive link between mtDNA depletion/somatic mutations and tumorigenesis/cancer progression is still missing.

Intriguingly, mouse models with a mtDNA mutator phenotype that display progeroid syndrome do not exhibit increased production of mitochondrial ROS [35], in contradiction with the core hypothesis of the mitochondrial theory of aging. In cancer, increase in ROS elicited by certain mtDNA mutations favors tumorigenesis and metastasis [56,57]. Recent studies have highlighted the role of alternative retrograde signaling transmitted by dysfunctional mitochondria to the nucleus that may modulate aging and cancer.

These signals include the UPRmt, relevant to the aging process, and $Ca^{2+}$-mediated signaling pathways, involved in the acquisition of some hallmarks of cancer cells. Mitochondrial dysfunction can also trigger telomere fragility and shortening, a common trait of aging and cancer. However, at variance with the aging process, cancer cells would not undergo cell cycle arrest because of the genetic/epigenetic upregulation of telomerase. These pathways are not mutually exclusive; rather they may intersect and contribute to the phenotype. Future studies, aimed at understanding the relative contribution of different mitochondrial retrograde signaling to aging and cancer, may open the road to the development of biologically active molecules targeting specific retrograde signaling pathways, in order to delay progression of age-related symptoms and/or to inhibit tumor growth and metastasis.

**Conflicts of Interest:** The author declares no conflict of interest.

## References

1. Lenaz, G.; Genova, M.L. Structure and organization of mitochondrial respiratory complexes: A new understanding of an old subject. *Antioxid. Redox Signal.* **2010**, *12*, 961–1008. [CrossRef]
2. Chen, H.; Chan, D.C. Mitochondrial dynamics—Fusion, fission, movement, and mitophagy—In neurodegenerative diseases. *Hum. Mol. Genet.* **2009**, *18*, R169–R176. [CrossRef] [PubMed]
3. Hoppins, S.; Lackner, L.; Nunnari, J. The machines that divide and fuse mitochondria. *Annu. Rev. Biochem.* **2007**, *76*, 751–780. [CrossRef] [PubMed]
4. Twig, G.; Graf, S.A.; Wikstrom, J.D.; Mohamed, H.; Haigh, S.E.; Elorza, A.; Deutsch, M.; Zurgil, N.; Reynolds, N.; Shirihai, O.S. Tagging and tracking individual networks within a complex mitochondrial web with photoactivatable GFP. *Am. J. Physiol. Cell Physiol.* **2006**, *291*, C176–C184. [CrossRef] [PubMed]
5. Smirnova, E.; Griparic, L.; Shurland, D.L.; van der Bliek, A.M. Dynamin-related protein Drp1 is required for mitochondrial division in mammalian cells. *Mol. Biol. Cell* **2001**, *12*, 2245–2256. [CrossRef]
6. Youle, R.J.; van der Bliek, A.M. Mitochondrial fission, fusion, and stress. *Science* **2012**, *337*, 1062–1065. [CrossRef]
7. Guantes, R.; Rastrojo, A.; Neves, R.; Lima, A.; Aguado, B.; Iborra, F.J. Global variability in gene expression and alternative splicing is modulated by mitochondrial content. *Genome Res.* **2015**, *25*, 633–644. [CrossRef]
8. Guaragnella, N.; Giannattasio, S.; Moro, L. Mitochondrial dysfunction in cancer chemoresistance. *Biochem. Pharmacol.* **2014**, *92*, 62–72. [CrossRef]
9. Guerra, F.; Guaragnella, N.; Arbini, A.A.; Bucci, C.; Giannattasio, S.; Moro, L. Mitochondrial Dysfunction: A Novel Potential Driver of Epithelial-to-Mesenchymal Transition in Cancer. *Front. Oncol.* **2017**, *7*, 295. [CrossRef]
10. DeBalsi, K.L.; Hoff, K.E.; Copeland, W.C. Role of the mitochondrial DNA replication machinery in mitochondrial DNA mutagenesis, aging and age-related diseases. *Ageing Res. Rev.* **2017**, *33*, 89–104. [CrossRef]
11. Soares, J.P.; Cortinhas, A.; Bento, T.; Leitao, J.C.; Collins, A.R.; Gaivao, I.; Mota, M.P. Aging and DNA damage in humans: A meta-analysis study. *Aging* **2014**, *6*, 432–439. [CrossRef] [PubMed]
12. Lopez-Otin, C.; Blasco, M.A.; Partridge, L.; Serrano, M.; Kroemer, G. The hallmarks of aging. *Cell* **2013**, *153*, 1194–1217. [CrossRef] [PubMed]
13. Harman, D. Aging: A theory based on free radical and radiation chemistry. *J. Gerontol.* **1956**, *11*, 298–300. [CrossRef] [PubMed]
14. Harman, D. Free radical theory of aging: Dietary implications. *Am. J. Clin. Nutr.* **1972**, *25*, 839–843. [CrossRef] [PubMed]
15. Alexeyev, M.F. Is there more to aging than mitochondrial DNA and reactive oxygen species? *FEBS J.* **2009**, *276*, 5768–5787. [CrossRef] [PubMed]
16. Kauppila, T.E.S.; Kauppila, J.H.K.; Larsson, N.G. Mammalian Mitochondria and Aging: An Update. *Cell Metab.* **2017**, *25*, 57–71. [CrossRef]

17. Wallace, D.C. Mitochondria and cancer. *Nat. Rev. Cancer* **2012**, *12*, 685–698. [CrossRef]
18. Gaude, E.; Frezza, C. Defects in mitochondrial metabolism and cancer. *Cancer Metab.* **2014**, *2*, 10. [CrossRef]
19. Vyas, S.; Zaganjor, E.; Haigis, M.C. Mitochondria and Cancer. *Cell* **2016**, *166*, 555–566. [CrossRef]
20. Anderson, S.; Bankier, A.T.; Barrell, B.G.; de Bruijn, M.H.; Coulson, A.R.; Drouin, J.; Eperon, I.C.; Nierlich, D.P.; Roe, B.A.; Sanger, F.; et al. Sequence and organization of the human mitochondrial genome. *Nature* **1981**, *290*, 457–465. [CrossRef]
21. Nicholls, T.J.; Minczuk, M. In D-loop: 40 years of mitochondrial 7S DNA. *Exp. Gerontol.* **2014**, *56*, 175–181. [CrossRef] [PubMed]
22. Gammage, P.A.; Frezza, C. Mitochondrial DNA: The overlooked oncogenome? *BMC Biol.* **2019**, *17*, 53. [CrossRef]
23. Mootha, V.K.; Bunkenborg, J.; Olsen, J.V.; Hjerrild, M.; Wisniewski, J.R.; Stahl, E.; Bolouri, M.S.; Ray, H.N.; Sihag, S.; Kamal, M.; et al. Integrated analysis of protein composition, tissue diversity, and gene regulation in mouse mitochondria. *Cell* **2003**, *115*, 629–640. [CrossRef]
24. Alexeyev, M.F.; Ledoux, S.P.; Wilson, G.L. Mitochondrial DNA and aging. *Clin. Sci.* **2004**, *107*, 355–364. [CrossRef] [PubMed]
25. Zeviani, M.; Antozzi, C. Defects of mitochondrial DNA. *Brain Pathol.* **1992**, *2*, 121–132. [CrossRef] [PubMed]
26. Parsons, T.J.; Muniec, D.S.; Sullivan, K.; Woodyatt, N.; Alliston-Greiner, R.; Wilson, M.R.; Berry, D.L.; Holland, K.A.; Weedn, V.W.; Gill, P.; et al. A high observed substitution rate in the human mitochondrial DNA control region. *Nat. Genet.* **1997**, *15*, 363–368. [CrossRef] [PubMed]
27. Kanki, T.; Nakayama, H.; Sasaki, N.; Takio, K.; Alam, T.I.; Hamasaki, N.; Kang, D. Mitochondrial nucleoid and transcription factor A. *Ann. N. Y. Acad. Sci.* **2004**, *1011*, 61–68. [CrossRef] [PubMed]
28. Alexeyev, M.; Shokolenko, I.; Wilson, G.; LeDoux, S. The maintenance of mitochondrial DNA integrity—Critical analysis and update. *Cold Spring Harb. Perspect. Biol.* **2013**, *5*, a012641. [CrossRef]
29. Chomyn, A.; Martinuzzi, A.; Yoneda, M.; Daga, A.; Hurko, O.; Johns, D.; Lai, S.T.; Nonaka, I.; Angelini, C.; Attardi, G. MELAS mutation in mtDNA binding site for transcription termination factor causes defects in protein synthesis and in respiration but no change in levels of upstream and downstream mature transcripts. *Proc. Natl. Acad. Sci. USA* **1992**, *89*, 4221–4225. [CrossRef]
30. Taylor, R.W.; Turnbull, D.M. Mitochondrial DNA mutations in human disease. *Nat. Rev. Genet.* **2005**, *6*, 389–402. [CrossRef]
31. Cortopassi, G.A.; Arnheim, N. Detection of a specific mitochondrial DNA deletion in tissues of older humans. *Nucleic Acids Res.* **1990**, *18*, 6927–6933. [CrossRef] [PubMed]
32. Bua, E.; Johnson, J.; Herbst, A.; Delong, B.; McKenzie, D.; Salamat, S.; Aiken, J.M. Mitochondrial DNA-deletion mutations accumulate intracellularly to detrimental levels in aged human skeletal muscle fibers. *Am. J. Hum. Genet.* **2006**, *79*, 469–480. [CrossRef] [PubMed]
33. Kennedy, S.R.; Salk, J.J.; Schmitt, M.W.; Loeb, L.A. Ultra-sensitive sequencing reveals an age-related increase in somatic mitochondrial mutations that are inconsistent with oxidative damage. *PLoS Genet.* **2013**, *9*, e1003794. [CrossRef] [PubMed]
34. Higuchi, M. Regulation of mitochondrial DNA content and cancer. *Mitochondrion* **2007**, *7*, 53–57. [CrossRef] [PubMed]
35. Trifunovic, A.; Wredenberg, A.; Falkenberg, M.; Spelbrink, J.N.; Rovio, A.T.; Bruder, C.E.; Bohlooly, Y.M.; Gidlof, S.; Oldfors, A.; Wibom, R.; et al. Premature ageing in mice expressing defective mitochondrial DNA polymerase. *Nature* **2004**, *429*, 417–423. [CrossRef]
36. Kujoth, G.C.; Hiona, A.; Pugh, T.D.; Someya, S.; Panzer, K.; Wohlgemuth, S.E.; Hofer, T.; Seo, A.Y.; Sullivan, R.; Jobling, W.A.; et al. Mitochondrial DNA mutations, oxidative stress, and apoptosis in mammalian aging. *Science* **2005**, *309*, 481–484. [CrossRef]
37. Vermulst, M.; Bielas, J.H.; Kujoth, G.C.; Ladiges, W.C.; Rabinovitch, P.S.; Prolla, T.A.; Loeb, L.A. Mitochondrial point mutations do not limit the natural lifespan of mice. *Nat. Genet.* **2007**, *39*, 540–543. [CrossRef]
38. Vermulst, M.; Wanagat, J.; Kujoth, G.C.; Bielas, J.H.; Rabinovitch, P.S.; Prolla, T.A.; Loeb, L.A. DNA deletions and clonal mutations drive premature aging in mitochondrial mutator mice. *Nat. Genet.* **2008**, *40*, 392–394. [CrossRef]
39. Kolesar, J.E.; Safdar, A.; Abadi, A.; MacNeil, L.G.; Crane, J.D.; Tarnopolsky, M.A.; Kaufman, B.A. Defects in mitochondrial DNA replication and oxidative damage in muscle of mtDNA mutator mice. *Free Radic. Biol. Med.* **2014**, *75*, 241–251. [CrossRef]

40. Safdar, A.; Annis, S.; Kraytsberg, Y.; Laverack, C.; Saleem, A.; Popadin, K.; Woods, D.C.; Tilly, J.L.; Khrapko, K. Amelioration of premature aging in mtDNA mutator mouse by exercise: The interplay of oxidative stress, PGC-1alpha, p53, and DNA damage. A hypothesis. *Curr. Opin. Genet. Dev.* **2016**, *38*, 127–132. [CrossRef]
41. Linford, N.J.; Schriner, S.E.; Rabinovitch, P.S. Oxidative damage and aging: Spotlight on mitochondria. *Cancer Res.* **2006**, *66*, 2497–2499. [CrossRef] [PubMed]
42. Schriner, S.E.; Linford, N.J.; Martin, G.M.; Treuting, P.; Ogburn, C.E.; Emond, M.; Coskun, P.E.; Ladiges, W.; Wolf, N.; Van Remmen, H.; et al. Extension of murine life span by overexpression of catalase targeted to mitochondria. *Science* **2005**, *308*, 1909–1911. [CrossRef] [PubMed]
43. Dai, D.F.; Chen, T.; Wanagat, J.; Laflamme, M.; Marcinek, D.J.; Emond, M.J.; Ngo, C.P.; Prolla, T.A.; Rabinovitch, P.S. Age-dependent cardiomyopathy in mitochondrial mutator mice is attenuated by overexpression of catalase targeted to mitochondria. *Aging Cell* **2010**, *9*, 536–544. [CrossRef] [PubMed]
44. Ross, J.M.; Coppotelli, G.; Hoffer, B.J.; Olson, L. Maternally transmitted mitochondrial DNA mutations can reduce lifespan. *Sci. Rep.* **2014**, *4*, 6569. [CrossRef] [PubMed]
45. Ross, J.M.; Stewart, J.B.; Hagstrom, E.; Brene, S.; Mourier, A.; Coppotelli, G.; Freyer, C.; Lagouge, M.; Hoffer, B.J.; Olson, L.; et al. Germline mitochondrial DNA mutations aggravate ageing and can impair brain development. *Nature* **2013**, *501*, 412–415. [CrossRef] [PubMed]
46. Gardner, K.; Hall, P.A.; Chinnery, P.F.; Payne, B.A. HIV treatment and associated mitochondrial pathology: Review of 25 years of in vitro, animal, and human studies. *Toxicol. Pathol.* **2014**, *42*, 811–822. [CrossRef]
47. Sohl, C.D.; Szymanski, M.R.; Mislak, A.C.; Shumate, C.K.; Amiralaei, S.; Schinazi, R.F.; Anderson, K.S.; Yin, Y.W. Probing the structural and molecular basis of nucleotide selectivity by human mitochondrial DNA polymerase gamma. *Proc. Natl. Acad. Sci. USA* **2015**, *112*, 8596–8601. [CrossRef]
48. DeBalsi, K.L.; Longley, M.J.; Hoff, K.E.; Copeland, W.C. Synergistic Effects of the in cis T251I and P587L Mitochondrial DNA Polymerase Gamma Disease Mutations. *J. Biol. Chem.* **2017**, *292*, 4198–4209. [CrossRef]
49. Hoff, K.E.; DeBalsi, K.L.; Sanchez-Quintero, M.J.; Longley, M.J.; Hirano, M.; Naini, A.B.; Copeland, W.C. Characterization of the human homozygous R182W POLG2 mutation in mitochondrial DNA depletion syndrome. *PLoS ONE* **2018**, *13*, e0203198. [CrossRef]
50. Chen, H.; Vermulst, M.; Wang, Y.E.; Chomyn, A.; Prolla, T.A.; McCaffery, J.M.; Chan, D.C. Mitochondrial fusion is required for mtDNA stability in skeletal muscle and tolerance of mtDNA mutations. *Cell* **2010**, *141*, 280–289. [CrossRef]
51. Chaudhari, S.N.; Kipreos, E.T. Increased mitochondrial fusion allows the survival of older animals in diverse C. elegans longevity pathways. *Nat. Commun.* **2017**, *8*, 182. [CrossRef]
52. Mengel-From, J.; Thinggaard, M.; Dalgard, C.; Kyvik, K.O.; Christensen, K.; Christiansen, L. Mitochondrial DNA copy number in peripheral blood cells declines with age and is associated with general health among elderly. *Hum. Genet.* **2014**, *133*, 1149–1159. [CrossRef]
53. Wachsmuth, M.; Hubner, A.; Li, M.; Madea, B.; Stoneking, M. Age-Related and Heteroplasmy-Related Variation in Human mtDNA Copy Number. *PLoS Genet.* **2016**, *12*, e1005939. [CrossRef] [PubMed]
54. O'Hara, R.; Tedone, E.; Ludlow, A.T.; Huang, E.; Arosio, B.; Mari, D.; Shay, J.W. Quantitative mitochondrial DNA copy number determination using droplet digital PCR with single cell resolution. *Genome Res.* **2019**, *29*, 1878–1888. [CrossRef] [PubMed]
55. Reznik, E.; Miller, M.L.; Senbabaoglu, Y.; Riaz, N.; Sarungbam, J.; Tickoo, S.K.; Al-Ahmadie, H.A.; Lee, W.; Seshan, V.E.; Hakimi, A.A.; et al. Mitochondrial DNA copy number variation across human cancers. *Elife* **2016**, *5*. [CrossRef] [PubMed]
56. Petros, J.A.; Baumann, A.K.; Ruiz-Pesini, E.; Amin, M.B.; Sun, C.Q.; Hall, J.; Lim, S.; Issa, M.M.; Flanders, W.D.; Hosseini, S.H.; et al. mtDNA mutations increase tumorigenicity in prostate cancer. *Proc. Natl. Acad. Sci. USA* **2005**, *102*, 719–724. [CrossRef]
57. Ishikawa, K.; Takenaga, K.; Akimoto, M.; Koshikawa, N.; Yamaguchi, A.; Imanishi, H.; Nakada, K.; Honma, Y.; Hayashi, J. ROS-generating mitochondrial DNA mutations can regulate tumor cell metastasis. *Science* **2008**, *320*, 661–664. [CrossRef]
58. Yu, M.; Shi, Y.; Wei, X.; Yang, Y.; Zhou, Y.; Hao, X.; Zhang, N.; Niu, R. Depletion of mitochondrial DNA by ethidium bromide treatment inhibits the proliferation and tumorigenesis of T47D human breast cancer cells. *Toxicol. Lett.* **2007**, *170*, 83–93. [CrossRef]
59. Cavalli, L.R.; Varella-Garcia, M.; Liang, B.C. Diminished tumorigenic phenotype after depletion of mitochondrial DNA. *Cell Growth Differ.* **1997**, *8*, 1189–1198.

60. Amuthan, G.; Biswas, G.; Zhang, S.Y.; Klein-Szanto, A.; Vijayasarathy, C.; Avadhani, N.G. Mitochondria-to-nucleus stress signaling induces phenotypic changes, tumor progression and cell invasion. *EMBO J.* **2001**, *20*, 1910–1920. [CrossRef]
61. Moro, L.; Arbini, A.A.; Yao, J.L.; di Sant'Agnese, P.A.; Marra, E.; Greco, M. Mitochondrial DNA depletion in prostate epithelial cells promotes anoikis resistance and invasion through activation of PI3K/Akt2. *Cell Death Differ.* **2009**, *16*, 571–583. [CrossRef] [PubMed]
62. Naito, A.; Cook, C.C.; Mizumachi, T.; Wang, M.; Xie, C.H.; Evans, T.T.; Kelly, T.; Higuchi, M. Progressive tumor features accompany epithelial-mesenchymal transition induced in mitochondrial DNA-depleted cells. *Cancer Sci.* **2008**, *99*, 1584–1588. [CrossRef] [PubMed]
63. Guha, M.; Srinivasan, S.; Ruthel, G.; Kashina, A.K.; Carstens, R.P.; Mendoza, A.; Khanna, C.; Van Winkle, T.; Avadhani, N.G. Mitochondrial retrograde signaling induces epithelial-mesenchymal transition and generates breast cancer stem cells. *Oncogene* **2014**, *33*, 5238–5250. [CrossRef] [PubMed]
64. Porporato, P.E.; Payen, V.L.; Perez-Escuredo, J.; De Saedeleer, C.J.; Danhier, P.; Copetti, T.; Dhup, S.; Tardy, M.; Vazeille, T.; Bouzin, C.; et al. A mitochondrial switch promotes tumor metastasis. *Cell Rep.* **2014**, *8*, 754–766. [CrossRef]
65. Srinivasan, S.; Guha, M.; Kashina, A.; Avadhani, N.G. Mitochondrial dysfunction and mitochondrial dynamics-The cancer connection. *Biochim. Biophys. Acta Bioenerg.* **2017**, *1858*, 602–614. [CrossRef] [PubMed]
66. Trotta, A.P.; Chipuk, J.E. Mitochondrial dynamics as regulators of cancer biology. *Cell Mol. Life Sci.* **2017**, *74*, 1999–2017. [CrossRef] [PubMed]
67. Gaude, E.; Frezza, C. Tissue-specific and convergent metabolic transformation of cancer correlates with metastatic potential and patient survival. *Nat. Commun.* **2016**, *7*, 13041. [CrossRef]
68. Ho, J.; de Moura, M.B.; Lin, Y.; Vincent, G.; Thorne, S.; Duncan, L.M.; Hui-Min, L.; Kirkwood, J.M.; Becker, D.; Van Houten, B.; et al. Importance of glycolysis and oxidative phosphorylation in advanced melanoma. *Mol. Cancer* **2012**, *11*, 76. [CrossRef]
69. Najjar, Y.G.; Menk, A.V.; Sander, C.; Rao, U.; Karunamurthy, A.; Bhatia, R.; Zhai, S.; Kirkwood, J.M.; Delgoffe, G.M. Tumor cell oxidative metabolism as a barrier to PD-1 blockade immunotherapy in melanoma. *JCI Insight* **2019**, *4*. [CrossRef]
70. Tan, A.S.; Baty, J.W.; Dong, L.F.; Bezawork-Geleta, A.; Endaya, B.; Goodwin, J.; Bajzikova, M.; Kovarova, J.; Peterka, M.; Yan, B.; et al. Mitochondrial genome acquisition restores respiratory function and tumorigenic potential of cancer cells without mitochondrial DNA. *Cell Metab.* **2015**, *21*, 81–94. [CrossRef]
71. Bohovych, I.; Khalimonchuk, O. Sending Out an SOS: Mitochondria as a Signaling Hub. *Front. Cell Dev. Biol.* **2016**, *4*, 109. [CrossRef] [PubMed]
72. Butow, R.A.; Avadhani, N.G. Mitochondrial signaling: The retrograde response. *Mol. Cell* **2004**, *14*, 1–15. [CrossRef]
73. Dillin, A.; Hsu, A.L.; Arantes-Oliveira, N.; Lehrer-Graiwer, J.; Hsin, H.; Fraser, A.G.; Kamath, R.S.; Ahringer, J.; Kenyon, C. Rates of behavior and aging specified by mitochondrial function during development. *Science* **2002**, *298*, 2398–2401. [CrossRef] [PubMed]
74. Yang, W.; Hekimi, S. A mitochondrial superoxide signal triggers increased longevity in Caenorhabditis elegans. *PLoS Biol.* **2010**, *8*, e1000556. [CrossRef] [PubMed]
75. Lapointe, J.; Hekimi, S. Early mitochondrial dysfunction in long-lived Mclk1+/− mice. *J. Biol. Chem.* **2008**, *283*, 26217–26227. [CrossRef] [PubMed]
76. Melber, A.; Haynes, C.M. UPR(mt) regulation and output: A stress response mediated by mitochondrial-nuclear communication. *Cell Res.* **2018**, *28*, 281–295. [CrossRef]
77. Martinus, R.D.; Garth, G.P.; Webster, T.L.; Cartwright, P.; Naylor, D.J.; Hoj, P.B.; Hoogenraad, N.J. Selective induction of mitochondrial chaperones in response to loss of the mitochondrial genome. *Eur. J. Biochem.* **1996**, *240*, 98–103. [CrossRef]
78. Zhao, Q.; Wang, J.; Levichkin, I.V.; Stasinopoulos, S.; Ryan, M.T.; Hoogenraad, N.J. A mitochondrial specific stress response in mammalian cells. *EMBO J.* **2002**, *21*, 4411–4419. [CrossRef]
79. Sun, N.; Youle, R.J.; Finkel, T. The Mitochondrial Basis of Aging. *Mol. Cell* **2016**, *61*, 654–666. [CrossRef]
80. Frezza, C. Mitochondrial metabolites: Undercover signalling molecules. *Interface Focus* **2017**, *7*, 20160100. [CrossRef]

81. Shaughnessy, D.T.; McAllister, K.; Worth, L.; Haugen, A.C.; Meyer, J.N.; Domann, F.E.; Van Houten, B.; Mostoslavsky, R.; Bultman, S.J.; Baccarelli, A.A.; et al. Mitochondria, energetics, epigenetics, and cellular responses to stress. *Environ. Health Perspect.* **2014**, *122*, 1271–1278. [CrossRef]
82. Pietrocola, F.; Galluzzi, L.; Bravo-San Pedro, J.M.; Madeo, F.; Kroemer, G. Acetyl coenzyme A: A central metabolite and second messenger. *Cell Metab.* **2015**, *21*, 805–821. [CrossRef] [PubMed]
83. Choudhary, C.; Weinert, B.T.; Nishida, Y.; Verdin, E.; Mann, M. The growing landscape of lysine acetylation links metabolism and cell signalling. *Nat. Rev. Mol. Cell Biol.* **2014**, *15*, 536–550. [CrossRef] [PubMed]
84. Sutendra, G.; Kinnaird, A.; Dromparis, P.; Paulin, R.; Stenson, T.H.; Haromy, A.; Hashimoto, K.; Zhang, N.; Flaim, E.; Michelakis, E.D. A nuclear pyruvate dehydrogenase complex is important for the generation of acetyl-CoA and histone acetylation. *Cell* **2014**, *158*, 84–97. [CrossRef]
85. Carrer, A.; Trefely, S.; Zhao, S.; Campbell, S.L.; Norgard, R.J.; Schultz, K.C.; Sidoli, S.; Parris, J.L.D.; Affronti, H.C.; Sivanand, S.; et al. Acetyl-CoA Metabolism Supports Multistep Pancreatic Tumorigenesis. *Cancer Discov.* **2019**, *9*, 416–435. [CrossRef]
86. Eisenberg, T.; Schroeder, S.; Andryushkova, A.; Pendl, T.; Kuttner, V.; Bhukel, A.; Marino, G.; Pietrocola, F.; Harger, A.; Zimmermann, A.; et al. Nucleocytosolic depletion of the energy metabolite acetyl-coenzyme a stimulates autophagy and prolongs lifespan. *Cell Metab.* **2014**, *19*, 431–444. [CrossRef]
87. Chung, H.Y.; Kim, D.H.; Lee, E.K.; Chung, K.W.; Chung, S.; Lee, B.; Seo, A.Y.; Chung, J.H.; Jung, Y.S.; Im, E.; et al. Redefining Chronic Inflammation in Aging and Age-Related Diseases: Proposal of the Senoinflammation Concept. *Aging Dis.* **2019**, *10*, 367–382. [CrossRef]
88. Mantovani, A.; Allavena, P.; Sica, A.; Balkwill, F. Cancer-related inflammation. *Nature* **2008**, *454*, 436–444. [CrossRef]
89. Nakahira, K.; Haspel, J.A.; Rathinam, V.A.; Lee, S.J.; Dolinay, T.; Lam, H.C.; Englert, J.A.; Rabinovitch, M.; Cernadas, M.; Kim, H.P.; et al. Autophagy proteins regulate innate immune responses by inhibiting the release of mitochondrial DNA mediated by the NALP3 inflammasome. *Nat. Immunol.* **2011**, *12*, 222–230. [CrossRef]
90. Mathew, A.; Lindsley, T.A.; Sheridan, A.; Bhoiwala, D.L.; Hushmendy, S.F.; Yager, E.J.; Ruggiero, E.A.; Crawford, D.R. Degraded mitochondrial DNA is a newly identified subtype of the damage associated molecular pattern (DAMP) family and possible trigger of neurodegeneration. *J. Alzheimers Dis.* **2012**, *30*, 617–627. [CrossRef]
91. Yu, J.; Nagasu, H.; Murakami, T.; Hoang, H.; Broderick, L.; Hoffman, H.M.; Horng, T. Inflammasome activation leads to Caspase-1-dependent mitochondrial damage and block of mitophagy. *Proc. Natl. Acad. Sci. USA* **2014**, *111*, 15514–15519. [CrossRef] [PubMed]
92. Tumurkhuu, G.; Shimada, K.; Dagvadorj, J.; Crother, T.R.; Zhang, W.; Luthringer, D.; Gottlieb, R.A.; Chen, S.; Arditi, M. Ogg1-Dependent DNA Repair Regulates NLRP3 Inflammasome and Prevents Atherosclerosis. *Circ. Res.* **2016**, *119*, e76–e90. [CrossRef] [PubMed]
93. Bronner, D.N.; Abuaita, B.H.; Chen, X.; Fitzgerald, K.A.; Nunez, G.; He, Y.; Yin, X.M.; O'Riordan, M.X. Endoplasmic Reticulum Stress Activates the Inflammasome via NLRP3- and Caspase-2-Driven Mitochondrial Damage. *Immunity* **2015**, *43*, 451–462. [CrossRef] [PubMed]
94. Zhong, Z.; Umemura, A.; Sanchez-Lopez, E.; Liang, S.; Shalapour, S.; Wong, J.; He, F.; Boassa, D.; Perkins, G.; Ali, S.R.; et al. NF-kappaB Restricts Inflammasome Activation via Elimination of Damaged Mitochondria. *Cell* **2016**, *164*, 896–910. [CrossRef] [PubMed]
95. Zhong, Z.; Liang, S.; Sanchez-Lopez, E.; He, F.; Shalapour, S.; Lin, X.J.; Wong, J.; Ding, S.; Seki, E.; Schnabl, B.; et al. New mitochondrial DNA synthesis enables NLRP3 inflammasome activation. *Nature* **2018**, *560*, 198–203. [CrossRef] [PubMed]
96. Coll, R.C.; Holley, C.L.; Schroder, K. Author Correction: Mitochondrial DNA synthesis fuels NLRP3 inflammasome. *Cell Res.* **2018**, *28*, 1202. [CrossRef]
97. Moossavi, M.; Parsamanesh, N.; Bahrami, A.; Atkin, S.L.; Sahebkar, A. Role of the NLRP3 inflammasome in cancer. *Mol. Cancer* **2018**, *17*, 158. [CrossRef]
98. Hahn, T.; Polanczyk, M.J.; Borodovsky, A.; Ramanathapuram, L.V.; Akporiaye, E.T.; Ralph, S.J. Use of anti-cancer drugs, mitocans, to enhance the immune responses against tumors. *Curr. Pharm. Biotechnol.* **2013**, *14*, 357–376. [CrossRef]
99. Guha, M.; Avadhani, N.G. Mitochondrial retrograde signaling at the crossroads of tumor bioenergetics, genetics and epigenetics. *Mitochondrion* **2013**, *13*, 577–591. [CrossRef]

100. Srinivasan, S.; Avadhani, N.G. Hypoxia-mediated mitochondrial stress in RAW264.7 cells induces osteoclast-like TRAP-positive cells. *Ann. N. Y. Acad. Sci.* **2007**, *1117*, 51–61. [CrossRef]
101. Srinivasan, S.; Koenigstein, A.; Joseph, J.; Sun, L.; Kalyanaraman, B.; Zaidi, M.; Avadhani, N.G. Role of mitochondrial reactive oxygen species in osteoclast differentiation. *Ann. N. Y. Acad. Sci.* **2010**, *1192*, 245–252. [CrossRef] [PubMed]
102. Arbini, A.A.; Guerra, F.; Greco, M.; Marra, E.; Gandee, L.; Xiao, G.; Lotan, Y.; Gasparre, G.; Hsieh, J.T.; Moro, L. Mitochondrial DNA depletion sensitizes cancer cells to PARP inhibitors by translational and post-translational repression of BRCA2. *Oncogenesis* **2013**, *2*, e82. [CrossRef] [PubMed]
103. Davis, F.M.; Azimi, I.; Faville, R.A.; Peters, A.A.; Jalink, K.; Putney, J.W., Jr.; Goodhill, G.J.; Thompson, E.W.; Roberts-Thomson, S.J.; Monteith, G.R. Induction of epithelial-mesenchymal transition (EMT) in breast cancer cells is calcium signal dependent. *Oncogene* **2014**, *33*, 2307–2316. [CrossRef] [PubMed]
104. Shammas, M.A. Telomeres, lifestyle, cancer, and aging. *Curr. Opin. Clin. Nutr. Metab. Care* **2011**, *14*, 28–34. [CrossRef] [PubMed]
105. Santos, J.H.; Meyer, J.N.; Skorvaga, M.; Annab, L.A.; Van Houten, B. Mitochondrial hTERT exacerbates free-radical-mediated mtDNA damage. *Aging Cell* **2004**, *3*, 399–411. [CrossRef] [PubMed]
106. Santos, J.H.; Meyer, J.N.; Van Houten, B. Mitochondrial localization of telomerase as a determinant for hydrogen peroxide-induced mitochondrial DNA damage and apoptosis. *Hum. Mol. Genet.* **2006**, *15*, 1757–1768. [CrossRef]
107. Haendeler, J.; Hoffmann, J.; Brandes, R.P.; Zeiher, A.M.; Dimmeler, S. Hydrogen peroxide triggers nuclear export of telomerase reverse transcriptase via Src kinase family-dependent phosphorylation of tyrosine 707. *Mol. Cell Biol.* **2003**, *23*, 4598–4610. [CrossRef]
108. Ahmed, S.; Passos, J.F.; Birket, M.J.; Beckmann, T.; Brings, S.; Peters, H.; Birch-Machin, M.A.; von Zglinicki, T.; Saretzki, G. Telomerase does not counteract telomere shortening but protects mitochondrial function under oxidative stress. *J. Cell Sci.* **2008**, *121*, 1046–1053. [CrossRef]
109. Haendeler, J.; Drose, S.; Buchner, N.; Jakob, S.; Altschmied, J.; Goy, C.; Spyridopoulos, I.; Zeiher, A.M.; Brandt, U.; Dimmeler, S.; et al. Mitochondrial telomerase reverse transcriptase binds to and protects mitochondrial DNA and function from damage. *Arterioscler Thromb. Vasc. Biol.* **2009**, *29*, 929–935. [CrossRef]
110. Indran, I.R.; Hande, M.P.; Pervaiz, S. hTERT overexpression alleviates intracellular ROS production, improves mitochondrial function, and inhibits ROS-mediated apoptosis in cancer cells. *Cancer Res.* **2011**, *71*, 266–276. [CrossRef]
111. Kovalenko, O.A.; Kaplunov, J.; Herbig, U.; Detoledo, S.; Azzam, E.I.; Santos, J.H. Expression of (NES-)hTERT in cancer cells delays cell cycle progression and increases sensitivity to genotoxic stress. *PLoS ONE* **2010**, *5*, e10812. [CrossRef] [PubMed]
112. Kovalenko, O.A.; Caron, M.J.; Ulema, P.; Medrano, C.; Thomas, A.P.; Kimura, M.; Bonini, M.G.; Herbig, U.; Santos, J.H. A mutant telomerase defective in nuclear-cytoplasmic shuttling fails to immortalize cells and is associated with mitochondrial dysfunction. *Aging Cell* **2010**, *9*, 203–219. [CrossRef] [PubMed]
113. Sharma, N.K.; Reyes, A.; Green, P.; Caron, M.J.; Bonini, M.G.; Gordon, D.M.; Holt, I.J.; Santos, J.H. Human telomerase acts as a hTR-independent reverse transcriptase in mitochondria. *Nucleic Acids Res.* **2012**, *40*, 712–725. [CrossRef] [PubMed]
114. Blackburn, E.H.; Epel, E.S.; Lin, J. Human telomere biology: A contributory and interactive factor in aging, disease risks, and protection. *Science* **2015**, *350*, 1193–1198. [CrossRef] [PubMed]
115. Xie, Z.; Jay, K.A.; Smith, D.L.; Zhang, Y.; Liu, Z.; Zheng, J.; Tian, R.; Li, H.; Blackburn, E.H. Early telomerase inactivation accelerates aging independently of telomere length. *Cell* **2015**, *160*, 928–939. [CrossRef]
116. Pereira, B.; Ferreira, M.G. Sowing the seeds of cancer: Telomeres and age-associated tumorigenesis. *Curr. Opin. Oncol.* **2013**, *25*, 93–98. [CrossRef]
117. Leao, R.; Apolonio, J.D.; Lee, D.; Figueiredo, A.; Tabori, U.; Castelo-Branco, P. Mechanisms of human telomerase reverse transcriptase (hTERT) regulation: Clinical impacts in cancer. *J. Biomed. Sci.* **2018**, *25*, 22. [CrossRef]
118. Hanahan, D.; Weinberg, R.A. Hallmarks of cancer: The next generation. *Cell* **2011**, *144*, 646–674. [CrossRef]
119. Okamoto, K.; Seimiya, H. Revisiting Telomere Shortening in Cancer. *Cells* **2019**, *8*, E107. [CrossRef]
120. Listerman, I.; Sun, J.; Gazzaniga, F.S.; Lukas, J.L.; Blackburn, E.H. The major reverse transcriptase-incompetent splice variant of the human telomerase protein inhibits telomerase activity but protects from apoptosis. *Cancer Res.* **2013**, *73*, 2817–2828. [CrossRef]

121. Qian, W.; Kumar, N.; Roginskaya, V.; Fouquerel, E.; Opresko, P.L.; Shiva, S.; Watkins, S.C.; Kolodieznyi, D.; Bruchez, M.P.; Van Houten, B. Chemoptogenetic damage to mitochondria causes rapid telomere dysfunction. *Proc. Natl. Acad. Sci. USA* **2019**, *116*, 18435–18444. [CrossRef]
122. mSahin, E.; Colla, S.; Liesa, M.; Moslehi, J.; Muller, F.L.; Guo, M.; Cooper, M.; Kotton, D.; Fabian, A.J.; Walkey, C.; et al. Telomere dysfunction induces metabolic and mitochondrial compromise. *Nature* **2011**, *470*, 359–365. [CrossRef]

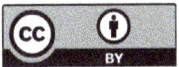

© 2019 by the author. Licensee MDPI, Basel, Switzerland. This article is an open access article distributed under the terms and conditions of the Creative Commons Attribution (CC BY) license (http://creativecommons.org/licenses/by/4.0/).

MDPI
St. Alban-Anlage 66
4052 Basel
Switzerland
Tel. +41 61 683 77 34
Fax +41 61 302 89 18
www.mdpi.com

*Journal of Clinical Medicine* Editorial Office
E-mail: jcm@mdpi.com
www.mdpi.com/journal/jcm

www.ingramcontent.com/pod-product-compliance
Lightning Source LLC
LaVergne TN
LVHW070211100526
838202LV00015B/2030